Dysphagia in Neurodevelopmental and Medical Disorders and Diseases:

A Lifespan Approach

Soultana Papadopoulou
https://orcid.org/0000-0002-0950-1456
University of Ioannina, Greece

IGI Global
Scientific Publishing
Publishing Tomorrow's Research Today

Published in the United States of America by
IGI Global Scientific Publishing
701 East Chocolate Avenue
Hershey, PA, 17033, USA
Tel: 717-533-8845 | Fax: 717-533-7115
Website: https://www.igi-global.com E-mail: cust@igi-global.com

Library of Congress Cataloging-in-Publication Data

LCCN: 2026932862 (CIP Data Pending)
ISBN13: 9798337364056
Isbn13Softcover: 9798337364063
EISBN13: 9798337364070

British Cataloguing in Publication Data
A Cataloguing in Publication record for this book is available from the British Library.

Table of Contents

Detailed Table of Contents

stimulation, neuromuscular electrical stimulation), and virtual reality (VR) and gamified interventions. The chapter emphasizes clinical applicability within multidisciplinary care pathways, while addressing ethical, accessibility, and cost-effectiveness challenges. By proposing a roadmap for combining these technologies with traditional approaches, it aims to enhance equitable access to dysphagia care for diverse populations, from pediatric to geriatric patients.

Dysphagia is a frequent and clinically significant complication in individuals with dementia, contributing to malnutrition, aspiration pneumonia, and reduced quality of life. Its prevalence and clinical presentation vary according to dementia subtype, disease stage, and underlying neuropathology. This chapter provides an overview of dysphagia across major dementia types, including Alzheimer's disease, vascular dementia, frontotemporal dementia, and Lewy body dementia. Dementia-specific swallowing profiles are discussed with emphasis on sensory, motor, and cognitive mechanisms affecting swallowing safety and efficiency. Current assessment approaches are reviewed, highlighting the limitations of self-report measures in cognitively impaired populations and the importance of caregiver input, clinical bedside evaluations, and instrumental assessments. Evidence-based management strategies—including postural techniques, diet modification, behavioral and environmental interventions, rehabilitative exercises, and enteral feeding—are also addressed.

Head and neck cancers comprise malignant tumors that arise in various sites, including the oral cavity, pharynx, larynx, nasal cavity, paranasal sinuses, and salivary glands. Surgical treatments for head and neck cancer can cause dysphagia and aspiration by compromising both anatomical and neurological functions. The type and severity of the resulting swallowing disorders depend on the tumor location, the extent of resection, and the reconstruction method used. Reconstruction involves repairing tissues removed during surgery with flaps, grafts, or prostheses, while aiming to preserve functional integrity. The risk of dysphagia after oral and/or oropharyngeal surgery is especially linked to resection of the tongue and related structures. A systematic assessment of dysphagia is essential to ensure safe swallowing in patients

Cerebral Palsy (CP) is a complex group of neurodevelopmental disorders characterized by postural and movement limitations resulting from a non-progressive lesion in the developing or immature brain, with a prevalence of 2 to 3 per 1,000 live births. Motor symptoms (spasticity, ataxia, dyskinesia) often combine with comorbid conditions such as sensory, cognitive, communication, and epilepsy, aggravating the clinical picture. Feeding and swallowing disorders in children with CP, namely oropharyngeal dysphagia (OPD), are a fairly common problem with a prevalence ranging from 22% to 99%.These feeding difficulties are directly related to Oral Motor Dysfunction (OMD) (tongue thrusting, weak sucking/swallowing), seen in over 90% of cases, and poor postural control; effective feeding depends on trunk and head stability. Dysphagia reduces the efficiency of food intake by causing impairments in the oral phase and pharyngeal phase (coughing, wet voice) of swallowing.

The practice of simulation-based learning now appears in dysphagia training because it enables healthcare professionals to practice their skills through controlled sessions which help them build their abilities while maintaining patient safety. Simulation provides essential value to competency-based training because traditional placement sites do not guarantee consistent availability of complex swallowing cases. Research findings show that participants who take part in simulated learning activities develop their diagnostic reasoning abilities and their assessment skills and their confidence levels and their communication abilities. The advantages of this technology have been documented in studies which used it for pediatric feeding, adult dysphagia assessment and treatments. The simulation environment enables students to receive directed feedback which enables them to develop their skills through multiple attempts before they interact with actual patients. Through simulation students can develop their clinical judgment while connecting theoretical knowledge to practical applications.

This chapter examines the diagnostic utility of Flexible Endoscopic Evaluation of Swallowing (FEES) in neurogenic dysphagia, focusing on pharyngeal phase impairments caused by neurological disorders such as stroke, traumatic brain injury (TBI), cerebral palsy (CP), multiple sclerosis (MS), Parkinson's disease (PD), and amyotrophic lateral sclerosis (ALS). FEES enables direct visualization of swallowing physiology, including secretion management, residue, penetration, and aspiration. Its portability, repeatability, and radiation-free nature make it ideal for acute and chronic settings. The chapter outlines standardized protocols using IDDSI-consistent bolus trials and validated tools like the Penetration–Aspiration Scale, Yale Pharyngeal Residue Severity Rating Scale, and the Murray Secretion Scale to support accurate diagnosis and individualized management.

This chapter per the authors conceptualizes swallowing as a cognitively mediated sensorimotor process rather than a purely brainstem reflex or peripheral biomechanical act. It synthesizes evidence from neuroimaging, electrophysiology, and dual-task paradigms to describe cortical, subcortical, and cerebellar networks supporting attentional control, executive regulation, and memory processes in swallowing. The chapter demonstrates how cognitive load, aging, and neurodegenerative conditions disrupt these networks, resulting in reduced swallowing safety, efficiency, and therapeutic adherence. An integrative assessment framework is presented, combining instrumental swallowing evaluations (VFSS, FEES, BRACS-Tr) with cognitive-linguistic measures (MoCA, TDQ-30/60 Tr, BECLA-Tr, DVAQ-30 Tr, DTLA-Tr), with emphasis on Turkish-adapted tools and cross-cultural normative data. Clinical implications focus on cognition-informed intervention planning, individualized cueing strategies, and multidisciplinary management, concluding with future directions for technology-assisted dysphagia care.

Autism Spectrum Disorders (ASD) are complex neurodevelopmental conditions marked by social communication difficulties, restricted interests, and repetitive behaviors. This chapter examines developmental trajectories, emphasizing genetic, neurobiological, and environmental influences on symptom emergence and progression. Comorbidities—including intellectual disabilities, ADHD, anxiety, epilepsy, gastrointestinal disorders, and dysphagia—are discussed regarding their prevalence, functional impact, and implications for diagnosis and intervention. The chapter also explores quality of life in ASD, highlighting the importance of adaptive skills, social support, educational inclusion, and access to individualized interventions. By integrating research and clinical insights, it provides a comprehensive overview of how developmental processes and comorbidities shape experiences of individuals with ASD and offers guidance for improving outcomes across the lifespan.

Charuwan Thanawiroon, Faculty of Pharmaceutical Sciences, Ubon Ratchathani University, Thailand
Rojjares Netthong, Faculty of Pharmaceutical Sciences, Ubon Ratchathani University, Thailand
Soultana Papadopoulou, Department of Speech and Language Therapy, University of Ioannina, Greece
Bancha Yingngam, Faculty of Pharmaceutical Sciences, Ubon Ratchathani University, Thailand

Dysphagia is common in children and elderly individuals, making conventional oral forms of medication such as tablets or capsules inappropriate for these patients. The inflexibility of these dosage forms is fraught with potential dangers; they cannot be altered without the potential for loss of their therapeutic effect. This rigidity of the systems can lead to dosing inaccuracies and potentially an insufficient therapeutic effect or aspiration. To overcome these limitations, several novel drug delivery systems have been proposed. These include rapidly dissolving films, gels with drugs, hydrogels and complex 3D-printed formulations, as well as a number of nanoengineering methodologies. These improvements lead to better swallowability and lung deposition. Moreover, the bioavailability of a given pharmaceutical and patient acceptance are maintained. This chapter concentrates on these new systems for drug delivery, their clinical implications and regulation considerations, specifically in compliance with medication errors in patients with dysphagia.

Swallowing, though often perceived as a simple, reflexive act, is in fact a highly complex sensorimotor process that relies on intricate coordination between the brain, cranial nerves, muscles, and cognitive mechanisms. Dysphagia, or difficulty in swallowing, is traditionally viewed as a disorder stemming from structural abnormalities, neuromuscular impairments, or damage to the swallowing reflex pathways. However, in recent decades, researchers and clinicians have come to recognize that cognitive functions such as attention, memory, executive functioning, and awareness play a significant role in initiating, regulating, and sustaining safe and effective swallowing. Understanding the cognitive influences on swallowing is essential not only for explaining why certain populations are more vulnerable to dysphagia but also for designing more effective diagnostic assessments and therapeutic interventions. The act of swallowing requires more than just mechanical muscle coordination; it demands conscious initiation, sustained attention to the task, and, in some cases, active problem-solving

Dysphagia, defined as difficulty in swallowing, is a multifaceted symptom that significantly affects patients with neurological conditions, particularly Parkinson's disease (PD). In clinical terms, dysphagia refers to any disruption in the normal swallowing mechanism, which involves coordinated muscular and neurological processes spanning the oral, pharyngeal, and esophageal phases. For individuals with Parkinson's disease, a progressive neurodegenerative disorder primarily associated with motor dysfunction due to dopaminergic neuronal loss in the substantia nigra, swallowing difficulties arise from both motor and non-motor impairments. The definition of dysphagia in the context of Parkinson's extends beyond a simple difficulty in swallowing food or liquids; it encompasses a spectrum of symptoms such as delayed initiation of swallowing, reduced pharyngeal clearance, impaired laryngeal elevation, and aspiration of food or fluids into the airway.

Dysphagia, a severe complication of neurological disorders, is now managed through advanced diagnostics and treatments that leverage technological innovation. Modern approaches utilize high-resolution manometry and endoscopic imaging for precise biomechanical assessment, moving beyond traditional strategies. The therapeutic focus has shifted towards harnessing neuroplasticity with interventions like pharyngeal electrical stimulation and biofeedback-aided exercises. These innovations enable targeted, mechanism-based rehabilitation that actively restores swallow function, significantly improving safety, reducing aspiration risk, and enhancing quality of life for patients. This integration of technology represents a new era in dysphagia care.

Preface

Dysphagia is not a singular symptom confined to one diagnosis, age group, or clinical setting. It is a complex, multifactorial condition that intersects with neurodevelopment, neurodegeneration, critical illness, oncology, cognition, pharmacology, and technological innovation. Across the lifespan, from the fragile coordination of neonatal feeding to the progressive challenges of neurodegenerative disease, swallowing disorders demand interdisciplinary insight, scientific rigor, and compassionate, person-centered care.

Dysphagia in Neurodevelopmental and Medical Disorders and Diseases: A Lifespan Approach brings together contemporary perspectives that reflect the expanding boundaries of dysphagia science and practice. This volume integrates foundational neurophysiology, developmental trajectories, and clinical reasoning with emerging diagnostic technologies, simulation-based education, formulation science, and digital health innovations. The result is a comprehensive reference designed to support clinicians, researchers, educators, and advanced students working in diverse healthcare contexts.

A defining strength of this book lies in its lifespan perspective. Swallowing is explored as a dynamic sensorimotor and cognitively mediated process that evolves from infancy through advanced age. The chapters collectively highlight how neurological, structural, developmental, cognitive, and systemic factors influence swallowing safety and efficiency. Importantly, they emphasize the essential role of multidisciplinary collaboration, uniting speech-language therapists, physicians, nurses, pharmacists, rehabilitation specialists, engineers, and researchers, in optimizing outcomes and quality of life.

This volume also reflects the transformation of dysphagia care in the twenty-first century. From instrumental diagnostics such as Flexible Endoscopic Evaluation of Swallowing to artificial intelligence–assisted assessments and advanced drug delivery systems, modern practice is increasingly data-driven, technology-enhanced, and patient-specific. At the same time, the human dimensions of care, ethics, communication, cognition, caregiver involvement, and quality of life, remain central themes throughout the text.

By bridging neonatal care, neurodevelopmental disorders, acute medical management, chronic neurological disease, oncology, dementia, and pharmacological innovation, this book seeks to provide an integrative framework for understanding dysphagia not as an isolated impairment, but as a condition deeply embedded within broader health and developmental systems.

CHAPTER OVERVIEW

Chapter 1: Development of a Protocol for Dysphagia Management in ICU Adults

This chapter presents an evidence-based, standardized protocol for identifying and managing dysphagia in critically ill adults. It emphasizes early bedside screening, timely instrumental assessment, and structured multidisciplinary collaboration. By integrating speech therapy within intensive care pathways, the chapter proposes a model designed to reduce aspiration risk, shorten hospitalization, and improve patient safety.

Chapter 2: Neonatal Swallowing Disorders

Focusing on the earliest stage of life, this chapter explores the neurodevelopmental and physiological foundations of neonatal swallowing. It reviews clinical and instrumental assessments and synthesizes evidence-based interventions used in neonatal intensive care units. Emphasis is placed on early detection, family-centered care, and interdisciplinary collaboration.

Chapter 3: Development and Disorders of Infant Sucking

Infant sucking is examined as a complex neurophysiological behavior shaped by sensory, motor, and environmental influences. The chapter discusses typical development, risk factors for dysfunction, and early biomarkers of neurological integrity. Clinical assessment tools and targeted intervention strategies are outlined to support safe feeding and developmental outcomes.

Chapter 4: Innovative Approaches in Dysphagia, from Assessment to Therapy

This chapter explores emerging technologies transforming dysphagia care, including artificial intelligence applications, tele-practice, neuromodulation, and virtual reality–based rehabilitation. Ethical considerations, accessibility, and cost-effectiveness are addressed, offering a roadmap for integrating innovation into routine clinical practice.

Chapter 5: Dysphagia in Dementia

Dysphagia across major dementia subtypes, including Alzheimer's disease, is examined through sensory, motor, and cognitive lenses. The chapter reviews assessment challenges in cognitively impaired populations and outlines management strategies that incorporate caregiver input, environmental modification, and individualized therapy planning.

Chapter 6: Dysphagia in Head and Neck Cancers

This chapter details how tumor location, surgical resection, and reconstructive techniques influence swallowing outcomes in head and neck cancer. It underscores the necessity of systematic assessment and rehabilitation to preserve functional integrity and quality of life.

Chapter 7: Post-Stroke Dysphagia

Addressing one of the most common neurological causes of swallowing disorders, this chapter reviews neurophysiology, screening protocols, instrumental diagnostics, and evidence-based interventions. The importance of early detection and coordinated multidisciplinary management in both acute and chronic stages is emphasized.

Chapter 8: Dysphagia in Parkinson's Disease

Swallowing impairments associated with Parkinson's disease are examined in relation to dopaminergic deficits and broader neurodegenerative mechanisms. The chapter discusses clinical presentation across swallowing phases, instrumental evaluation, medical optimization, and rehabilitative strategies.

Chapter 9: Feeding and Swallowing Disorders in Cerebral Palsy

This chapter explores oropharyngeal dysphagia in individuals with Cerebral Palsy, highlighting the interaction between oral motor dysfunction, posture, and comorbid conditions. Assessment frameworks and intervention models are presented within a developmental and functional context.

Chapter 10: Simulation-Based Learning in Dysphagia Training

Recognizing the growing need for competency-based education, this chapter examines simulation as a training tool in dysphagia assessment and intervention. It discusses how structured simulation enhances diagnostic reasoning, clinical judgment, and patient safety.

Chapter 11: Flexible Endoscopic Evaluation in Neurogenic Dysphagia

Dedicated to Flexible Endoscopic Evaluation of Swallowing, this chapter outlines standardized protocols, validated rating scales, and clinical decision-making processes. The portability and repeatability of FEES are highlighted as key advantages across acute and chronic care settings.

Chapter 12: The Cognitive Dimension of Swallowing Disorders Assessment and Clinical Implications

This chapter conceptualizes swallowing as a cognitively mediated process involving attentional control, executive function, and memory systems. It proposes integrative assessment models that combine instrumental evaluation with cognitive-linguistic measures to guide individualized intervention planning.

Chapter 13: Developmental Processes, Comorbidities, and Quality of Life in Autism Spectrum Disorders

Focusing on Autism Spectrum Disorder, this chapter examines developmental trajectories, associated comorbidities, including feeding and swallowing challenges, and quality of life considerations. It integrates neuropsychological insights with clinical guidance for lifespan support.

Chapter 14: Formulation Science in Dysphagia Care

This chapter explores innovative oral drug delivery systems designed for individuals with swallowing difficulties. Rapidly dissolving films, hydrogels, and 3D-printed formulations are discussed in relation to safety, bioavailability, and regulatory considerations.

Chapter 15: The Cognitive Dimension of Swallowing Disorders

Expanding on cognitive influences in dysphagia, this chapter analyzes how attention, executive functioning, and awareness shape swallowing performance. It provides theoretical foundations and clinical implications for cognition-informed therapeutic approaches.

Chapter 16: A Comprehensive Overview of Dysphagia in Parkinson's Disease

Offering an additional perspective on Parkinson's disease, this chapter explores the multifaceted motor and non-motor contributors to swallowing impairment and highlights advances in diagnosis and rehabilitation.

Chapter 17: Modern Approaches to Dysphagia, From Neurological Disorders to Technological Innovations

The concluding chapter synthesizes advances in high-resolution diagnostics, neuroplasticity-based therapies, and biofeedback-driven rehabilitation. It reflects the evolving landscape of dysphagia care and underscores the integration of neurological science and technological innovation in shaping future practice.

Together, these chapters provide a cohesive and forward-looking examination of dysphagia across populations, disciplines, and care environments. By integrating developmental science, clinical expertise, and technological advancement, this book aspires to contribute meaningfully to improved safety, function, and quality of life for individuals living with swallowing disorders worldwide.

Chapter 1
Development of a Protocol for Dysphagia Management in ICU Adults Integrating Speech Therapy and Multidisciplinary Approaches

Soultana I Papadopoulou
http://orcid.org/0000-0002-0950-1456
University of Ioannina, Greece

ABSTRACT

Dysphagia is a common and serious complication in critically ill patients in Intensive Care Units, typically following prolonged intubation or mechanical ventilation. It is linked to dehydration, malnutrition, and aspiration pneumonia, prolonging hospitalization and impairing quality of life. Despite affecting up to 60% of this population, dysphagia remains underdiagnosed due to limited screening and the absence of standardized management protocols. This chapter presents an evidence-based protocol for ICU dysphagia management, integrating clinical and instrumental assessment methods. Bedside screening enables early identification of swallowing deficits, followed by targeted instrumental examinations such as FEES or VFSS when required. The framework supports individualized therapy planning

DOI: 10.4018/979-8-3373-6405-6.ch001

led by speech-language therapists within a multidisciplinary team. Implementing this standardized approach may reduce complications and costs, while improving safety, recovery, and overall quality of dysphagia care in critical settings.

1. INTRODUCTION

Feeding and swallowing constitute essential physiological processes that are inherently safe, efficient, and pleasurable. These functions play a critical role not only in maintaining systemic homeostasis but also in facilitating social participation and significantly enhancing overall quality of life. Recent studies highlight ICU-acquired dysphagia's impact across age groups, with pediatric cohorts showing 29% prevalence post-extubation, linked to prolonged intubation (>7 days) and extended PICU stays (up to 27 days longer), emphasizing neuroplastic differences versus geriatric presbyphagia. A 2025 narrative review confirms 3-62% incidence in adults, with persistent deficits mirroring neurodevelopmental patterns in young patients, underscoring lifespan surveillance needs (Bertschi et al. 2025).

Pediatric ICU cohorts demonstrate 29% post-extubation dysphagia prevalence, with >7-day intubation delaying suck-swallow-breathe maturation by 21-27 days versus adult muscle atrophy patterns. NICU sensory deprivation induces chronic oral aversion in 35% of preterm infants, contrasting geriatric presbyphagia and necessitating lifespan-differentiated protocols (da Silva et al. 2023).

Dysphagia is defined as the delayed or misdirected transfer of saliva, food of any consistency, and/or medication from the oral cavity to the stomach, increasing morbidity and mortality rates (McCarty and Chao 2021; Papadopoulou et al. 2013). It is observed in all age groups and can occur at any stage of swallowing (Hamdy et al. 1998; Meuret, Dietz, and Fuchs 2014). It is listed under code MD93 in the International Classification of Diseases (ICD), 11th revision (Bertschi et al. 2025).

The normal swallowing process is a complex neuromuscular, dynamic, semi-autonomous, sensory-kinetics, cognitive function regulated by the central nervous system, involving coordinated sensory and motor pathways and significant cortical activation, as demonstrated by recent neuroimaging studies (Cheng et al. 2022; Ludlow 2015). Various conditions can disrupt this intricate mechanism, leading to dysphagia, particularly in ICU patients where the underlying pathophysiology remains poorly understood and optimal management strategies are still debated (Brodsky, Nollet, et al. 2020; Zuercher et al. 2019). Accurate diagnosis and multidisciplinary intervention are therefore essential priorities in dysphagia care.

ICU-acquired dysphagia manifests in up to 60% of critically ill adults post-prolonged endotracheal intubation, precipitating adverse sequelae including aspiration pneumonia, malnutrition, protracted mechanical ventilation dependence, and extended hospitalization (Brodsky et al. 2021; Zuercher, Dziewas, and Schefold 2020). Contemporary epidemiological data delineates incidence at 3-62% across cohorts, surging to 85-90% in neuro-ICUs, with 22% exhibiting protracted impairment at 10-17 months post-discharge; protocolized SLP screening attenuates pneumonia risk and fosters decannulation (Bertschi et al. 2025; Reitz et al. 2024). Multidisciplinary paradigms, emphasizing temporal optimization, efficaciously abrogate these sequelae (Clavé and Shaker 2015; Speyer et al. 2019). Recent expert consensus recommends clinical algorithms for systematic screening and Management of swallowing disorders in ICU patients (Likar et al. 2024).

The structured protocol presented herein emphasizes systematic screening, comprehensive clinical assessment, and coordinated management primarily led by speech and language therapists in collaboration with allied healthcare professionals. This protocol facilitates critical decision-making and continuous evaluation throughout the therapeutic process, while embedding essential temporal and financial planning to ensure efficient resource utilization and enhanced patient safety (Muhle et al. 2021; Zuercher et al. 2019). By fostering an evidence-based, coordinated care pathway, this framework aims to reduce secondary complications and improve clinical outcomes among this vulnerable population (Likar et al. 2024).

This approach aligns with current evidence highlighting that early intervention, targeted therapeutic techniques, and collaborative care significantly improve outcomes in ICU-acquired dysphagia (Hongo et al. 2022; Reitz et al. 2024; Turra et al. 2021; Yang et al. 2023).

1.1. Central Control of Swallowing

The neuromuscular organization of swallowing is orchestrated by the central pattern generator (CPG) for swallowing, which is in the brainstem, specifically within the medulla oblongata. It encompasses the hypoglossal nucleus, the nucleus tractus solitarius (NTS), the nucleus ambiguous, and the reticular formation. The CPG coordinates the sequential, rhythmic contractions of the oral, pharyngeal, and laryngopharyngeal musculature, including the upper esophageal sphincter, thus generating a highly organized motor sequence required for the physiological execution of swallowing (Jean 2001; Neuhuber and Bieger 2013). Although the brainstem serves as the pivotal neural hub, higher cortical regions, including the primary motor cortex, supplementary motor area, and premotor cortex, regulate the functioning of the swallowing CPG. From these cortical centers, the initiation of swallowing is triggered, while sensory feedback and cognitive processes allow for modulation and adaptation of the motor sequence. Subcortical structures, such as the basal ganglia and thalamus, contribute to motor control through the cortico–basal ganglia thalamo–cortical loop, further refining voluntary and automatic aspects of swallowing control

(Ghaemi et al. 2016; Hamdy 2006; Wilmskoetter, Daniels, and Miller 2020). The cerebellum also plays a critical role, enhancing temporal precision, coordination, and fine-tuning of the motor sequence through its reciprocal connections with the cortex and brainstem. Furthermore, the brainstem receives continuous sensory input from peripheral receptors via cranial nerves (V, VII, IX, X) that converge at the NTS. Here, afferent information is integrated with cortical efferent commands to ensure safe and synchronized swallowing (Bieger and Neuhuber 2006; Sasegbon and Hamdy 2017; Steele and Miller 2010). This dynamic, multi-level interaction guarantees adaptation of swallowing behaviors according to bolus properties and contextual demands (Humbert and German 2013; Jean 2001; Peyron et al. 2011).

1.2. Peripheral Control of Swallowing

Peripheral control relies on the coordinated action of cranial nerves (V, VII, IX, X, XII), which transmit descending motor signals to the oral, pharyngeal, and laryngeal musculature while simultaneously conveying sensory input from these regions back to the central nervous system. These cranial nerves possess either motor, sensory, or mixed functions, collectively contributing not only to swallowing but also to speech. Through their precise interaction, these nerves ensure bolus preparation, propulsion, and transit from the oral cavity to the esophagus, while safeguarding the airway via epiglottic closure and laryngeal adduction. Pathology affecting any of these cranial nerves or their target muscles results in impaired swallowing or dysphagia (Sasegbon and Hamdy 2017; Shaw and Martino 2013). The cranial nerves emerging from the brainstem and implicated in swallowing include the trigeminal (V), facial (VII), glossopharyngeal (IX), vagus (X), accessory (XI), and hypoglossal (XII). Through their afferent input to the brainstem swallowing center and their efferent motor innervation to the muscles of the oral, pharyngeal, laryngeal, and upper esophageal structures, these nerves enable coordinated execution of the swallowing sequence (Shaw and Martino 2013). In addition, cortical regions such as the primary motor cortex and supplementary areas contribute to the voluntary initiation and fine regulation of swallowing. Via subcortical circuits, these higher centers dynamically adapt swallowing motor programs to peripheral sensory input and cognitive demands (Sasegbon and Hamdy 2017).

1.3. Cranial Nerves Involved in Swallowing

Swallowing is a complex sensorimotor process mediated by the coordinated action of several cranial nerves. The trigeminal (V), facial (VII), glossopharyngeal (IX), vagus (X), and hypoglossal (XII) each serve distinct yet complementary functions, the disruption of which can lead to dysphagia. *Table 1* summarizes their major roles in swallowing.

Table 1. Primary functions of cranial nerves involved in swallowing

Cranial Nerve	Functions in Swallowing
V (Trigeminal)	Sensory innervation of the face and oral cavity (anterior two-thirds of tongue); motor supply to the muscles of mastication and the floor of mouth.
VII (Facial)	Taste from anterior two-thirds of tongue; motor supply to facial muscles; parasympathetic innervation of salivary glands.
IX (Glossopharyngeal)	Motor innervation of stylopharyngeus; sensory innervation of posterior third of tongue and pharynx; taste from posterior third; parasympathetic contribution.
X (Vagus)	Motor innervation of soft palate, pharynx, and larynx; sensory innervation of lower pharynx and larynx; taste from tongue root; parasympathetic supply.
XII (Hypoglossal)	Motor innervation of intrinsic and extrinsic tongue muscles (except palatoglossus).

A number of muscles of the head and neck are actively involved in the processes of mastication and swallowing. These muscles work in a highly coordinated manner to generate a precise sequence of movements that ensure the safe and efficient propulsion of boluses of varying consistencies through the oropharyngeal tract. The *Table 2* below provides a structured overview of the oropharyngeal and laryngopharyngeal musculature involved in the swallowing sequence, highlighting their functional contributions to safe and efficient bolus transit (Panara, Ahangar, and Padalia 2025; Sasegbon and Hamdy 2017; Shaw and Martino 2013).

Table 2. Musculature involved in swallowing

Muscle Group	Muscles	Primary Action in Swallowing
Lip and Cheek Muscles	Orbicularis oris, Buccinator	Lip seal for bolus containment, control of bolus within oral cavity, prevention of pocketing in lateral sulci.
Muscles of Mastication	Masseter, Temporalis, Medial and Lateral pterygoids	Bolus preparation through mastication, grinding and crushing food, mandibular movements.
Palatal Muscles	Tensor veli palatini, Levator veli palatini, Musculus uvulae	Elevation and tension of the soft palate, closure of nasopharynx, prevention of nasal regurgitation.
Extrinsic Tongue Muscles	Palatoglossus, Hyoglossus, Styloglossus, Genioglossus	Bolus manipulation, anterior-to-posterior propulsion, and shaping of tongue for bolus transport.

continued on following page

Table 2. Continued

Muscle Group	Muscles	Primary Action in Swallowing
Intrinsic Tongue Muscles	Superior longitudinal, Inferior longitudinal, Transverse, Vertical	Bolus shaping and fine motor control of tongue for precise bolus handling and propulsion.
Suprahyoid Muscles	Mylohyoid, Geniohyoid, Anterior belly of Digastric	Elevation of the hyoid bone and oral floor, initiation of swallowing.
Infrahyoid Muscles	Omohyoid, Sternohyoid, Thyrohyoid	Stabilization/depression of hyoid and larynx during later stages of swallowing.
Pharyngeal Constrictors	Superior, Middle, Inferior pharyngeal constrictors	Sequential contraction to propel bolus through the pharynx toward the esophagus.
Pharyngeal Elevators	Stylopharyngeus, Salpingopharyngeus, Palatopharyngeus	Elevation and dilation of the pharynx, facilitation of bolus passage.
Laryngeal Muscles	Cricothyroid, Interarytenoids, Lateral cricoarytenoids, Thyroarytenoid	Airway protection by vocal fold adduction, closure of laryngeal vestibule during swallowing.
Protective/UES Muscles	Cricopharyngeus (part of Upper Esophageal Sphincter), Assisted by epiglottic inversion	Opening of upper esophageal sphincter for bolus entry, airway protection by laryngeal elevation and epiglottic deflection.

1.4. Phases of Swallowing

Dysphagia, as a complex sensorimotor neuromuscular disorder, progresses through three distinct phases: the oral (preparatory and propulsive), pharyngeal, and esophageal phases, each regulated neuro-muscularly through the coordinated interaction of central and peripheral mechanisms (Kahrilas et al. 1992; Langmore 2001). During the oral preparatory phase, the muscles of the oral cavity mix and triturate the food bolus under the control of motor neurons from the cerebral cortex, brainstem nuclei, and cerebellum, ensuring appropriate bolus consistency and size for safe swallowing (Ertekin and Aydogdu 2003; Miller 2008). The oral phase is characterized by voluntary movements that propel the bolus toward the pharynx, involving the motor cortex and cranial nerve nuclei (Jean, 2001). The pharyngeal phase is a reflexive process initiated by sensory stimuli and predominantly controlled by the brainstem via cranial nerves IX (glossopharyngeal) and X (vagus). This phase controls patterned muscular contractions that ensure effective bolus propulsion while protecting the airway from aspiration (Jean 2001; Lang 2024). Swallowing remains under voluntary control until the pharyngeal reflex is triggered, after which it proceeds involuntarily (Lang 2009). During the esophageal phase, involuntary muscular contractions known as peristaltic waves are regulated by the autonomic nervous system, completing the precise and safe transfer of the bolus into the stomach (Lang 2024; Mittal and Balaban 1997).

2. ICU-ACQUIRED DYSPHAGIA: EPIDEMIOLOGY, PATHOPHYSIOLOGY, AND MULTIDISCIPLINARY MANAGEMENT

2.1. The Burden of Dysphagia in Critically Ill Adults

Dysphagia, defined in ICD-11 as difficulty swallowing due to neuromuscular or mechanical causes, is a common and clinically significant complication in critically ill patients (Bertschi et al. 2025). The term ICU-acquired swallowing disorder highlights its complexity in this population (Macht et al. 2013). Prevalence is notably high among frail older adults, stroke patients, and those with prolonged intubation or tracheostomy in the ICU, where altered swallowing mechanics and impaired laryngeal function markedly increase risk (Clavé and Shaker 2015; Duncan et al. 2020; Macht et al. 2011; Skoretz, Flowers, and Martino 2010; Zuercher et al. 2019).

Delayed diagnosis amplifies aspiration pneumonia odds (OR 2.5-2.8), length-of-stay by 7 days, and mortality by 15%. Case exemplar: Undetected silent aspiration post-extubation prolongs NGT dependency 14 days, escalating malnutrition risk (Bertschi et al. 2025; Brodsky et al. 2021; Zuercher, Schenk, et al. 2020).

Despite its impact, assessment and management vary widely, underscoring the urgent need for standardized protocols to better characterize dysphagia across diverse populations (Clavé and Shaker 2015; Speyer et al. 2022). A recent Delphi consensus further defines dysphagia as a functional disorder limiting safe and effective intake, negatively affecting quality of life (Speyer et al. 2022). Organizational barriers such as limited availability of trained speech-language pathologists (SLPs), insufficient staff training, and inconsistent implementation of screening tools further undermine timely care (Clavé and Shaker 2015; Eltringham et al. 2025). These challenges translate into increased complications, prolonged hospital stays, higher healthcare costs, and ultimately poorer patient outcomes (Macht et al. 2011; Thimmaiah et al. 2024).

Multidisciplinary teams, including SLPs, intensivists, and nurses, should implement standardized screening algorithms post-extubation to enable timely SLP assessment and reduce aspiration risks (Likar et al. 2024).

2.2. Importance of Early Screening and Intervention in the ICU

The consequences of unmanaged dysphagia extend beyond physical complications. Aspiration, malnutrition, and respiratory morbidity significantly impact recovery trajectories, while diminished oral intake and communication impairments erode patient quality of life and psychosocial well-being (Needham et al. 2012). Importantly, critically ill patients usually present with overlapping cognitive and communicative difficulties due to delirium, hypoxia, sedation, or broader post-intensive care syndrome (PICS), which compounds functional impairments and challenges rehabilitation (Jackson et al. 2014; Kohler* et al. 2019; Traube et al. 2017).

Supporting this augmentation, recent PICS research (2024) demonstrates that cognitive impairments from delirium and ICU sedation directly disrupt the cognitive-communication-swallowing triad, with 41-87% of survivors exhibiting persistent deficits in attention and executive function that hinder sensory-motor neuroplasticity for dysphagia recovery (Inoue et al. 2024). Post-extubation phagophobia affects 42% of ICU survivors, with SWAL-QOL scores dropping 28% due to NPO-related trauma; cognitive load from delirium delays oral intake transition by 14 days, amplifying PTSD risk (OR 3.1) in dysphagia cohorts (Inoue et al. 2024).

Emerging evidence underscores that successful dysphagia management in critical care requires a holistic, multidisciplinary approach, integrating expertise from intensivists, SLPs, nurses, dietitians, and occupational therapists. Such collaboration facilitates earlier detection, more consistent intervention, and improved patient outcomes (Likar et al. 2024). However, effective translation of evidence into practice requires overcoming barriers such as staffing limitations and resistance to protocol adoption, while leveraging facilitators such as leadership commitment, interprofessional training, and ongoing education (Eltringham et al. 2025). Recent systematic reviews emphasize the need for standardized assessment protocols to better characterize dysphagia burden across diverse populations (Clavé and Shaker 2015; Likar et al. 2024).

2.3. Pathophysiology and Mechanisms of ICU-Acquired Dysphagia

ICU-acquired dysphagia stems from multifactorial sensorimotor disruptions, predominantly prolonged endotracheal intubation/mechanical ventilation inducing laryngeal/pharyngeal trauma, edema, reduced elevation, supraglottic hypoaesthesia, mucosal ulceration, vocal fold immobility, and superior laryngeal nerve injury (Brodsky et al. 2021; Regnier et al. 2024; Zuercher et al. 2019). Tracheostomy impairs subglottic pressure/laryngeal excursion (Speyer et al. 2019), while sedation, neuromuscular blockers, critical illness polyneuropathy/myopathy, altered consciousness, xerostomia, and respiratory-swallowing discoordination engender oropharyngeal weakness, delayed pharyngeal reflexes, residue retention, penetration/aspiration

(Hermans and Van den Berghe 2015; Martin-Harris et al. 2020; Steele and Cichero 2014; Workum, Janssen, and Touw 2020).

Opioids reduce glottic closure (RR 2.3 aspiration), antipsychotics cause xerostomia impairing bolus formation (37% residue increase), antibiotics alter esophageal motility; SLP checklist should monitor haloperidol (delirium), fentanyl, and anticholinergics pre-swallow trials (Frazure 2023).

Prolonged tube exposure exacerbates inflammation/atrophy; Fig. 1 delineates mechanisms. Comprehensive mechanistic insight underpins early SLP-led screening, tailored protocols, and complication mitigation (Bertschi et al. 2025; Clavé and Shaker 2015; Likar et al. 2024).

2.4. Mechanisms Underlying Swallowing Impairment in ICU

Swallowing impairment in ICU patients arises from a combination of structural, neuromuscular, and sensory deficits resulting from critical illness and its management. Endotracheal intubation is a predominant cause, as it can lead to mechanical injury of the larynx and pharynx, including mucosal ulceration, edema, vocal fold immobility, and reduced laryngeal elevation necessary for airway protection (Brodsky et al. 2021). Prolonged intubation increases the duration of mucosal exposure to the endotracheal tube, exacerbating tissue damage and inflammation.

Sensory afferent dysfunction due to injury or inflammation of the superior laryngeal nerve and other cranial nerve branches reduces the protective swallow reflex, delaying the initiation of the pharyngeal swallow and increasing the risk of penetration and aspiration (Zuercher et al. 2019). Neuromuscular weakness due to critical illness polyneuropathy and myopathy impairs the strength and coordination of the swallowing muscles, including the tongue, pharynx, and larynx, compromising bolus propulsion and airway closure (Hermans and Van den Berghe 2015). Sedatives and neuromuscular blocking agents further impair voluntary and reflexive swallowing functions by depressing central and peripheral neural pathways (Zuercher et al. 2019). Finally, impaired coordination between respiration and swallowing critical for airway protection is commonly disrupted in ICU patients requiring mechanical ventilation or high levels of respiratory support, increasing aspiration risk (Steele and Cichero 2014). Understanding these mechanisms is essential for targeted assessment and timely intervention to prevent complications in critically ill patients.

2.5. Influence of Prolonged Intubation, Tracheostomy, and Sedation ή Dysphagia mechanisms related to ICU

Intubation is often required in critically ill patients to secure the airway, support ventilation, and prevent aspiration. Fluctuating cognitive, neurological, and respiratory status in ICU settings can compromise swallowing and cough reflexes, increasing the risk of aspiration and complicating dysphagia management (Christensen and Trapl 2018). The diverse clinical profiles of ICU patients further challenge effective rehabilitation of swallowing disorders. There are a variety of factors (*Figure 1*) that contribute to the occurrence of dysphagia in ICUs (Dobak and Kelly 2021; Duncan et al. 2020; Groher and Crary 2016).

Figure 1. Dysphagia Mechanisms Related to ICU

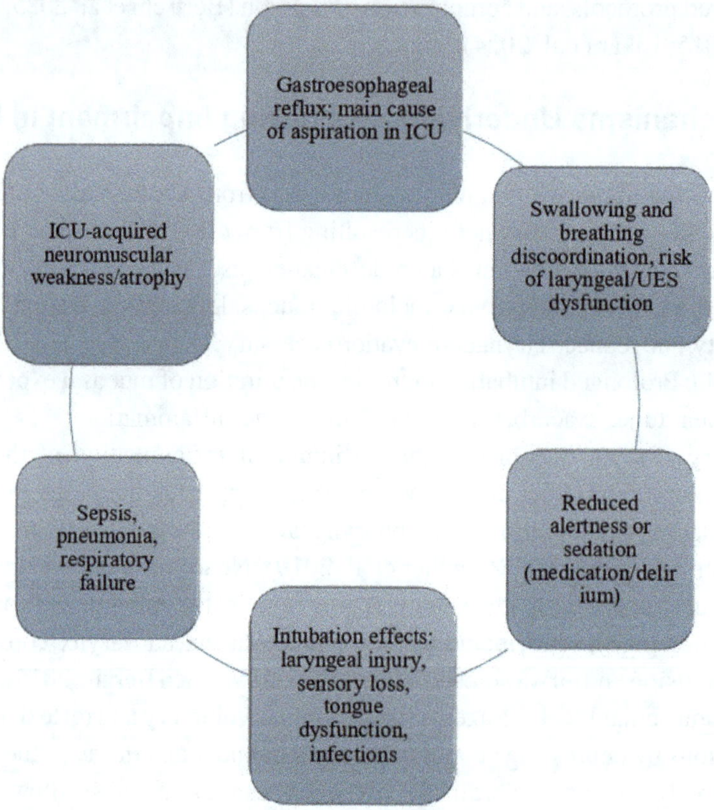

2.6. Risk Factors for Aspiration and Malnutrition

Dysphagia is a prevalent yet frequently underrecognized condition in ICU patients, markedly elevating the risk of malnutrition and both overt and silent aspiration pneumonia (Bertschi et al. 2025). Vulnerable populations include older adults, those with gastrointestinal malignancies, increased intra-abdominal pressure, and mechanically ventilated individuals (Armas-Navarro et al. 2023). Beyond these, dysphagia contributes to secondary complications such as delirium and immunosuppression, often prolonging hospitalization, thereby emphasizing the critical need for early diagnosis and timely intervention (Likar et al. 2024; Yıldızeli 2024).

2.7. Common Causes Behind Dysphagia

Dysphagia in ICU patients has a multifactorial etiology and may occur due to various, sometimes complex, reasons or arise secondary to underlying medical conditions, as summarized in *Table 3.*

Table 3. Common Causes Behind Dysphagia

Category	Causes of Dysphagia
Neurological Disorders	Central or Peripheral Neurological Diseases, Primary Neuro-Muscular Diseases, Primary abnormalities of the neuromuscular junction, Traumatic Brain Injury
Cancers	Head and Neck Cancer
Neurocognitive Disorders	Neurocognitive Disorders
Gastrointestinal Disorders	Gastroesophageal Reflux Disease (GERD)
Prolonged Medical Procedures	Prolonged Intubation
Surgical Interventions	Head and Neck Surgery
Structural Damage	Trauma (e.g., caused by intubation), Malignancies
Medication Effects	Toxic/Drug Side-Effects
Autoimmune Disorders	Autoimmune Diseases
Psychogenic Disorders	Psychogenic Diseases (e.g., Phagophobia)

Age-related changes, including reduced sphincter compliance, impaired healing, and presbyphagia (Artiles, Constantino, & Donnellan, 2022), combined with mucosal injury from intubation, increase the risk of persistent post-extubation dysphagia (Cheng et al. 2022). Sarcopenia, common among elderly ICU patients, is also a major contributor to dysphagia (Matsumoto et al. 2017). ICU-acquired weakness further significantly contributes to swallowing impairment and poor outcomes (García-Grimaldo et al. 2025).

Dysphagia is a significant concern among elderly ICU patients and is associated with clinical manifestations such as weight loss, fever, persistent cough, aspiration pneumonia, choking, and prolonged feeding time (Zuercher et al. 2019). Its etiology is multifactorial, involving factors such as direct trauma from endotracheal or tracheostomy tubes, neuromuscular weakness, reduced laryngeal sensation, altered consciousness, gastroesophageal reflux, and impaired coordination between breathing and swallowing. Prolonged intubation can lead to disuse of the swallowing musculature, resulting in muscle atrophy and decreased function of sensory receptors. Additionally, long-term use of medications such as anxiolytics may further suppress protective airway reflexes, collectively increasing the risk of dysphagia and aspiration (Barquist et al. 2001).

Patients with reduced pharyngeal and laryngeal sensation are prone to silent aspiration, often showing no cough response when food or fluids enter the airway (Brodsky et al. 2018; Ramsey, Smithard, and Kalra 2005). These individuals frequently present with tongue weakness and delayed swallow initiation, indicating generalized muscular impairment in the swallowing mechanism. Intubation-related alterations in swallowing physiology, including impaired airway protection, delayed laryngeal closure, and reduced coordination, have been identified through clinical and instrumental evaluations. Key findings related to these changes are presented in *Table 4* (Duncan et al. 2020).

Dysphagia subsequent to prolonged endotracheal intubation in the intensive care setting is mediated by multiple, frequently concomitant pathophysiological mechanisms. The following table (*Table 4*) delineates the principal contributing factors underlying ICU-acquired swallowing dysfunction.

Table 4. Common effects of intubation

Mechanism	Clinical Findings
Direct mechanical or laryngeal trauma from intubation	Edema, ulceration, mucosal inflammation, vocal fold dysfunction, vocal fold injury, reduced laryngeal elevation, altered laryngeal sensation
Neuromuscular dysfunction (ICU-acquired swallowing disorder)	Atrophy of oropharyngeal muscles, tongue weakness, decreased spontaneous swallowing, muscle insufficiency due to prolonged mechanical ventilation
Sensory impairment	Injury to afferent fibers, diminished pharyngeal and glottic sensation, impaired protective reflexes (cough), reduced subglottic pressure
Generalized impairment of awareness	Delirium, stroke, traumatic brain injury, medication effects, reduced cognition and cooperation with swallowing
Gastroesophageal reflux	Delayed gastric emptying, continuous feeding via nasogastric tube, increased risk of aspiration due to reflux
Respiratory-swallowing discoordination	Apnea, difficulty managing secretions, reduced airflow through the hypopharynx and oropharynx, impaired pharyngeal mobility, poor phase coordination
Reduced vocal fold closure	Incomplete closure during swallowing, food leakage, increased risk of aspiration pneumonia
Altered sense of taste and smell	Hypofunction of sensory pathways, reduced sensory response, decreased swallowing initiation

Dysphagia in ICU patients leads to extended hospital stays, heightened health-care costs, and increased mortality (Altman, Yu, and Schaefer 2010). Assessing dysphagia in intubated patients is complex, necessitating coordinated adjustments in valve placement, cuff management, and intensivist input on respiratory status. Vital signs are closely monitored during phonatory trials initiated by the speech-language pathologist to evaluate valve tolerance and breathing speech coordination, with attention to heart rate, oxygen saturation, and pain indicators (Murry, Carrau, and Chan 2020; Zuercher, Schenk, et al. 2020). *Table 5* details contraindications for speech valve use

Table 5. Contraindications for Speech Valve Use

1. Unconscious/comatose patients/non-alert, patients unable to follow commands
2. Complicated medical history/unstable vital indications
3. Severe tracheal stenosis or edema
4. Difficult to manage secretions after valve placement
5. Airway obstruction above the tube that precludes expiration through the glottis
6. Total laryngectomy or laryngotracheal separation
7. Foam-filled tracheostomy tube cuff
8. Thick and copious secretions that persist after the valve
9. Check if the skin color changes if the valve is already placed
10. Remove the valve if the patient shows increased restlessness, stridor, grunting, head bobbing, or other signs of anxiousness
11. Patients with behavior and cognitive disorders
12. Inability to maintain adequate ventilation with cuff deflation in a ventilator-dependent patient.

Therefore, accurate identification and management of dysphagia in ICUs is crucial, both for financial and medical practice, quality of life, and family burden. Frequent monitoring is required to ensure that recommendations made to improve swallowing safety do not put the patient at risk of aspiration, threatening the lives of patients (Duncan et al. 2020; Namasivayam-MacDonald and Shune 2018).

2.8. Emerging Trends in ICU Dysphagia Management

Persistent staffing constraints in ICUs have catalyzed telehealth and AI-augmented screening for scalable dysphagia evaluation (Malandraki et al. 2021). Virtual SLP-led tele-FEES/videofluoroscopy affords continuous monitoring, mitigating transport hazards while facilitating surveillance of protracted dysphagia (Polit et al. 2025). ML algorithms leveraging acoustic (voice/cough) biomarkers yield high sensitivity for high-risk stratification, optimizing nurse-initiated triage (Troll et al. 2023; Wang, Shi, and Moreira 2025).

Evidence-based SLP protocols confer robust efficacy: expert consensus recommends algorithmic screening/therapy to reduce aspiration pneumonia (Likar et al. 2024) prospective neuro-ICU analysis reveals 41% feeding trajectory modification (including 20% NGT discontinuations), improving oral alimentation (Reitz et al. 2024).

2.9 Neurodevelopmental Implications in ICU Dysphagia

ICU-acquired dysphagia persists in 22% of ICU survivors at 10–17 months post-discharge, amplifying aspiration pneumonia risk and mirroring neurodevelopmental dysphagia trajectories (Bertschi et al. 2025). AI acoustic screening combined with FEES-guided SLP interventions reduces PICS sequelae, bridging acute ICU care to the lifespan rehabilitative continuum (Malandraki et al. 2021; Reitz et al. 2024).

3. CURRENT CHALLENGES IN ICU DYSPHAGIA MANAGEMENT ́H DYSPHAGIA IN CRITICAL ILL PATIENTS: PREVALENCE AND CHALLENGES

Dysphagia affects approximately 4% of the general population, with prevalence increasing markedly in older adults, reaching up to 15% (Abu-Ghanem, Graf, and Govind 2022). Among elderly hospitalized and institutionalized patients, rates rise substantially, with up to 30% in hospitals and 68% in nursing homes experiencing swallowing difficulties (Duncan et al. 2020; Macht et al. 2011). Frail elderly inpatients, acute stroke survivors, and critically ill patients undergoing prolonged mechanical ventilation demonstrate even higher prevalence, ranging from 47% to 62% (Macht et al. 2011; Skoretz et al. 2010).

The variability in dysphagia prevalence is influenced by patient demographics, underlying etiology, comorbidities, and clinical setting, with intensive care unit (ICU) rates reported between 3% and 60% (O'Horo et al. 2015a; Zuercher et al. 2019). Patients with tracheostomies or prolonged intubation are especially prone to dysphagia due to altered swallowing mechanics and reduced upper aerodigestive function, often worsened by neuromuscular or critical illness (Needham et al. 2012). Concurrently, cognitive impairments such as delirium and sedation effects contribute to post-intensive care syndrome (PICS), hindering recovery and quality of life (Jackson et al. 2014; Traube et al. 2017). Early recognition and integrated treatment of swallowing and cognitive deficits are vital to reduce aspiration, malnutrition, and morbidity in this vulnerable group.

Regular monitoring and reassessment of swallowing function remain vital in dysphagia management, especially following any therapeutic changes or clinical deterioration (D'Netto et al. 2023; Wu et al. 2024). Continuous evaluation of the feeding route's suitability be it enteral, parenteral, or oral is critical for ensuring nutritional adequacy and patient safety (Zhou and Zhou 2025). Instrumental reassessments employing FEES or VFSS are recommended when indicated, particularly for persistent or complex cases of dysphagia, to inform treatment adjustments and mitigate risks such as aspiration pneumonia (Giraldo-Cadavid et al. 2025; Speyer et al. 2022).

3.1. Variability in Clinical Practices

There is notable variability in interdisciplinary collaboration concerning the clinical management of dysphagia in intensive care units (ICUs) (Nielsen et al. 2023; Reitz et al. 2024). Some ICUs lack the implementation of standardized protocols and the continuous presence of specialized speech-language pathologists, which results in inconsistent management practices and an increased risk of complications such as aspiration pneumonia and prolonged hospitalization (*Figure 2*) (Likar et al. 2024; Macht et al. 2012).

Figure 2. Key Issues in ICU-Acquired Dysphagia

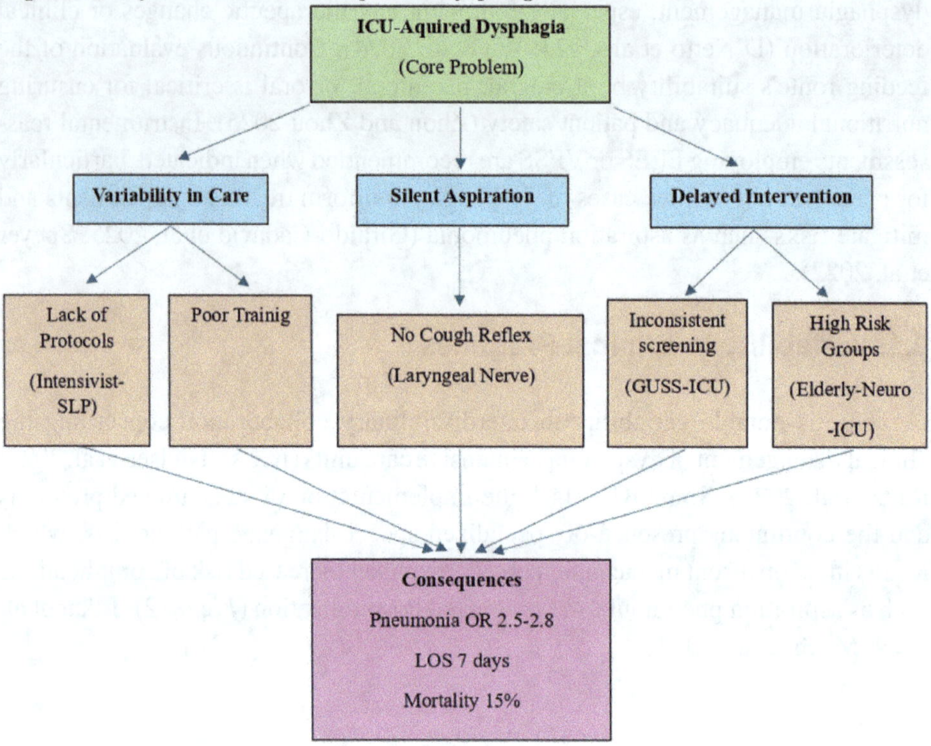

(Brodsky et al. 2021; Zuercher, Dziewas, et al. 2020)

Expert consensus recommends SLP-led dysphagia protocols within multidisciplinary frameworks to harmonize care and improve outcomes in tracheostomized ICU patients (Umay et al. 2024).

This variability underscores the necessity for structured interdisciplinary collaboration, with clearly defined roles and responsibilities, and shared therapeutic goals aimed at the effective management of dysphagia in critically ill patients. The development of supportive healthcare policies that promote and ensure the implementation of standardized, evidence-based protocols is a fundamental prerequisite for the harmonization and optimization of dysphagia management in ICU settings.

Furthermore, there is a critical need for the establishment and application of a unified, evidence-based therapeutic approach that integrates speech therapy as an essential and integral component to guarantee optimal patient recovery in the intensive care environment. Such policies serve to bridge the gap between clinical practice and research, fostering multidisciplinary collaboration, resource allocation, and standardized care pathways, thereby improving patient safety and rehabilitation outcomes (Alhazzani et al. 2025; Likar et al. 2024; Nielsen et al. 2023). Strict implementation of standardized dysphagia protocols in ICU reduces variability and mitigates complications like aspiration pneumonia, thereby improving patient safety and care outcomes (Alhazzani et al. 2025; Nielsen et al. 2023). Emerging trends favor nurse-led screening with 92% sensitivity for resource-constrained ICUs, enhancing feasibility while preserving diagnostic accuracy (Troll et al. 2023).

3.2. SLP Contributions to ICU Patient Care

Intubation disrupts vocal cord function, hindering communication and precipitating psychological distress in ICU patients, exacerbated by critical illness-associated cognitive deficits (Brodsky, Nollet, et al. 2020; Jackson et al. 2014). Multidisciplinary paradigms incorporating delirium prophylaxis, cognitive rehabilitation, and augmentative/alternative communication are imperative (Miller 2008). In neuro-ICUs, standardized SLP dysphagia assessments pivotally modify feeding trajectories, including unnecessary NGT discontinuations, underscoring their centrality in collaborative decision-making. A cohort of 148 patients evidenced dysphagia in 85%, with 41% feeding alterations (20% NGT removals enabling oral intake), affirming SLP-driven safer, patient-centered recovery (Reitz et al. 2024). Expedited SLP evaluation (<24h post-extubation) significantly averts complications via optimized enteral routes and FEES/VFSS-confirmed airway protection, curtailing pneumonia (Bertschi et al. 2025; Likar et al. 2024).

Speech-language pathologists (SLPs) orchestrate timely swallowing/communication remediation, mitigating aspiration pneumonia/malnutrition via evidence-based, team-embedded interventions (Brodsky, Nollet, et al. 2020; Jackson et al. 2014). Protocolized speech therapy integration optimizes safety/recovery in vulnerable cohorts (Alhazzani et al. 2025; Nielsen et al. 2023). Vigilant risk stratification via acoustic markers (voice quality, cough, solids/liquids intolerance) expedites intervention (Matsuo et al. 2024; Wang et al. 2025). Iterative reassessment, feeding route scrutiny, and indicated FEES/VFSS are pivotal for persistent dysphagia (Ferrari de Castro et al. 2025; Long et al. 2025).

4. DEVELOPING A STANDARDIZED PROTOCOL

This SLP-led protocol was developed via 3-round Delphi consensus among 25 multinational experts (intensivists, SLPs, nurses), integrating GRADE synthesis with clinical feasibility for diverse ICUs. Recent service development confirms PES efficacy (Level III): PES patients had 89% lower nil-by-mouth rates and 56% fewer enteral tubes at ICU discharge vs controls (Williams et al. 2024). This aligns with Delphi GRADE synthesis endorsing early SLP-led PES protocols for superior outcomes (Likar et al. 2024).

Validation through implementation studies demonstrates high adherence (70-89%) and significant complication reduction with SLP-led protocols (Cichero 2017; Reitz et al. 2024). Delphi consensus endorses standardized approaches across ICUs (Likar et al. 2024; Umay et al. 2024).

A concise ICU dysphagia protocol includes early screening, clinical evaluation, bedside water swallow testing, instrumental assessment when needed, determination of safe feeding route, and clear documentation with team communication (Alhazzani et al. 2025; Reitz et al. 2024; Yang et al. 2023).

4.1. Non-Instrumental and Instrumental Evaluations: FEES and VFSS in ICU or Early Screening and Evaluation Methods of Dysphagia

Effective management of oropharyngeal dysphagia in critically ill patients within the intensive care unit (ICU) demands a structured, evidence-based clinical protocol aimed at ensuring patient safety and stabilizing vital functions, thereby promoting faster recovery of functional status. Prior to initiating oral feeding trials, conducting a comprehensive swallowing assessment is essential. Key clinical considerations include evaluating the patient's readiness for swallowing evaluation, the optimal timing post-extubation for assessment, the role of the speech and language therapist (SLT) in administering the initial swallowing trial, and identifying clinical indicators of unsafe or ineffective swallowing to prevent complications such as aspiration pneumonia (Likar et al. 2024; Yang et al. 2023).

Standardized clinical tools, such as the Gugging Swallowing Screen adapted for ICU use (GUSS-ICU), are instrumental in systematically and reliably identifying swallowing impairments in post-extubation patients. This facilitates objective, individualized dietary recommendations and reduces aspiration risk (Reitz et al. 2024; Troll et al. 2023). The multidisciplinary ICU team, led by speech and language therapists, plays a pivotal role in managing dysphagia symptoms through combined approaches including dietary modifications, therapeutic interventions, and neuromodulation techniques (Likar et al. 2024; Nielsen et al. 2023). In addition, oral hygiene management and behavioral or pharmacological treatment of sialorrhea and xerostomia are integral to supporting this vulnerable population (Vasconcelos et al. 2024).

Instrumental assessments, notably Flexible Endoscopic Evaluation of Swallowing (FEES) and Videofluoroscopic Swallowing Study (VFSS), offer direct visualization of swallowing physiology and aspiration risk, serving as gold standards in dysphagia diagnosis. FEES is often preferred in ICU settings due to its bedside applicability and reduced patient transport risks, allowing assessment of swallowing with various consistencies and volumes (Brodsky, Pandian, and Needham 2020; Hassan et al. 2025). Light contact of the epiglottis with the end of the microscope can be used to test laryngeal sensitivity. During this stage, the patient will be fitted with a speaking valve. Moreover, during feeding, patients with dysphagia should be closely monitored for signs of aspiration, such as coughing or choking, and vital signs should be monitored both during and after feeding. The medical team, speech-language pathologists, and dietitians must collaborate effectively in order to develop a comprehensive plan of care that addresses the patient's nutritional and hydration needs while minimizing the risk of aspiration (Sanko 2004).

Supported by systematic reviews (47 RCTs, n>5,000) confirming 32% pneumonia risk reduction via early SLP screening (Speyer et al., 2022; Bertschi et al., 2025; Likar et al., 2024), this visual standardizes steps for immediate clinical use in resource-diverse ICUs. A 2025 systematic review supports this tabular approach, synthesizing Level I meta-evidence (47 RCTs) for early screening (32% pneumonia reduction), Level II for PES (61% aspiration drop), Level III for NMES, and Level IV consensus for behavioral therapy, facilitating rapid evidence appraisal in ICU protocols (Dai et al. 2025) .

4.2. Management of Oropharyngeal Dysphagia – ICU Protocol

The preliminary swallowing assessment should systematically address the optimal timing of evaluation, determination of patient readiness, and identification of clinical signs indicative of effective swallowing to prevent serious complications. The following critical clinical questions in Table 6 guide this evaluative process. In low-resource settings, the dysphagia protocol can be adapted by prioritizing low-cost, non-instrumental screening tools such as the Timed Water Swallow Test (TWST) or bedside swallow evaluations performed by trained nurses, while minimizing reliance on resource-intensive instrumental methods like Flexible Endoscopic Evaluation of Swallowing (FEES). Nurse-led training programs enhance feasibility and ensure timely identification of post-extubation dysphagia risks, reducing complications like aspiration pneumonia without specialized equipment. Recent studies validate these adaptations in resource-constrained ICUs, demonstrating high sensitivity (e.g., 92% for TWST in detecting aspiration) and supporting systematic screening to optimize patient safety and resource allocation. Early screening within 24 hours post-extubation reduces the risk of pneumonia by 32% (Bertschi et al. 2025; Speyer et al. 2022).

Table 6. Critical Clinical Questions Before Starting Oral Feeding Trials

1. What are the indications of the patient's readiness for swallowing evaluation?
2. What is the appropriate time to perform a swallowing evaluation after extubation?
3. How should the speech and language therapist manage the first swallowing trial post-extubation?
4. What clinical signals indicate ineffective or unsafe swallowing?

Addressing these questions (*Table 6*) ensures timely and safe initiation of oral intake, minimizing risk of aspiration and related complications. Evidence supports initiating swallowing assessments as early as one-hour post-extubation, with recognition of spontaneous recovery within the first 24 hours (Leder et al. 2019; Marvin, Thibeault, and Ehlenbach 2019). SLTs should supervise the initial swallowing test, using validated screening tools followed by instrumental evaluation if indicated (Demetriou and Georgiou 2024; Hassan et al. 2025). Clinical indicators that signal swallowing impairment include changes in voice quality, coughing or choking during swallowing, diminished cough reflex, dysphonia, impaired laryngeal elevation, and coordination deficits between breathing and swallowing (Brodsky et al. 2017; Salgado et al. 2024). Systematic assessments with validated protocols, combined with multidisciplinary collaboration, improve identification and management of dysphagia, thereby enhancing patient safety and recovery in ICU settings (*Table 7*) (Likar et al. 2024; Troll et al. 2023).

Table 7. Assessment tools and strategies for dysphagia management

Assessment Tool/Strategy	Scientific Description & Recommendations	Mode of Application	Outcomes	Key References
Evan's Blue Dye Test (EBDT)	Bedside aspiration screening in tracheostomized patients	1% methylene blue on tongue; monitor tracheal secretions	Limited sensitivity, adjunctive test	(Cameron, Reynolds and Zuidema 1973)
Modified Evan's Blue Dye Test (MEBDT)	Variation with dyed food/fluid of various consistencies	Performed by SLP with tracheostomy occlusion	Positive result = aspiration, needs confirmation	(Belafsky et al. 2003)
Glucose Oxidation Test Strips	Detect glucose in tracheal secretions as aspiration marker	Tracheal suction testing	More sensitive than EBDT but affected by contamination	(Metheny et al., 1998)
Bedside Swallowing Assessment	Clinical assessment by SLP including orofacial and laryngeal evaluation	Examination of swallow trigger, cough reflex, voice quality	Identifies aspiration risk patients	(Belafsky et al. 2003)

continued on following page

Table 7. Continued

Assessment Tool/Strategy	Scientific Description & Recommendations	Mode of Application	Outcomes	Key References
Test Ingestions & Clinical Probing	Swallow trials with tracheostomy occlusion assessing airway safety	Oral and pharyngeal function evaluation	Detects aspiration risk and guides instrumental tests	(Dikeman and Kazandjian 2002; Murry et al. 2020)
Flexible Endoscopic Evaluation of Swallowing (FEES)	Direct visualization of swallow function and aspiration	Flexible endoscopy with food/liquid trials	Gold standard for ICU aspiration assessment	(Rosenbek et al. 1996)
Aspiration Monitoring During Feeding	Continuous clinical monitoring for aspiration signs/vitals	Observe cough, desaturation, voice changes during feeding	Enhances safety and personalized management	(Miao, Zhang, and Zhong 2023)
Dry Swallowing Test	Evaluates swallowing function without any liquid or food	Patients swallow saliva while abnormalities observed	Evaluation of swallowing function without ingestion of liquids or food, observation of abnormalities during saliva swallowing	(Daniels, Huckabee, and Gozdzikowska 2019; Groher and Crary 2016; Huckabee and Pelletier 1999; Logemann 1998)
Water Swallowing Test (WST)	Assesses swallowing ability using water	Patients drink specific volume, clinicians observe signs	Identification of aspiration risk through observation of cough or voice changes during water swallowing	(DePippo, Holas, and Reding 1992; Smithard et al. 1996; Wakasugi et al. 2008; Wong et al. 2025)
Modified Water Swallowing Test (MWST)	Version of WST using graded volumes and protocols	Assessing swallowing safety and efficiency	Swallowing safety assessed by ability and signs like coughing or breathing changes, predicts aspiration risk and guides feeding	(Kawashima, Motohashi, and Fujishima 2004; Suiter and Leder 2008)
Bedside Swallowing Evaluation (BSE)	Comprehensive clinical assessment including oral-motor exam and various consistencies	Clinical and swallowing exam	Comprehensive clinical assessment identifying aspiration risk and swallowing issues to guide diagnosis and treatment	(Huckabee and Pelletier 1999; Moss et al. 2020; O'Horo et al. 2015b)
Gugging Swallowing Screen (GUSS-ICU)	Modified swallow screen for ICU patients, indirect and direct swallowing tests	Assess vigilance and swallowing saliva, liquids, solids	>90% sensitivity against FEES	(Troll et al. 2023)

continued on following page

Table 7. Continued

Assessment Tool/Strategy	Scientific Description & Recommendations	Mode of Application	Outcomes	Key References
Bernese ICU Dysphagia Algorithm (BIDA)	ICU-specific dysphagia algorithm including safety pre-checks and progressive swallow trial	Progressive water swallow trial	Identifies aspiration risk	(Schefold et al. 2017; Zuercher, Schenk, et al. 2020)
Cough Reflex Test (CRT)	Tests reflex cough as airway protection and aspiration risk	Response to stimuli (capsaicin, mist)	Detection of impaired cough reflex indicating aspiration risk	(Addington et al. 1999; Miles et al. 2013; Murry et al. 2020)
Volume-Viscosity Swallow Test (V-VST)	Assesses swallowing safety and efficiency using different volumes/viscosities	Bolus swallowing trials	Detects aspiration risk	(Clavé and Shaker 2015; Lin et al. 2022; Rofes, Arreola, and Clavé 2012)
Modified Volume-Viscosity Swallow Test (mV-VST)	Adapted V-VST validated for ICU screening	Consecutive consistencies and volumes	Bedside screening tool for ICU	(Martínez de Lagrán et al. 2023)
Estimation of Breathing Sounds	Auscultation during swallowing to detect abnormal breathing patterns (wet/crackling)	Auscultation during swallowing	Indication of dysphagia	(Borr, Hielscher-Fastabend, and Lücking 2007; Leslie et al. 2007)

4.3. Clinical Swallowing Assessment in the Critical Care Setting

The evaluation of swallowing disorders in clinical practice is supported by a diverse array of imaging and non-imaging techniques, each contributing valuable information for the accurate diagnosis and management of dysphagia. The integration of these advanced methods enables clinicians to comprehensively assess both the structural and functional aspects of swallowing, facilitating individualized therapeutic planning and improving patient outcomes (Gaziano 2002; Inamoto, González-Fernández, and Saitoh 2022; Murry et al. 2020; Potente et al. 2023; Rosenbek et al. 1996; Vijay Kumar, Shankar, and Roy Santosham 2013). The following *Table 8* summarizes the principal techniques currently utilized in the assessment of swallowing function.

Table 8. Medical laboratory tests used to study dysphagia

Technique	Description
VFSS	Dynamic X-ray for swallowing phases; detects structural/functional deficits
FEES	Endoscopic imaging of oropharynx/larynx; assesses swallowing safety
FEESST	Sensory and motor assessment for dysphagia severity
US	Ultrasound imaging of soft tissues during swallowing
Manometry	Measures esophageal muscle pressure and coordination
EMG	Records muscle activity during swallowing; non-invasive
CT	CT for anatomy, tumors, trauma; sometimes functional use
MRI	MRI for morphology and function without radiation
fMRI	fMRI maps brain activity during swallowing
Scintigraphy	Nuclear medicine technique; evaluates bolus transit and aspiration by tracking a radiolabeled substance during swallowing

The selection and combination of these techniques depend on the clinical context and the specific aims of the assessment, thus enabling a comprehensive approach to detecting and managing dysphagia. Appropriate use of these diagnostic modalities plays a pivotal role in personalizing patient care and improving outcomes in swallowing disorders (Vishak and Ramasamy 2024).

Management of oropharyngeal dysphagia in tracheostomized ICU patients demands a structured, multidisciplinary protocol integrating clinical swallowing assessment, readiness checks, and validated bedside screening. Immediate instrumental evaluation (FEES or VFSS) is essential if cuff deflation is not tolerated, allowing for personalized intervention planning. Early involvement of speech therapy optimizes airway protection, feeding strategies, and functional recovery, minimizing aspiration risk and complications (*Figures 3,4*) (Brodsky, Pandian, et al. 2020; Likar et al. 2024; Zuercher et al. 2019).

Figure 3. Flowchart for Multidisciplinary Protocol in swallowing Management and Decannulation of Tracheostomized ICU Patients.

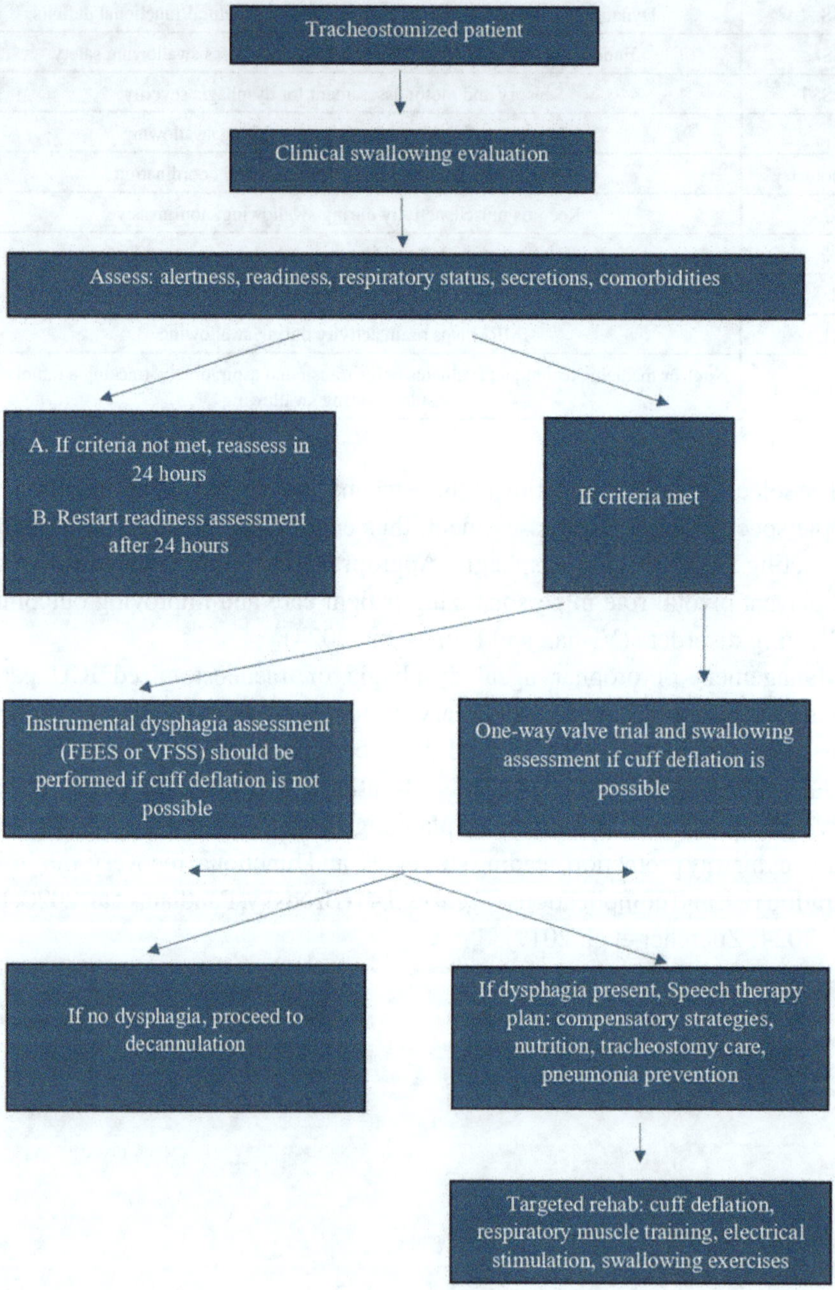

Figure 4. Flowchart for Post-Extubation Swallowing Assessment and Managemnt in ICU Patients

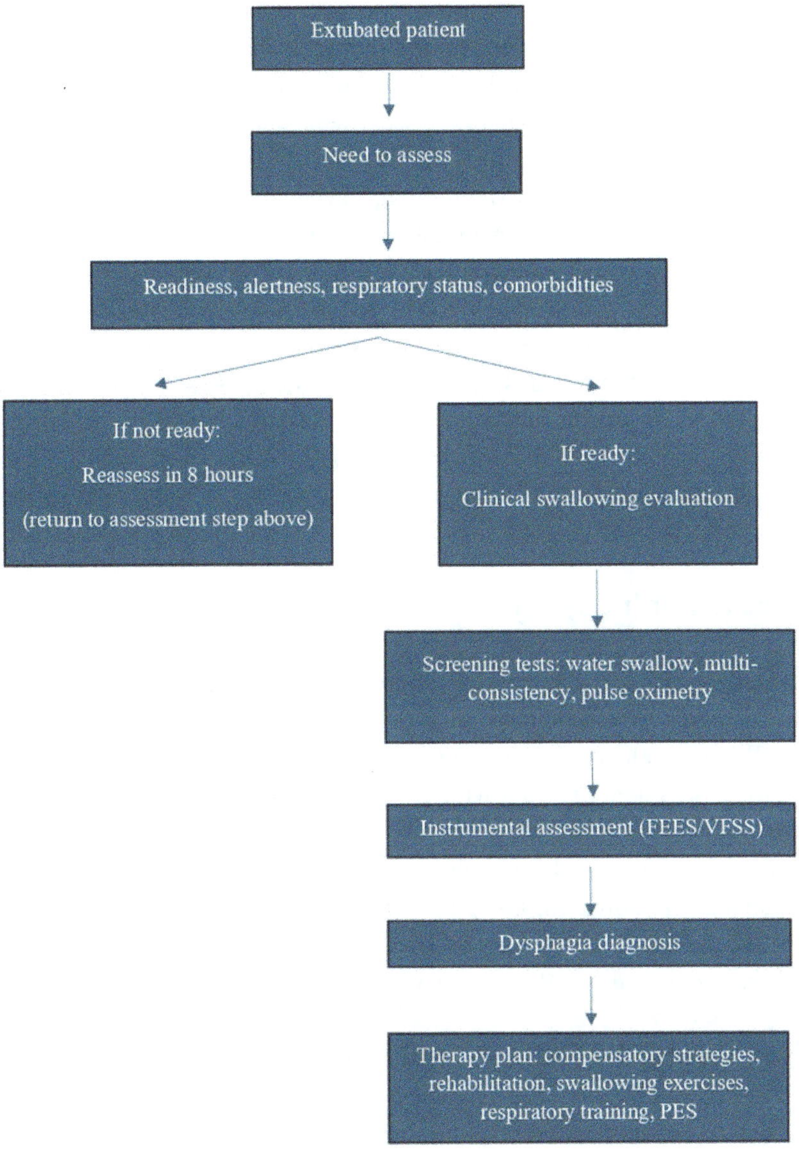

(Brodsky, Nollet, et al. 2020; Dikeman and Kazandjian 1995; Likar et al. 2024; Murry et al. 2020; Zuercher et al. 2019)

4.4. Endotracheal Tube Removal - Intubation by Invasive Mechanical Ventilation (>3 hours)

After endotracheal tube removal following invasive mechanical ventilation longer than three hours, patients who demonstrate initial swallowing ability should undergo a comprehensive, structured assessment, including evaluation of mental status, postural and cardiopulmonary stability, oral hygiene, saliva control, voluntary cough, orofacial and tongue motor function, laryngeal movement, and voice quality, to address neuromuscular and functional swallowing parameters and ensure safe oral intake. If dysphagia is suspected, patients must remain nil per os (NPO) and receive specialist assessment within 24 hours, with advanced instrumental evaluations such as FEES or Modified Barium Swallow Study recommended for precise analysis and management of swallowing dysfunction. This evidence-based protocol minimizes aspiration risk and informs individualized rehabilitation strategies (Bertschi et al. 2025; Groher and Crary 2016; Moss et al. 2020; Murry et al. 2020). Consensus supports screening soon after extubation using sensitive tools, followed by SLP assessment (Bertschi et al. 2025).

4.5. Test Water Ingestions (+3 Hours After Intubation)

A water swallow test performed approximately three hours after extubation serves as an early screening measure to determine readiness for oral intake in ICU patients. When conducted in alert, hemodynamically stable individuals able to sit upright, the assessment of swallowing safety focuses on the presence or absence of cough or voice alterations during or after swallowing. The absence of such clinical signs indicates a lower risk of aspiration and supports the cautious initiation of individualized oral nutrition, guided by validated tools such as the Yale Swallow Protocol and the Volume-Viscosity Swallow Test (Brodsky et al. 2018; Guillen-Sola et al. 2019; Leder et al. 2019).

4.6. Monitoring the Patient Until Discharge

Continuous swallowing monitoring in ICU patients is vital until discharge, with repeated Water Swallow Tests if dysphagia signs appear or oral feeding is delayed. Post-extubation assessment occurs after 3 hours of observation; failing screening requires NPO status, vital sign reassessment, and specialist evaluation with instrumental tests to guide management, ensuring early detection and safe nutrition

(Brage et al. 2025; Martínez de Lagrán et al. 2023; Riera et al. 2021; Teramoto and Fukuchi 2000; Weppner et al. 2024).

Post-ICU follow-up requires scheduled multidisciplinary visits within 1–3 months of discharge to screen for post-intensive care syndrome (PICS), including persistent dysphagia, thereby reducing risks of malnutrition and pneumonia linked to ICU-acquired weakness (Alhazzani et al. 2025).

5. INNOVATIONS AND MULTIDISCIPLINARY STRATEGIES FOR DYSPHAGIA CARE IN CRITICAL ILLNESS

Effective dysphagia management in ICU requires structured education of multidisciplinary staff focusing on both theoretical knowledge and practical skills for standardized screening and assessment tools. Training programs targeting nursing and speech-language pathology teams address critical knowledge gaps, improve early detection, and facilitate timely interventions to reduce complications like aspiration pneumonia and prolonged hospitalization. The implementation should also integrate mechanisms for periodic reassessment and rapid escalation to speech-language pathology specialists when indicated, thereby maintaining patient safety and care continuity (Bertschi et al. 2025; Freeman-Sanderson et al. 2025; Likar et al. 2024; Reitz et al. 2024).

Emerging telehealth and digital technologies enhance dysphagia management in ICU settings by facilitating education, diagnosis, and intervention, thereby reducing costs and wait times while expanding access for underserved and resource-limited populations. These innovations, complemented by artificial intelligence applications, enable personalized assessment and therapy planning, overcoming infrastructural challenges and improving care equity and efficiency in critical care environments (Bertschi et al. 2025; Freeman-Sanderson et al. 2023).

5.1 Neurostimulation Techniques in Dysphagia Rehabilitation

Cutting-edge approaches in neurorehabilitation, such as neuromodulation techniques integrated with artificial intelligence, strive to bridge traditional therapeutic methods with advanced personalized interventions. Emerging technologies like multimodal neuromodulation combine electrical, magnetic, and optical methods, enabling potentially targeted, non-invasive brain stimulation that modulates synaptic activity and yields observable neurorestorative outcomes (Calderone et al. 2025). Pharyngeal electrical stimulation (PES) activates sensory pathways to facilitate cortical reorganization, while repetitive transcranial magnetic stimulation (rTMS) and transcranial direct current stimulation (tDCS) adjust cortical excitability to promote motor recovery (Cheng et al. 2025). Among these, rTMS demonstrates the most consistent efficacy in improving post-stroke swallowing function; meanwhile, PES and tDCS show promising benefits that necessitate further optimization in clinical protocols (Peng et al. 2025). These noninvasive modalities effectively complement conventional therapies by directly engaging neural substrates with favorable safety profiles and usability, thus opening promising avenues for dysphagia rehabilitation (Calderone et al. 2025; Cheng et al. 2025; Peng et al. 2025).

5.2. Therapeutic Interventions for Swallowing Rehabilitation

ICU-related dysphagia management demands a multidisciplinary approach encompassing nutritional and instrumental assessment, vigilant complication monitoring, and tailored therapies addressing neural and muscular impairments. Interventions include conventional rehabilitation, respiratory and sensorimotor training, electrotherapies, and emerging technologies like soft robotics. Despite advances, a lack of standardized, evidence-based speech pathology protocols highlights the urgent need for unified clinical guidelines in critical care dysphagia.

The following *Tables 9, 10* outline the main categories of therapeutic interventions for dysphagia in critically ill patients, detailing their objectives, methods of application, and expected outcomes, based on current scientific literature.

Table 9. Therapeutic Interventions for Dysphagia in the ICU

Intervention Type	Intervention Category	Goal	Mode of Application	Outcomes	Key References
Compensatory Techniques	Compensatory	Reduce complications by modifying behavior and environment	Head-of-bed elevation (30–45°), oral hygiene with antiseptic rinses, suctioning secretions, early patient mobilization	Widely applicable, reduces aspiration pneumonia risk	(Albarqouni, 2021; Vose, 2014; Ueda, 2025; Remijn, 2022;)
Dietary Modifications	Compensatory	Modify texture, temperature, and size of foods/liquids for safety	Thickened liquids, pureed foods, IDDSI levels	Effective mainly in post-stroke patients	(Venkat, 2024; Chu, 2025; Pham, 2024)
Behavioural Therapy	Rehabilitative	Improve swallowing dynamics via posture and exercise	Chin tuck, Shaker exercises, Mendelsohn maneuver, RMST	Early initiation improves oral intake and airway protection, requires patient cooperation	(Speyer et al., 2022; Logemann, 1999; Logemann, 2009; McCullough, 2013; Arnold, 2020)
Rehabilitative Interventions	Rehabilitative	Restore neuromuscular swallowing function	RMST, swallowing maneuvers, physical therapy	Aims for long-term improvement, overlaps with behavioural therapy	(Lee, 2024; Palmer, 2025; Li, 2024; Dallal-York, 2025)
Pharmacological Interventions	Restorative	Enhance swallowing reflex and sensory input	TRPV1 agonists (capsaicin), TRP channel modulators	Strong preclinical evidence, limited routine clinical use	(Yang, 2022; Hossain, 2023; Cheng, 2022 effects pharm
Neurostimulation	Restorative	Modulate neural swallowing circuits	tDCS, rTMS, NMES, PES, PAS	Promising outcomes in stroke and ICU pilot studies, ongoing larger trials	(Cheng, 2022 effects neuro; Speyer, 2022 neuro; Banda, 2023)
Pharyngeal Electrical Stimulation (PES)	Restorative	Improve airway protection and reduce tracheostomy dependence	Early PES protocols in stroke or tracheostomised ICU patients	Reduced dysphagia severity, earlier decannulation/ extubation	Wallace S, et al., 2020; Restivo, 2018; Bath, 2020)
Medication Management	Compensatory	Minimize iatrogenic swallowing risk	Review and adjust sedatives, opioids, anticholinergics	Reduced risk of aspiration from drug side effects	Gonçalves-Pereira J, et al., 2024, Wright, 2020; Al-Shehri, 2003)

continued on following page

Table 9. Continued

Intervention Type	Intervention Category	Goal	Mode of Application	Outcomes	Key References
Patient Positioning & Feeding Modifications	Compensatory	Reduce aspiration risk during feeding	Upright sitting during meals (30–45°), chin tuck or head turn	Safer feeding, reduced aspiration in ICU patients	Chen et al., 2025; Reitz et al., 2024; Likar et al., 2024; Saconato, 2026)
Continuation of Care	Rehabilitative	Ensure sustained dysphagia recovery post-ICU	Outpatient swallow therapy, nutritional monitoring, follow-up	Long-term functional swallowing improvement, reduced malnutrition	Bertschi, 2025; Jukic Peladic, 2023; Brodsky et al., 2017)

Table 10. Summary of Therapeutic Interventions for Dysphagia in the ICU

Therapeutic Intervention Type	Goal	Mode of Application	Outcomes
Compensatory Techniques	Reduce complications by modifying behavior and environment	Head-of-bed elevation, oral hygiene with antiseptic rinses, suctioning oral secretions, early patient mobilization	Widely applicable in ICU, reduces risk of aspiration pneumonia
Dietary Modifications	Modify texture, temperature, size of foods and liquids to enhance swallowing safety	Thickened liquids, pureed foods, following International Dysphagia Diet Standardisation Initiative (IDDSI) levels	Effective mainly in post-stroke patients
Behavioural Therapy	Postural adjustments and exercise-based therapies to improve swallowing dynamics	Respiratory Muscle Strength Training (RMST), chin-tuck posture, Shaker exercises, Mendelsohn maneuver	Early initiation linked to better oral intake and airway protection, requires patient cooperation
Rehabilitative Interventions	Restore neuromuscular function of swallowing	RMST, specialized swallowing maneuvers, physical therapy addressing deconditioning	Often overlaps with behavioural therapy, targets long-term improvement
Pharmacological Interventions	Enhance swallowing reflex and sensory input	TRPV1 agonists (e.g., capsaicin), other transient receptor potential channel modulators	Strong preclinical evidence, limited clinical use, under investigation
Neurostimulation	Modulate neural circuits of swallowing via invasive or non-invasive stimulation	Transcranial Direct Current Stimulation (tDCS), Repetitive Transcranial Magnetic Stimulation (rTMS), Neuromuscular Electrical Stimulation (NMES), Pharyngeal Electrical Stimulation (PES), Paired Associative Stimulation (PAS)	Promising results in stroke and pilot ICU studies, ongoing larger clinical trials

5.3. ICU Teamwork and Patient-Centered Engagement

Constructive communication and effective coordination within ICU teams are essential for optimizing patient outcomes. Structured interdisciplinary rounds, standardized communication tools such as SBAR (Situation-Background-Assessment-Recommendation), and closed-loop communication systems minimize information transfer errors and foster a shared mental model among team members, facilitating timely, high-stakes decision-making (Leonard, Graham, and Bonacum 2004; Manser 2009). This systematic approach enhances collaboration, mitigates misunderstandings, and strengthens team resilience in the complex ICU environment (Reader et al. 2007).

Patient-centered care in the ICU requires active involvement of both patients and their families in shared decision-making to enhance transparency and trust while addressing psychosocial needs (Curtis and White 2008).

Family involvement in dysphagia care is critical, as relatives often assume the role of caregivers, experiencing significant psychosocial impacts. Training families in safe feeding techniques and recognition of complication signs is recommended, incorporating family-centered care models to enhance system adaptation and resilience (Noë et al. 2021).

Family engagement supports individualized care planning by incorporating patient values and preferences, which correlates with improved satisfaction, reduced anxiety, and better adherence to therapeutic goals (Davidson et al. 2017). Emphasizing communication strategies that prioritize empathy and clarity ensures holistic care respecting patient autonomy in the critical care environment (Azoulay et al. 2000).

Systematic training of families in safe feeding techniques such as food consistency control, posture, and supervision is advised, as it improves compliance and reduces risks. Educational programs increase compliance from 58% to over 80%, with long-term retention (Noë et al. 2021).

Incorporating family-centered care models, based on family systems theory and biopsychosocial-spiritual frameworks, strengthens family system resilience and improves adaptation. Such models promote interdisciplinary collaboration and caregiver support, reducing third-party disability (Ninfa et al. 2025; Noë et al. 2021; Rangira et al. 2022; Shune, Linville, and Namasivayam-MacDonald 2022; Tabor Gray et al. 2025).

5.4. Global Perspectives and Harmonization of Guidelines

Global practices in ICU dysphagia management demonstrate marked variability in screening protocols, access to speech-language pathology services, and instrumental assessments such as FEES. Recent international expert consensus and studies emphasize the critical need to implement standardized, evidence-based guidelines to enhance early identification and management of dysphagia in critically ill patients (Alhazzani et al. 2025; Likar et al. 2024; Reitz et al. 2024). Harmonization of protocols across diverse healthcare systems is essential to improve patient safety, optimize feeding strategies, and reduce complications associated with dysphagia in ICU settings (Bertschi et al. 2025; Nielsen et al. 2023).

DISCUSSION

Despite the limited methodological rigor of existing protocols, accumulating evidence demonstrates that speech therapy interventions in intensive care units (ICUs) are feasible and yield significant improvements in swallowing function, effectively mitigating oropharyngeal dysphagia, particularly in mechanically ventilated patients. Comprehensive dysphagia management in critical care necessitates the assessment of both structural and functional parameters, prioritizing functionally relevant metrics such as tongue propulsion for bolus transit and laryngeal elevation for airway protection. Methodologies should integrate daily assistance during the transition from enteral to oral feeding. Within multidisciplinary teams, speech-language therapists (SLTs) occupy a central role, bringing specialized expertise to the evaluation and management of swallowing and communication impairments. Their contributions encompass advanced interventions including Above Cuff Vocalization (ACV), cuff management, and the utilization of speaking valves as well as instrumental assessments such as Fibreoptic Endoscopic Evaluation of Swallowing (FEES) and Videofluoroscopy (VFS) to determine dysphagia severity and silent aspiration risk. The involvement of SLTs is crucial to optimizing recovery trajectories, guiding structured oral intake reassessment, and ensuring that treatments are both effective and well-tolerated. Future research should prioritize the systematic refinement of evaluation methodologies and investigate novel therapeutic approaches, such as neuromodulation and soft robotics, to further advance the field.

CONCLUSION

In the ICU, speech-language therapists are pivotal in the early detection and targeted management of communication and swallowing disorders particularly oropharyngeal dysphagia following extubation or tracheostomy. Their practice is characterized by the use of instrumental diagnostics to inform individualized interventions and promote efficient rehabilitation outcomes. Effective care in critical settings is underpinned by multidisciplinary collaboration, enabling the integration of contemporary modalities like neuromodulation and soft robotics with traditional therapeutic strategies. Furthermore, SLTs advocate for non-verbal patients by implementing augmentative and alternative communication (AAC) systems, thereby supporting comprehensive decision-making and capacity assessments. Through interdisciplinary cooperation with a broader healthcare team including occupational and physiotherapists, speech-language therapy delivers holistic, patient-centered care. The systematic review and continued refinement of swallowing management algorithms are fundamental for enhancing the design of future clinical trials and improving protocols for dysphagia treatment in intensive care environments.

REFERENCES

Abu-Ghanem, S., Graf, A., & Govind, J. (2022). 'Diagnosis of Sarcopenic Dysphagia in the Elderly: Critical Review and Future Perspectives'. *Dysphagia*, *37*(5), 1093–1102. DOI: 10.1007/s00455-021-10371-8 PMID: 34535803

Addington, W. R., Stephens, R. E., Gilliland, K., & Rodriguez, M. (1999). 'Assessing the Laryngeal Cough Reflex and the Risk of Developing Pneumonia after Stroke'. *Archives of Physical Medicine and Rehabilitation*, *80*(2), 150–154. DOI: 10.1016/s0003-9993(99)90112-0 PMID: 10025488

Alhazzani, W., Lewis, K., Selan, J., Alotaibi, H. F., Alnasser, S., Alrwais, A., Alhomoud, A., Alsayer, R. M., & Tamim, H. (2025). 'Post-Critical Illness Dysphagia in the Intensive Care Unit (the Dysphagia-ICU Study): Protocol for a Prospective Cohort Study'. *JMIR Research Protocols*, *14*, e68053. DOI: 10.2196/68053 PMID: 40812780

Altman, K. W., Yu, G.-P., & Schaefer, S. D. (2010). 'Consequence of Dysphagia in the Hospitalized Patient: Impact on Prognosis and Hospital Resources'. *Archives of Otolaryngology—Head & Neck Surgery*, *136*(8), 784–789. DOI: 10.1001/archoto.2010.129 PMID: 20713754

Armas-Navarro, L. P., Santana-Padilla, Y. G., Mendoza-Segura, L., Ramos-Díaz, M., Santana-López, B. N., Alcaraz-Jiménez, J. A., Rico-Rodríguez, J., & Santana-Cabrera, L. (2023). 'Dysphagia in Intensive Care, a Real Problem: Analysis of Risk Factors'. *Enfermeria Intensiva*, *34*(3), 115–125. DOI: 10.1016/j.enfie.2022.08.001 PMID: 36935305

Artiles, E., Constantino, J. R., & Donnellan, C. (2022). 'Physiological Mechanisms and Associated Pathophysiology of Dysphagia in Older Adults'. *Gerontology & Geriatric Medicine*, *8*, 23337214221142949. DOI: 10.1177/23337214221142949 PMID: 36582660

Azoulay, E., Chevret, S., Leleu, G., Pochard, F., Barboteu, M., Adrie, C., Canoui, P., Le Gall, J. R., & Schlemmer, B. (2000). 'Half the Families of Intensive Care Unit Patients Experience Inadequate Communication with Physicians'. *Critical Care Medicine*, *28*(8), 3044–3049. DOI: 10.1097/00003246-200008000-00061 PMID: 10966293

Barquist, E., Brown, M., Cohn, S., Lundy, D., & Jackowski, J. (2001). 'Postextubation Fiberoptic Endoscopic Evaluation of Swallowing after Prolonged Endotracheal Intubation: A Randomized, Prospective Trial'. *Critical Care Medicine*, *29*(9), 1710–1713. DOI: 10.1097/00003246-200109000-00009 PMID: 11546969

Belafsky, P. C., Blumenfeld, L., LePage, A., & Nahrstedt, K. (2003). 'The Accuracy of the Modified Evan's Blue Dye Test in Predicting Aspiration'. *The Laryngoscope*, *113*(11), 1969–1972. DOI: 10.1097/00005537-200311000-00021 PMID: 14603057

Bertschi, D., Rotondo, F., Waskowski, J., Venetz, P., Pfortmueller, C. A., & Schefold, J. C. (2025). 'Post-Extubation Dysphagia in the ICU–a Narrative Review: Epidemiology, Mechanisms and Clinical Management (Update 2025)'. *Critical Care*, *29*(1), 244. DOI: 10.1186/s13054-025-05492-7 PMID: 40524213

Bieger, D., & Neuhuber, W. (2006). *Neural Circuits and Mediators Regulating Swallowing in the Brainstem*. GI Motility Online., DOI: 10.1038/gimo74

Borr, C., Hielscher-Fastabend, M., & Lücking, A. (2007). 'Reliability and Validity of Cervical Auscultation'. *Dysphagia*, *22*(3), 225–234. DOI: 10.1007/s00455-007-9078-3 PMID: 17457548

Brage, L., Nylén, F., Hägglund, P., & Holmlund, T. (2025). 'eTWST: An Extension to the Timed Water Swallow Test for Increased Dysphagia Screening Accuracy'. *Dysphagia*, *40*(4), 801–810. DOI: 10.1007/s00455-024-10778-z PMID: 39521747

Brodsky, M. B., Akst, L. M., Jedlanek, E., Pandian, V., Blackford, B., Price, C., Cole, G., Mendez-Tellez, P. A., Hillel, A. T., Best, S. R., & Levy, M. J. (2021). 'Laryngeal Injury and Upper Airway Symptoms After Endotracheal Intubation During Surgery: A Systematic Review and Meta-Analysis'. *Anesthesia and Analgesia*, *132*(4), 1023–1032. DOI: 10.1213/ANE.0000000000005276 PMID: 33196479

Brodsky, M. B., De, I., Chilukuri, K., Huang, M., Palmer, J. B., & Needham, D. M. (2018). 'Coordination of Pharyngeal and Laryngeal Swallowing Events During Single Liquid Swallows After Oral Endotracheal Intubation for Patients with Acute Respiratory Distress Syndrome'. *Dysphagia*, *33*(6), 768–777. DOI: 10.1007/s00455-018-9901-z PMID: 29713897

Brodsky, M. B., Huang, M., Shanholtz, C., Mendez-Tellez, P. A., Palmer, J. B., Colantuoni, E., & Needham, D. M. (2017). 'Recovery from Dysphagia Symptoms after Oral Endotracheal Intubation in Acute Respiratory Distress Syndrome Survivors. A 5-Year Longitudinal Study'. *Annals of the American Thoracic Society*, *14*(3), 376–383. DOI: 10.1513/AnnalsATS.201606-455OC PMID: 27983872

Brodsky, M. B., Nollet, J. L., Spronk, P. E., & González-Fernández, M. (2020). 'Prevalence, Pathophysiology, Diagnostic Modalities, and Treatment Options for Dysphagia in Critically Ill Patients'. *American Journal of Physical Medicine & Rehabilitation*, *99*(12), 1164–1170. DOI: 10.1097/PHM.0000000000001440 PMID: 32304381

Brodsky, M. B., Pandian, V., & Needham, D. M. (2020). 'Post-Extubation Dysphagia: A Problem Needing Multidisciplinary Efforts'. *Intensive Care Medicine*, *46*(1), 93–96. DOI: 10.1007/s00134-019-05865-x PMID: 31768568

Calderone, A., Latella, D., La Fauci, E., Puleo, R., Sergi, A., De Francesco, M., Mauro, M., Foti, A., Salemi, L., & Calabrò, R. S. (2025). 'Artificial Intelligence-Driven Neuromodulation in Neurodegenerative Disease: Precision in Chaos, Learning in Loss'. *Biomedicines*, *13*(9), 2118. DOI: 10.3390/biomedicines13092118 PMID: 41007681

Cameron, J. L., Reynolds, J., & Zuidema, G. D. (1973). 'Aspiration in Patients with Tracheostomies'. *Surgery, Gynecology & Obstetrics*, *136*(1), 68–70. PMID: 4682266

Cheng, I., Bath, P. M., Hamdy, S., Muhle, P., Mistry, S., Dziewas, R., & Suntrup-Krüger, S. (2025). 'Clinical Predictors of Outcome after Pharyngeal Electrical Stimulation (PES) in Non-Stroke Related Neurogenic Dysphagia after Mechanical Ventilation and Tracheotomy: Results from Subgroup Analysis of PHADER Study'. *Neurological Research and Practice*, *7*(1), 23. DOI: 10.1186/s42466-025-00380-5 PMID: 40189593

Cheng, I., Hamad, A., Sasegbon, A., & Hamdy, S. (2022). 'Advances in the Treatment of Dysphagia in Neurological Disorders: A Review of Current Evidence and Future Considerations'. *Neuropsychiatric Disease and Treatment*, *18*, 2251–2263. DOI: 10.2147/NDT.S371624 PMID: 36268265

Christensen, M., & Trapl, M. (2018). 'Development of a Modified Swallowing Screening Tool to Manage Post-Extubation Dysphagia'. *Nursing in Critical Care*, *23*(2), 102–107. DOI: 10.1111/nicc.12333 PMID: 29285846

Cichero, J. A. Y. (2017). 'Unlocking Opportunities in Food Design for Infants, Children, and the Elderly: Understanding Milestones in Chewing and Swallowing across the Lifespan for New Innovations'. *Journal of Texture Studies*, *48*(4), 271–279. DOI: 10.1111/jtxs.12236 PMID: 28766752

Clavé, P., & Shaker, R. (2015). 'Dysphagia: Current Reality and Scope of the Problem'. *Nature Reviews. Gastroenterology & Hepatology*, *12*(5), 259–270. DOI: 10.1038/nrgastro.2015.49 PMID: 25850008

Curtis, J. R., & White, D. B. (2008). 'Practical Guidance for Evidence-Based ICU Family Conferences'. *Chest*, *134*(4), 835–843. DOI: 10.1378/chest.08-0235 PMID: 18842916

D'Netto, P., Rumbach, A., Dunn, K., & Finch, E. (2023). 'Clinical Predictors of Dysphagia Recovery After Stroke: A Systematic Review'. *Dysphagia, 38*(1), 1–22. DOI: 10.1007/s00455-022-10443-3 PMID: 35445366

da Silva, P. S. L., Reis, M. E., Fonseca, T. S. M., Kubo, E. Y., & Fonseca, M. C. M. (2023). 'Postextubation Dysphagia in Critically Ill Children: A Prospective Cohort Study'. *Pediatric Pulmonology, 58*(1), 315–324. DOI: 10.1002/ppul.26202 PMID: 36226514

Dai, M., Cheng, I., Sasegbon, A., Li, W., & Hamdy, S. (2025). 'A Meta-Analysis and Systematic Review of the Effects of Sensory Modulation Treatments for Neurogenic Oropharyngeal Dysphagia'. *CNS Neuroscience & Therapeutics, 31*(7), e70452. DOI: 10.1111/cns.70452 PMID: 40625241

Daniels, S. K., Huckabee, M.-L., & Gozdzikowska, K. (2019). *Dysphagia Following Stroke* (3rd ed.). Plural Publishing.

Davidson, J. E., Aslakson, R. A., Long, A. C., Puntillo, K. A., Kross, E. K., Hart, J., Cox, C. E., Wunsch, H., Wickline, M. A., Nunnally, M. E., Netzer, G., Kentish-Barnes, N., Sprung, C. L., Hartog, C. S., Coombs, M., Gerritsen, R. T., Hopkins, R. O., Franck, L. S., Skrobik, Y., & Randall Curtis, J. (2017). 'Guidelines for Family-Centered Care in the Neonatal, Pediatric, and Adult ICU'. *Critical Care Medicine, 45*(1), 103–128. DOI: 10.1097/CCM.0000000000002169 PMID: 27984278

Ferrari de Castro, Mario Augusto, Rogério Aparecido Dedivitis, Leandro Luongo de Matos, José Carlos Baraúna, Luiz Paulo Kowalski, Kauê de Carvalho Moura, and Daniel Herman Partezani. 2025. 'Endoscopic and Videofluoroscopic Evaluations of Swallowing for Dysphagia: A Systematic Review'. *Brazilian Journal of Otorhinolaryngology* 91 Suppl 1(Suppl 1):101598. doi:.DOI: 10.1016/j.bjorl.2025.101598

Demetriou, M., & Georgiou, A. M. (2024). 'Perspective on Dysphagia Screening, Assessment Methods, and Protocols in Intensive Care Units: An Opinion Article'. *Frontiers in Human Neuroscience, 18*. Advance online publication. DOI: 10.3389/fnhum.2024.1375408 PMID: 38655373

DePippo, K. L., Holas, M. A., & Reding, M. J. (1992). 'Validation of the 3-Oz Water Swallow Test for Aspiration Following Stroke'. *Archives of Neurology, 49*(12), 1259–1261. DOI: 10.1001/archneur.1992.00530360057018 PMID: 1449405

Dikeman, Karen, and Marta Kazandjian. 2002. *Communication and Swallowing Management of Tracheostomized and Ventilator Dependent Adults.*

Dikeman, K. J., & Kazandjian, M. S. (1995). *Communication & Swallowing Management Of Tracheostomized & Ventilator Dependent Adults*. Cengage Learning.

Dobak, S., & Kelly, D. (2021). 'Tough Pill to Swallow: Postextubation Dysphagia and Nutrition Impact in the Intensive Care Unit'. *Nutrition in Clinical Practice*, *36*(1), 80–87. DOI: 10.1002/ncp.10602 PMID: 33242222

Duncan, S., McAuley, D. F., Walshe, M., McGaughey, J., Anand, R., Fallis, R., & Blackwood, B. (2020). 'Interventions for Oropharyngeal Dysphagia in Acute and Critical Care: A Systematic Review and Meta-Analysis'. *Intensive Care Medicine*, *46*(7), 1326–1338. DOI: 10.1007/s00134-020-06126-y PMID: 32514597

Eltringham, S. A., Martindale, N., Lightbody, E., Pownall, S., Booth, A., & Smith, C. J. (2025). 'Barriers and Facilitators to Implementation of the Free Water Protocol in the Acute Stroke Unit Setting: A Mixed Methods Systematic Review'. *Dysphagia*. Advance online publication. DOI: 10.1007/s00455-025-10805-7 PMID: 39907731

Ertekin, C., & Aydogdu, I. (2003). 'Neurophysiology of Swallowing'. *Clinical Neurophysiology*, *114*(12), 2226–2244. DOI: 10.1016/s1388-2457(03)00237-2 PMID: 14652082

Frazure, M. (2023). *Swallow, Breathing and Survival: Sex-Specific Effects of Opioids*. Electronic Theses and Dissertations., DOI: 10.18297/etd/4145

Freeman-Sanderson, A., Clayton, N. A., Zaga, C. J., Sutt, A.-L., & Brodsky, M. B. (2025). 'Navigating Nutrition Complexity in Critical Care: A Focus on Swallowing Function and Rehabilitation'. *Critical Care Clinics*, *41*(2), 327–344. DOI: 10.1016/j.ccc.2024.11.001 PMID: 40021283

Freeman-Sanderson, A., Hemsley, B., Thompson, K., Rogers, K. D., Knowles, S., & Hammond, N. E.George Institute for Global Health and the Australian and New Zealand Intensive Care Society Clinical Trials Group. (2023). 'Dysphagia in Adult Intensive Care Patients: Results of a Prospective, Multicentre Binational Point Prevalence Study'. *Australian Critical Care: Official Journal of the Confederation of Australian Critical Care Nurses*, *36*(6), 961–966. DOI: 10.1016/j.aucc.2023.01.004 PMID: 36868933

García-Grimaldo, A., Rodríguez-Moguel, N. C., Godínez-Victoria, M., Rodríguez-Llamazares, S., Ríos-Ayala, M. A., Cadeza-Aguilar, J. D., & Osuna-Padilla, I. A. (2025). 'Associations between Intensive Care Unit Acquired Weakness with Post-Extubation Dysphagia and Other Clinical Outcomes-a Cohort Study in Critically Ill Respiratory Patients'. *Clinical Nutrition ESPEN*, *66*, 194–201. DOI: 10.1016/j.clnesp.2025.01.044 PMID: 39864521

Gaziano, J. E. (2002). 'Evaluation and Management of Oropharyngeal Dysphagia in Head and Neck Cancer'. *Cancer Control : Journal of the Moffitt Cancer Center*, *9*(5), 400–409. DOI: 10.1177/107327480200900505 PMID: 12410179

Ghaemi, H., Sobhani-Rad, D., Arabi, A., Saifpanahi, S., & Anaraki, Z. G. (2016). 'Role of Basal Ganglia in Swallowing Process: A Systematic Review'. *Iranian Rehabilitation Journal, 14*(4), 239–245. DOI: 10.18869/nrip.irj.14.4.239

Giraldo-Cadavid, L. F., Insignares, D., Velasco, V., Londoño, N., Galvis, A. M., Rengifo, M. L., & Bastidas-Goyes, A. R. (2025). 'Fiberoptic Endoscopy Evaluation of Swallowing (FEES) Findings Associated with High Pneumonia Risk in a Cohort of Patients at Risk of Dysphagia'. *Dysphagia, 40*(1), 282–291. DOI: 10.1007/s00455-024-10727-w PMID: 38958706

Gray, T., Lauren, S. S., Perry, S., Kosty, D., & Namasivayam-MacDonald, A. (2025). 'Dysphagia Symptoms Contribute to Greater Care Partner Burden in Neurodegenerative Disease'. *American Journal of Speech-Language Pathology, 34*(4), 2053–2061. DOI: 10.1044/2025_AJSLP-24-00529 PMID: 40324158

Groher, M. E., & Crary, M. A. (2016). *Dysphagia: Clinical Management in Adults and Children* (2nd ed.). Elsevier.

Guillen-Sola, A., Soler, N. B., Marco, E., Pera-Cegarra, O., & Foro, P. (2019). 'Effects of Prophylactic Swallowing Exercises on Dysphagia and Quality of Life in Patients with Head and Neck Cancer Receiving (Chemo) Radiotherapy: The Redyor Study, a Protocol for a Randomized Clinical Trial'. *Trials, 20*(1), 503. DOI: 10.1186/s13063-019-3587-x PMID: 31412947

Hamdy, S. (2006). *Role of Cerebral Cortex in the Control of Swallowing*. GI Motility Online., DOI: 10.1038/gimo8

Hamdy, S., Aziz, Q., Rothwell, J. C., Power, M., Singh, K. D., Nicholson, D. A., Tallis, R. C., & Thompson, D. G. (1998). 'Recovery of Swallowing after Dysphagic Stroke Relates to Functional Reorganization in the Intact Motor Cortex'. *Gastroenterology, 115*(5), 1104–1112. DOI: 10.1016/s0016-5085(98)70081-2 PMID: 9797365

Hassan, A. M. M., Shah, S., Bustamante, N., Solano, J., Hassan, A. M. M., Shah, S., Bustamante, N., & Solano, J. (2025). 'Post-Resuscitation Critical Illness Dysphagia: A Case Report'. *Cureus, 17*(6). Advance online publication. DOI: 10.7759/cureus.86640 PMID: 40718190

Hermans, G., & Van den Berghe, G. (2015). 'Clinical Review: Intensive Care Unit Acquired Weakness'. *Critical Care (London, England), 19*(1), 274. DOI: 10.1186/s13054-015-0993-7 PMID: 26242743

Hongo, T., Yamamoto, R., Liu, K., Yaguchi, T., Dote, H., Saito, R., Masuyama, T., Nakatsuka, K., Watanabe, S., Kanaya, T., Yamaguchi, T., Yumoto, T., Naito, H., & Nakao, A. (2022). 'Association between Timing of Speech and Language Therapy Initiation and Outcomes among Post-Extubation Dysphagia Patients: A Multicenter Retrospective Cohort Study'. *Critical Care*, *26*(1), 98. DOI: 10.1186/s13054-022-03974-6 PMID: 35395802

Huckabee, M. L., & Pelletier, C. A. (1999). *Management of Adult Neurogenic Dysphagia*. Cengage Learning.

Humbert, Ianessa A., and Rebecca Z. German. (2013). 'New Directions for Understanding Neural Control in Swallowing: The Potential and Promise of Motor Learning'. *Dysphagia*, *28*(1), 1–10. DOI: 10.1007/s00455-012-9432-y PMID: 23192633

Inamoto, Y., González-Fernández, M., & Saitoh, E. (2022). '3D-CT Evaluation of Swallowing: Metrics of the Swallowing Response Using Swallowing CT'. *Dysphagia*, *37*(2), 237–249. DOI: 10.1007/s00455-021-10288-2 PMID: 33818630

Inoue, S., Nakanishi, N., Amaya, F., Fujinami, Y., Hatakeyama, J., Hifumi, T., Iida, Y., Kawakami, D., Kawai, Y., Kondo, Y., Liu, K., Nakamura, K., Nishida, T., Sumita, H., Taito, S., Takaki, S., Tsuboi, N., Unoki, T., Yoshino, Y., & Nishida, O. (2024). 'Post-Intensive Care Syndrome: Recent Advances and Future Directions'. *Acute Medicine & Surgery*, *11*(1), e929. DOI: 10.1002/ams2.929 PMID: 38385144

Jackson, James C., Pandharipande, Pratik P., Girard, Timothy D., Brummel, Nathan E., Thompson, Jennifer L., Hughes, Christopher G., Pun, Brenda T., Vasilevskis, Eduard E., Morandi, Alessandro, Shintani, Ayumi K., Hopkins, Ramona O., Bernard, Gordon R., & Dittus, Robert S., E. Wesley Ely, and Bringing to light the Risk Factors And Incidence of Neuropsychological dysfunction in ICU survivors (BRAIN-ICU) study investigators. (2014). 'Depression, Post-Traumatic Stress Disorder, and Functional Disability in Survivors of Critical Illness in the BRAIN-ICU Study: A Longitudinal Cohort Study'. *The Lancet. Respiratory Medicine*, *2*(5), 369–379. DOI: 10.1016/S2213-2600(14)70051-7 PMID: 24815803

Jean, A. (2001). 'Brain Stem Control of Swallowing: Neuronal Network and Cellular Mechanisms'. *Physiological Reviews*, *81*(2), 929–969. DOI: 10.1152/physrev.2001.81.2.929 PMID: 11274347

Kahrilas, P. J., Logemann, J. A., Lin, S., & Ergun, G. A. (1992). 'Pharyngeal Clearance during Swallowing: A Combined Manometric and Videofluoroscopic Study'. *Gastroenterology*, *103*(1), 128–136. DOI: 10.1016/0016-5085(92)91105-D PMID: 1612322

Kawashima, K., Motohashi, Y., & Fujishima, I. (2004). 'Prevalence of Dysphagia among Community-Dwelling Elderly Individuals as Estimated Using a Questionnaire for Dysphagia Screening'. *Dysphagia*, *19*(4), 266–271. DOI: 10.1007/s00455-004-0013-6 PMID: 15667063

Kohler*, Joel, Friedrich Borchers*, Matthias Endres, Björn Weiss, Claudia Spies, and Julius Valentin Emmrich. 2019. 'Cognitive Deficits Following Intensive Care'. *Deutsches Ärzteblatt International* 116(38):627–34. doi:.DOI: 10.3238/arztebl.2019.0627

Lang, I. M. (2009). 'Brain Stem Control of the Phases of Swallowing'. *Dysphagia*, *24*(3), 333–348. DOI: 10.1007/s00455-009-9211-6 PMID: 19399555

Lang, I. M. (2024). 'Coordination of Pharyngeal and Esophageal Phases of Swallowing'. *Journal of Neurogastroenterology and Motility*, *30*(4), 397–406. DOI: 10.5056/jnm24003 PMID: 39397618

Langmore, S. E. (2001). *Endoscopic Evaluation and Treatment of Swallowing Disorders*. Thieme.

Leder, S. B., Warner, H. L., Suiter, D. M., Young, N. O., Bhattacharya, B., Siner, J. M., Davis, K. A., Maerz, L. L., Rosenbaum, S. H., Marshall, P. S., Pisani, M. A., Siegel, M. D., Brennan, J. J., & Schuster, K. M. (2019). Evaluation of Swallow Function Post-Extubation: Is It Necessary to Wait 24 Hours? *The Annals of Otology, Rhinology, and Laryngology*, *128*(7), 619–624. DOI: 10.1177/0003489419836115 PMID: 30841709

Leonard, M., S. Graham, and D. Bonacum. 2004. 'The Human Factor: The Critical Importance of Effective Teamwork and Communication in Providing Safe Care'. *Quality & Safety in Health Care* 13 Suppl 1(Suppl 1):i85-90. doi:.DOI: 10.1136/qhc.13.suppl_1.i85

Leslie, P., Drinnan, M. J., Zammit-Maempel, I., Coyle, J. L., Ford, G. A., & Wilson, J. A. (2007). 'Cervical Auscultation Synchronized with Images from Endoscopy Swallow Evaluations'. *Dysphagia*, *22*(4), 290–298. DOI: 10.1007/s00455-007-9084-5 PMID: 17554472

Likar, R., Aroyo, I., Bangert, K., Degen, B., Dziewas, R., Galvan, O., Grundschober, M. T., Köstenberger, M., Muhle, P., Schefold, J. C., & Zuercher, P. (2024). 'Management of Swallowing Disorders in ICU Patients - A Multinational Expert Opinion'. *Journal of Critical Care*, *79*, 154447. DOI: 10.1016/j.jcrc.2023.154447 PMID: 37924574

Lin, Y., Wan, G., Wu, H., Shi, J., Zhang, Y., Chen, H., Wei, X., Tang, Z., Dai, M., Dou, Z., & Wen, H. (2022). 'The Sensitivity and Specificity of the Modified Volume-Viscosity Swallow Test for Dysphagia Screening among Neurological Patients'. *Frontiers in Neurology, 13*. Advance online publication. DOI: 10.3389/fneur.2022.961893 PMID: 36188363

Logemann, J. A. (1998). *Evaluation and Treatment of Swallowing Disorders*. Pro Ed.

Long, H., Lu, B., Tan, Q., Dai, D., & Zeng, F. (2025). 'Correction: Swallowing Function Management in Patients with Disorders of Consciousness: A Scoping Review'. *Frontiers in Neuroscience, 19*, 1665746. DOI: 10.3389/fnins.2025.1665746 PMID: 40778356

Ludlow, C. L. (2015). 'Central Nervous System Control of Voice and Swallowing'. *Journal of Clinical Neurophysiology : Official Publication of the American Electroencephalographic Society, 32*(4), 294–303. DOI: 10.1097/WNP.0000000000000186 PMID: 26241238

Macht, M., Wimbish, T., Bodine, C., & Moss, M. (2013). 'ICU-Acquired Swallowing Disorders'. *Critical Care Medicine, 41*(10), 2396–2405. DOI: 10.1097/CCM.0b013e31829caf33 PMID: 23939361

Macht, M., Wimbish, T., Clark, B. J., Benson, A. B., Burnham, E. L., Williams, A., & Moss, M. (2011). 'Postextubation Dysphagia Is Persistent and Associated with Poor Outcomes in Survivors of Critical Illness'. *Critical Care : the Official Journal of the Critical Care Forum, 15*(5), R231. DOI: 10.1186/cc10472 PMID: 21958475

Macht, M., Wimbish, T., Clark, B. J., Benson, A. B., Burnham, E. L., Williams, A., & Moss, M. (2012). 'Diagnosis and Treatment of Post-Extubation Dysphagia: Results from a National Survey'. *Journal of Critical Care, 27*(6), 578–586. DOI: 10.1016/j.jcrc.2012.07.016 PMID: 23084136

Malandraki, G. A., Arkenberg, R. H., Mitchell, S. S., & Malandraki, J. B. (2021). 'Telehealth for Dysphagia Across the Life Span: Using Contemporary Evidence and Expertise to Guide Clinical Practice During and After COVID-19'. *American Journal of Speech-Language Pathology, 30*(2), 532–550. DOI: 10.1044/2020_AJSLP-20-00252 PMID: 33555933

Manser, T. (2009). 'Teamwork and Patient Safety in Dynamic Domains of Healthcare: A Review of the Literature'. *Acta Anaesthesiologica Scandinavica, 53*(2), 143–151. DOI: 10.1111/j.1399-6576.2008.01717.x PMID: 19032571

Martin-Harris, B., Canon, C. L., Bonilha, H. S., Murray, J., Davidson, K., & Lefton-Greif, M. A. (2020). 'Best Practices in Modified Barium Swallow Studies'. *American Journal of Speech-Language Pathology*, *29*(2, Suppl), 1078–1093. DOI: 10.1044/2020_AJSLP-19-00189 PMID: 32650657

Martínez de Lagrán, Z., Itziar, L. B. L., Soria, C. V., Guisasola, C. P., & Marcos-Neira, P. (2023). 'Utility of the Modified Volume-Viscosity Swallow Test for Bedside Screening of Dysphagia in Critically Ill Patients'. *Clinical Nutrition ESPEN*, *53*, 214–223. DOI: 10.1016/j.clnesp.2022.12.021 PMID: 36657916

Marvin, S., Thibeault, S., & Ehlenbach, W. J. (2019). Post-Extubation Dysphagia: Does Timing of Evaluation Matter? *Dysphagia*, *34*(2), 210–219. DOI: 10.1007/s00455-018-9926-3 PMID: 30043081

Matsumoto, H., Tanimura, C., Tanishima, S., Osaki, M., Noma, H., & Hagino, H. (2017). 'Sarcopenia Is a Risk Factor for Falling in Independently Living Japanese Older Adults: A 2-Year Prospective Cohort Study of the GAINA Study'. *Geriatrics & Gerontology International*, *17*(11), 2124–2130. DOI: 10.1111/ggi.13047 PMID: 28517243

Matsuo, K., Yoneki, K., Tamiya, S., Mibu, K., Furuzono, K., Kobayashi, K., Yasuda, S., Onoda, D., Tatsuki, H., & Iseki, H. (2024). 'Impact of Sarcopenia and Malnutrition on Swallowing Function Utilizing Ultrasonography in Patients with Acute Heart Failure: A Retrospective Cohort Study'. *Clinical Nutrition ESPEN*, *59*, 296–306. DOI: 10.1016/j.clnesp.2023.12.021 PMID: 38220390

McCarty, E. B., & Chao, T. N. (2021). 'Dysphagia and Swallowing Disorders'. *The Medical Clinics of North America*, *105*(5), 939–954. DOI: 10.1016/j.mcna.2021.05.013 PMID: 34391544

Metheny, N. A., St John, R. E., & Clouse, R. E. (1998). 'Measurement of Glucose in Tracheobronchial Secretions to Detect Aspiration of Enteral Feedings'. *Heart & Lung: The Journal of Cardiopulmonary and Acute Care*, *27*(5), 285–292. DOI: 10.1016/S0147-9563(98)90047-4 PMID: 9777373

Meuret, S., Dietz, A., & Fuchs, M. (2014). 'Dysphagie'. *Laryngo- Rhino- Otologie*, *93*(2), 121–137. DOI: 10.1055/s-0033-1363679 PMID: 24477436

Miao, P., Zhang, Y., & Zhong, A. (2023). 'Risk Factors of Aspiration Occurrence with Different Feeding Patterns in Elderly Intensive Care Unit Patients: A Cross-Sectional Study'. *Journal of Thoracic Disease*, *15*(5), 2585–2600. DOI: 10.21037/jtd-23-430 PMID: 37324079

Miles, A., Moore, S., McFarlane, M., Lee, F., Allen, J., & Huckabee, M.-L. (2013). 'Comparison of Cough Reflex Test against Instrumental Assessment of Aspiration'. *Physiology & Behavior, 118*, 25–31. DOI: 10.1016/j.physbeh.2013.05.004 PMID: 23672854

Miller, A. J. (2008). 'The Neurobiology of Swallowing and Dysphagia'. *Developmental Disabilities Research Reviews, 14*(2), 77–86. DOI: 10.1002/ddrr.12 PMID: 18646019

Mittal, R. K., & Balaban, D. H. (1997). 'The Esophagogastric Junction'. *The New England Journal of Medicine, 336*(13), 924–932. DOI: 10.1056/NEJM199703273361306 PMID: 9070474

Moss, M., White, S. D., Warner, H., Dvorkin, D., Fink, D., Gomez-Taborda, S., Higgins, C., Krisciunas, G. P., Levitt, J. E., McKeehan, J., McNally, E., Rubio, A., Scheel, R., Siner, J. M., Vojnik, R., & Langmore, S. E. (2020). 'Development of an Accurate Bedside Swallowing Evaluation Decision Tree Algorithm for Detecting Aspiration in Acute Respiratory Failure Survivors'. *Chest, 158*(5), 1923–1933. DOI: 10.1016/j.chest.2020.07.051 PMID: 32721404

Muhle, P., Labeit, B., Wollbrink, A., Claus, I., Warnecke, T., Wolters, C. H., Gross, J., Dziewas, R., & Suntrup-Krueger, S. (2021). 'Targeting the Sensory Feedback within the Swallowing Network-Reversing Artificially Induced Pharyngolaryngeal Hypesthesia by Central and Peripheral Stimulation Strategies'. *Human Brain Mapping, 42*(2), 427–438. DOI: 10.1002/hbm.25233 PMID: 33068056

Murry, T., Carrau, R. L., & Chan, K. (2020). *Clinical Management of Swallowing Disorders*. Plural Publishing, Inc.

Namasivayam-MacDonald, A. M., & Shune, S. E. (2018). 'The Burden of Dysphagia on Family Caregivers of the Elderly: A Systematic Review'. *Geriatrics (Basel, Switzerland), 3*(2), 30. DOI: 10.3390/geriatrics3020030 PMID: 31011068

Needham, D. M., Davidson, J., Cohen, H., Hopkins, R. O., Weinert, C., Wunsch, H., Zawistowski, C., Bemis-Dougherty, A., Berney, S. C., Bienvenu, O. J., Brady, S. L., Brodsky, M. B., Denehy, L., Elliott, D., Flatley, C., Harabin, A. L., Jones, C., Louis, D., Meltzer, W., & Harvey, M. A. (2012). 'Improving Long-Term Outcomes after Discharge from Intensive Care Unit: Report from a Stakeholders' Conference'. *Critical Care Medicine, 40*(2), 502–509. DOI: 10.1097/CCM.0b013e318232da75 PMID: 21946660

Neuhuber, W., & Bieger, D. (2013). Brainstem Control of Deglutition: Brainstem Neural Circuits and Mediators Regulating Swallowing. In Shaker, R., Belafsky, P. C., Postma, G. N., & Easterling, C. (Eds.), *Principles of Deglutition: A Multidisciplinary Text for Swallowing and its Disorders* (pp. 89–113). Springer.

Nielsen, A. H., Kaldan, G., Nielsen, B. H., Kristensen, G. J., Shiv, L., & Egerod, I. (2023). 'Intensive Care Professionals' Perspectives on Dysphagia Management: A Focus Group Study'. *Australian Critical Care: Official Journal of the Confederation of Australian Critical Care Nurses, 36*(4), 528–535. DOI: 10.1016/j.aucc.2022.04.004 PMID: 35610091

Ninfa, A., Morandi, G., Schindler, A., & Delle Fave, A. (2025). 'The Daily Experience of Family Members Caring for Persons With Chronic Oropharyngeal Dysphagia: A Qualitative Investigation'. *International Journal of Language & Communication Disorders, 60*(5), e70094. DOI: 10.1111/1460-6984.70094 PMID: 40709912

Noë, S., Goeleven, A., Brouwers, H., Meurrens, T., De Cock, A., Kos, D., & Vanhaecht, K. (2021). 'Training for Caregivers and Compliance with Dysphagia Recommendations in a Tertiary Multiple Sclerosis Rehabilitation Center'. *International Journal of MS Care, 23*(5), 223–228. DOI: 10.7224/1537-2073.2020-019 PMID: 34720762

O'Horo, John C., Rogus-Pulia, Nicole, & Garcia-Arguello, Lisbeth, JoAnne Robbins, and Nasia Safdar. (2015a). 'Bedside Diagnosis of Dysphagia: A Systematic Review'. *Journal of Hospital Medicine, 10*(4), 256–265. DOI: 10.1002/jhm.2313 PMID: 25581840

Panara, K., Ahangar, E. R., & Padalia, D. (2025). Physiology, Swallowing. In *StatPearls*. StatPearls Publishing.

Papadopoulou, S., Exarchakos, G., Beris, A., & Ploumis, A. (2013). 'Dysphagia Associated with Cervical Spine and Postural Disorders'. *Dysphagia, 28*(4), 469–480. DOI: 10.1007/S00455-013-9484-7 PMID: 23959456

Peng, X.-M., Gong, C., Xiao, M.-X., Chen, L.-S., Li, Y., Chen, J., Wang, M.-Y., & Luo, Y. (2025). 'Effect of Repetitive Transcranial Magnetic Stimulation with Different Stimulation Parameters on Post-Stroke Dysphagia: A Systematic Review and Meta-Analysis of Randomized Controlled Trials'. *Frontiers in Neurology, 16*. Advance online publication. DOI: 10.3389/fneur.2025.1586734 PMID: 40474922

Peyron, M.-A., Gierczynski, I., Hartmann, C., Loret, C., Dardevet, D., Martin, N., & Woda, A. (2011). 'Role of Physical Bolus Properties as Sensory Inputs in the Trigger of Swallowing'. *PLoS One, 6*(6), e21167. DOI: 10.1371/journal.pone.0021167 PMID: 21738616

Polit, M., Chmielewska-Walczak, J., Sobol, M., Domitrz, I., & Niemczyk, K. (2025). 'Safety of FEES Performed by Speech-Language Pathologists and Physicians-Evidence Supporting Task Sharing from a Retrospective Observational Study of 964 Consecutive Examinations'. *Nutrients*, *17*(20), 3193. DOI: 10.3390/nu17203193 PMID: 41156446

Potente, P., Stella, A. B., Vidotto, M., Passerini, M., Furlanis, G., Naccarato, M., & Manganotti, P. (2023). 'Application of Ultrasonography in Neurogenic Dysphagia: A Systematic Review'. *Dysphagia*, *38*(1), 65–75. DOI: 10.1007/s00455-022-10459-9 PMID: 35556172

Ramsey, D., Smithard, D., & Kalra, L. (2005). Silent Aspiration: What Do We Know? *Dysphagia*, *20*(3), 218–225. DOI: 10.1007/s00455-005-0018-9 PMID: 16362510

Rangira, D., Najeeb, H., Shune, S. E., & Namasivayam-MacDonald, A. (2022). 'Understanding Burden in Caregivers of Adults With Dysphagia: A Systematic Review'. *American Journal of Speech-Language Pathology*, *31*(1), 486–501. DOI: 10.1044/2021_AJSLP-21-00249 PMID: 34962832

Reader, T. W., Flin, R., Mearns, K., & Cuthbertson, B. H. (2007). 'Interdisciplinary Communication in the Intensive Care Unit'. *British Journal of Anaesthesia*, *98*(3), 347–352. DOI: 10.1093/bja/ael372 PMID: 17272386

Regnier, A., Mélotte, E., Aubinet, C., Alnagger, N., Fischer, D., Lagier, A., Thibaut, A., Laureys, S., Kaux, J.-F., & Gosseries, O. (2024). 'Swallowing Dysfunctions in Patients with Disorders of Consciousness: Evidence from Neuroimaging Data, Assessment, and Management'. *NeuroRehabilitation*, *54*(1), 91–107. DOI: 10.3233/NRE-230135 PMID: 38217621

Reitz, S. C., Marly, J., Neef, V., Konczalla, J., Czabanka, M., Grefkes-Hermann, C., Foerch, C., & Lapa, S. (2024). 'Intensive Care Unit-Acquired Dysphagia - Change in Feeding Route after a Standardized Dysphagia Assessment in Neurocritical Care Patients'. *Scientific Reports*, *14*(1), 29993. DOI: 10.1038/s41598-024-81529-1 PMID: 39622919

Riera, S. A., Marin, S., Serra-Prat, M., Tomsen, N., Arreola, V., Ortega, O., Walshe, M., & Clavé, P. (2021). 'A Systematic and a Scoping Review on the Psychometrics and Clinical Utility of the Volume-Viscosity Swallow Test (V-VST) in the Clinical Screening and Assessment of Oropharyngeal Dysphagia'. *Foods*, *10*(8), 1900. DOI: 10.3390/foods10081900 PMID: 34441677

Rofes, L., Arreola, V., & Clavé, P. (2012). 'The Volume-Viscosity Swallow Test for Clinical Screening of Dysphagia and Aspiration'. *Nestlé Nutrition Institute Workshop Series*, *72*, 33–42. DOI: 10.1159/000339979 PMID: 23051998

Rosenbek, J. C., Robbins, J. A., Roecker, E. B., Coyle, J. L., & Wood, J. L. (1996). 'A Penetration-Aspiration Scale'. *Dysphagia, 11*(2), 93–98. DOI: 10.1007/BF00417897 PMID: 8721066

Salgado, T. T., Magna dos Santos Oliveira, C., Gatti, M., Gonçalves da Silva, R., Marques Honório, H., & Berretin-Felix, G. (2024). 'Degree of Swallowing Impairment in the Elderly: Clinical and Instrumental Assessment'. *Brazilian Journal of Otorhinolaryngology, 90*(4), 101426. DOI: 10.1016/j.bjorl.2024.101426 PMID: 38608636

Sanko, J. S. (2004). 'Aspiration Assessment and Prevention in Critically Ill Enterally Fed Patients: Evidence-Based Recommendations for Practice'. *Gastroenterology Nursing: The Official Journal of the Society of Gastroenterology Nurses and Associates, 27*(6), 279–285. DOI: 10.1097/00001610-200411000-00007 PMID: 15632762

Sasegbon, A., & Hamdy, S. (2017). 'The Anatomy and Physiology of Normal and Abnormal Swallowing in Oropharyngeal Dysphagia'. *Neurogastroenterology and Motility, 29*(11). Advance online publication. DOI: 10.1111/nmo.13100 PMID: 28547793

Schefold, J. C., Berger, D., Zürcher, P., Lensch, M., Perren, A., Jakob, S. M., Parviainen, I., & Takala, J. (2017). 'Dysphagia in Mechanically Ventilated ICU Patients (DYnAMICS): A Prospective Observational Trial'. *Critical Care Medicine, 45*(12), 2061–2069. DOI: 10.1097/CCM.0000000000002765 PMID: 29023260

Shaw, S. M., & Martino, R. (2013). 'The Normal Swallow: Muscular and Neurophysiological Control'. *Otolaryngologic Clinics of North America, 46*(6), 937–956. DOI: 10.1016/j.otc.2013.09.006 PMID: 24262952

Shune, S. E., Linville, D., & Namasivayam-MacDonald, A. (2022). 'Integrating Family-Centered Care Into Chronic Dysphagia Management: A Tutorial'. *Perspectives of the ASHA Special Interest Groups, 7*(3), 795–806. DOI: 10.1044/2022_PERSP-21-00314

Skoretz, S. A., Flowers, H. L., & Martino, R. (2010). 'The Incidence of Dysphagia Following Endotracheal Intubation: A Systematic Review'. *Chest, 137*(3), 665–673. DOI: 10.1378/chest.09-1823 PMID: 20202948

Smithard, D. G., O'Neill, P. A., Parks, C., & Morris, J. (1996). Complications and Outcome after Acute Stroke. Does Dysphagia Matter? *Stroke, 27*(7), 1200–1204. DOI: 10.1161/01.str.27.7.1200 PMID: 8685928

Speyer, R., Cordier, R., Farneti, D., Nascimento, W., Pilz, W., Verin, E., Walshe, M., & Woisard, V. (2022). 'White Paper by the European Society for Swallowing Disorders: Screening and Non-Instrumental Assessment for Dysphagia in Adults'. *Dysphagia*, *37*(2), 333–349. DOI: 10.1007/s00455-021-10283-7 PMID: 33787994

Speyer, R., Cordier, R., Kim, J.-H., Cocks, N., Michou, E., & Wilkes-Gillan, S. (2019). 'Prevalence of Drooling, Swallowing, and Feeding Problems in Cerebral Palsy across the Lifespan: A Systematic Review and Meta-analyses'. *Developmental Medicine and Child Neurology*, *61*(11), 1249–1258. DOI: 10.1111/dmcn.14316 PMID: 31328797

Steele, C. M., & Cichero, J. A. Y. (2014). 'Physiological Factors Related to Aspiration Risk: A Systematic Review'. *Dysphagia*, *29*(3), 295–304. DOI: 10.1007/s00455-014-9516-y PMID: 24562507

Steele, C. M., & Miller, A. J. (2010). 'Sensory Input Pathways and Mechanisms in Swallowing: A Review'. *Dysphagia*, *25*(4), 323–333. DOI: 10.1007/s00455-010-9301-5 PMID: 20814803

Suiter, D. M., & Leder, S. B. (2008). 'Clinical Utility of the 3-Ounce Water Swallow Test'. *Dysphagia*, *23*(3), 244–250. DOI: 10.1007/s00455-007-9127-y PMID: 18058175

Teramoto, S., & Fukuchi, Y. (2000). 'Detection of Aspiration and Swallowing Disorder in Older Stroke Patients: Simple Swallowing Provocation Test versus Water Swallowing Test'. *Archives of Physical Medicine and Rehabilitation*, *81*(11), 1517–1519. DOI: 10.1053/apmr.2000.9171 PMID: 11083358

Thimmaiah, G., Pandey, N., Prinja, S., Jain, K., Biswal, M., Agarwal, R., Koushal, V., & Sethi, S. (2024). Ventilator-Associated Pneumonia - What Price Does the Public Health System Pay? *Lung India : Official Organ of Indian Chest Society*, *41*(4), 278–283. DOI: 10.4103/lungindia.lungindia_597_23 PMID: 38953191

Traube, C., Silver, G., Gerber, L. M., Kaur, S., Mauer, E. A., Kerson, A., Joyce, C., & Greenwald, B. M. (2017). 'Delirium and Mortality in Critically Ill Children: Epidemiology and Outcomes of Pediatric Delirium'. *Critical Care Medicine*, *45*(5), 891–898. DOI: 10.1097/CCM.0000000000002324 PMID: 28288026

Troll, C., Trapl-Grundschober, M., Teuschl, Y., Cerrito, A., Compte, M. G., & Siegemund, M. (2023). 'A Bedside Swallowing Screen for the Identification of Post-Extubation Dysphagia on the Intensive Care Unit – Validation of the Gugging Swallowing Screen (GUSS)—ICU'. *BMC Anesthesiology*, *23*(1), 122. DOI: 10.1186/s12871-023-02072-6 PMID: 37055724

Turra, G. S., Ida, V. D. S., Tamanini de Almeida, S., Martinez, C. C., Bridi, M., & Sérgio, S. M. B. (2021). 'Efficacy of Speech Therapy in Post-Intubation Patients with Oropharyngeal Dysphagia: A Randomized Controlled Trial'. *CoDAS, 33*(2), e20190246. DOI: 10.1590/2317-1782/20202019246 PMID: 33909759

Umay, E., Eyigor, S., Demirag, K., Karatas, G. K., Gundogdu, I., Giray, E., Ates, M. P., Kocer, B. G., Gurcay, E., Unlu, Z., Bengisu, S., Karaahmet, F., Bagcier, F., Vural, M., Aydeniz, B., Kullukcu, H., Oztekin, F., Alicura, S., Uz, C., & Adiguzel, E. (2024). 'Best Practice Recommendations for Dysphagia Management in Intensive Care Unit (ICU): A Delphi Study from Multidisciplinary Experts in Turkey'. *Dysphagia, 39*(2), 241–254. DOI: 10.1007/s00455-023-10606-w PMID: 37542552

Vasconcelos, Manuela Leitão de, Divany Guedes Pereira da Cunha, Giorvan Ânderson Dos Santos Alves, Tatiana Carneiro da Cunha Almeida Santos, Luiz Medeiros de Araujo Lima-Filho, Karinna Veríssimo Meira Taveira, Cristiano Miranda de Araújo, and Leandro Pernambuco. (2024). 'Management of Sialorrhea in Children: A Systematic Review'. *Revista da Associação Médica Brasileira, 70*(3), e20230971. DOI: 10.1590/1806-9282.20230971

Vijay Kumar, K. V., & Shankar, V., and Roy Santosham. (2013). 'Assessment of Swallowing and Its Disorders-a Dynamic MRI Study'. *European Journal of Radiology, 82*(2), 215–219. DOI: 10.1016/j.ejrad.2012.09.010 PMID: 23068561

Vishak, M. S., and Ramasamy, K. (2024). 'Swallowing Rehabilitation: Tracing the Evolution of Assessment and Intervention Approaches for Dysphagia over 30 Years'. *Indian Journal of Otolaryngology and Head and Neck Surgery : Official Publication of the Association of Otolaryngologists of India, 76*(2), 2171–2175. DOI: 10.1007/s12070-023-04325-9 PMID: 38566735

Wakasugi, Y., Tohara, H., Hattori, F., Motohashi, Y., Nakane, A., Goto, S., Ouchi, Y., Mikushi, S., Takeuchi, S., & Uematsu, H. (2008). 'Screening Test for Silent Aspiration at the Bedside'. *Dysphagia, 23*(4), 364–370. DOI: 10.1007/s00455-008-9150-7 PMID: 18594914

Wang, Z., Shi, R., & Moreira, P. (2025). 'Post-Stroke Dysphagia: Identifying the Evidence Missing'. *Frontiers in Medicine, 12*. Advance online publication. DOI: 10.3389/fmed.2025.1494645 PMID: 40078394

Weppner, J., Senol, S., Larick, R., & Jackson, S. (2024). 'Diagnostic Accuracy of the Yale Swallow Protocol in Moderate-to-Severe Traumatic Brain Injury: A Prospective Blinded Videofluoroscopic Investigation'. *The Journal of Head Trauma Rehabilitation, 39*(5), E393–E398. DOI: 10.1097/HTR.0000000000000929 PMID: 38453631

Williams, T., Walkden, E., Patel, K., Cochrane, N. E., McGrath, B. A., & Wallace, S. (2024). 'Research Report: Management of Dysphagia Using Pharyngeal Electrical Stimulation in the General Intensive Care Population - A Service Development'. *The Journal of the Intensive Care Society*, *25*(4), 374–382. DOI: 10.1177/17511437241270244 PMID: 39524066

Wilmskoetter, J., Daniels, S. K., & Miller, A. J. (2020). Cortical and Subcortical Control of Swallowing-Can We Use Information From Lesion Locations to Improve Diagnosis and Treatment for Patients With Stroke? *American Journal of Speech-Language Pathology*, *29*(2S), 1030–1043. DOI: 10.1044/2019_AJSLP-19-00068 PMID: 32650664

Wong, D. W.-C., Wang, J., Cheung, S. M.-Y., Lai, D. K.-H., Chiu, A. T.-S., Pu, D., Cheung, J. C.-W., & Kwok, T. C.-Y. (2025). 'Current Technological Advances in Dysphagia Screening: Systematic Scoping Review'. *Journal of Medical Internet Research*, *27*(1), e65551. DOI: 10.2196/65551 PMID: 40324167

Workum, J. D., Janssen, S. H. V., & Touw, H. R. W. (2020). 'Considerations in Neuromuscular Blockade in the ICU: A Case Report and Review of the Literature'. *Case Reports in Critical Care*, *8780979*. Advance online publication. DOI: 10.1155/2020/8780979 PMID: 32206357

Wu, Y., Guo, K., Chu, Y., Wang, Z., Yang, H., & Zhang, J. (2024). 'Advancements and Challenges in Non-Invasive Sensor Technologies for Swallowing Assessment: A Review'. *Bioengineering (Basel, Switzerland)*, *11*(5), 430. DOI: 10.3390/bioengineering11050430 PMID: 38790297

Yang, W., Du, Y., Chen, M., Li, S., Zhang, F., Yu, P., & Xu, X. (2023). 'Effectiveness of Home-Based Telerehabilitation Interventions for Dysphagia in Patients With Head and Neck Cancer: Systematic Review'. *Journal of Medical Internet Research*, *25*, e47324. DOI: 10.2196/47324 PMID: 37682589

Yıldızeli, Ş. O. (2024). 'Determinants of Hospital Stay, Mortality, and Readmission in Aspiration Pneumonia Patients'. *European Journal of Geriatrics and Gerontology*. Advance online publication. DOI: 10.4274/ejgg.galenos.2024.2024-2-1

Zhou, Z., & Zhou, J. (2025). 'Intermittent vs. Continuous: A Comparative Narrative Review of Enteral and Parenteral Nutrition Support Strategies in the Perioperative Setting'. *European Journal of Clinical Nutrition*. Advance online publication. DOI: 10.1038/s41430-025-01669-z PMID: 41034630

Zuercher, P., Dziewas, R., & Schefold, J. C. (2020). 'Dysphagia in the Intensive Care Unit: A (Multidisciplinary) Call to Action'. *Intensive Care Medicine*, *46*(3), 554–556. DOI: 10.1007/s00134-020-05937-3 PMID: 31996956

Zuercher, P., Moret, C. S., Dziewas, R., & Schefold, J. C. (2019). 'Dysphagia in the Intensive Care Unit: Epidemiology, Mechanisms, and Clinical Management'. *Critical Care*, *23*(1), 103. DOI: 10.1186/s13054-019-2400-2 PMID: 30922363

Zuercher, P., Schenk, N. V., Moret, C., Berger, D., Abegglen, R., & Schefold, J. C. (2020). 'Risk Factors for Dysphagia in ICU Patients After Invasive Mechanical Ventilation'. *Chest*, *158*(5), 1983–1991. DOI: 10.1016/j.chest.2020.05.576 PMID: 32525018

Zuercher, P., Moret, C. S., Dziewas, R., & Schefold, J. C. (2019). Dysphagia in the Intensive Care Unit: Epidemiology, Mechanisms, and Clinical Management. Critical Care, 23(1), 103. DOI: 10.1186/s13054-019-2400-2 PMID: 30922363

Zuercher, P., Schenk, N. V., Moret, C., Berger, D., Abegglen, R., & Schefold, J. C. (2020). Risk Factors for Dysphagia in ICU Patients After Invasive Mechanical Ventilation. Chest, 158(5), 1983–1991. DOI: 10.1016/j.chest.2020.05.576 PMID: 32525018

Chapter 2
Neonatal Swallowing Disorders:
Early Diagnosis, Assessment, and Interventional Approaches

Hilal Berber Çiftci
http://orcid.org/0000-0002-6577-837X
Tarsus University, Turkey

ABSTRACT

Swallowing disorders in newborns are characterized by sensory-motor coordination disorders and/or early-stage problems with physiological regulation. This section will address swallowing disorders in newborns, which are an important component of developmental and medical dysphagia. The primary objective of this section is to provide a comprehensive overview of the pathophysiological, neurodevelopmental, and clinical characteristics of swallowing function in newborns. In addition to fundamental clinical information, the section will also cover instrumental methods such as early assessment, standardized feeding evaluations, and videofluoroscopic and endoscopic studies. Evidence-based interventions used in neonatal intensive care, including oral-motor stimulation, cue-based feeding, compensatory strategies, and some device-assisted methods, will also be discussed. The chapter aims to guide neonatology professionals towards safe, efficient, and family-centered feeding outcomes by integrating current research, developmental neuroscience, and clinical knowledge. Finally, it is emphasized that current research, as well as neonatal dysphagia research, lacks technological innovations, interdisciplinary collaboration, and standardized outcome measures.

DOI: 10.4018/979-8-3373-6405-6.ch002

1. INTRODUCTION

Swallowing, a crucial aspect of neonatal medicine and developmental rehabilitation, is one of the first complex motor behaviors a newborn must master for survival. However, for premature or medically fragile infants, achieving swallowing function safely and efficiently is not so easy. Dysphagia, particularly in early development, indicates impairments in several systems, including neuromuscular, sensory, respiratory, and autonomic. It can also manifest as an early biomarker in neurologically fragile infants (Jadcherla et al., 2009; Lau, 2015).

During swallowing, a rhythmic movement, reflexive and voluntary phases work synergistically. Swallowing function, controlled by central pattern generators (CPGs) in the brainstem, is modulated by higher cortical centers including the insula, anterior cingulate, and somatosensory cortex. Any damage or underdevelopment in the neural networks that control this process disrupts the coordination of sucking, swallowing, and breathing, resulting in an increased risk of aspiration and impaired food intake (Barlow et al., 2014; Amaizu et al., 2008).

Swallowing disorders in newborns are most commonly observed in premature infants. On average, 25% to 50% of infants born before the 34th week of gestation experience impaired swallowing function. Most preterm infants experience difficulties transitioning to oral feeding. As a result, they require long-term enteral feeding (Thoyre et al., 2005; Jadcherla, 2016). Swallowing and feeding difficulties can also occur in full-term infants due to medical complications. Regardless of the cause, early diagnosis and intervention are essential to minimize respiratory complications, support neuroplasticity, and ensure safe oral intake.

Clinical and Developmental Significance

Feeding difficulties in the neonatal period do not stem solely from malnutrition. The feeding experience also leads to significant adverse outcomes regarding growth, brain development, and the parent-infant bond. This is because the feeding experience is linked to the sensory, motor, and emotional systems involved in early learning and attachment. Consequently, repeated negative feeding experiences due to aspiration or choking can lead to maladaptive sensory responses and negative conditioning (Lau & Smith, 2011; ASHA, undated).

The mother-infant bond is one of the most important opportunities for attachment during the feeding process. However, the feeding process can become stressful or medical in nature due to tubes, monitors, or inconsistent routines. Adverse conditions negatively impact the delicate structure of trust and bonding between parent and child. At this point, implementing family-centered approaches can be beneficial.

This allows for gains not only in terms of clinical outcomes but also in terms of emotional and developmental well-being (Filippa & Kuhn, 2024; Murthy et al., 2023).

From a systemic perspective, feeding difficulties in newborns prolong hospital stays and increase healthcare costs. Infants discharged without achieving safe and efficient oral feeding often require readmission due to aspiration pneumonia or growth failure. These situations typically lead to prolonged outpatient care or readmission (Kamity et al., 2021). Consequently, feeding performance remains a critical indicator in terms of both the newborn's medical condition and discharge criteria.

Scope and Aims of the Chapter

This chapter provides a comprehensive overview of the developmental, clinical and management aspects of swallowing disorders in newborns. Furthermore, it addresses current research, evidence-based clinical frameworks and practical strategies applicable in neonatal intensive care units (NICUs).

The objectives of this chapter are as follows:

1. To summarise the developmental physiology and neurobiological foundations of neonatal swallowing
2. To introduce aetiological mechanisms and at-risk groups
3. To explain structured clinical and instrumental assessment protocols
4. To convey evidence-based therapeutic interventions, including oral-motor, sensory-motor, cue-based, compensatory and device-assisted approaches
5. To discuss the feasibility of interventions in clinical settings and within multidisciplinary care frameworks.
6. To introduce technological innovations, ethical considerations and family-centred models, and to provide guidance for future research

This section aims to enhance the understanding of swallowing difficulties in newborns by integrating developmental science with clinical practice. It also aims to provide a comprehensive and lifelong knowledge base for the management of neonatal dysphagia.

2. ETIOLOGY AND NEURODEVELOPMENTAL BASIS

Neonatal dysphagia arises from the interaction of neurological issues, physiological imbalances and adverse environmental factors. The swallowing function, which involves more than 26 muscle pairs and six cranial nerves, requires the coordination of a complex neural network. A dysfunction at any level of this complex nervous system can lead to swallowing difficulties.

2.1 Developmental Foundations

The ontogenesis of swallowing begins in the early stages of fetal life. Primitive pharyngeal swallowing, observable by the 11th week of gestation, matures alongside sucking-swallowing-breathing patterns between the 32nd and 34th weeks of post-conception age (Lau, 2015). Maturation in these developmental processes also parallels rapid brainstem myelination and the maturation of the respiratory and gastrointestinal systems. During the sucking-swallowing-breathing (SSB) sequence, which operates in an extremely delicate balance, physiological events work synergistically. Indeed, while negative intraoral pressure is generated during sucking, airway protection is ensured during swallowing, and oxygenation occurs via respiration. If any immaturity or neurological dysfunction occurs during the sequence, feeding efficiency decreases and the risk of aspiration increases (Amaizu et al., 2008; Jadcherla et al., 2017).

In preterm infants, shortened sucking movements, delayed swallowing reflexes and prolonged breathing pauses are frequently observed. The abnormalities observed may stem not only from structural abnormalities but also from a failure to achieve neural synchronisation. With targeted stimulation, many babies can develop regular behavioural patterns equivalent to those of full-term babies of the same age. What enables this is, in fact, the brain's capacity for adaptive reorganisation (Barlow et al., 2014).

2.2 Epidemiology and Risk Groups

Feeding and swallowing difficulties are one of the most common causes of delayed discharge from the neonatal intensive care unit. The prevalence of dysphagia, which may vary depending on diagnostic criteria, is approximately 35–45% in very low birth weight infants (Lau, 2015; Jadcherla, 2017). It is known that the prevalence is higher in high-risk infants with bronchopulmonary dysplasia, hypoxic-ischaemic encephalopathy, congenital heart disease, or those who have been intubated for a prolonged period. The risk of dysphagia increases further when environmental and iatrogenic factors are taken into account. For example, prolonged mechanical ventilation can negatively affect oral sensory experiences, thereby delaying the development of coordinated sucking skills. Similarly, orogastric tube feeding can negatively impact oral sensory-motor development because it prevents exploration of the oral region (Krüger & Kritzinger, 2019).

Inequalities within healthcare systems can lead to delays in diagnosis and treatment. For example, in facilities lacking trained nutritionists or standardized assessment protocols, dysphagia often goes undiagnosed. Late diagnosis of swallowing disorders leads to delayed intervention. To address this inequality, training in neonatal feeding care can be provided for speech-language pathologists (SLPs) and occupational therapists (OTs). Global initiatives promoting professional and interprofessional training are working to bridge this gap (Weber & Voos, 2022).

2.3 Neurophysiologic and Sensory-Motor Mechanisms

Swallowing is primarily coordinated by the nucleus tractus solitarius (NTS) and nucleus ambiguus, which together form the central pattern generator (CPG) of the brainstem nuclei. Sensory inputs from cranial nerves V, VII, IX, and X trigger the swallowing reflex. Afferent feedback is provided to modulate the trigger, while motor commands execute the movement via cranial nerves IX, X, and XII (Jean, 2001).

Functional neuroimaging studies also confirm that cortical regions including the insular cortex, sensorimotor cortex, and additional motor area control the voluntary phases of swallowing (Variane et al., 2022). In newborns, however, the immaturity of these descending connections leads to decreased sensitivity in swallowing triggering. This, in turn, leads to increased delay in swallowing. During the neonatal period, the oropharyngeal structures and the somatosensory system are of vital importance for swallowing. This is because orofacial mechanoreceptors receive sensory stimuli from the nipple or pacifier. These sensory stimuli trigger the rhythmic motor response necessary for sucking. However, in situations of sensory deprivation, such as prolonged intubation, the cortical representation of oral movements may be disrupted. Consequently, delays may occur in the process of becoming ready for feeding (Barlow et al., 2014; Lau & Smith, 2011).

Recent research has shown that early-stage tactile, gustatory, and auditory inputs (including the mother's voice and scent) strengthen brainstem-cortex connections. It is proposed that early-stage inputs improve feeding coordination (Filippa & Kuhn, 2024; Variane et al., 2022). Therefore, sensory-rich, developmentally sensitive care environments are recommended to promote neural integration.

2.4 Pathophysiologic Mechanisms in High-Risk Infants

The pathophysiology of neonatal dysphagia is multifactorial. In some premature infants whose CPGs in the brainstem are not yet fully mature, a temporal incoordination between swallowing and breathing occurs. In infants with neurological damage, such as hypoxic-ischaemic encephalopathy, delayed swallowing and pharyngeal residuals are observed as a result of cortical and subcortical damage (Jadcherla & Stoner, 2009; Rommel et al., 2003).

Respiratory comorbidities, however, affect not only swallowing-drinking coordination but also endurance and alertness. For example, in infants with chronic lung disease or pulmonary hypertension, priority is given to breathing over feeding. Naturally, this leads to shorter swallowing times and incomplete clearance of the bolus (Amaizu et al., 2008; Lau & Smith, 2011; Jadcherla, 2017). Stress and negative experiences related to feeding can exacerbate existing functional impairments. Forced feeding without considering behavioral cues causes the infant to associate oral stimuli with distress. Indeed, repetition of this leads to autonomic dysregulation and reinforces maladaptive behaviors (Marshall et al., 2025). Behavioral adaptations associated with negativity may persist even if physiological stability is achieved. Therefore, positive sensory experiences related to feeding and the caregiver's responsiveness are of utmost importance in the early stages.

2.5 Developmental and Environmental Modifiers

Feeding naturally occurs not in an isolated environment, but within a relational and environmental context. Today, developmental care principles such as clustered care, noise reduction, and skin-to-skin contact are adopted to support autonomic balance and feeding. In particular, the perception of a parent's presence through the mother's voice and scent has measurable effects on the baby's heart rate and feeding patterns (Filippa & Kuhn, 2024).

However, negative factors such as overstimulation, inconsistent routines or the carer's stress adversely affect feeding development. Although feeding practices vary across societies, culturally sensitive interventions that respect family values and caregiving styles are increasingly recommended (Velasco Arias et al., 2025).

In conclusion, achieving newborn feeding skills is multifactorial. First, the infant must have reached a certain level of neurological and physiological maturity. In addition to biological readiness, sensory regulation and developmental care are also important environmental factors in terms of support. In addition, the caregiver should interpret the baby's feeding behaviors and make adjustments accordingly. Feeding skills involve multiple factors, and all these situations can influence each other.

3. CLINICAL ASSESSMENT

3.1 Principles of Early Clinical Evaluation

When evaluating newborn swallowing, a developmental perspective is considered, including the baby's physiological stability, behavioral organization, and neurodevelopmental stage. Clinical evaluation is generally based on observing the baby's feeding performance. However, how the baby responds to sensory and caregiver inputs, and how it regulates its breathing and oromotor control during this performance should also be continuously interpreted (Jadcherla et al., 2017; Thoyre et al., 2013).

The first step in clinical feeding evaluation should always be pre-feeding observation. The baby's wakefulness level, muscle tone, postural control, color changes, and baseline respiratory rate are important at this stage. A prerequisite for initiating oral stimulation or feeding attempts is that the infant is physiologically and respiratorily stable. If oral feeding is initiated before stability has been achieved, conditions such as physiological stress, bradycardia or reluctance to feed may arise. For this reason, it is recommended that a developmental assessment be carried out prior to both stimulation and feeding. The developmental assessment generally consists of four sections:

1. Oral Structure Assessment: The assessment examines symmetry, palate contour, range of tongue movement and jaw alignment. Subtle findings such as a high-arched palate or a restricted tongue tie may negatively affect sucking volume and quality (Krüger & Kritzinger, 2019).
2. Reflex Testing: Sucking, gag, and swallowing reflexes provide information about neurological status. The absence or weakness of reflexes indicates immaturity of the brainstem or involvement of cranial nerves.
3. Non-Nutritive Sucking (NNS) Assessment: Rhythm, amplitude, and endurance are tested using a pacifier or a gloved finger. This provides reliable preliminary information about oral-motor coordination without the risk of aspiration (Lau & Smith, 2011).
4. Feeding Observation: The clinician observes the infant's swallowing timing, breathing pattern, and signs of fatigue or stress (e.g., arching the back, spreading the toes, decreased oxygen saturation) during feeding. Modern neonatal feeding observation emphasizes cue-based and infant-centered approaches. In baby-centered approaches, the caregiver is not required to follow a fixed schedule during feeding. Instead, they initiate, accelerate, and conclude feeding by following the baby's cues (Marshall et al., 2025). This approach focuses on quality

rather than quantity. The goal is to support trust-based feeding interactions by improving physiological regulation.

3.2 Standardized Tools and Scoring Systems

Various standardized tools have been developed for objective and reproducible oral feeding assessments in newborns. The tools used comprehensively evaluate the infant's readiness, motor organization, and physiological stability. The use of standardized tools also supports consistent interdisciplinary communication among speech-language pathologists, neonatologists, occupational therapists, and nurses. Some standardized assessment tools are mentioned below:

Early Feeding Skills (EFS) Assessment — Originally developed by Thoyre et al. (2005), this scale was later updated by the same Thoyre et al. in 2018. (Thoyre et al., 2018) The EFS scale assesses three areas: readiness for oral feeding, organization of sucking-swallowing-breathing coordination, and resilience during feeding sessions. Infants are categorized as "ready," "in transition," or "not ready." The aim is to help clinicians determine the suitability for initiating oral feeding and to identify intervention goals.

Neonatal Oral Motor Assessment Scale (NOMAS) — Developed by Palmer et al. in 1993, NOMAS assesses infants based on observable jaw-tongue movements and rhythm regularity. Based on observations, it differentiates between irregular and dysfunctional sucking patterns. NOMAS is particularly used to classify neuromotor deficits in premature infants. It is also commonly used to monitor improvements after therapies.

Oral Motor Assessment Program (SOMA) — Designed for older infants, SOMA allows for the measurement of oral-motor skills with different food textures and consistencies (Reilly et al., 1995). This scale is useful for monitoring feeding during the transition from liquid to semi-solid foods. Furthermore, it can identify abnormalities in fine motor skills that may not be detected during routine clinical observations. In addition to the basic tools, various supplementary scales are also used in feeding assessments. The Premature Infant Oral Feeding Readiness Assessment Scale (POFRAS) (Fujinaga et al., 2013) is a standardised measure used to assess whether a premature infant is ready for oral feeding. It assesses the infant's neuromotor tone, oxygen saturation, postural control and non-feeding sucking patterns. According to the scale's results (Lau et al., 2015), feeding efficiency is categorised into four performance levels. POFRAS is also valuable for monitoring the feeding process and reporting treatment outcomes objectively.

The Neonatal Feeding Assessment Scale (NFAS) (Viviers et al., 2019), a relatively recent scale, assesses both behavioural and physiological parameters such as posture, sucking quality and oxygen stability. The NFAS, which facilitates interdisciplinary communication in the neonatal intensive care unit, is used as a reliable bedside tool. However, rather than relying on a single tool, the use of multiple purpose-specific tools is recommended. This provides a comprehensive framework that integrates behavioural observation with physiological monitoring, thereby enhancing diagnostic sensitivity. It is also beneficial in standardising what may appear to be complex terminology. Furthermore, it supports collaborative decision-making in feeding care processes.

3.3 Physiologic and Behavioral Feeding Cues

It is important to understand the signals babies give during feeding. The subtle cues they use to indicate they are ready to feed or are experiencing stress during feeding should be observed. A baby who breathes regularly, moves in a coordinated manner, can focus their gaze, and exhibits rhythmic sucking movements is generally considered ready to feed. However, symptoms such as changes in skin color, tongue thrusting, coughing, and apnea are associated with stress. Early recognition of these symptoms allows caregivers to make adjustments during feeding (Shaker, 2013; Thoyre et al., 2013; Marshall et al., 2025). In addition to behavioral observation, incorporating physiological data such as heart rate and oxygen saturation into the assessment provides a multidimensional perspective on feeding safety. It also helps clinicians adjust their actions based on symptoms. Depending on the infant's assessment results, they can adjust the flow rate, position, or duration as needed (Shaker, 2017; Lau, 2015).

Table 1. Summary of Key Insights – Clinical Assessment

Key Point	Clinical Application
Feeding readiness is determined by stability and state, not gestational age.	Prevents aspiration and negative conditioning.
Standardized tools (EFS, NOMAS, POFRAS etc.) improve objectivity.	Enables shared decision-making in NICU teams.
Cue-based models reduce stress and enhance caregiver engagement.	Supports neurobehavioral regulation.

4. INSTRUMENTAL ASSESSMENT

Instrumental evaluations allow for the visualization of swallowing physiology. Clinical hypotheses can be validated using the results obtained from instrumental evaluations. Instrumental evaluation is recommended when the risk of aspiration, pharyngeal timing, or structural integrity cannot be determined through clinical bedside assessment (Kamity et al., 2021).

4.1 Videofluoroscopic Swallowing Study (VFSS)

The Videofluoroscopic Swallowing Study (VFSS), also known as modified barium swallow, is the gold standard for understanding bolus flow, airway protection, and the phases of swallowing. Real-time imaging visualizes penetration, aspiration, delayed swallowing onset, and post-swallow residues. Studies involving infants have demonstrated that VFSS is effective in understanding the physiology and pathophysiology of swallowing. In a cohort comprising both preterm and term infants, common abnormalities were also identified using VFSS. Evaluations have found that VFSS diagnostically confirms delayed swallowing onset, nasopharyngeal reflux, and signs of aspiration (Uhm et al., 2013).

Recent studies emphasize the use of VFSS in both the diagnosis and clinical management of neonatal dysphagia. In addition to measuring the severity of aspiration, it is also used to determine individualized treatment strategies such as acceleration, flow regulation, and compensatory positioning (Shih et al., 2022).

Overall, VFSS is of critical importance both for understanding the mechanisms of swallowing disorders and for guiding safe, evidence-based feeding management in the neonatal intensive care unit.

4.2 Fiberoptic Endoscopic Evaluation of Swallowing (FEES)

FEES allows for the visualization of laryngeal and pharyngeal functions during feeding without exposing the patient to radiation. Since it can be performed using flexible endoscopes suitable for infants, its use in Neonatal Intensive Care Units (NICUs) is becoming increasingly widespread (Pizzorni et al., 2024).

With FEES, airway obstruction, secretion management, and reflex responses can be observed. In addition to assessment, feeding strategies can be tested in real time during intervention using FEES. Adjusting these strategies to synchronize with swallowing enhances clinical efficiency.

However, the brief “loss of image” period during swallowing limits the visualization of the bolus. Nevertheless, FEES remains an ideal option for repeated monitoring, bedside access, and for fragile infants where VFSS cannot be used.

4.3 Integration of Findings Across Modalities

If findings from instrumental evaluations are interpreted in isolation, the patient may be misguided. Therefore, findings from these evaluations must be combined with clinical data. For example, an infant who shows a delay in the onset of swallowing on VFSS but exhibits a strong, non-nutritive sucking movement may benefit more from sensory-motor stimulation than from flow regulation.

In addition to FEES and VFSS, high-resolution pharyngeal manometry and oropharyngeal ultrasound allow for the noninvasive measurement of pressure and timing during swallowing. These tools, which provide information about the swallowing mechanism, hold promise for future research (Variane et al., 2022).

5. EVIDENCE-BASED INTERVENTIONS

In a comprehensive intervention plan, numerous strategies are designed to suit the infant's medical condition and developmental level. Generally, interventions are divided into five complementary areas: oral-motor/sensory, cue-based, compensatory, device-assisted, and pathway integration.

5.1 Oral-Motor and Sensory-Motor Approaches

Structured oral stimulation programs are frequently used in the early rehabilitation of premature infants with feeding difficulties. The aim of these interventions is to improve oral sensory awareness, muscle tone, and coordination. The goal is to ensure safe and effective feeding by improving coordination.

The most comprehensively studied evidence-based oral stimulation program is the Oral Motor Intervention for Premature Infants (PIOMI) program. Designed by Brenda Knoll, PIOMI is typically administered once daily, approximately 15 minutes before a feeding session. The entire program, which includes tactile and oral motor stimulation, lasts five minutes. Stimulation is applied to perioral and intraoral structures to improve neuromuscular coordination and oral sensory integration. Stimulation consists of stroking and gentle pressure techniques. The final step of the protocol is the encouragement of non-feeding sucking. Numerous randomized controlled trials have been conducted on the effectiveness of the PIOMI program in various clinical settings, including Thailand, Iran, Turkey, and India. These studies have shown that premature infants experience shorter time to achieve complete oral feeding, improved sucking efficiency, and shorter discharge times (Knoll, Daramas, and Drake, 2019; Ghomi et al., 2019; Guler et al., 2022; Sasmal et al., 2023).

A recent systematic review found that PIOMI accelerates the feeding process, increases weight gain, and shortens the length of stay in the neonatal intensive care unit (Sivasanker et al., 2025). Based on these findings, it can be said that PIOMI is a standard, time-efficient, and safe protocol for neonatal intensive care units.

In addition to PIOMI, the Fucile protocol (Fucile, Gisel, McFarland, and Lau) is one of the first programs developed for oral-sensorimotor stimulation in preterm infants. Within the program, tactile stimulation is applied to oral structures such as the lips, cheeks, gums, and tongue. As with other programs, the final step of the intervention is to encourage non-nutritive sucking. Studies have found that the Fucile approach accelerates the transition from tube feeding to oral feeding, improves sucking organization, and supports the early development of swallowing-breathing coordination (Fucile et al., 2002; Fucile et al., 2005).

Both the PIOMI and Fucile protocols are structured, evidence-based oral-motor stimulation programs implemented as part of early intervention. Clinicians can support infants' neurodevelopmental maturation by integrating these approaches into NICU care. Additionally, it is known that interventions such as PIOMI and Fucile reduce hospital length of stay and improve long-term feeding outcomes.

In addition to oral stimulation programs, non-nutritive sucking (NNS) performed with a pacifier or a gloved finger provides rhythmic stimulation. NNS stimulation aids in CPG synchronization and autonomic regulation. When combined with oral stimulation, NNS may create synergistic effects on feeding endurance and oxygen stability (Barlow et al., 2014; Song et al., 2019).

Additionally, thermal-tactile stimulation and stimulation with breast milk (e.g., small drops of breast milk) may facilitate the initiation of the swallowing process in infants with neurological disorders (Arvedson & Brodsky, 2019). However, excessive stimulation should be avoided during these applications. It should be remembered that excessive tactile input can trigger defense reflexes in newborns, who have a very fragile and sensitive constitution.

5.2 Cue-Based and Infant-Driven Feeding

Today, the traditional program-based approach is beginning to be replaced by cue-based feeding. In cue-based feeding, the baby's physiological and behavioral signals are taken into account in initiating and adjusting the rate of feeding. In this infant-led approach, feeding sessions are only initiated when the baby indicates readiness. Infant readiness is characterized by a stable heart rate, regular posture, and rhythmic non-feeding sucking (Thoyre et al., 2013; Shaker, 2013).

Clinical studies and randomized controlled trials have shown that cue-based programs shorten the time to achieve full oral feeding and reduce apnea and bradycardia events (Shaker, 2017; Marshall et al., 2025). Involving parents in cue interpretation further increases family participation, continuity of care, and post-discharge feeding success. Self-regulation is also encouraged when caregiver responses are aligned with infant cues. For all these reasons, cue-based feeding, where the family is the primary element, can be adopted as a central element of neonatal intensive care unit care. This approach embraces developmental care principles that emphasize infant-centered pacing, physiological stability, and caregiver engagement. Cue-based feeding administered in the neonatal intensive care unit (NICU) has the potential to improve neurocognitive development. Studies have also shown that it supports energy conservation and shortens the length of hospital stay (Campbell-Yeo et al., 2021; Thoyre et al., 2013).

5.3 Compensatory Strategies and Positioning

Compensatory interventions optimize safety rather than retraining the underlying physiology. The benefits of elevated lateral and semi-upright positions to facilitate airway protection and reduce flow rate have been indicated in scientific studies (Crossley et al., 2022).

Providing short pauses every 3-5 feedings can prevent fatigue and ensure synchronization with breathing. Varying the flow rate using special nipples used in premature infants allows for individual adjustment according to the baby's endurance (Shaker, 2017; Thoyre et al., 2013).

Mouth support techniques, including chin and cheek support, stabilize chin movement. They also increase sucking efficiency in infants with hypotonia [Dewi et al., 2024].

Environmental modifications such as dim lighting, swaddling, and reduced noise support autonomic stability and attention focus. Environmental modifications have a complementary effect when applied in conjunction with the other interventions mentioned above (Campbell-Yeo et al., 2021).

5.4 Device-Assisted and Neurostimulation-Based Therapies

In addition to the traditional therapy approaches mentioned above, innovations such as the NTrainer® system and the Supplementary Breastfeeding System (SNS) are used as device-based approaches.

NTrainer® provides patterned orocutaneous pneumatic stimulation by mimicking natural sucking rhythms. Scientific studies have reported that infants using NTrainer achieve oral feeding earlier and experience improvements in CNS coordination (Song et al., 2019).

On the other hand, SNS enables simultaneous breastfeeding for infants who have difficulty transitioning to breastfeeding. This supports the mother-child bond by providing natural sensory feedback (Krüger & Kritzinger, 2019).

Beyond these, neurostimulation technologies with vibratory tactile, transcutaneous, and proprioceptive features are developing in this field. The aim of these new technologies is to activate trigeminal and glossopharyngeal afferents with the given stimuli and potentially increase cortical connectivity (Martens & Melkonian, 2024).

5.5 Integrating Interventions into Clinical Pathways

The most effective approach to newborn care undoubtedly involves a combination of various strategies and their individual structuringIn clinics, personalized, holistic treatment approaches determined by a multidisciplinary team are applied. The Individualized Nutrition Care Plan (INC) takes into account medical, developmental, and behavioral characteristics. Goals are set based on all data, and patients' progress is monitored (Jadcherla et al., 2012).

Team collaboration is crucial in the nutrition care plan:

- Speech and Language Therapists (SLPs) conduct assessments and develop therapy plans.
- Neonatologists ensure the maintenance of medical stability.
- Occupational therapists provide support with positioning and sensory regulation.
- Dietitians determine nutritional adequacy.
- Nurses provide bedside care and interventions.

Models such as the Movement-Oriented Feeding Approach (Jadcherla et al., 2012) and the COVES Framework (Campbell-Yeo et al., 2021) increase nutritional efficiency and parental satisfaction. Studies have shown that applying these models results in measurable improvements in infants at discharge.

Table 2. Summary of Key Insights – Intervention Section

Intervention Domain	Key Mechanism	Evidence-Based Outcome
Oral-motor & sensory stimulation	Activates mechanoreceptors, enhances CPG maturation	Shorter transition to full oral feeding
Cue-based feeding	Aligns feeding with behavioral and physiologic readiness	Fewer desaturation and apnea events
Positioning & pacing	Optimizes airway protection, improves endurance	Reduces aspiration and fatigue
Device-assisted therapies	Provides patterned stimulation for neural entrainment	Earlier oral feeding and discharge
Integrated care pathways	Synchronize interventions across disciplines	Consistent, family-centered feeding success

6. FUTURE RESEARCH DIRECTIONS

Significant progress has been made in the field of neonatal dysphagia in recent years. However, there are still gaps in standardization of care, integration of new technologies, and global equity. Future research should focus on neuroscientific discoveries, technological innovations, and family-centered care.

6.1 Technological Innovations in Assessment and Monitoring

The integration of artificial intelligence (AI) and machine learning (ML) into neonatal care has opened up new possibilities in real-time feeding analysis. AI algorithms trained on video, respiratory, and pressure sensor data can detect abnormal suck-swallow-breathe (SSB) sequences that clinicians might overlook (Keles & Bagci, 2023). AI algorithms have the potential to predict aspiration risk or fatigue thresholds in advance. This enables personalized and early intervention.

Wearable biosensors and microfluidic pressure patches are currently available for use during feeding. New technologies allow for the continuous and non-invasive monitoring of swallowing activity and oxygen saturation (Sullivan & Beam, 2023). When used in conjunction with cloud-based dashboards, they allow clinicians and parents to receive automatic alerts when signs of stress or irregularities are detected in infants. Looking at the last decade in the field of neonatal dysphagia, it is clear that significant progress has been made. However, differences in practice between clinics make it difficult to integrate new technologies into the clinical setting. At the same time, the lack of standardization presents significant challenges in ensuring global equity in clinical care. Therefore, future research in the neonatology field may focus more on combining neuroscientific discoveries and technological innovations with clinical applications. However, it should aim to close these gaps by emphasizing both multicenter and family-center practices.

6.1 Technological Innovations in Assessment and Monitoring

Real-time feeding analysis has come to the fore thanks to the integration of artificial intelligence (AI) and machine learning (ML) into neonatal care. Clinicians can identify and concretize abnormal sucking-swallowing-breathing (SSB) sequences using AI algorithms trained on video, respiratory, and pressure sensor data (Keles & Bagci, 2023).

The use of trained algorithms can predict feeding readiness, aspiration risk, or fatigue thresholds in advance. This allows for individualized pace adjustment and early intervention specific to the baby.

Swallowing activity and oxygen saturation are monitored non-invasively during feeding thanks to wearable biosensors and microfluidic pressure patches (Sullivan & Beam, 2023). It seems possible to receive automated alerts about the baby's condition with these cloud-based devices. Alerts can be transmitted to clinicians and parents, especially when signs of stress or irregularity occur in babies.

Furthermore, telehealth and virtual neonatal intensive care unit (NICU) care pathways, which have become more prevalent in our lives with the COVID-19 pandemic, have proven applicable for parent education and post-discharge follow-up. Studies by Holm et al. (2019) and Campbell-Yeo et al. (2021) found that tele-home care programs for premature babies improved feeding outcomes and reduced parental anxiety. The use of AI-powered tele-coaching, where machine learning systems provide real-time visual feedback during home feeding sessions, is also a potential research topic for the future.

Another promising area is neuroimaging-based biofeedback. By combining functional near-infrared spectroscopy (fNIRS) with EEG, clinicians can visualise cortical activation during eating tasks. This enables them to link eating behaviours to the underlying neural processes (Variane et al., 2022). These multimodal systems also provide therapeutic biofeedback by directing targeted stimulation. Consequently, neuroplasticity can be enhanced through stimulus management.

6.2 Standardisation of Clinical Studies and Outcomes

Although scientific evidence in the field of neonatal feeding disorders is growing, heterogeneity in study designs limits the synthesis of results. The lack of focus on a standard outcome measure in studies makes it difficult to systematically evaluate the effectiveness of interventions. Measures typically vary from the time to transition to full oral feeding to the length of hospital stay. There is a clear and urgent need for core outcome sets (COS) from both physiological and developmental perspectives. The recommended areas are as follows:

- Feeding safety (aspiration incidents, frequency of desaturation),
- Feeding efficiency (volume per minute, fatigue scores),
- Neurodevelopmental outcomes (Bayley Scales, sensory-motor integration),
- Family well-being (parental stress and self-confidence).

To ensure consistency, a standard classification system for the severity of dysphagia should be adopted in neonatal intensive care units (NICUs). Just as the Penetration-Aspiration Scale (PAS) is used during videofluoroscopic swallowing studies (VFSS), the use of a newborn-specific scale during instrumental or clinical swallowing assessments may be beneficial (Kamity et al., 2021).

Multicentre randomised controlled trials (RCTs) comparing oral-motor programmes, cue-based feeding and neurostimulation may be effective in defining best practice.

Another important point is the need for longitudinal follow-up studies to fully understand the effectiveness of the intervention. As many studies end at discharge, long-term developmental and feeding outcomes remain unknown. Integrating early intervention and outpatient nutritional follow-up into the study design will better reflect the real-world impact from a practical perspective (Jose et al., 2024).

6.3 Integration of Neuroscience and Developmental Physiology

Advances in neonatal neuroimaging have accelerated research into the neural mechanisms underlying the swallowing process. Methods such as diffusion tensor imaging (DTI) and resting-state functional magnetic resonance imaging (fMRI) are particularly useful in providing concrete evidence. For example, research by Variane et al. (2022) demonstrated correlations between thalamocortical connectivity and feeding coordination. The research findings are important for understanding interventions targeting sensory feedback and arousal regulation. Consequently, a biological rationale can be provided when planning intervention programmes based on the information obtained. Neurostimulation studies involving orodermal, vibrotactile and non-invasive electrical stimulation offer promising insights for improving sensorimotor integration. Preliminary findings suggest that these interventions may accelerate cortical maturation and improve SSB synchronisation (Martens & Melkonian, 2024; Song et al., 2019). Combining these methods with neuroimaging may assist in identifying response biomarkers. This could pave the way for personalised nutritional therapy.

6.4 Ethical, Cultural and Practical Considerations

The rapid pace of technological advancement undoubtedly brings with it ethical responsibilities. When using artificial intelligence or remote monitoring with vulnerable groups, attention must always be paid to data privacy, algorithmic transparency and parental consent. As algorithms trained on patient groups in neonatal intensive care units are predominantly used in Western societies, generalising the results on a global scale may not yield accurate outcomes. Therefore, there is a need for diverse and inclusive datasets that encompass other global communities (Sullivan & Beam, 2023).

Equity and accessibility should guide future innovations. Unfortunately, many neonatal intensive care units worldwide lack access to VFSS or paediatric dietitians.

The global care gap can be bridged through low-cost solutions such as simplified cue-based protocols, smartphone-based coaching, and sensorless feeding analytics.

Finally, research design must incorporate family participation for both ethical and scientific reasons. Parents should not merely give consent; they should also collaborate as co-researchers and be involved as stakeholders in design, interpretation and implementation. Models in which all stakeholders play an active role offer both an innovative perspective and results that are applicable in the real world.

7. CONCLUSION

7.1 Synthesis of Key Insights

Swallowing disorders in newborns arise from a combination of physiological, neurological and environmental factors. The key findings derived from the examination of all these factors are as follows:

- Swallowing disorders observed in the neonatal period reflect both biological immaturity and environmental influences.
- Developmental assessment is the first step in early intervention. Combining bedside clinical assessment with imaging provides the most accurate diagnosis.
- Holistic interventions, including sensory stimulation, cue-based feeding and neurostimulation, yield the best results when applied systematically.
- A family-centred approach and multidisciplinary collaboration are essential for safe, efficient and emotionally supportive feeding care.

7.2 Integrating Research and Practice

The gap between scientific discoveries and clinical practice still appears to be a significant problem. As Weber and Voos (2022) also point out, collaboration between academic centres and clinical neonatal intensive care units is of vital importance. Through such collaborations, existing evidence can be further developed and rapidly implemented in clinical settings. Another key issue in the field of neonatology is knowledge transfer initiatives (Estrem et al., 2022). Education, structural support, leadership and family involvement are crucial for standardising practices.

Using Plan-Do-Check-Act (PDSA) cycles, neonatal teams can test feeding protocols under real-world conditions. In clinical practice, quality can be improved and datasets for evidence-based practices can be created through routine data collection (Campbell-Yeo et al., 2021).

7.3 Towards the Future of Neonatal Feeding Care

Technological advancements should be integrated with both clinical applications and human interaction. AI-powered monitoring, biosensors, and neurostimulation technologies have great potential in neonatology, as in all other application areas. However, it is important to ensure that interventions are always relationship-focused and family-centered. Every feeding interaction is a developmental opportunity as well as a clinical event. When caregivers and parents approach the baby's cues with patience and sensitivity, they do much more than just prevent aspiration. They lay a solid foundation for secure attachment and lifelong neurodevelopmental health. In short, feeding difficulties in newborns should be understood as an intervenable developmental issue. Early diagnosis, evidence-based intervention, and ongoing collaboration are crucial in this process. Through early intervention, the neonatal intensive care unit team can transform feeding from a risky experience into a healing and growth-supporting experience for both the baby and the family.

Note from Publisher

Correction Notice: A correction to the manuscript has been implemented.

Reason: Concerns/Issues About Article

Revisions have been made to enhance the clarity and readability of the text. No changes have been made to the scientific content, data, or references.

Correction Date: April 17, 2026

REFERENCES

Amaizu, N., Shulman, R. J., Schanler, R. J., & Lau, C. (2008). Maturation of oral feeding skills in preterm infants. *Acta Paediatrica (Oslo, Norway)*, *97*(1), 61–67.

American Speech-Language-Hearing Association. (n.d.). Pediatric feeding and swallowing [Practice Portal]. Retrieved December 3, 2025, from https://www.asha.org/practice-portal/clinical-topics/pediatric-feeding-and-swallowing/

Arvedson, J. C., Brodsky, L., & Lefton-Greif, M. A. (Eds.). (2019). *Pediatric swallowing and feeding: Assessment and management* (Vol. 1). Plural publishing.

Barlow, S. M., Lee, J., Wang, J., Oder, A., Hall, S., Knox, K., & Thompson, D. (2014). Frequency-modulated orocutaneous stimulation promotes non-nutritive suck development in preterm infants with respiratory distress syndrome or chronic lung disease. *Journal of Perinatology*, *34*(2), 136–142.

Campbell-Yeo, M., Dol, J., Richardson, B., McCulloch, H., Hundert, A., Foye, S., & Whitehead, L. (2021). A co-design of clinical virtual care pathways to engage and support families requiring neonatal intensive care in response to the COVID-19 pandemic (COVES study). *Journal of Neonatal Nursing*, *27*(6), 463–470.

Crossley, S. L., Duthie, K., Newton, M., & Harding, C. (2022). Investigation into the flow rate of bottle teats typically used on an Australian neonatal unit. *Speech, Language and Hearing (London, England)*, *25*(1), 29–36.

Dewi, D. J., Rachmawati, E. Z. K., Wahyuni, L. K., Hsu, W. C., Tamin, S., Yunizaf, R., & Iskandar, R. A. T. P. (2024). Risk of dysphagia in a population of infants born pre-term: Characteristic risk factors in a tertiary NICU. *Jornal de Pediatria*, *100*(2), 169–176.

Estrem, H. H., Park, J., Thoyre, S., McComish, C., & McGlothen-Bell, K. (2022). Mapping the gaps: A scoping review of research on pediatric feeding disorder. *Clinical Nutrition ESPEN*, *48*, 45–55.

Filippa, M., & Kuhn, P. (2024). Early parental vocal contact in neonatal units: Rationale and clinical guidelines for implementation. *Frontiers in Neurology*, *15*, 1441576.

Fucile, S., Gisel, E., & Lau, C. (2002). Oral stimulation accelerates the transition from tube to oral feeding in preterm infants. *The Journal of Pediatrics*, *141*(2), 230–236.

Fucile, S., Gisel, E. G., McFarland, D. H., & Lau, C. (2011). Oral and non-oral sensorimotor interventions enhance oral feeding performance in preterm infants. *Developmental Medicine and Child Neurology*, *53*(9), 829–835.

Fujinaga, C. I., Moraes, S. A. D., Zamberlan-Amorim, N. E., Castral, T. C., Silva, A. D. A., & Scochi, C. G. S. (2013). Clinical validation of the preterm oral feeding readiness assessment scale. *Revista Latino-Americana de Enfermagem, 21*, 140–145.

Ghomi, H., Yadegari, F., Soleimani, F., Knoll, B. L., Noroozi, M., & Mazouri, A. (2019). The effects of premature infant oral motor intervention (PIOMI) on oral feeding of preterm infants: A randomized clinical trial. *International Journal of Pediatric Otorhinolaryngology, 120*, 202–209.

Guler, S., Cigdem, Z., Knoll, B. S. L., Ortabag, T., & Yakut, Y. (2022). Effect of the Premature Infant Oral Motor Intervention on sucking capacity in preterm infants in Turkey: A randomized controlled trial. *Advances in Neonatal Care, 22*(6), E196–E206.

Holm, K. G., Clemensen, J., Brødsgaard, A., Smith, A. C., Maastrup, R., & Zachariassen, G. (2019). Growth and breastfeeding of preterm infants receiving neonatal tele-homecare compared to hospital-based care. *Journal of Neonatal-Perinatal Medicine, 12*(3), 277–284.

Jadcherla, S. R. (2017). Advances with neonatal aerodigestive science in the pursuit of safe swallowing in infants: Invited review. *Dysphagia, 32*(1), 15–26.

Jadcherla, S. R., Dail, J., Malkar, M. B., McClead, R., Kelleher, K., & Nelin, L. (2016). Impact of process optimization and quality improvement measures on neonatal feeding outcomes at an all-referral neonatal intensive care unit. *JPEN. Journal of Parenteral and Enteral Nutrition, 40*(5), 646–655.

Jadcherla, S. R., Peng, J., Moore, R., Saavedra, J., Shepherd, E., Fernandez, S., & DiLorenzo, C. (2012). Impact of personalized feeding program in 100 NICU infants: Pathophysiology-based approach for better outcomes. *Journal of Pediatric Gastroenterology and Nutrition, 54*(1), 62–70.

Jadcherla, S. R., Stoner, E., Gupta, A., Bates, D. G., Fernandez, S., Di Lorenzo, C., & Linscheid, T. (2009). Evaluation and management of neonatal dysphagia: Impact of pharyngoesophageal motility studies and multidisciplinary feeding strategy. *Journal of Pediatric Gastroenterology and Nutrition, 48*(2), 186–192.

Jean, A. (2001). Brain stem control of swallowing: Neuronal network and cellular mechanisms. *Physiological Reviews, 81*(2), 929–969.

Jose, M., Krishnamurthy, R., Venkatesh, L., Kamath, N., Bhat, K. G., & Balasubramanium, R. K. (2024). Assessment and management of dysphagia in the neonatal intensive care units in India: A survey report. *Clinical Epidemiology and Global Health, 29*, 101683.

Kamity, R., Kapavarapu, P. K., & Chandel, A. (2021). Feeding problems and long-term outcomes in preterm infants—A systematic approach to evaluation and management. *Children (Basel, Switzerland)*, *8*(12), 1158.

Kaspy, K. R., Burg, G., Garrison, A. P., Miller, C. K., Pentiuk, S., Smith, M. M., & Benscoter, D. (2022). The follow up of complex infants in an aerodigestive clinic. *Paediatric Respiratory Reviews*, *44*, 3–10.

Keles, E., & Bagci, U. (2023). The past, current, and future of neonatal intensive care units with artificial intelligence: A systematic review. *NPJ Digital Medicine*, *6*(1), 220.

Knoll, B. S. L., Daramas, T., & Drake, V. (2019). Randomized controlled trial of a prefeeding oral motor therapy and its effect on feeding improvement in a Thai NICU. *Journal of Obstetric, Gynecologic, and Neonatal Nursing : JOGNN*, *48*(2), 176–188.

Krüger, E., Kritzinger, A., & Pottas, L. (2019). Oropharyngeal dysphagia in breastfeeding neonates with hypoxic-ischemic encephalopathy on therapeutic hypothermia. *Breastfeeding Medicine*, *14*(10), 718–723.

Lau, C. (2015a). Development of suck and swallow mechanisms in infants. *Annals of Nutrition & Metabolism*, *66*(Suppl. 5), 7–14.

Lau, C., Bhat, K., Potak, D., & Schanler, R. J. (2015b). Oral feeding assessment predicts length of hospital stay in late preterm infants. *Journal of Pediatrics and Mother Care*, *1*(1), 102.

Lau, C., & Smith, E. O. (2011). A novel approach to assess oral feeding skills of preterm infants. *Neonatology*, *100*(1), 64–70.

Marshall, J., Gosa, M. M., & Dodrill, P. (2025). (in press). A systematic review of clinical assessment tools that evaluate the feeding skills domain for paediatric feeding disorder. *International Journal of Speech-Language Pathology*, •••, 1–11.

Martens, A., Melkonian, A., Shaughnessy, S., & Zimmerman, E. (2024). Perspectives on Device-Facilitated Therapy in Management of Pediatric Dysphagia in the Neonatal Intensive Care Unit. *Perspectives of the ASHA Special Interest Groups*, *9*(1), 228–237.

Murthy, S., Yan, S. D., Alam, S., Kumar, A., Rangarajan, A., Sawant, M., & Semrau, K. E. (2023). Improving neonatal health with family-centered, early postnatal care: A quasi-experimental study in India. *PLOS Global Public Health*, *3*(5), e0001240.

Palmer, M. M., Crawley, K., & Blanco, I. A. (1993). Neonatal Oral-Motor Assessment scale: a reliability study. Journal of perinatology: official journal of the California Perinatal Association, 13(1), 28-35.

Pizzorni, N., Rocca, S., Eplite, A., Monticelli, M., Rama, S., Mozzanica, F., & Schindler, A. (2024). Fiberoptic endoscopic evaluation of swallowing (FEES) in pediatrics: A systematic review. *International Journal of Pediatric Otorhinolaryngology, 181*, 111983.

Reilly, S., Skuse, D., Mathisen, B., & Wolke, D. (1995). The objective rating of oral-motor functions during feeding. *Dysphagia, 10*(3), 177–191.

Rommel, N., De Meyer, A. M., Feenstra, L., & Veereman-Wauters, G. (2003). The complexity of feeding problems in 700 infants and young children presenting to a tertiary care institution. *Journal of Pediatric Gastroenterology and Nutrition, 37*(1), 75–84.

Sasmal, S., Shetty, A. P., Saha, B., Knoll, B., & Mukherjee, S. (2023). Effect of prefeeding oromotor stimulation on oral feeding performance of preterm neonates during hospitalization and at corrected one month of age: A randomized controlled trial. *Journal of Neonatology, 37*(2), 149–158.

Shaker, C. S. (2013). Cue-based feeding in the NICU: Using the infant's communication as a guide. *Neonatal Network, 32*(6), 404.

Shaker, C. S. (2017, April). Infant-guided, co-regulated feeding in the neonatal intensive care unit. Part II: Interventions to promote neuroprotection and safety. [Thieme Medical Publishers]. *Seminars in Speech and Language, 38*(02), 106–115.

Shih, M. C., Rappazzo, C., Hudson, C., & Ongkasuwan, J. (2022). Videofluoroscopic Swallow Studies and Diagnostic Outcomes in Otherwise Healthy Infants With Dysphagia. *The Annals of Otology, Rhinology, and Laryngology, 131*(8), 892–896.

Sivasanker, A. A., Koul, P., Paul, D. R., & Kumar, S. R. (2025). Preterm Infant Oral Motor Intervention (PIOMI) on feeding progression, length of stay, and gain in weight: A systematic review and meta-analysis. *Journal of Scientific & Technical Research, 15*(1), 1–12.

Song, D., Jegatheesan, P., Nafday, S., Ahmad, K. A., Nedrelow, J., Wearden, M., & Govindaswami, B. (2019). Patterned frequency-modulated oral stimulation in preterm infants: A multicenter randomized controlled trial. *PLoS One, 14*(2), e0212675.

Sullivan, B. A., Beam, K., Vesoulis, Z. A., Aziz, K. B., Husain, A. N., Knake, L. A., & McAdams, R. M. (2024). Transforming neonatal care with artificial intelligence: Challenges, ethical consideration, and opportunities. *Journal of Perinatology*, *44*(1), 1–11.

Thoyre, S., Park, J., Pados, B., & Hubbard, C. (2013). Developing a co-regulated, cue-based feeding practice: The critical role of assessment and reflection. *Journal of Neonatal Nursing*, *19*(4), 139–148.

Thoyre, S. M., Pados, B. F., Shaker, C. S., Fuller, K., & Park, J. (2018). Psychometric properties of the early feeding skills assessment tool. *Advances in Neonatal Care*, *18*(5), E13–E23.

Thoyre, S. M., Shaker, C. S., & Pridham, K. F. (2005). The early feeding skills assessment for preterm infants. Neonatal network: NN, 24(3), 7.

Uhm, K. E., Yi, S. H., Chang, H. J., Cheon, H. J., & Kwon, J. Y. (2013). Videofluoroscopic swallowing study findings in full-term and preterm infants with dysphagia. *Annals of Rehabilitation Medicine*, *37*(2), 175–182.

Variane, G. F. T., Camargo, J. P. V., Rodrigues, D. P., Magalhães, M., & Mimica, M. J. (2022). Current status and future directions of neuromonitoring with emerging technologies in neonatal care. *Frontiers in Pediatrics*, *9*, 755144.

Velasco Arias, J. M., Peres, A. M., Escandell Rico, F. M., Solano-Ruiz, M. C., Gil-Guillen, V. F., & Noreña-Peña, A. (2025). Developmental-Centered Care in Preterm Newborns: Scoping Review. *Children (Basel, Switzerland)*, *12*(6), 783.

Viviers, M., Kritzinger, A., & Graham, M. (2019). Reliability and validity of the neonatal feeding assessment scale (NFAS) for the early identification of dysphagia in moderate to late preterm neonates. *African Health Sciences*, *19*(3), 2718–2727.

Weber, A. M., Voos, K. C., Bakas, T. M., Rice, J. B., Blatz, M. A., Ribeiro, A. P. D., & Kaplan, H. C. (2022). A clinical-academic partnership to develop a family management intervention for parents of preterm infants. *Journal of Clinical Nursing*, *31*(3-4), 390–405.

ADDITIONAL READING

Browne, J. V. (2013). Early relationship environments: Physiology of skin-to-skin contact, breastfeeding, and development of the parent–infant relationship. *Clinics in Perinatology*, *40*(4), 493–511.

Dodrill, P., & Gosa, M. M. (2015). Pediatric dysphagia: Physiology, assessment, and management. *Annals of Nutrition & Metabolism*, *66*(Suppl. 5), 24–31.

Gewolb, I. H., & Vice, F. L. (2006). Maturation of rhythmic suckle and swallow in preterm infants. *Developmental Medicine and Child Neurology*, *48*(7), 589–594.

Jadcherla, S. R. (2019). Challenges to eating, swallowing, and aerodigestive functions in infants: A burning platform that needs attention! *The Journal of Pediatrics*, *211*, 7–9.

Lau, C. (2018). Developmental physiology of feeding and swallowing. *Current Opinion in Gastroenterology*, *34*(3), 195–201.

McGrattan, K. E., McFarland, D. H., & Fucile, S. (2021). Neural control of swallowing and feeding in preterm infants. *Frontiers in Pediatrics*, *9*, 627985.

Philbin, M. K., & Ross, E. S. (2011). The influence of environmental factors on feeding and sleeping behaviors of preterm infants. *Newborn and Infant Nursing Reviews; NAINR*, *11*(4), 228–233.

Shaker, C. S. (2020). Cue-based feeding in the NICU: A neurodevelopmental framework for supporting infants. *Neonatal Network*, *39*(2), 77–83.

Silverman, A. H., & Arvedson, J. C. (2022). Developmental feeding and swallowing disorders: A multidisciplinary perspective. *Seminars in Speech and Language*, *43*(1), 1–15.

Zimmerman, E., & Barlow, S. M. (2012). The effects of environmental noise on the development of suck–swallow–breathe coordination in preterm infants. *Journal of Speech, Language, and Hearing Research: JSLHR*, *55*(2), 519–531.

KEY TERMS AND DEFINITIONS

The following key terms summarize essential concepts discussed throughout this chapter and are defined in the author's own words to support clarity and reader comprehension.

Aspiration: The entry of material such as milk or liquid into the airway below the level of the vocal folds, often caused by delayed swallow initiation or poor airway protection mechanisms in neonates.

Central Pattern Generator (CPG): A neural network located in the brainstem that coordinates the rhythmic sequence of sucking, swallowing, and breathing required for safe feeding.

Compensatory Feeding Strategies: Adaptive clinical techniques—such as pacing, positioning, and flow control—used to maintain safe and efficient feeding when swallowing deficits are present.

Cue-Based Feeding: A responsive feeding approach guided by the infant's physiologic and behavioral signals, emphasizing co-regulation, self-pacing, and individualized readiness rather than rigid schedules.

Dysphagia: A disorder characterized by difficulty or inefficiency in swallowing, which may involve the oral, pharyngeal, or esophageal stages and can lead to feeding challenges and aspiration risk.

Fiberoptic Endoscopic Evaluation of Swallowing (FEES): An instrumental method that uses a flexible endoscope to visualize swallowing function and detect penetration or aspiration events during feeding.

Neonatal Intensive Care Unit (NICU): A specialized hospital unit providing intensive medical and developmental care to premature and medically fragile newborns, including feeding and swallowing management.

Non-Nutritive Sucking (NNS): Repetitive sucking movements performed without fluid intake, such as on a pacifier, which support the development of oral-motor coordination and readiness for nutritive feeding.

Oral-Motor Stimulation: A structured therapeutic approach targeting oral structures (lips, tongue, cheeks) through tactile and sensory input to enhance coordination, strength, and feeding readiness.

Preterm Infant Oral Motor Intervention (PIOMI): A brief, structured oral stimulation program developed for preterm infants to improve oral-motor function, shorten transition to full oral feeding, and promote neurodevelopmental maturation.

Suck–Swallow–Breathe Coordination: The sequential motor pattern integrating oral, pharyngeal, and respiratory systems to ensure safe, rhythmic feeding without aspiration or fatigue.

Videofluoroscopic Swallow Study (VFSS): A radiographic imaging technique that captures dynamic swallowing movements to evaluate bolus transit, airway protection, and the timing of swallowing events.

Chapter 3
Development and Disorders of Infant Sucking:
Clinical Perspectives and Intervention Strategies

Göksu Tarakçı
http://orcid.org/0000-0001-6123-8395
Üsküdar University, Turkey

Ceren Söğüt
http://orcid.org/0000-0003-0610-2764
Üsküdar University, Turkey

Özlem Oğuz
http://orcid.org/0000-0001-7590-0028
Üsküdar University, Turkey

Büşra Çınar
http://orcid.org/0000-0002-9844-4659
Üsküdar University, Turkey

Ayşe Buse Saraç
http://orcid.org/0000-0003-0170-8775
Üsküdar University, Turkey

Ahmet Konrot
Üsküdar University, Turkey

ABSTRACT

Infant sucking is one of the earliest organized motor behaviors essential for safe oral feeding, growth, and survival. Beyond a simple nutritive action, it emerges from the integration of brainstem pattern generators, cranial nerves, respiratory–cardiovascular functions, craniofacial structures, and the infant's sensory and relational environment. Prematurity, neurological injury, craniofacial anomalies, medical comorbidities, genetic syndromes, or adverse environmental conditions can disrupt this sequence, leading to aspiration risk, feeding refusal, prolonged hospitalization, and developmental concerns. Advances in neurophysiology, clinical scales, and pressure-based measurement systems have positioned non-nutritive sucking as an

DOI: 10.4018/979-8-3373-6405-6.ch003

early biomarker of nervous system integrity. This chapter summarizes typical sucking and feeding development, multifactorial determinants of sucking disorders, and evidence-based assessment and early intervention approaches.

The American Academy of Pediatrics has recognized the *"ability of the newborn to feed orally independently"* as one of the criteria necessary for discharge from the hospital (Committee on Fetus and Newborn, 2008). Therefore, the transition of infants to independent oral feeding and sucking ability is an important factor affecting hospital stay duration (Lau, 2016).

The early diagnosis and treatment of health problems in newborns related to sucking skills is an important issue not only in terms of the money spent on health services, but also for mother-infant interaction and the physiological and neurological development of the infant. In this context, a widely used scale that shows the condition of the newborn immediately after birth is *the APGAR score* which is developed by Dr. Virginia Apgar (1953). The parameters evaluated consist of five components: *skin color, heart rate, respiratory rate, reflexes and responsiveness*, and *muscle tone* in order to obtain APGAR score (Apgar, 1953). Each of these components is scored between zero and two and the total score obtained indicates the newborn's condition immediately after birth. An Apgar score between 8 and 10 indicates that *normal care is sufficient for the newborn.* A score between 4 and 7 indicates that *the newborn needs oxygen* and a total score below 4 indicates *severe oxygen deficiency and the need for resuscitation* (Letko, 1996). In addition, screening tests developed to enable the early diagnosis of certain diseases during the newborn period are also available through the national newborn screening program. Some of these tests are *"Congenital Hypothyroidism Screening", "Phenylketonuria", "Biotinidase Deficiency, "Cystic Fibrosis Screening, "Hearing Screening", "Congenital Heart Disease Screening, "Developmental Hip Dysplasia Screening"* and *"Red Reflex Test-Vision Screening"* (Erçin and Ovalı, 2019). However, since there is no such service as newborn sucking screening and the APGAR method cannot directly measure a newborn's sucking ability, failing to consider sucking ability when evaluating a newborn's condition may result in an incomplete assessment of the newborn's general health. Additionally, newborns who struggle with feeding are more likely to be readmitted for feeding-related problems including failure to thrive, which raises the expense of medical treatment (Underwood et al., 2007). Therefore, oral feeding is not only a fundamental requirement for most infants before discharge from the neonatal intensive care unit, but the underdevelopment of these skills may influence future growth and developmental stages of the infant (Azuma and Maron, 2020). Considering all these factors together, this section will address the importance, development, assessment and strategies related to infant sucking ability.

ORAL FEEDING IN INFANTS

Oral feeding for newborns is a complex neurodevelopmental process andalso a skill that requires integration of the senses and the coordination of motor movements (sucking, swallowing, breathing) (Azuma and Maron, 2020).

Due to the rhythmic nature of the sucking-swallowing-breathing process, these motor functions are controlled by Central Pattern Generators (CPGs) (Shandley et al., 2021; Matsuo et al., 2008; Barlow, 2009; Maynard et al., 2020). It has been demonstrated that the interneurons of CPGs are located in the brainstem, particularly in the upper medulla and pons regions and can generate a basic swallowing pattern without any other input (Mistry et al., 2008; Barlow, 2009). One level of regulation of CPGs is situated in subcortical structures, such as the basal ganglia, hypothalamus, cerebellum, amygdala, and midbrain tegmentum, whereas another level of control operates in the suprabulbar cortical swallowing area. (Mistry et al., 2008). Researchers indicate that the integration of these control levels in the brain is necessary to coordinate the (i) oral, (ii) pharyngeal and (iii) esophageal phases of feeding (Mistry et al., 2008; Matsuo et al., 2008; Barlow, 2009; Maynard et al., 2020).

Development of Normal Sucking Behavior

Premature infants are defined as babies born before the 37th week of gestation. Delivery occurring before 32–34 weeks is associated with infants whose physiological and neurological development is not yet complete(Tenhaaf, 2008; Akbarzadeh et al., 2020). Consequently, premature infants typically have long-term health complications including negative hearing and vision problems, high risk of infection, low immunity and digestive problems (Akbarzadeh et al., 2020). Furthermore, they cannot fully coordinate the necessary activities of sucking, swallowing and breathing when it comes to feeding (Boiron et al., 2007). Until sucking, swallowing and breathing coordination is fully developed, the *gavage method* is used to feed these infants; however, prolonged feeding by gavage may lead to digestive problems and jeopardize the calorie intake necessary for growth (Hwang et al., 2010; Fucile et al., 2002). Therefore, oral feeding difficulties are considered one of the most important problems in premature infants (Hwang et al., 2010; Fucile et al., 2002).

Oral feeding skills in infants develop step by step from birth. *In the newborn period*, the infant is fed with the breast or bottle and parental interaction plays an important role in this process. *From the sixth month onwards*, the infant transitions to being fed with a smooth spoon and sucking-swallowing coordination gradually increases. *Around the ninth month*, behaviors such as drinking from a cup and chewing mashed foods are observed. *After the 12th month*, the child begins to hold the spoon themselves, drink from a cup with both hands and take sips in succession. *From the 18th month onwards*, swallowing with lip closure and the ability to chew foods of different textures develop. *Between the ages of 2 and 3*, mature movements such as jaw rotation, chewing with lip closure and drinking from a cup without spilling are observed. This is the period whenhe child achieves complete independence in feeding (Arvedson & Brodsky, 2002).

Sucking and swallowing skills develop in utero because they play a role in regulating fetal amniotic fluid levels (Poore and Barlow, 2009; Mistry et al., 2008). These skills alsoneed to be further developed in the ex utero period to incorporate breathing after birth (Shandley et al., 2021). It is stated that the development of sucking, swallowing and breathing skills is more related to postmenstrual age (PMA) than to postnatal age (Gewolb et al., 2001). In this context, it is stated that 28 weeks PMA is sufficient for sucking and swallowing to begin oral feeding, but that infants can usually coordinate sucking with breathing by 32-34 weeks PMA (Cunha et al., 2009; Bertoncelli et al., 2012). Therefore, newborn infants need to develop both physiologically (gestational age and PMA) and experientially in order to achieve a safe and coordinated suck-swallow-breathe rhythm in all three phases: oral, pharyngeal and esophageal. (Cunha et al., 2009; Bertoncelli et al., 2012; Shandley et al., 2021). Regarding this, sucking ability in infants is divided into two categories: *nutritive sucking (NS)* and *non-nutritive sucking (NNS)* (da Costa et al., 2008). Feeding sucking is the newborn's primary means of obtaining nutrition while non-feeding sucking is considered to have a calming effect on the newborn and to serve as an initial method for exploring the environment(Palmer et al., 1993; Lau and Kusnierczyk, 2001). Nutritive and non-nutritive sucking differ not only in purpose but also in pattern. As stated by Wolff (1968),nutritive sucking occurs at 1 cycle/second while non-nutritive sucking occurs at 2 cycles/second. Both nutritive and non-nutritive sucking provide information about a newborn's oral-motor skills and both sucking patterns are reported to consist of rhythmic, sequential movements of suction and expression (da Costa et al., 2008). Specifically, expression is characterized by the tongue pressing against the hard palate to expel fluid from the breast. Sucking, on the other hand, is characterized by intraoral negative pressure that draws fluid into the mouth (Shandley et al., 2021). Sucking also requires lowering the jaw to increase the volume of the mouth, closing the nasal passage with the soft palate and tightly closing the lips to prevent air from entering (Shandley et al., 2021).

Research indicates that preterm infants have lower sucking frequency, volume and negative oral pressure during nutritive sucking compared to their term counterparts (Zimmerman and Barlow, 2008). Furthermore, similar to feeding suckling, non-feeding suckling is also present around 28 weeks PMA and it is stated that as the preterm infant matures, the frequency, duration, periodicity and negative pressure amplitude observed in suckling bursts increase (Pineda et al., 2019; Hafstrom et al., 2000).

Martens et al. (2024) examined the relationship between NNS behaviors observed in infancy and neurodevelopmental processes in later years. According to the research results, infants who exhibited a more mature and rhythmic NNS pattern at three months of age achieved higher cognitive and overall development scores at 12 months. These findings suggest that early sucking behaviors may be an indicator of neuromotor maturity and could be used for the early detection of developmental risks. Therefore, NNS reflects neurodevelopmental maturity and may serve as a simple, noninvasive predictor of infants' neuromotor development. Taken together, these findings suggest that the biorhythms of sucking and swallowing follow a predictable maturation pattern, and that disruptions to this process may represent important diagnostic clues.

Regarding sucking development, Lau and Kusnierczyk (2001) divided the typical maturation process of feeding and non-feeding sucking into five main stages based on the presence or absence of sucking and expression patterns (Table 1). Lau and Kusnierczyk (2001) used this scale to demonstrate the relationship between sucking development and oral feeding skills in premature infants.

Table 1. Five-stage descriptive scale of sucking and expression component development (Lau and Kusnierczyk, 2001).

Stage	Sucking and Expression Characteristics	Description / Clinical Explanation	Biorythm Pattern
1A	No sucking, only arrhythmic expression movements	Sucking is not observed; irregular muscle contractions are seen.	Irregular and low-amplitude waves on the time axis
1B	Irregular changes in sucking and expression	Sucking attempts begin but there is no pattern; aspiration risk is present.	Signals starting at short intervals with irregular amplitude
2A	No sucking, rhythmic expression	Expressive movements become regular, but sucking is still absent.	Rhythmic, repetitive low-amplitude waves
2B	Aritmic changes in sucking and expression; sucking bursts begin	First sucking bursts are observed; synchronization of sucking and expression begins to develop.	Interwave order is partially established, short sucking clusters
3A	No sucking, rhythmic expression	Sucking is weak but regular; rhythmic expression is dominant.	Rhythmic small-amplitude waves
3B	Rhythmic suction and expression; amplitude increases, wide intervals and prolonged bursts	Coordination becomes more pronounced; the power of the suction increases, and longer-lasting suction clusters are observed.	Increasingly high-amplitude, regularly repeating waves
4	Rhythmic and defined sucking-expression; decreased amplitude range	Mature sucking pattern develops; movements are more stable and controlled.	Smooth, medium-amplitude, and regularly repeating waves
5	Rhythmic and well-defined sucking-expression; increased amplitude	Mature rhythm similar to term infant sucking pattern; strong, consistent sucking and swallowing coordination.	Regular, high-amplitude, typical mature sucking traces

Neurodevelopmental Significance and Prognostic Value of Sucking Behavior

Considering the interaction between the central nervous system (CNS) and the neuromuscular system required for oral feeding, preterm infants are therefore expected to experience feeding difficulties.Indeed, feeding difficulties and potential sucking problems extend beyond preterm infants to include those with orofacial anomalies (Caron et al., 2018), respiratory insufficiency related to congenital heart disease (Indramohan et al., 2017), genetic or neurological disorders affecting muscle tone (Stanley et al., 2019; van den Engel-Hoek et al., 2015), and hyperbilirubinemia (Bromiker et al., 2016).

Pineada et al. (2019) found that premature infants with more variability and less stability in their NNS sucking patterns had more medical complications., Notably, these findings are consistent with other studies showing variable NNS patterns in infants with comorbidities such as respiratory distress syndrome (Poore et al., 2008) and preterm birth (da Costa et al., 2010). Additionally, infants of mothers with gestational diabetes represent another population at risk for impaired oral feeding. Researchers observed that infants born to mothers receiving insulin therapy exhibited fewer suckling bursts, reflecting an immature sucking pattern, along with a reduced number of sucks within each sucking burst. Researchers believe this situation stems from neuroimmaturity in babies born to diabetic mothers (Bromiker et al., 2006).

Zimmerman et al. (2023), who examined the effect of environmental exposures in utero on sucking patterns, investigated the relationship between *prenatal maternal stress (PREMS)* and NNS in newborn infants and observed that higher PREMS differentiated infant NNS patterns. The researchers suggest that this differentiation in NNS patterns may serve as an early indicator of subsequent neurobiological problems. In parallel, Zimmerman et al. (2021) observed that, in conjunction with environmental exposure to phthalates in utero, introoral negative pressure waves in newborn NNS had a lower frequency and higher amplitude compared to the control group. Indeed, studies linking phthalate exposure during pregnancy to lower scores in language development in male children also exist (Olesen et al. 2018; Bornehag et al. 2018). Additionally, it has been suggested that increased oxidative stress levels during pregnancy (Ferguson et al., 2014) may also affect fetal neurodevelopment. In this context, defining NNS as a sensitive indicator of neurotoxicity is thought to provide a tool for the early detection of exposure-related changes in neurodevelopment (Zimmerman et al., 2021; 2023).

Moreover, Medoff-Cooper (2005) conducted a study on 19 very low birth weight infants to determine predictive factors for development in the neonatal period. The average pressure generated by sucking and the duration of sucking bursts were found to show a positive correlation with the scores of the Psychomotor Scale administered at 6 months of age.

Numerous studies have investigated the association between sucking patterns and developmental stages in children. Palmer and Heyman (1999) reassessed 18 children, whom they had evaluated shortly after birth (using *Neonatal Oral-Motor Assessment Scale [NOMAS]* and the *Bayley Scales* of Infant Development), at 24 to 36 months of age and found that all seven children who had an ineffective sucking pattern in infancy showed developmental delay, two children with a normal sucking pattern showed normal development and four of the nine children with an irregular sucking pattern did not show normal development. Mizuno and Ueda (2003) also examined the relationship between the feeding behavior (measured with a pressure transducer device) of 65 newborns (average 37.8 weeks) and their neurological development at 18 months (measured using the Bayley-II Scale). The researchers found a positive correlation between sucking and expression patterns and Bayley-II scores.

However, although standardized tests are useful for assessing newborns developmentally, they can be influenced by many factors such as the practitioner's experience, training and other individual variables. Therefore, there is a urgent need to develop quantitative, early-stage physiological-based measurements related to subsequent development and non-nutritive sucking (NNS) may serve as an early measure of newborn brain function (Slattery et al., 2012).

One of the requirements for safe oral feeding is adequate oxygenation. The respiratory rate of preterm infants averages 1-1.5 breaths/second. However, given that a swallowing event can last between 0.35 and 0.7 seconds (Koenig et al., 1990) and that the expiratory phase lengthens while the inspiratory phase shortens during oral feeding, some infants may not have sufficient time to breathe adequately between successive swallows, potentially compromising the balance between oxygenation and ventilation (Mathew et al., 1985; Miller & Difiore, 1995). Consequently, some preterm infants may have difficulty tolerating prolonged oral feeding, and in some cases, oxygen desaturation may occur.

Gewolb et al. (2001) investigated sucking and swallowing development in premature infants with severe bronchopulmonary dysplasia and observed that sucking and swallowing developed up to 35 weeks (PMA) as in healthy premature infants. However, it was later observed that these infants struggled to coordinate breathing and sucking. The researchers stated that this was due to difficulties in coordinating breathing with sucking and swallowing (Gewolb et al., 2001). Therefore, it is thought that coordination of breathing, swallowing and sucking rhythms may be a predictor of feeding, respiratory and/or neurodevelopmental abnormalities (da Costa et al., 2008).

In light of all this evidence, understanding NNS pattern which varies according to the environmental exposures, may help to predict potential developmental differences early after birth and guide intervention process in early infancy and childhood. In other words, the ability to assess the NNS pattern in newborns using objective tools may expand the curreny limited the scope of the objective neurofunctional assessments in this population.

Tools for Assessing Infant Readiness for Oral Feeding

Neonate may be at risk of aspiration and hypoxia if they are fed before developing the necessary coordination between sucking, swallowing and breathing required for safe swallowing (Delaney et al., 2008). To address this issue, different feeding assessment tools have been developed to identify and evaluate babies who are ready for oral feeding. These assessments involve *behavioral observations* by caregivers of sucking, swallowing and breathing coordination for oral feeding skills during the five minutes following feeding (da Costa et al., 2008). Several tools are commonly used for this purpose, including the *"Evidence-Based Guide for Initiating Oral Feeding in Healthy Preterm Infants (McCain, 2003)"*, the "*Early Feeding Skills Assessment (EFS)* for Preterm Infants (Thoyre et al., 2005)" and the *"Preterm Oral Feeding Readiness Assessment Scale (POFRAS) (Fujinaga et al., 2013)"*.

Subjective and Objective Tools for Assessing Feeding and Non-Feeding Sucking Skills

Standardized assessments are available to evaluate nutritive sucking or oral feeding. The most commonly used standardized tool for this purpose is the *"Neonatal Oral-Motor Assessment Scale (NOMAS)"* (Palmer et al., 1993). NOMAS is a non-invasive tool used for breastfeeding and bottle feeding. The tool includes *checklists* for feeding behavior and allows for the analysis of sucking patterns by evaluating the oral-motor components of the tongue and jaw during newborn sucking. Additionally, it identifies the *type of sucking pattern* used by the infant and defines two abnormal patterns have been defined: *"irregular sucking pattern"* and *"dysfunctional sucking pattern"*.

An *irregular sucking pattern* means a lack of rhythm in total sucking activity. It means that the infant cannot coordinate sucking and swallowing with breathing. In this context, when a newborn's sucking pattern is irregular, the newborn may not feed well and have difficulty breathing with color changes and/or episodes of apnea and bradycardia (Palmer et al., 1993).

A *dysfunctional sucking pattern* is characterized by abnormalities in orofacial tone. In cases of orofacial hypertonia, there may be a restriction in the range of motion of the temporomandibular joint, which can lead to minimal jaw movement and/or tongue retraction. In cases of orofacial hypotonia, a drooping tongue and/or excessive jaw movements are present during sucking. ;It is suggested that infants with dysfunctional sucking patterns are likely to benefit from therapeutic interventions targeting compensatory strategies during oral feeding (Palmer et al., 1993). Although a dysfunctional pattern is thought to be a sign of neurological disorder (Palmer and Heyman, 1999), there are also a study that do not support this evidence (Zhang et al., 2017). However, one significant limitation of the NOMAS assessment is that the scores and evaluation may be influenced by the evaluator's training, experience and individual characteristics. This is because the NOMAS assessment relies solely on observation without an objective evaluation (Shandley et al., 2021).

There is no standard method for assessing NNS. A common approach used to assess NNS is to place the person's little finger halfway into the infant's mouth with an expected non-nutritive sucking rate of approximately two sucks per second (da Costa et al., 2008). However, it should be noted that an infant exhibiting a normal NNS pattern may not yet be ready for oral feeding because, unlike *NNS*, nutritive sucking (NS) involves a sucking-swallowing pattern that also includes breathing and the coordination between these three patterns is a prerequisite for oral feeding. Related current research focuses on electronic systems based on intraoral pressure changes during sucking (NS or NNS), which allow for both NS and NNS assessment and are intended to be used as an objective measurement tool.

Numerous studies have investigated NNS patterns using objective measurement tools. Kron et al. (1963) were the first researchers to record negative intraoral pressure values during active sucking using a pressure transducer *(KRON apparatus)* and define certain parameters based on the waveform obtained (defined parameters: *number of sucks per minute, volume consumed per minute, and average pressure change per minute*). Based on the parameters examined, the researchers concluded that full-term infants change their sucking rates on the second and third days of life to increase the amount of fluid consumed (Kron et al., 1963).

Medoff-Cooper et al. (2002) observed the feeding sucking behavior of a total of 213 infants divided into three different age groups (*24-29 weeks*, *30-32 weeks* and *38-42 weeks*) during a 5-minute sucking session using the KRON apparatus. As a result, they obtained parameters showing differences between the three groups in terms of sucking bursts, time between bursts, number of sucks per burst and average maximum pressure. The researchers attributed the differences in NNS patterns to maturity at birth.

Medoff-Cooper et al. (2009) examined the correlation between a 5-minute non-nutritive sucking assessment using a modified version of the KRON apparatus and scores obtained from the Bayley Developmental Scale. The researchers' findings are consistent with the suggestion that regulating sucking behavior in the neonatal period may be an early risk indicator for neurodevelopmental delays in preterm infants (Mizuno and Ueda, 2001). Based on manual review of sucking pressure recordings, Mizuno and Ueda (2001) confirmed that sucking performance at 40 weeks PMA was a significant and independent predictor of developmental status as assessed by the Bayley scale at 1 year. In this context, the researchers stated that a tool developed for neonatal sucking assessment could offer a cost-effective early screening strategy for preterm infants at highest risk for developmental delay (Mizuno and Ueda, 2001). Ongoing modifications to the KRON apparatus have been published under the name of the feeding sucking apparatus (M-CNSA) (Medoff-Cooper et al., 2015). The final form of the apparatus is marketed under the device name *"NeoSUCK-NTraniner"*.

To better understand the relationship between sucking, swallowing and breathing, Mizuno and Ueda (2003) modified newborn bottle nipples which are routinely used to measure negative intraoral pressure. Similar to their findings, Bromiker et al. (2005) found that sucking pressure, frequency and duration matured with age in healthy preterm infants. They also reported that breathing and swallowing coordination matured with age (Mizuno and Ueda, 2003).

Fucile et al. (2009) observed sucking and expression performance in *vacuum-free bottle systems* compared to commercial standard bottles. Sucking and expression components were monitored using two pressure transducers. For sucking, one transducer was passed through a polyethylene tube aligned with the nipple tip without entering the infant's mouth. Expression was monitored via a second transducer attached to a catheter made of soft plastic tubing with the compressible plastic section extending beyond the nipple tip. To ensure accurate recording of the expression component, the catheter was positioned upward against the hard palate. The study results showed that vacuum-free bottle use improved oral feeding performance compared to standard bottle use in infants born between 26 and 29 weeks of gestation, characterized by greater total intake, milk transfer rate, and shorter feeding time.

Lang et al. (2011) developed *a system (the Orometer). to monitor intraoral pressure* during feeding. The sucking ability of all infants was assessed using the same type of bottle and nipple (Orometer) and recordings were continued for up to 15 minutes or as long as the infant continued feeding. However, analyses were limited to the first 8 minutes of feeding. A sucking burst was defined as a group of suckling events separated from adjacent groups by intervals longer than three seconds. Interburst intervals were defined as time periods exceeding four seconds, measured from the peak of the final suck in one burst to the peak of the first suck in the subsequent burst. The parameters examined in this context are: the number of suction bursts in the analyzed time interval, the number of suction peaks, the number of suctions per minute, the average number of suction peaks, the average ratio of the number of suction bursts to the number of suction peaks, the average suction burst duration, the average pause duration, the average amplitude variability (standard deviation of successive suction amplitudes within a burst), the average variability of pause durations (standard deviation of pause durations between bursts) and the coefficient of variation of sucking amplitudes (standard deviation divided by the mean). The 8-minute analysis interval in the study was divided into 2-minute segments and pairwise comparisons of the parameters at time points were performed. Most of these comparisons showed statistically significant changes in the basic parameters of infant feeding. In this context, the number of sucks per time sub-interval decreased from an average of 118 sucks in the first 2 minutes to an average of 58 sucks in the last 2 minutes and the amplitude related to the average suck pressure decreased by 7% after the first 2 minutes and by 14% after 6 minutes. The researchers interpreted this as possibly indicating increased satiety or fatigue over time. However, they observed that the suckling frequency (suckles per second) did not show any significant change during a feeding. Finally, they observed that the coefficient of variation of sucking amplitudes increased after the first 2 minutes and predicted that this could be a useful parameter for characterizing irregular sucking patterns during feeding (Lang et al., 2011).

To measure both sucking and expression, Tamilia et al. (2016) also developed *a portable sucking monitoring device (SuMOD)* designed to be easily integrated into any standard bottle and an analytical automated system for data analysis.Capilouto et al. (2014) produced a pacifier containing strategically placed piezoelectric crystals to enable direct measurement of nipple kinematics during non-nutritive and nutritive sucking. However, the researchers stated that this system was impractical for the evaluation process and developed the system further, creating a system called *Infant ® Feeding Solution* (nFS; NFANT Labs, Marietta GA, USA). This system is FDA-approved for use in evaluating infants' sucking performance in neonatal intensive care units and has research demonstrating its validity (Capilouto et al., 2019a; 2019b).

Ebrahimi et al. (2019) developed *a portable pacifier* to evaluate non-nutritive sucking in infants. A commercial sensor was used to measure the negative pressure of sucking. The parameters examined in the study were the ratio of suckling peaks per minute (suckling frequency), number of suckles per minute, number of suckling bursts per minute and average duration of bursts, number of pauses per minute and average duration of pauses and peak amplitude during suckling (mbar) (Ebrahimi et al., 2019). It was observed that as gestational age increased, the average sucking burst duration, number of sucks per minute, average suck peak amplitude and average suck frequency increased while the average suck duration and average pause duration decreased with GA. Therefore, researchers state that non-nutritive sucking ability develops as the infant matures (Ebrahimi et al., 2019).

Akbarzadeh et al. (2020) used a system *(SUMOD)* that could record both feeding and non-feeding sucking patterns. The researchers were able to record expression pressure (positive pressure created by the palate and tongue compressing the closed-tip rubber catheter) and intraoral (negative) pressure occurring during sucking using the system they developed. Two different pressure sensors were used to record both patterns. All data were recorded for 2 minutes and analyses were performed based on this time period. The parameters analyzed were: sucking frequency per minute, average sucking duration (calculated by summing all intervals during which sucking occurred) and the average of pressure amplitudes during sucking. Researchers examined the relationship between infants' *APGAR* scores and sucking patterns and found that those with lower APGAR scores had lower pressure amplitudes during sucking (Akbarzadeh et al., 2020).

Cunha et al. (2019) recorded and analyzed a 1-minute sucking pattern for NS and a 10-minute sucking pattern for NNS using a pressure sensor. The parameters examined for feeding and non-feeding suckles were; the number of suckling bursts observed during the analysis periods, the number of sucking bursts per minute, the average duration of suckling bursts, the number of pauses, the average duration of pauses, the average sucking frequency and the average suckling pressure (mmHg). Differences were observed between the sucking patterns of preterm and term infants. Term infants showed longer non-nutritive sucking durations with more sucking per burst, lower sucking pressure amplitude and significantly lower frequency for non-nutritive sucking. For nutritive sucking, when considering the fixed amount of milk (1 ml) delivered per minute, preterm infants exhibited significantly shorter burst durations and greater sucking pressure with fewer sucks per burst (Cunha et al., 2019). Indeed, these findings are consistent with the developmental process of NNS and NS models reported by Lau et al. (2012).

Zimmerman et al. (2021) investigated whether exposure to phthalate metabolites during pregnancy affects non-nutritive sucking parameters. The researchers recorded non-nutritive sucking using a pacifier equipped with a pressure sensor and stored the data in a data acquisition system (Power Lab, ADInstruments, Dunedin, New Zealand). They then analyzed the data using LabChart software (ADInstruments) on a laptop-connected system. The recording period lasted for 5 minutes but the researchers selected the most active 2 minutes for analysis. The researchers manually selected NNS bursts using the following criteria. The selection criteria were: sucking bursts must contain two or more sucking cycles; the amplitude of each sucking cycle must be above 1 cmH_2O; if there is an interval of >1,000 ms between sucking cycles, this is considered a new sucking burst. These criteria are similar to those used in previous studies examining NNS in infants (Barlow et al., 2012; Estep et al., 2008; Poore et al., 2008a; Poore et al., 2008b). Exposure to phthalate metabolites during pregnancy was observed to reduce the infant's non-nutritive sucking frequency and cause higher pressure amplitude. Relatedly, studies have linked phthalate exposure during pregnancy to lower scores in language development in male children (Olesen et al. 2018; *Bornehag et al. 2018*). In this context, researchers have concluded that knowledge of the NNS model, which varies in relation to environmental exposures, may help guide treatment in early infancy and childhood to reduce subsequent developmental delays.

Zimmerman et al. (2023) also used a methodology similar to the above study to examine the relationship between *prenatal maternal stress (PREMS)* and non-nutritive sucking (NNS) and concluded that higher PREMS values were associated with fewer but longer NNS bursts per minute.

Martens et al. (2020) observed non-nutritive sucking patterns longitudinally between three and 12 months. The system and variables used for measurement were the same as in previous studies (Zimmerman et al., 2021; 2023). The best two minutes of suckling from each five-minute recording were selected and analyzed. The researchers concluded that full-term infants exhibited significant changes in NNS duration, amplitude and number of suckling bursts between 3 and 12 months, though NNS frequency remained unchanged. The researchers emphasized the need to define how sucking characteristics change in different infant populations, such as preterm infants and infants with Down syndrome, in addition to healthy full-term infants.

In another longitudinal study, Pineda et al. (2019) evaluated the NNS of 50 preterm infants born at 32 weeks of gestation weekly from 32 weeks onwards using the *NTrainer System*. They examined the following parameters: NNS bursts per minute, NNS sucks per minute, NNS per burst and NNS peak pressure. According to the results of the study, as postmenstrual age progressed, there was an increase in NNS bursts per minute, the number of NNS within a burst, and intraoral pressure values. Additionally, the level of development was found to be related to NNS measurements. The researchers predicted that variability in NNS scores could reflect maturity.

Lee et al. (2023) developed a *flexible pressure sensor based on silver nanowires (AgNWs)* coated with polydimethylsiloxane (PDMS) for NNS assessment and integrated it with a pacifier. The study included 31 preterm infants aged 25-36 weeks and the researchers compared each infant's sucking pressure and NOMAS scores. The findings showed that the average sucking pressure was significantly higher in infants who could achieve full oral feeding. The researchers predicted that the developed sensor could objectively reflect readiness for oral feeding in infants.

Lobos et al. (2025) developed a *low-cost, portable, sterilizable device* for clinical use. This dual-sensor system can measure NNS behavior independently and simultaneously during suction and expression phases. Data were collected via an ATmega328P microcontroller and wirelessly transmitted to a computer via Bluetooth. The measurements clearly distinguished the pressure changes in both phases. Pressure values ranging from -20 to -120 mmHg were obtained during the suction phase and from 80 to 280 mmHg during the expression phase. Consequently, the researchers concluded that their device could provide a cost-effective means of reliably measuring NNS skills.

Advances in sensor technology have enabled systems originally designed to assess sucking in newborns to be applied to the evaluation of swallowing function in adults, through accurate measurement of negative intraoral pressure (Grassi et al., 2016). In related studies, assessments of the oral phase of swallowing have been made by measuring the intraoral pressure generated during the intake of active or passive boluses of different consistencies. These systems, which are generally commercial pressure sensors and are connected to a computer-operated manometer, are useful for evaluating the oral phase of swallowing, particularly in cases of neurological or structural abnormalities in the mouth and face region (Adamske et al., 2021; Fuentes et al., 2015; Engelke et al., 2014; Engelke et al., 2011; Santander et al., 2013; Knösel et al., 2016).

In conclusion, various tools are available for the objective assessment of sucking ability (NS and NNS) in newborns, which are both scientifically proven and commercially available. These tools are primarily based on pressure or bending sensors and are systems that measure intraoral pressure changes or the bending measurements created by tongue movements on the sensor. This section compiles the methods and scientific outputs of current assessment tools and presents them to the reader. In conclusion, objective sucking assessment tools available for both commercial and scientific use and the technological systems they employ have been compiled based on accessible sources, and answers to the question *"why is newborn sucking assessment important"* have been attempted.

FACTORS INFLUENCING THE DEVELOPMENT OF SUCKING

Sucking is not merely a motor skill that provides nourishment in the first months of life; it is also one of the fundamental building blocks of oral-motor development, sensory integration, respiratory regulation, and parent-infant interaction. The healthy functioning of this skill depends on the safe and rhythmic maintenance of the sucking-swallowing-breathing cycle, that is, the *simultaneous and coordinated functioning of the central and peripheral nervous systems, craniofacial structures, cardiopulmonary and gastrointestinal functions and environmental-psychosocial factors* (Goday et al., 2019). Therefore, it is often impossible to attribute a sucking disorder to a single cause. Biological, structural and environmental factors usually play a role together and the interaction of these factors determines how and how severely the disorder manifests itself. This section addresses the main factors affecting sucking developmentin terms of neurological, structural, medical, genetic-syndromic and environmental-psychosocial dimensions.

Neurological Causes

The ability to suck rhythmically and in a controlled manner depends on the integrated functioning of the sucking-swallowing centers in the brainstem, the cranial nerves and the central pattern generators. Developmental immaturity, structural damage or functional disorders in these neurological networks can lead to irregular sucking patterns, insufficient intraoral pressure and impaired integration between breathing and swallowing. In preterm infants, due to delayed neurological and physiological maturation, both non-nutritive and nutritive sucking are reported to be short, irregular and of low efficiency; coordination between sucking, swallowing, and breathing is particularly impaired (Dewi et al., 2024). Neonatal brain damage also negatively affects oral-motor functions in the early period.ıt is stated that sucking and swallowing difficulties are common in these infants and that early feeding problems may be an important clinical sign in terms of neurodevelopmental outcomes (Slattery et al., 2012). In neuromuscular diseases, hypotonia, muscle weakness and inadequate motor unit activation make it difficult to close the lips and create negative intraoral pressure; bulbar muscle involvement weakens the swallowing trigger and increases the risk of aspiration. Weakness of the respiratory muscles also disrupts the safe coordination of the sucking-swallowing-breathing sequence, reducing the efficiency of oral feeding (van den Engel-Hoek et al., 2015).

Structural Reasons

Sucking is a fundamental oromotor process based on the anatomical integrity of oral and craniofacial structures and the coordinated movement of muscles. Coordination between the tongue, lips, palate, cheeks and mandible creates intraoral negative pressure.Therefore, congenital anomalies in these structures can directly disrupt the integrity of the sucking-swallowing-breathing sequence (Arvedson, 2008). Among structural causes, the most common condition is cleft lip and/or palate (CLP). An opening in the palate creates an open passage between the oral and nasal cavities, leading to loss of negative pressure, nasal regurgitation and inadequate direction of food within the mouth (Green & Resnick, 2021). Therefore, short and rapid sucking bursts, a high sucking-swallowing ratio, increased air swallowing and rapid fatigue during feeding are common in infants with CLP. As the cleft widens, oral intake may decrease further and weight gain may be negatively affected (Reid., 2004).

Pierre Robin Sequence (PRS) is characterized by a triad of micrognathia, glossoptosis and often accompanying cleft palate. The small size of the lower jaw and the backward displacement of the tongue reduce the oral cavity volume making it difficult to generate negative pressure; glossoptosis significantly impairs bolus control and airway patency (Green and Resnick, 2021). As a result, apnea, oxygen desaturation, aspiration risk and inadequate oral intake are common in infants with PRS.

In addition to CLP and PRS, other craniofacial anomalies such as *Treacher Collins syndrome, hemifacial microsomia, Crouzon and Apert syndromes, Moebius syndrome* and *22q11.2 deletion* can also affect sucking function. Mandibular or maxillary hypoplasia, midface retrusion, perioral muscle weakness and cranial nerve involvement seen in these syndromes reduce feeding efficiency by weakening the mechanisms of grasping, sealing and creating intraoral pressure (Miller & Madhoun, 2016; Cooper-Brown et al., 2008).

Medical Causes

The respiratory, muscular and gastrointestinal systems must work together for sucking behavior to be maintained in a healthy manner in newborns,. Dysfunction in any of these systems disrupts the coordination of the sucking-swallowing-breathing sequence which can lead to feeding problems. Premature infants often experience respiratory problems such as *bronchopulmonary dysplasia (BPD)* and *chronic lung disease (CLD)* which indirectly affect sucking performance. These diseases disrupt the coordination of sucking, swallowing and breathing, thereby reducing feeding efficiency and oxygenation (Kao et al., 2010; Martin & Shaw, 1997). Similarly, *congenital heart disease (CHD)* significantly limits the coordination of sucking, swallowing and breathing by affecting parameters related to respiration and oxygenation (Norman et al., 2022). Furthermore, intestinal problems such as *gastroesophageal reflux disease (GERD)* are considered primary factors affecting sucking ability stability due to the pain, regurgitation and swallowing difficulties they can cause (Puccini & Berretin-Felix, 2015).

Genetic and Syndromic Causes

Sucking development in infants with genetic syndromes is often at risk because differences that occur simultaneously in structural, neuromotor and physiological systems affect the natural flow of the sucking process. Hypotonia, craniofacial anomalies, cardiac and gastrointestinal problems, sensory regulation difficulties, and neurological differences may coexist with these syndromes. For example, in *Down syndrome*, sucking may be weak and irregular due to hypotonia, macroglossia and sensory-motor deficiencies; feeding time is prolonged and the infant tires quickly (Cooper-Brown et al., 2008). In *Prader-Willi syndrome,* the sucking reflex is markedly weak due to severe hypotonia in the early period of life and most infants are fed with enteral support. In *CHARGE, DiGeorge, Mowat-Wilson* and other syndromes, differences in craniofacial structure, laryngeal anomalies, cardiac problems and neurodevelopmental impairments further complicate the sucking and feeding process (Cooper-Brown et al., 2008; Green & Resnick, 2021). In this context, since the profile of each syndrome is different, intervention plans for the stages of sucking and transition to full oral feeding should be tailored to the specific needs of the syndrome.

Environmental and Psychosocial Effects

Although the newborn's sucking behavior is biologically based, *parent-infant interaction* is one of the fundamental psychosocial components that determine the quality of the feeding process. The caregivers ability to recognize the infant's signals, respond to them in a timely and effective manner, adjust the feeding pace to the infant's rhythm and correctly interpret signs of satiety and fatigue are covariates that can affect the coordination of the entire suck-swallow-breathe cycle. *Conversely, anxious, overly controlling* or *inconsistent caregiving styles* can increase the infant's stress levels and lead to disruptions in sucking coordination (Brown & Arnot, 2014; Shaker, 2013). Relatedly, it has been reported that *mothers experiencing depression, anxiety* and *postpartum stress* have difficulty making eye contact, interpret infant signals later or incorrectly and perceive feeding interactions as a more mechanical task (Field, 2010).

The *physical environment* can also be a determining factor in sucking performance. In this regard, *excessively noisy* or *stimulating environments* can distract the newborn and weaken the coordination between sucking, swallowing and breathing. *Choosing an inappropriate nipple, flow rates that do not match the infant's capacity, incorrect positioning* or *feeding attempts when the infant is sleepy* can disrupt the natural development of sucking (Shaker, 2013). Furthermore, *environmental toxins such as secondhand smoke* have been shown to impair respiratory function in premature and BPD infants, negatively affecting the rhythm of the sucking-swallowing-breathing cycle (Collaco et al., 2014).

APPROACHES SUPPORTING NUTRITIVE SUCKING

NS and NNS have been described in detail in previous sections. This section will discuss strategies used to support NS. It is thought that NNS helps develop NS skills by supporting physiological development (Harding et al., 2018). Ithas been shown that very low birth weight premature infants as long as they are clinically stable, benefit from oral stimulation and NNS applications, leading to earlier initiation of oral feeding and earlier discharge from the hospital (Rocha et al., 2007; Pimenta et al., 2008; Boiron et al., 2007; Harding et al., 2014). *NNS applications are generally performed using a pacifier or thumb while oral stimulation applications are techniques involving a series of procedures performed by a clinician.* In addition to these, the literature also includes practices that involve *stimulating swallowing with milk (by dripping a few drops of milk onto the center of the tongue)* before transitioning to oral breastfeeding (Lau & Smith, 2012). The aim of these approaches is to strengthen the muscles used in NS, which is the main goal, or to support NS development through neurological stimulation. In this context, it is thought that the babies who benefit most from NNS, as an approach that appears to aid the development of oral feeding, are those without significant additional medical problems (Harding et al., 2018). According to the findings of a recent meta-analysis, the *combined use of oral stimulation and NNS* is reported to be much more effective in supporting NS than NNS alone (Tsai et al., 2023). Another important point to remember is that these types of interventions should be performed when the infant is in a calm, awake state and when cardiopulmonary parameters are optimal (i.e., without bradycardia and/or desaturation) (Boiron et al., 2007). In this context, some oral stimulation procedures defined by the have been summarized in the table below (Table 2).

Table 2. Oral Stimulation Protocols

Target	Stimulation Technique	Dosage	Therapeutic Purpose
Hwang et al., 2010			
Cheeks (Perioral)	Light touches to the cheeks with the index finger; stroking from the base of the nose towards the ear and returning to the corner of the lips	8 repetitions/cheek (two different maneuvers)	Perioral sensory stimulation
Lips (Perioral)	Gently stretching the upper and lower lips outward from the center line; circular stroking around the lips	Stretching: 8 repetitions/ lip; Circular: 4 repetitions/lip	Lip muscle activation
Gums (Intraoral)	Pressure massage from the center to the back of the upper and lower gums using a suction device	4 repetitions/side	Oral motor organization
Tongue (Intraoral)	Pressure with the pacifier towards the front and downwards; if there is tongue protrusion, only downward pressure	8 repetitions	Tongue control and NNS

continued on following page

Table 2. Continued

Target	Stimulation Technique	Dosage	Therapeutic Purpose
Hwang et al., 2010			
Pacifier	Stroking forward from the center of the hard palate, followed by suction	2 min	Non-nutritive sucking (NNS)
Harding et al., 2014			
Cheeks (Perioral)	Bilateral cheek stimulation from the perioral region	x4 repetitions - 2 min	Muscle excitability
Upper / Lower Lip	Perioral lip stimulation	x4 repetitions - 1 min (each)	Lip strength
Lip Curl	Curl movements on the upper and lower lips	x2/lip - 1 min	Lip coordination
Upper/Lower Gums	Gum stimulation	x2 - 1 min (each)	Swallowing and sucking
Internal cheek	Stimulation of the cheek mucosa from inside the mouth	x2/cheek - 2 min	Oral sensory input
Tongue (Lateral and Midline)	Stimulation of the edges and midline of the tongue	Lateral: x2; Median: x4	Swallowing and sucking
Sucking – Finger / Pacifier	Initiating sucking with finger; pacifier with NNS	Finger: 1 min; Pacifier: 3 min	Soft palate activation
Boiron et al., 2007			
Cheeks (Perioral)	Pressure stimulation from the ear to the corner of the mouth	2 min	Perioral muscle activation
Upper Lip	Pressure from the base of the nose to the upper, the midline of the lip, and the corners	1 min	Lip sensory input
Lower Lip	Pressure from the chin base toward the midline and corners of the lower lip.	1 min	Lip control
Orientation reflex	Upper lip midline, left corner of the mouth, lower lip midline, right corner of the mouth	2 min	Orientation and reflex integration
Tongue (Intraoral)	Pressure in the posterior–anterior direction	3 repetitions	Tongue movement pattern
Palate	Pressure from the hard palate to the soft palate	3 repetitions	Oral phase organization

continued on following page

Table 2. Continued

Target	Stimulation Technique	Dosage	Therapeutic Purpose
Hwang et al., 2010			
Gums	Pressure from the midline of the upper jaw toward the corners of the mouth	3 repetitions	Oral stability
Application Note	Perioral: index finger; Intraoral: little finger	All maneuvers x3	Standard application technique

In addition to these methods, it has been reported that *"oral support"* defined as supporting effective sucking during bottle feeding or breastfeeding, provides stability to the mandible and pressure under the mandible to achieve optimal sucking behavior, thereby increasing/facilitating sucking efficiency (Boiron et al., 2007). The stages of oral support defined by Boiron et al. (2007) are as follows:

- The thumb gently compresses the cheek toward the lips to minimize fluid loss.
- The bottle is held with the therapist's other hand using the thumb, index finger and middle finger.
- The little finger stabilizes the chin upward to support the oral cavity under the chin and facilitate swallowing.
- The ring finger presses the cheek toward the lips to prevent fluid loss on the opposite side of the mouth cavity.
- The sucking-swallowing cycle is interrupted at regular intervals by sliding the nipple toward the corner of the mouth after six to eight consecutive swallows to facilitate breathing.
- During feeding, the pacifier is removed from the mouth at regular intervals and two to three long breaks are taken to allow breathing to regulate.

In conclusion, oral stimulation, non-nutritive sucking and oral support approaches used during feeding to support the development of nutritive sucking contribute significantly to the maturation of the sucking-swallowing-breathing coordination. The interventions described in the literature have been shown to shorten the transition time to oral feeding and increase feeding efficiency, particularly in clinically stable preterm infants without additional medical problems. Future studies focusing on standardizing these approaches and determining their effects on long-term feeding outcomes will contribute significantly to the development of clinical guidelines.

SUMMARY

Oral feeding in infants must be efficient and safe enough to allow for the intake of calories necessary for growth (it should not cause aspiration or compromise breathing) and this can only be achieved if sucking, swallowing and breathing are properly coordinated. In this context, it is stated that a condition that could compromise normal breathing, sucking and swallowing coordination may stem from congenital or acquired damage to the central nervous system (da Costa et al., 2008). Therefore, it is thought that the sucking ability of newborns is an important biomarker for providing insight into areas that may be damaged (Reilly and Skuse, 1992). Indeed, scales developed to assess sucking ability exist, but they may lack sufficient objectivity as they depend on the assessor's training, skill and other individual characteristics. Therefore, user-friendly and cost-effective objective assessment devices are needed to evaluate sucking ability.

Newborn sucking ability requires coordinated sucking-swallowing-breathing actions and is divided into two basic types: *non-nutritive* (NNS)and *nutritive*. NNS is the newborn's sucking ability without any food intake and was first characterized by Wolff in 1968. NNS has a burst-pause pattern consisting of 6-12 sucking cycles per sucking burst and a burst-internal sucking frequency of 2 Hz. It has been suggested that NNS is a potentially predictive factor for subsequent neurodevelopment in various domains (e.g., motor skills, balance, intelligence, and language) (Wolthuis-Stigter et al., 2015; 2017).

Clinical manifestations associated with impaired sucking function vary depending on the underlying etiology but some are described below:

- Irregular sucking movements, weak lip closure, low intraoral pressure, short and frequent sucking bursts
- Coughing during feeding, choking, color changes or recurrent pneumonias indicating silent aspiration
- Deviation from the growth curve and slow weight gain due to inadequate oral intake and prolonged feeding times
- Feeding refusal due to negative feeding experiences or feeding demands that exceed the newborn's physiological capacity

These symptoms often indicate an underlying neurological, structural or medical condition and require evaluation and follow-up by a multidisciplinary team including speech-language pathologists, neonatologists, pediatric gastroenterologists, cardiologists and dietitians (Arvedson, 2008).

The most important strategy used to make NS safer or to develop this skill is *oral stimulation* and *supporting NNS skills*. It is stated that stimulating the sucking reflex of premature infants with oral stimulation and NNS is quite beneficial in terms of shortening feeding time, maturing the sucking reflex and accelerating weight gain (Bernbaum et al., 1983; Pinelli et al., 2011). In this way, the transition to oral feeding can be carried out in a controlled manner and the newborn's hospital stay can also be shortened (Noori et al., 2018). The newborn's ability to transition to full oral feeding independently is critical for the infant's discharge from the hospital. Infants with severe feeding problems often require readmission to the hospital and tube feeding (Sullivan et al., 2000). Therefore, feeding problems contribute significantly to increased healthcare costs (March of Dimes, 2008). Relatedly, delayed sucking and feeding have been reported in approximately 35-48% of infants with different types of neonatal brain damage (Slattery et al., 2012). Therefore, NNS may be a sensitive indicator of central nervous system (CNS) dysfunction in infants (Medoff-Cooper and Ray, 1995). In this context, the assessment of NNS can provide valuable information about the infant's sucking pattern, readiness for oral feeding, integrity of the CNS and anatomical and physiological integrity related to the oral phase (Lau, 2006; Barlow et al., 2006; Lau and Kusnierczyk, 2001). Therefore, an objective assessment of the newborn's suckling and non-suckling behavior may have prognostic value for the early diagnosis of possible neurological problems and/or other problems that may affect sucking ability. Consequently, considering that sucking ability is one of the discharge criteria for preterm infants, monitoring the sucking ability of both preterm and term newborns is important.

REFERENCES

Adamske, D., Heyduck, A., Weidenmüller, M., Göricke, B., Frank, T., & Olthoff, A. (2021). Dysphagia in amyotrophic lateral sclerosis: Quantification of bulbar motor dysfunction. *Journal of Oral Rehabilitation, 48*(9), 1044–1049. PMID: 34185922

Akbarzadeh, S., Farhoodi, R., Lyu, T., Awais, M., Zhao, X., Abbasi, S. F., & Chen, W. (July 2020). Evaluation of Apgar scores and non-nutritive sucking skills in infants using a novel sensitized non-nutritive sucking system. In *2020 42nd Annual International Conference of the IEEE Engineering in Medicine & Biology Society (EMBC)* (pp. 4282-4285).

Apgar, V. (1953). A proposal for a new method of evaluation of the newborn infant. *Anesthesia and Analgesia, 32*(4), 260–267. PMID: 13083014

Arvedson, J. C. (2008). Assessment of pediatric dysphagia and feeding disorders: Clinical and instrumental approaches. *Developmental Disabilities Research Reviews, 14*(2), 118–127. PMID: 18646015

Arvedson, J. C., & Brodsky, L. (2002). *Pediatric Swallowing and Feeding: Assessment and Management* (2nd ed.). Singular–Thomson Learning.

Azuma, D., & Maron, J. L. (2020). Individualizing oral feeding assessment and therapies in the newborn. *Research and Reports in Neonatology, 10*, 23.

Barlow, S. M. (2009). Central pattern generation involved in oral and respiratory control for feeding in the term infant. *Current Opinion in Otolaryngology & Head & Neck Surgery, 17*(3), 187–193. PMID: 19417662

Barlow, S. M., Burch, M., Venkatesan, L., Harold, M., & Zimmerman, E. (2012). Frequency modulation and spatiotemporal stability of the sCPG in preterm infants with RDS. *International Journal of Pediatrics, 2012*(1), 581538. PMID: 22888359

Barlow, S. M., & Estep, M. (2006). Central pattern generation and the motor infrastructure for suck, respiration, and speech. *Journal of Communication Disorders, 39*(5), 366–380. PMID: 16876186

Bernbaum, J. C., Pereira, G. R., Watkins, J. B., & Peckham, G. J. (1983). Non-nutritive sucking during gavage feeding enhances growth and maturation in premature infants. *Pediatrics, 71*(1), 41–45. PMID: 6401358

Bertoncelli, N., Cuomo, G., Cattani, S., Mazzi, C., Pugliese, M., Coccolini, E., & Ferrari, F. (2012). Oral feeding competences of healthy preterm infants: A review. *International Journal of Pediatrics, 2012*(1), 896257. PMID: 22675368

Boiron, M., Nobrega, L. D., Roux, S., Henrot, A., & Saliba, E. (2007). Effects of oral stimulation and oral support on non-nutritive sucking and feeding performance in preterm infants. *Developmental Medicine and Child Neurology*, *49*(6), 439–444. PMID: 17518930

Bornehag, C. G., Lindh, C., Reichenberg, A., Wikström, S., Hallerback, M. U., Evans, S. F., & Swan, S. H. (2018). Association of prenatal phthalate exposure with language development in early childhood. *JAMA Pediatrics*, *172*(12), 1169–1176. PMID: 30383084

Bromiker, R., Arad, I., Loughran, B., Netzer, D., Kaplan, M., & Medoff-Cooper, B. (2005). Comparison of sucking patterns at introduction of oral feeding and at term in Israeli and American preterm infants. *Acta Paediatrica (Oslo, Norway)*, *94*(2), 201–204. PMID: 15984087

Bromiker, R., Medoff-Cooper, B., Flor-Hirsch, H., & Kaplan, M. (2016). Influence of hyperbilirubinemia on neonatal sucking. *Early Human Development*, *99*, 53–56. PMID: 27391573

Bromiker, R., Rachamim, A., Hammerman, C., Schimmel, M., Kaplan, M., & Medoff-Cooper, B. (2006). Immature sucking patterns in infants of mothers with diabetes. *The Journal of Pediatrics*, *149*(5), 640–643. PMID: 17095335

Brown, A., & Arnott, B. (2014). Breastfeeding duration and early parenting behavior: The importance of an infant-led, responsive style. *PLoS One*, *9*(2), e83893. PMID: 24533046

Capilouto, G. J., Cunningham, T., Frederick, E., Dupont-Versteegden, E., Desai, N., & Butterfield, T. A. (2014). Comparison of tongue muscle characteristics of preterm and full-term infants during nutritive and nonnutritive sucking. *Infant Behavior and Development*, *37*(3), 435–445. PMID: 24956503

Capilouto, G. J., Cunningham, T. J., & Desai, N. (2019b). Quantifying the impact of common feeding interventions on nutritive sucking performance using a commercially available smart bottle. *The Journal of Perinatal & Neonatal Nursing*, *33*(4), 331–339. PMID: 31651627

Capilouto, G. J., Cunningham, T. J., Giannone, P. J., & Grider, D. (2019a). A comparison of the nutritive sucking performance of full-term and preterm neonates at hospital discharge: A prospective study. *Early Human Development*, *134*, 26–30. PMID: 31128389

Caron, C. J., Pluijmers, B. I., Joosten, K. F., Dunaway, D., Padwa, B. L., Wolvius, E. B., & Koudstaal, M. J. (2018). Feeding difficulties in craniofacial microsomia: A multicenter retrospective analysis of 755 patients. *Journal of Cranio-Maxillo-Facial Surgery*, *46*(10), 1777–1782. PMID: 30158061

Collaco, J. M., Aherrera, A. D., Ryan, T., & McGrath-Morrow, S. A. (2014). Secondhand smoke exposure in preterm infants with bronchopulmonary dysplasia. *Pediatric Pulmonology*, *49*(2), 173–178. PMID: 23804596

Committee on Fetus and Newborn. (2008). Hospital discharge of the high-risk neonate. *Pediatrics*, *122*(5), 1119–1126. PMID: 18977994

Cooper-Brown, L., Copeland, S., Dailey, S., Downey, D., Petersen, M. C., Stimson, C., & Van Dyke, D. C. (2008). Feeding and swallowing dysfunction in genetic syndromes. *Developmental Disabilities Research Reviews*, *14*(2), 147–157. PMID: 18646013

Cunha, M., Barreiros, J., Gonçalves, I., & Figueiredo, H. (2009). Nutritive sucking pattern-from very low birth weight preterm to term newborn. *Early Human Development*, *85*(2), 125–130. PMID: 18768269

Cunha, M., Barreiros, J., Pereira, J. M., Viegas, V., Banha, C., Diniz, A., & Carreiro, H. (2019). A promising and low-cost prototype to evaluate the motor pattern of nutritive and non-nutritive suction in newborns. [JPNIM]. *Journal of Pediatric and Neonatal Individualized Medicine*, *8*(2), e080220–e080220.

da Costa, S. P., van Den Engel–Hoek, L., & Bos, A. F. (2008). Sucking and swallowing in infants and diagnostic tools. *Journal of Perinatology*, *28*(4), 247–257. PMID: 18200022

da Costa, S. P., van der Schans, C. P., Zweens, M. J., Boelema, S. R., van der Meij, E., Boerman, M. A., & Bos, A. F. (2010). The development of sucking patterns in preterm, small-for-gestational age infants. *The Journal of Pediatrics*, *157*(4), 603–609. PMID: 20542296

Delaney, A. L., & Arvedson, J. C. (2008). Development of swallowing and feeding: Prenatal through first year of life. *Developmental Disabilities Research Reviews*, *14*(2), 105–117. PMID: 18646020

Dewi, D. J., Rachmawati, E. Z. K., Wahyuni, L. K., Hsu, W. C., Tamin, S., Yunizaf, R., & Iskandar, R. A. T. P. (2024). Risk of dysphagia in a population of infants born pre-term: Characteristic risk factors in a tertiary NICU. *Jornal de Pediatria*, *100*(2), 169–176. PMID: 37848170

Ebrahimi, Z., Moradi, H., & Ashtiani, S. J. (2019). A compact pediatric portable pacifier to assess non-nutritive sucking of premature infants. *IEEE Sensors Journal*, *20*(2), 1028–1034.

Engelke, W., Glombek, J., Psychogios, M., Schneider, S., Ellenberger, D., & Santander, P. (2014). Displacement of oropharyngeal structures during suction-swallowing cycles. *European Archives of Oto-Rhino-Laryngology*, *271*, 1987–1997. PMID: 24510235

Engelke, W., Jung, K., & Knösel, M. (2011). Intra-oral compartment pressures: A biofunctional model and experimental measurements under different conditions of posture. *Clinical Oral Investigations*, *15*, 165–176. PMID: 20127264

Erçin, S., & Ovali, F. (2019). Newborn Screenings. *Journal of Clinical Medicine Pediatrics*, *11*(4), 193–199.

Estep, M., Barlow, S. M., Vantipalli, R., Finan, D., & Lee, J. (2008). Non-nutritive suck parameters in preterm infants with RDS. *Journal of Neonatal Nursing*, *14*(1), 28–34. PMID: 19190723

Ferguson, K. K., McElrath, T. F., Chen, Y. H., Mukherjee, B., & Meeker, J. D. (2014). Urinary phthalate metabolites and biomarkers of oxidative stress in pregnant women: A repeated measures analysis. *Environmental Health Perspectives*, *123*(3), 210. PMID: 25402001

Field, T. (2010). Effects of postpartum depression on early interactions, parenting, and safety practices: A review. *Infant Behavior and Development*, *33*(1), 1–6. PMID: 19962196

Fucile, S., Gisel, E., & Lau, C. (2002). Oral stimulation accelerates the transition from tube to oral feeding in preterm infants. *The Journal of Pediatrics*, *141*(2), 230–236. PMID: 12183719

Fucile, S., Gisel, E., Schanler, R. J., & Lau, C. (2009). A controlled-flow vacuum-free bottle system enhances preterm infants' nutritive sucking skills. *Dysphagia*, *24*, 145–151. PMID: 18836778

Fuentes, R., Engelke, W., Flores, T., Navarro, P., Borie, E., Curiqueo, A., & Salamanca, C. (2015). Description of intraoral pressures on the sub-palatal space in young adult patients with normal occlusion. *International Journal of Clinical and Experimental Medicine*, *8*(7), 11208. PMID: 26379925

Fujinaga, C. I., Moraes, S. A. D., Zamberlan-Amorim, N. E., Castral, T. C., Silva, A. D. A., & Scochi, C. G. S. (2013). Clinical validation of the preterm oral feeding readiness assessment scale. *Latin American Journal of Nursing*, *21*, 140–145. PMID: 23459901

Gewolb, I. H., Vice, F. L., Schweitzer-Kenney, E. L., Taciak, V. L., & Bosma, J. F. (2001). Developmental patterns of rhythmic suck and swallow in preterm infants. *Developmental Medicine and Child Neurology*, *43*(1), 22–27. PMID: 11201418

Goday, P. S., Huh, S. Y., Silverman, A., Lukens, C. T., Dodrill, P., Cohen, S. S., & Phalen, J. A. (2019). Pediatric feeding disorder: Consensus definition and conceptual framework. *Journal of Pediatric Gastroenterology and Nutrition*, *68*(1), 124–129. PMID: 30358739

Grassi, A., Cecchi, F., Sgherri, G., Guzzetta, A., Gagliardi, L., & Laschi, C. (2016). Sensorized pacifier to evaluate non-nutritive sucking in newborns. *Medical Engineering & Physics*, *38*(4), 398–402. PMID: 26830270

Green, M. A., & Resnick, C. M. (2021, December). Feeding considerations for infants with craniofacial malformations. []). WB Saunders.]. *Seminars in Fetal & Neonatal Medicine*, *26*(6), 101280. PMID: 34561178

Harding, C., Cockerill, H., Cane, C., & Law, J. (2018). Using non-nutritive sucking to support feeding development for premature infants: A commentary on approaches and current practice. *Journal of Pediatric Rehabilitation Medicine*, *11*(3), 147–152. PMID: 29125505

Harding, C., Frank, L., Van Someren, V., Hilari, K., & Botting, N. (2014). How does non-nutritive sucking support infant feeding? *Infant Behavior and Development*, *37*(4), 457–464. PMID: 24974134

Hwang, Y. S., Vergara, E., Lin, C. H., Coster, W. J., Bigsby, R., & Tsai, W. H. (2010). Effects of prefeeding oral stimulation on feeding performance of preterm infants. *Indian Journal of Pediatrics*, *77*(8), 869–873. PMID: 20814844

Indramohan, G., Pedigo, T. P., Rostoker, N., Cambare, M., Grogan, T., & Federman, M. D. (2017). Identification of risk factors for poor feeding in infants with congenital heart disease and a novel approach to improve oral feeding. *Journal of Pediatric Nursing*, *35*, 149–154. PMID: 28169036

Kao, H. M., Lin, C. H., & Chang, Y. J. (2010). Feeding with cross-cut teats has better sucking effects and oxygenation in preterm infants with chronic lung disease. *Journal of Clinical Nursing*, *19*(21-22), 3016–3022. PMID: 21040008

Knösel, M., Nüser, C., Jung, K., Helms, H. J., Engelke, W., & Sandoval, P. (2016). Interaction between deglutition, tongue posture, and malocclusion: A comparison of intraoral compartment formation in subjects with neutral occlusion or different types of malocclusion. *The Angle Orthodontist*, *86*(5), 697–705. PMID: 26894981

Koenig, J. S., Davies, A. M., & Thach, B. T. (1990). Coordination of breathing, sucking, and swallowing during bottle feedings in human infants. *Journal of Applied Physiology*, *69*(5), 1623–1629. PMID: 2272953

Kron, R. E., Stein, M., & Goddard, K. E. (1963). A method of measuring sucking behavior of newborn infants. *Psychosomatic Medicine*, *25*(2), 181–191. DOI: 10.1097/00006842-196303000-00010 PMID: 13927027

Lang, W. C., Buist, N. R., Geary, A., Buckley, S., Adams, E., Jones, A. C., & Rogers, B. R. (2011). Quantification of intraoral pressures during nutritive sucking: Methods with normal infants. *Dysphagia*, *26*, 277–286. PMID: 20853119

Lau, C. (2006). Oral feeding in the preterm infant. *NeoReviews*, *7*(1), e19–e27.

Lau, C. (2016). Development of infant oral feeding skills: What do we know? *The American Journal of Clinical Nutrition*, *103*(2), 616S–621S. PMID: 26791183

Lau, C., Geddes, D., Mizuno, K., & Schaal, B. (2012). The development of oral feeding skills in infants. *International Journal of Pediatrics*, *2012*, 572341. PMID: 23193413

Lau, C., & Kusnierczyk, I. (2001). Quantitative evaluation of infant's nonnutritive and nutritive sucking. *Dysphagia*, *16*(1), 58–67. PMID: 11213247

Lau, C., & Smith, E. O. (2012). Interventions to improve the oral feeding performance of preterm infants. *Acta Paediatrica (Oslo, Norway)*, *101*(7), e269–e274. PMID: 22404221

Lee, K. J., Shin, Y. B., Park, H. E., Choi, S., de Oliveira, J. G., Hong, D., Kim, S., & Yoon, J. A. (2023). Quantitative non-nutritive sucking measurement as a predictor of oral feeding readiness in newborns. *Frontiers in Pediatrics*, *11*, 1143416. DOI: 10.3389/fped.2023.1143416 PMID: 37635795

Letko, M. D. (1996). Understanding the Apgar score. *Journal of Obstetric, Gynecologic, and Neonatal Nursing : JOGNN*, *25*(4), 299–303. PMID: 8708830

Lobos, S., Spencer, E., Reyes, P., Weinstein, A., Stojanova, J., & Retamal-Walter, F. (2025). A low-cost device for measuring non-nutritive sucking in newborns. *Sensors (Basel)*, *25*(16), 5080. DOI: 10.3390/s25165080 PMID: 40871943

March of Dimes. (2008). *New report from the March of Dimes about the cost of pre-term birth.* March of Dimes.

Martens, A., Hines, M., & Zimmerman, E. (2020). Changes in non-nutritive suck between 3 and 12 months. *Early Human Development, 149*, 105141. PMID: 32784100

Martens, A., Phillips, H., Hines, M., & Zimmerman, E. (2024). An examination of the association between infant non-nutritive suck and developmental outcomes at 12 months. *PLoS One, 19*(2), e0298016. DOI: 10.1371/journal.pone.0298016 PMID: 38315689

Martin, M., & Shaw, N. J. (1997). Feeding problems in infants and young children with chronic lung disease. *Journal of Human Nutrition and Dietetics, 10*(5), 271–275.

Mathew, O. P., Clark, M. L., & Pronske, M. H. (1985). Apnea, bradycardia, and cyanosis during oral feeding in term neonates. *The Journal of Pediatrics, 106*(5), 857. PMID: 3998930

Matsuo, K., & Palmer, J. B. (2008). Anatomy and physiology of feeding and swallowing: Normal and abnormal. *Physical Medicine and Rehabilitation Clinics of North America, 19*(4), 691–707. PMID: 18940636

Maynard, T. M., Zohn, I. E., Moody, S. A., & LaMantia, A. S. (2020). Suckling, feeding, and swallowing: Behaviors, circuits, and targets for neurodevelopmental pathology. *Annual Review of Neuroscience, 43*(1), 315–336. PMID: 32101484

McCain, G. C. (2003). An evidence-based guideline for introducing oral feeding to healthy preterm infants. *Neonatal Network: NN, 22*(5), 45–50. PMID: 14598979

Medoff-Cooper, B. (2005). Nutritive sucking research: From clinical questions to research answers. *The Journal of Perinatal & Neonatal Nursing, 19*(3), 265–272. PMID: 16106235

Medoff-Cooper, B., McGrath, J. M., & Shults, J. (2002). Feeding patterns of full-term and preterm infants at forty weeks postconceptional age. *Journal of Developmental and Behavioral Pediatrics, 23*(4), 231–236. PMID: 12177569

Medoff-Cooper, B., Rankin, K., Li, Z., Liu, L., & White-Traut, R. (2015). Multisensory intervention for preterm infants improves sucking organization. *Advances in Neonatal Care, 15*(2), 142–149. PMID: 25822519

Medoff-Cooper, B., & Ray, W. (1995). Neonatal sucking behaviors. *Image—the Journal of Nursing Scholarship, 27*(3), 195–200. PMID: 7590801

Medoff-Cooper, B., Shults, J., & Kaplan, J. (2009). Sucking behavior of preterm neonates as a predictor of developmental outcomes. *Journal of Developmental and Behavioral Pediatrics*, *30*(1), 16–22. PMID: 19194323

Meyer Palmer, M., & Heyman, M. B. (1999). Developmental outcome for neonates with dysfunctional and disorganized sucking patterns: Preliminary findings. *Infant-Toddler Intervention*, *9*, 299–308.

Miller, C. K., & Madhoun, L. (2016). Feeding in infants with craniofacial anomalies. *Perspectives of the ASHA Special Interest Groups*, *1*(13), 12–28.

Miller, M. J., & Difiore, J. M. (1995). A comparison of swallowing during apnea and periodic breathing in premature infants. *Pediatric Research*, *37*(6), 796–799. PMID: 7651766

Mistry, S., & Hamdy, S. (2008). Neural control of feeding and swallowing. *Physical Medicine and Rehabilitation Clinics of North America*, *19*(4), 709–728. PMID: 18940637

Mizuno, K., & Ueda, A. (2001). Development of sucking behavior in infants who have not been fed for 2 months after birth. *Pediatrics International*, *43*(3), 251–255. PMID: 11380918

Mizuno, K., & Ueda, A. (2003). The maturation and coordination of sucking, swallowing, and respiration in preterm infants. *The Journal of Pediatrics*, *142*(1), 36–40. PMID: 12520252

Noori, F., Nariman, S., Rahmiaan, H., Sadat, H. A. S., & Ravarian, A. (2018). The effect of non-nutritive sucking by mothers on full oral feeding attainment in preterm neonates. *Journal of Comprehensive Pediatrics*, *9*(1), e59657.

Norman, V., Zühlke, L., Murray, K., & Morrow, B. (2022). Prevalence of feeding and swallowing disorders in congenital heart disease: A scoping review. *Frontiers in Pediatrics*, *10*, 843023. PMID: 35450100

Olesen, T. S., Bleses, D., Andersen, H. R., Grandjean, P., Frederiksen, H., Trecca, F., & Jensen, T. K. (2018). Prenatal phthalate exposure and language development in toddlers from the Odense Child Cohort. *Neurotoxicology and Teratology*, *65*, 34–41. PMID: 29198963

Palmer, M. M., Crawley, K., & Blanco, I. A. (1993). Neonatal Oral-Motor Assessment scale: A reliability study. *Journal of Perinatology: Official Journal of the California Perinatal Association*, *13*(1), 28–35. PMID: 8445444

Pimenta, H. P., Moreira, M. E., Rocha, A. D., Gomes, S. C.Junior, Pinto, L. W., & Lucena, S. L. (2008). Effects of non-nutritive sucking and oral stimulation on breastfeeding rates for preterm, low birth weight infants: A randomized clinical trial. *The Journal of Pediatrics, 84*, 423–427. PMID: 18923786

Pineda, R., Dewey, K., Jacobsen, A., & Smith, J. (2019). Non-nutritive sucking in the preterm infant. *American Journal of Perinatology, 36*(03), 268–276. PMID: 30081403

Pinelli, J., & Symington, A. J. (2011). Cochrane Review: Non-nutritive sucking for promoting physiological stability and nutrition in preterm infants. *Evidence-Based Child Health: A Cochrane Review Journal, 6*(4), 1134–1169.

Poore, M., Barlow, S. M., Wang, J., Estep, M., & Lee, J. (2008). Respiratory treatment history predicts suck pattern stability in preterm infants. *Journal of Neonatal Nursing, 14*(6), 185–192. PMID: 19956344

Poore, M., Zimmerman, E., Barlow, S. M., Wang, J., & Gu, F. (2008b). Patterned orocutaneous therapy improves sucking and oral feeding in preterm infants. *Acta Paediatrica (Oslo, Norway), 97*(7), 920–927. PMID: 18462468

Poore, M. A., & Barlow, S. M. (2009). Suck predicts neuromotor integrity and developmental outcomes. *Perspectives on Speech Science and Orofacial Disorders, 19*(1), 44–51.

Puccini, F. R. S., & Berretin-Felix, G. (2015). Gastroesophageal reflux and swallowing in newborns and infants: Integrative review of literature. *Revista CEFAC, 17*, 1664–1673.

Reid, J. (2004). A review of feeding interventions for infants with cleft palate. *The Cleft Palate-Craniofacial Journal, 41*(3), 268–278. PMID: 15151444

Reilly, S., & Skuse, D. (1992). Characteristics and management of feeding problems of young children with cerebral palsy. *Developmental Medicine and Child Neurology, 34*(5), 379–388. PMID: 1592191

Rocha, A. D., Moreira, M. E. L., Pimenta, H. P., Ramos, J. R. M., & Lucena, S. L. (2007). A randomized study of the efficacy of sensory-motor-oral stimulation and non-nutritive sucking in very low birthweight infants. *Early Human Development, 83*(6), 385–388. PMID: 16979854

Santander, P., Engelke, W., Olthoff, A., & Völter, C. (2013). Intraoral pressure patterns during swallowing. *European Archives of Oto-Rhino-Laryngology, 270*, 1019–1025. PMID: 23238701

Shaker, C. S. (2013). Cue-based feeding in the NICU: Using the infant's communication as a guide. *Neonatal Network*, *32*(6), 404. PMID: 24195800

Shandley, S., Capilouto, G., Tamilia, E., Riley, D. M., Johnson, Y. R., & Papadelis, C. (2021). Abnormal nutritive sucking as an indicator of neonatal brain injury. *Frontiers in Pediatrics*, *8*, 599633. PMID: 33511093

Slattery, J., Morgan, A., & Douglas, J. (2012). Early sucking and swallowing problems as predictors of neurodevelopmental outcome in children with neonatal brain injury: A systematic review. *Developmental Medicine and Child Neurology*, *54*(9), 796–806. PMID: 22607330

Stanley, M. A., Shepherd, N., Duvall, N., Jenkinson, S. B., Jalou, H. E., Givan, D. C., & Roper, R. J. (2019). Clinical identification of feeding and swallowing disorders in 0–6-month-old infants with Down syndrome. *American Journal of Medical Genetics. Part A*, *179*(2), 177–182. PMID: 30588741

Sullivan, P. B., Lambert, B., Rose, M., Ford-Adams, M., Johnson, A., & Griffiths, P. (2000). Prevalence and severity of feeding and nutritional problems in children with neurological impairment: Oxford Feeding Study. *Developmental Medicine and Child Neurology*, *42*(10), 674–680. PMID: 11085295

Tamilia, E., Formica, D., Scaini, A., & Taffoni, F. (2015). An automated system for the analysis of newborns' oral-motor behavior. *IEEE Transactions on Neural Systems and Rehabilitation Engineering*, *24*(12), 1294–1303. PMID: 26540691

Tenhaaf, J. J. (2008). Critical review: The effects of oral stimulation on feeding behaviors in preterm infants. *School of Communication Sciences and Disorders, the University of Western Ontario*, 230-236.

Thoyre, S. M., Shaker, C. S., & Pridham, K. F. (2005). The early feeding skills assessment for preterm infants. *Neonatal Network: NN*, *24*(3), 7. PMID: 15960007

Tsai, Y. L., Hsieh, P. C., Chen, T. Y., & Lin, Y. C. (2023). Effects of complete oral motor intervention and nonnutritive sucking alone on the feeding performance of premature infants: A systematic review and meta-analysis. *Children (Basel, Switzerland)*, *11*(1), 4. PMID: 38275425

Underwood, M. A., Danielsen, B., & Gilbert, W. M. (2007). Cost, causes and rates of rehospitalization of preterm infants. *Journal of Perinatology*, *27*(10), 614–619. PMID: 17717521

van den Engel-Hoek, L., de Groot, I. J., de Swart, B. J., & Erasmus, C. E. (2015). Feeding and swallowing disorders in pediatric neuromuscular diseases: An overview. *Journal of Neuromuscular Diseases*, *2*(4), 357–369. PMID: 27858755

Wolff, P. H. (1968). The serial organization of sucking in the young infant. *Pediatrics, 42*(6), 943–956. PMID: 4235770

Wolthuis-Stigter, M. I., Da Costa, S. P., Bos, A. F., Krijnen, W. P., Van Der Schans, C. P., & Luinge, M. R. (2017). Sucking behavior in infants born preterm and developmental outcomes at primary school age. *Developmental Medicine and Child Neurology, 59*(8), 871–877. PMID: 28432690

Wolthuis-Stigter, M. I., Luinge, M. R., da Costa, S. P., Krijnen, W. P., van der Schans, C. P., & Bos, A. F. (2015). The association between sucking behavior in preterm infants and neurodevelopmental outcomes at 2 years of age. *The Journal of Pediatrics, 166*(1), 26–30. PMID: 25311711

Zhang, X., Zhou, M., Yin, H., Dai, Y., & Li, Y. (2017). The predictive value of early oral motor assessments for neurodevelopmental outcomes of moderately and late preterm infants. *Medicine, 96*(50), e9207. PMID: 29390342

Zimmerman, E., Aguiar, A., Aung, M. T., Geiger, S. D., Hines, M., & Woodbury, M. L. & Program Collaborators for Environmental Influences on Child Health Outcomes. (2023). Examining the association between prenatal maternal stress and infant non-nutritive suck. *Pediatric Research, 93*(5), 1285–1293. PMID: 34916626

Zimmerman, E., & Barlow, S. M. (2008). Pacifier stiffness alters the dynamics of the suck central pattern generator. *Journal of Neonatal Nursing, 14*(3), 79–86. PMID: 19492006

Zimmerman, E., Watkins, D. J., Huerta-Montanez, G., Pabon, Z. R., Feric, Z., Manjourides, J., & Meeker, J. D. (2021). Associations of gestational phthalate exposure and non-nutritive suck among infants from the Puerto Rico Testsite for Exploring Contamination Threats (PROTECT) birth cohort study. *Environment International, 152*, 106480. PMID: 33740674

Chapter 4
Innovative Approaches in Dysphagia:
From Assessment to Therapy

Seren Düzenli Öztürk
http://orcid.org/0000-0003-3630-173X
Department of Speech and Language Therapy, Izmir Bakircay University, İzmir, Turkey

Cansu Yildirim
http://orcid.org/0000-0002-9957-3006
Department of Speech and Language Therapy, Izmir Bakircay University, İzmir, Turkey

Emre Cengiz
http://orcid.org/0000-0001-9224-6742
Department of Physical Therapy and Rehabilitation, Faculty of Health Sciences, Usak University, Usak, Turkey

ABSTRACT

This chapter explores emerging technological innovations in the assessment and rehabilitation of dysphagia across the lifespan, addressing the limitations of conventional methods and proposing a framework for integrating advanced solutions into clinical practice. It synthesizes evidence on artificial intelligence (AI) for automated swallowing assessments, mobile health (mHealth) and tele-practice models, neuromodulation techniques (e.g., transcranial direct current stimulation, neuromuscular electrical stimulation), and virtual reality (VR) and gamified interventions. The chapter emphasizes clinical applicability within multidisciplinary care pathways, while addressing ethical, accessibility, and cost-effectiveness challenges. By pro-

DOI: 10.4018/979-8-3373-6405-6.ch004

posing a roadmap for combining these technologies with traditional approaches, it aims to enhance equitable access to dysphagia care for diverse populations, from pediatric to geriatric patients.

INTRODUCTION

Dysphagia, a prevalent condition affecting individuals from premature infancy through older adulthood, is associated with severe consequences, including malnutrition, aspiration pneumonia, increased healthcare costs, and reduced quality of life (Pisegna et al., 2016). Traditional assessment methods, such as videofluoroscopic swallowing studies (VFSS; also termed the modified barium swallow study, MBSS) and fiberoptic endoscopic evaluation of swallowing (FEES), and rehabilitation techniques, such as manual swallowing exercises, are resource-intensive, heavily reliant on clinician expertise, and often inaccessible in low-resource settings. These limitations necessitate innovative solutions to improve diagnostic precision, therapeutic efficacy, and access to care.

Recent advances in biomedical engineering, neuroscience, and digital health technologies are transforming dysphagia management. Artificial intelligence enables automated analysis of instrumental assessments, improving efficiency and objectivity (Silva et al., 2025; Wong et al., 2025). Surface electromyography (sEMG) is also a key tool; sEMG devices record the electrical activity of swallowing muscles via skin-surface electrodes, providing real-time information on muscle activation and contraction (Perlman, 2006; Ye-Lin et al., 2022). Mobile health applications and telepractice platforms extend care to underserved populations, supporting continuous monitoring and the remote delivery of evidence-based interventions (Malandraki et al., 2021). Neuromodulation techniques, including transcranial direct current stimulation (tDCS), repetitive transcranial magnetic stimulation (rTMS), and neuromuscular electrical stimulation (NMES), promote neuroplasticity and enhance swallowing outcomes (Carnaby-Mann & Crary, 2007; Miller, Peters, & Ptok, 2022; Simons & Hamdy, 2017). Virtual reality and gamified interventions further enrich rehabilitative experiences by increasing patient engagement and adherence (Hwang et al., 2025). Importantly, these emerging technologies differ substantially in clinical readiness, evidentiary support, and implementation feasibility, underscoring the need for careful clinical integration rather than uniform adoption.

This chapter synthesizes recent advances in dysphagia assessment and rehabilitation into a lifespan-oriented, translational framework to support clinical interpretation and implementation. The chapter is organized into four sections: Section 1 summarizes AI applications in dysphagia assessment and therapy; Section 2 reviews peripheral and central neuromodulation techniques; Section 3 focuses on sEMG for assessment and biofeedback; and Section 4 discusses digital technologies for home- and remote-based rehabilitation across the lifespan.

1. ARTIFICIAL INTELLIGENCE IN DYSPHAGIA MANAGEMENT

Artificial intelligence (AI) has the potential to be a transformative tool in speech-language therapy (SLT) and dysphagia intervention. AI refers to the development of computational models that mimic cognitive functions such as learning, reasoning, and decision-making (Kumar et al., 2025). AI in healthcare includes a wide range of methods, from rule-based systems and traditional machine learning (ML) to more advanced deep learning (DL) and generative AI models (Alowais et al., 2023; Maleki Varnosfaderani & Forouzanfar, 2024). Traditional statistical methods concentrate on inferential analysis and structured datasets. In contrast, AI techniques can process extensive, unstructured, and multimodal data, including audio recordings, acoustic waveforms, and real-time speech monitoring (Cordella et al., 2025). Lack of timely diagnosis and treatment of dysphagia leads to prolonged hospital stays, extended rehabilitation needs, increased mortality, and increased healthcare costs. Technological advances play a critical role in the diagnosis and intervention of dysphagia; artificial intelligence, big data analysis, and deep learning methods offer effective solutions in this area. From a clinical standpoint, AI should be viewed primarily as a decision-support technology that augments clinician expertise, enhances efficiency, and reduces variability, rather than as an autonomous replacement for clinical judgment. AI-assisted intervention approaches offer significant benefits in the delivery of medical services to populations with inadequate access to dysphagia specialists, especially in aging societies (Weng et al., 2022). The role of AI in dysphagia intervention can be divided into two primary areas: (1) AI-assisted dysphagia screening and assessment; and (2) AI-assisted swallowing rehabilitation (Figure 1) (Gallano et al., 2025). At present, the greatest clinical readiness is observed in clinician-supervised applications that support assessment interpretation and monitoring (e.g., AI-assisted VFSS/FEES analysis). In contrast, fully autonomous screening and therapeutic systems remain largely investigational and require further validation.

Figure 1. Applications of artificial intelligence in dysphagia management (Gallano et al., 2025).

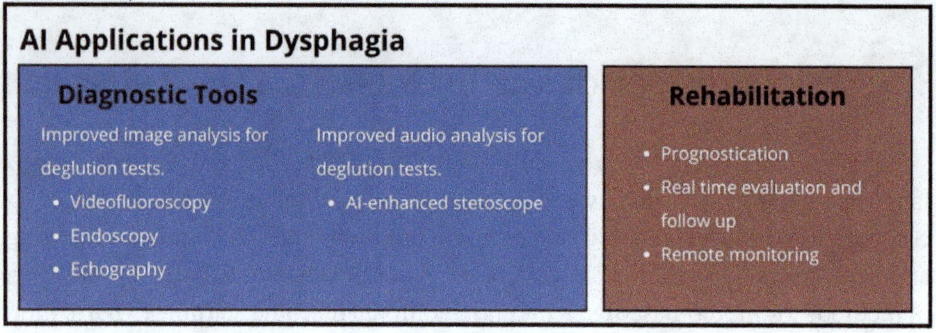

This subsection synthesizes current evidence on AI applications in dysphagia diagnosis and therapy, with emphasis on clinically feasible, clinician-supervised use. While AI can facilitate radiation-free alternatives, remote monitoring, and automated pattern recognition for dysphagia diagnosis, its integration into routine therapy is still in an early phase. It is most appropriately implemented alongside established behavioral and clinician-led interventions.

1.1. Artificial Intelligence in Dysphagia Diagnosis

The benefits of dysphagia diagnosis with AI-assisted tools include higher accuracy and efficiency, shorter diagnosis time, and the potential for remote diagnosis and monitoring (Heo et al., 2024; Kim, Kim, Choi, & Ryu, 2024). These benefits can lead to earlier interventions and better outcomes for patients with dysphagia. AI-assisted dysphagia diagnosis can address some limitations of traditional diagnostic methods, such as the videofluoroscopic swallowing study (VFSS) and the fiberoptic endoscopic evaluation of swallowing (FEES). Although these methods meet gold standards, they can be time-consuming and expensive, require specialized equipment, and pose risks such as radiation exposure (Khalifa et al., 2023; Kim, Kim, Choi, Lee, et al., 2024). AI algorithms can automatically detect dysphagia symptoms by analyzing images and videos obtained from these procedures, potentially leading to earlier and more accurate diagnoses (C.-W. Jeong et al., 2024; Weng et al., 2022).

The FEES method, developed by Langmore et al. (1998), offers advantages such as no radiation exposure, no time limitation on examination length, the ability to assess the patient's endurance during eating, direct visualization of the larynx and pharynx, and sensory assessment. However, accurately diagnosing aspiration and penetration with FEES remains a clinical challenge for inexperienced therapists because the swallowing movement is very rapid, typically lasting only 0.3 seconds.

Furthermore, the interpretation of FEES results can vary among therapists with different levels of experience (Weng et al., 2022). One possible solution is to detect aspiration and penetration with AI-assisted FEES. Weng et al. (2022) examined the performance of AI-supported computerized diagnostic systems in detecting aspiration and penetration during FEES. The study used 25,630 labelled images obtained from 199 patients who underwent FEES for suspected oropharyngeal dysphagia and trained an AI model using a deep learning algorithm. As a result of their study, they developed the first AI-supported diagnostic tool that achieved accuracy comparable to experts in detecting aspiration and penetration during FEES (Weng et al., 2022).

VFSS provides functional and structural information and is the only method to visualize the bolus throughout the three phases of swallowing. Also known as the modified barium swallow study (MBSS), VFSS involves instructing the patient to swallow food mixed with barium sulfate (Sanjeevi et al., 2025). VFSS videos include a sagittal view of the oropharynx, pharynx, and upper esophagus, capturing all relevant swallowing structures. This allows clinicians to assess the physiological function of the swallowing process and determine the severity of dysphagia by visualizing bolus flow and structural movement through the upper aerodigestive tract (Martin-Harris & Jones, 2008). SLTs require frame-by-frame or repeated analyses to interpret VFSS results. This assessment method requires years of training and involves inter- and intra-rater variability. This time-consuming process involves evaluating each component of the swallowing action multiple times (Sejdic et al., 2019; 2020). In recent years, deep learning (DL), a subset of AI proposed as a solution to this problem, has become an important tool for diagnostics, assisting clinicians. AI frameworks offer promising results in diagnosing complex diseases by analyzing and extracting biomarkers and patterns from medical data (Girardi et al., 2023; Sejdic et al., 2020). Jeong et al. (2023) aimed to develop a DL-based model for automatic measurement of various temporal swallowing parameters. Multiple indicators, including oral phase duration, pharyngeal delay time, pharyngeal response time, pharyngeal transit time, laryngeal vestibule closure reaction time, laryngeal vestibule closure duration, and upper esophageal sphincter opening duration, were used in the study. The average accuracy of the proposed model was reported to range from 0.901 to 0.981. Jeong et al. (2024) presented a pilot artificial intelligence application using DL to analyze VFSS swallowing videos. The developed model demonstrated successful results in the testing phase, specifically identifying the most serious complication, aspiration, with 96% accuracy, and penetration with 92% accuracy. Accuracy in the detection of swallowing phases was 90% for the oral phase, 82% for the pharyngeal phase, and 79% for the esophageal phase. Kwak et al. (2025) aimed to investigate whether machine learning could predict the long-term prognosis of post-stroke dysphagia using early VFSS data. The study retrospectively collected data from dysphagia patients who had their first acute stroke, from VFSSs performed within 1 month of onset, and from swallowing status at 6 months. Five machine learning algorithms were used to analyze whether long-term prognosis could be predicted from VFSS data. As a result of the study, machine learning models using early VFSS data demonstrated high accuracy and predictive power in predicting the long-term prognosis of patients with post-stroke dysphagia. In their review, Girardi, Cardell, and Bird (2023) examined the applications of AI in VFSS and its implications for SLTs. They emphasized that AI has revolutionary potential for dysphagia intervention by transforming VFSSs and supporting SLTs' diagnostic processes, but careful steps should be taken for integration.

Cervical auscultation is the recording of the sounds and vibrations produced by the human body in the throat during swallowing. Compared with videofluoroscopy and video endoscopy, cervical auscultation is a simple, minimally invasive method for assessing swallowing function that can be performed in the patient's normal eating environment. However, because cervical auscultation with an analogue stethoscope depends on the practitioner's report, evaluations can be subjective and difficult to quantify. Swallow sounds are generally quite brief, lasting approximately 0.7 seconds from the beginning to the end of swallowing, and are heard as a single sound block (Dudik et al., 2015; Morinière et al., 2008). In this context, Suzuki et al. (2022) combined electronic stethoscope techniques with AI to create a system that uses sound recognition to quantify swallowing sounds. Within the scope of their study, 20 fifth-year dental students volunteered to participate in the study; each participant drank 10 ml and then 20 ml of water in different positions (sitting and supine). They developed an AI-based algorithm to index bolus-entry sounds by comparing swallowing sounds to generate a new index. In a neurological context, Nakamori et al. (2023) investigated the usefulness of swallowing-sound assessment in patients with amyotrophic lateral sclerosis (ALS) using a novel AI analysis tool for electronic stethoscopes. Their study found that AI analysis of swallowing sounds recorded with an electronic stethoscope correlated with established swallowing assessment indicators in ALS, demonstrating its usefulness as a new method.

Surface electromyography (sEMG) has increasingly been integrated into AI-assisted diagnostic research as a complementary, non-invasive source of electrophysiological information related to swallowing function. By providing indirect, quantitative analysis of dynamic muscle activation patterns during swallowing, sEMG contributes to the objective characterization of dysphagia-related impairments (Alfonsi et al., 2013; Sejdic et al., 2019). sEMG signals have been recorded to assess the electrophysiological effects of volume and consistency in patients (Koyama et al., 2021). Roldan-Vasco et al. (2023) evaluated 31 healthy and 29 dysphagic patients performing swallowing tasks with water, yoghurt, saliva, and crackers. sEMG activity was recorded using bilateral channels for the masseter, suprahyoid, and infrahyoid muscle groups. As the main conclusion of the study, they proposed a set of sEMG-related biomarkers and classification approaches suitable for automated dysphagia screening, thereby enabling the implementation of noninvasive, objective strategies for swallowing assessment.

Across diagnostic applications, the clinical utility of AI systems depends on high-quality training data, clinician supervision, and validation within specific patient populations. From a clinical decision-making perspective, AI-assisted diagnostic tools should therefore be interpreted as structured decision-support systems that reduce inter- and intra-rater variability and accelerate analysis, while final diagnostic judgments remain clinician-led.

The expanding use of AI in dysphagia diagnostics also raises ethical and data-governance considerations. VFSS and FEES recordings, swallowing acoustics, and home-based monitoring data constitute sensitive audiovisual health information that requires secure storage, transparent data-handling policies, and explicit informed consent. Algorithm transparency and ongoing clinician oversight are essential to prevent inappropriate reliance on automated outputs, especially in high-risk clinical decisions such as aspiration management.

Equity and feasibility considerations further shape clinical implementation. Although AI-assisted diagnostic workflows may enhance access through remote triage and screening in low-resource or underserved settings, their effectiveness depends on the availability of infrastructure, clinician training, and contextual validation. Without deliberate implementation strategies, AI-driven solutions may inadvertently widen existing disparities in dysphagia care.

Cross-technology synthesis of assessment-oriented innovations, including AI-assisted diagnostics and sEMG-based evaluation, is presented later in the chapter (Section 3) to support integrated clinical interpretation and decision-making.

1.2. Artificial Intelligence in Dysphagia Therapy

AI algorithms analyze patient data, including medical history, diagnostic results, and treatment responses, to create personalized therapy plans. This personalized approach can increase therapy effectiveness and patient compliance (Gugatschka et al., 2024; Saab et al., 2023). Studies have also demonstrated the value of real-time feedback during swallowing exercises, helping patients adjust their techniques and monitor progress. This interactive approach increases motivation and supports motor learning (Khalifa et al., 2023).

Biofeedback is a technique that represents physiological processes in different ways. Visual, auditory, or tactile representation allows the patient to gain voluntary control over physiological processes that occur automatically under healthy conditions. Feedback learning supports operant conditioning by providing information and motivation about progress in physiological abilities and raises awareness of unconscious processes (Frank et al., 2010). Studies on biofeedback in dysphagia therapy use electromyography (EMG) measurements with electrodes placed in the submental region. Riebold, Seidl, and Schauer (2024) examined the EMG and BI measurements of 41 dysphagia patients to compare timing and performance in the Detection of Swallow Onsets (DoSO) using EMG alone versus combined Bioimpedance (BI) and EMG measurements. They also used BI-based data segmentation of potential swallow onsets and a machine learning-based classifier to distinguish swallow onsets from non-swallow events. The study found that BI/EMG-based DoSO had better timing and detection performance compared to EMG-based DoSO and could be used as biofeedback in dysphagia therapy.

Advanced interactive technologies such as AI-based video games (AI-VG) offer promising new directions for the rehabilitation of patients with dysphagia after stroke. The use of video games for rehabilitation visualization can increase patient motivation, improve patient retention, and provide transparent measurement of the objective outcomes of patient education (Burdea et al., 2021). Video games incorporating artificial intelligence can be more adaptive to a participant's behavior, accurately capture their movements, and enhance the overall gaming experience (Swar Gujrania et al., 2019). Zhang et al. (2025) investigated the effectiveness of an AI-VG intervention in improving swallowing function in stroke patients with dysphagia. A prospective, single-blind, randomized controlled trial (RCT) was conducted in a rehabilitation hospital from October 2023 to July 2024. Participants were randomly assigned to the AI-VG system group or the control group and received training in 30-minute sessions, five times a week, for 4 weeks. The study provides promising evidence for the effectiveness of AI-VG interventions in improving swallowing function, quality of life, and nutritional status in patients with post-stroke dysphagia. The high level of patient satisfaction further supports the potential of this approach. However, it emphasizes the need for larger, more diverse studies to define the role of AI-VG in dysphagia rehabilitation definitively and to guide its implementation in clinical settings.

From a clinical perspective, current AI-assisted diagnostic and therapeutic applications should be regarded as adjunctive tools that support clinician-guided dysphagia management rather than autonomous systems. In conclusion, integrating AI into dysphagia assessment and therapy has great potential to improve diagnostic accuracy and professional efficiency. Traditional methods such as VFSS and FEES face challenges related to accessibility and human interpretation. Machine learning and deep learning algorithms offer solutions to standardize and automate assessments, making them more objective. These same AI applications are also expanding into patient monitoring, rehabilitation, and education. As AI technologies advance, more innovative applications spanning the full spectrum of dysphagia intervention are expected.

2. NEUROMODULATION TECHNIQUES IN NEUROGENIC DYSPHAGIA

The management of neurogenic dysphagia requires interventions that promote adaptive neuroplasticity across both peripheral and central levels of the swallowing network. Patient-specific impairment profiles, recovery stage, safety considerations, and available clinical resources should guide the selection of neuromodulation techniques. This subsection briefly summarizes the core mechanisms and clinical relevance of peripheral techniques, including PES, NMES, transcutaneous auricular vagus nerve stimulation (taVNS), and central neuromodulation methods such as tDCS and rTMS.

2.1 Pharyngeal Electrical Stimulation

Pharyngeal Electrical Stimulation (PES) is a peripheral neuromodulation technique that targets the sensory–motor swallowing network by directly stimulating the pharyngeal mucosa. The procedure uses an intraluminal catheter with embedded electrodes that deliver controlled electrical pulses to the pharyngeal wall, thereby activating pharyngeal sensory afferents in a highly localized manner (Cheng et al., 2022; Sasegbon et al., 2020; Stampanoni Bassi et al., 2025). PES activates mucosal afferent fibers primarily transmitted by the glossopharyngeal (IX) and vagus (X) cranial nerves. These afferent signals project to the nucleus tractus solitarius (NTS), which serves as the main sensory integration center of the swallowing network. From the NTS, signaling engages the brainstem central pattern generator. This activity then propagates to higher-order cortical regions involved in swallowing. As a result, PES provides both peripheral sensory facilitation and central excitatory modulation (Sasegbon et al., 2020; Stampanoni Bassi et al., 2025). Experimental studies support these neurophysiological effects. For example, seminal studies indicate that PES enhances cortical excitability within pharyngeal motor regions (Cheng et al., 2022; Sasegbon et al., 2020). Specifically, a 10-minute PES session produces a significant increase in pharyngeal motor-evoked potential (PMEP) amplitudes immediately after stimulation and again at 30 minutes post-exposure (Hamdy et al., 1998). Frequency optimization studies have identified 5 Hz stimulation at 75% of the maximum tolerated intensity as most effective for cortical facilitation (Fraser et al., 2002). The functional importance of these neurophysiological modifications is highlighted in experimental models (Cheng et al., 2022; Sasegbon et al., 2020). In the 'virtual lesion' model, low-frequency rTMS transiently suppresses cortical regions involved in swallowing. Notably, PES has been shown to reverse both neurophysiological suppression and the associated delays in swallowing reaction time (Jayasekeran et al., 2010). These findings underscore PES's ability to restore impaired sensorimotor integration and offer a mechanistic explanation for its therapeutic effects (Sasegbon et al., 2020).

Clinically, PES has been most thoroughly studied in post-stroke dysphagia (Stampanoni Bassi et al., 2025). Randomized controlled trials have shown that PES improves pharyngeal transit times, lowers Penetration–Aspiration Scale (PAS) scores, and supports the resumption of oral feeding (Fraser et al., 2002; Jayasekeran et al., 2010). Dose–response studies indicate that a single daily session over three consecutive days is the most effective protocol, whereas higher dosing yields diminishing returns, likely reflecting a neuroplasticity threshold (Jayasekeran et al., 2010). However, other studies (Bath et al., 2016; Vasant et al., 2016) have not demonstrated significant improvements compared with sham stimulation. To contextualize these variable trial-level findings, meta-analytic evidence offers a broader perspective on the potential therapeutic benefits of PES. Cheng et al.'s meta-analysis (2021), which synthesized data from 852 stroke patients across 26 randomized controlled trials, reported that PES was associated with a significant, moderate effect size on swallowing outcomes (Hedges' $g = 0.68$; 95% CI = 0.22–1.14; $p = 0.004$). Subsequently, Liu et al. (2024), in a systematic review of 6 RCTs involving 341 patients, similarly found that PES improved swallowing function, reduced dysphagia severity, and increased the rate of nasogastric tube removal, while effects on hospitalization duration were less consistent.

Beyond stroke-related dysphagia, PES has been investigated in several other neurogenic conditions, though the evidence base is smaller. In multiple sclerosis, an RCT showed significant improvements in swallowing safety up to four weeks after treatment (Restivo et al., 2013). Preliminary work also suggests potential benefit in dysphagia associated with Parkinson's disease, traumatic brain injury (TBI), and polyneuropathy (Sasegbon et al., 2020; Stampanoni Bassi et al., 2025). The most consistent findings come from tracheostomized patients in intensive care units. Both the Suntrup et al. (2015) study and the multicenter PHAST-TRAC trial (Dziewas et al., 2018) demonstrated higher decannulation rates with PES than with sham, while registry data indicate lower pneumonia and reintubation rates (Koestenberger et al., 2020). Overall, early evidence supports the broader applicability of PES, although larger condition-specific trials are needed (Sasegbon et al., 2020; Stampanoni Bassi et al., 2025).

In summary, PES's ability to engage pharyngeal afferent pathways and support central reorganization within the swallowing network positions it as a sensory-oriented, targeted neuromodulation approach. Its capacity to pair localized peripheral stimulation with measurable cortical effects suggests that PES may serve as a helpful adjunct in the rehabilitation of neurogenic dysphagia. As the evidence base continues to expand, PES is likely to maintain its role within comprehensive neurorehabilitation programs aimed at promoting safe, efficient, and physiologically coordinated swallowing function (Sasegbon et al., 2020; Stampanoni Bassi et al., 2025).

2.2. Neuromuscular Electrical Stimulation

Neuromuscular electrical stimulation (NMES) is an increasingly recognized peripheral neuromodulation approach used as an adjunct in dysphagia management. Electrical impulses delivered through surface electrodes over the suprahyoid and/or infrahyoid muscles stimulate muscle and nerve tissue, producing motor contractions and strong sensorimotor feedback (Cheng et al., 2022; Ebdah & Searl, 2024; Wang et al., 2024). The therapeutic effects of NMES are thought to arise not only from improvements in muscle strength and coordination but also from re-education of neural pathways associated with the swallowing reflex and prevention of muscle atrophy (Ebdah & Searl, 2024). At a neurophysiological level, NMES lowers the threshold for triggering the swallowing reflex by simultaneously activating low-threshold afferent fibers and motor pathways, thereby exerting a sensorimotor neuromodulatory influence that supports the reorganization of neural circuits involved in swallowing. Involuntary activation of the suprahyoid muscles facilitates hyoid elevation and enhances airway protection, while afferent stimulation increases the excitability of the central pattern generator via the nucleus tractus solitarius (Miller, Peters, and Ptok, 2022).

High-level evidence for the efficacy of NMES is primarily derived from meta-analyses. Wang et al. (2024) reviewed nine randomized controlled trials and found that NMES improves Functional Oral Intake Scale (FOIS) scores, reduces PAS scores, and enhances SWAL-QoL outcomes. These results support both the physiological and functional benefits of NMES. However, the analysis found no significant effects on the Water Swallow Test (WST), the Repetitive Saliva Swallowing Test (RSST), or the Dysphagia Outcome and Severity Scale (DOSS), suggesting that NMES efficacy varies across outcome domains and assessment tools.

A major limitation in NMES research is the substantial variability in stimulation parameters. Reported frequencies range from 25 to 120 Hz, and pulse widths from 300 to 1000 μs. Intensity criteria are inconsistently defined as 'sensory threshold,' 'motor threshold,' or 'maximum tolerable intensity.' Electrode placement also varies (suprahyoid, infrahyoid, or combined), and stimulation may be applied at rest, during voluntary swallowing, or with swallowing maneuvers. These factors substantially influence therapeutic outcomes (Miller, Peters, and Ptok, 2022).

This variability is also evident in clinical practice. An international survey of 122 clinicians across 19 countries found that NMES is used in approximately half of clinical settings, but only one-third of clinicians employ it consistently (Ebdah & Searl, 2024). Most clinicians reported that NMES receives limited attention during academic training (90%) and identified protocol heterogeneity (85%) and lack of expert consensus (86%) as major barriers. Among clinicians who routinely use NMES, 80% reported integrating it with behavioral therapies, most commonly strengthening exercises, swallowing maneuvers, and compensatory strategies.

Taken together, these data indicate that NMES is a valuable peripheral neuromodulation technique, demonstrating efficacy in reducing aspiration risk, enhancing hyoid elevation, and facilitating oral intake. However, current evidence strongly supports the use of NMES within multimodal therapeutic frameworks, particularly when combined with behavioral swallowing interventions to optimize neuroplastic outcomes. Looking forward, with refined stimulation parameters, increased standardization, and improved clinical training, NMES is expected to remain a key component of comprehensive rehabilitation for neurogenic dysphagia (Cheng et al., 2022; Wang et al., 2024).

2.3. Transcutaneous Auricular Vagus Nerve Stimulation

Transcutaneous auricular vagus nerve stimulation (taVNS) is a distinct form of peripheral neuromodulation that indirectly targets the swallowing network by stimulating the auricular branch of the vagus nerve (ABVN). Unlike PES and NMES, which deliver stimulation directly to the pharyngeal mucosa or swallowing-related musculature, taVNS engages vagal afferent pathways at the level of the external ear, providing a noninvasive gateway to brainstem and suprabrainstem swallowing circuits (Badran et al., 2018; Gerges et al., 2024; Pikov, 2025; Prabhu et al., 2024). Anatomically, the ABVN projects centrally to the NTS, the primary sensory integration hub of the swallowing network. From the NTS, afferent signaling propagates to the parabrachial nucleus, locus coeruleus, raphe nuclei, cerebellum, thalamus, insula, cingulate cortex, and frontal opercular regions, all of which play critical roles in sensorimotor integration and autonomic modulation of swallowing (Badran et al., 2018; Gerges et al., 2024; Pikov, 2025; Prabhu et al., 2024; Sun et al., 2025) (Figure 2). This widespread connectivity positions taVNS as a peripheral intervention capable of inducing system-level modulation of swallowing-related neural networks rather than merely localized sensory facilitation.

Neuroimaging studies provide strong mechanistic support for this model. Concurrent taVNS–fMRI investigations have consistently demonstrated activation of multiple cortical and subcortical regions. These regions—including the insula, anterior and mid-cingulate cortices, cerebellum, basal ganglia, and prefrontal cortex—are implicated in sensorimotor integration and neuroplastic mechanisms relevant to swallowing rehabilitation (Badran et al., 2018; Gerges et al., 2024). Importantly, stimulation of auricular sites with dense ABVN innervation—particularly the tragus and cymba conchae—produces significantly greater engagement of vagal afferent networks than stimulation of non-vagal ear regions. This finding indicates that taVNS is not merely a form of somatosensory stimulation but represents a biologically active mode of vagal neuromodulation (Badran et al., 2018; Gerges et al., 2024; Pikov, 2025).

Clinical evidence for the therapeutic efficacy of taVNS in neurogenic dysphagia is most robust in post-stroke populations. In a sham-controlled, double-blind, randomized trial, taVNS combined with conventional swallowing therapy resulted in significantly greater improvements in swallowing function than sham stimulation, as measured by the Modified Mann Assessment of Swallowing Ability (MASA), the Functional Communication Measure (FCM), and the PAS (Wang et al., 2023). Notably, these improvements persisted for at least 4 weeks after treatment, suggesting durable neuromodulatory effects rather than transient facilitation. Subdomain analyses further demonstrated improvements in tongue movement and strength, saliva control, cough reflex, and soft palate function, highlighting taVNS's capacity to influence multiple physiological components of swallowing (Gerges et al., 2024; Wang et al., 2023).

From a mechanistic perspective, taVNS appears to promote adaptive neuroplasticity by modulating ascending neuromodulatory systems. These include noradrenergic and serotonergic pathways originating in the locus coeruleus and raphe nuclei, which are known to facilitate learning-dependent plasticity and motor recovery (Badran et al., 2018; Gerges et al., 2024; Pikov, 2025). These mechanisms suggest that taVNS may enhance the effects of task-specific swallowing therapy when paired with behavioral training. Accordingly, taVNS may be conceptualized as a peripheral–central hybrid intervention that links bottom-up sensory afferent stimulation with top-down cortical reorganization (Gerges et al., 2024; Pikov, 2025; Sun et al., 2025).

Taken together, taVNS broadens the scope of peripheral neuromodulation in dysphagia rehabilitation by providing a noninvasive, well-tolerated approach to engage central swallowing networks via vagal afferent pathways. Evidence synthesized from clinical trials and scoping reviews indicates that taVNS is safe and feasible. When integrated into multimodal rehabilitation frameworks, taVNS is also associated with sustained functional gains in post-stroke dysphagia (Gerges et al., 2024; Pikov, 2025; Wang et al., 2023).

Figure 2. Brain network activation associated with transcutaneous auricular vagus nerve stimulation (NTS: the nucleus tractus solitarius; PB: parabrachial nucleus; LC: locus coeruleus; CB: cerebellum; Hip: hippocampus; Amg: amygdala; BG: basal ganglia; Cing: cingulate cortex; PFC: prefrontal cortex) (Sun et al., 2025).

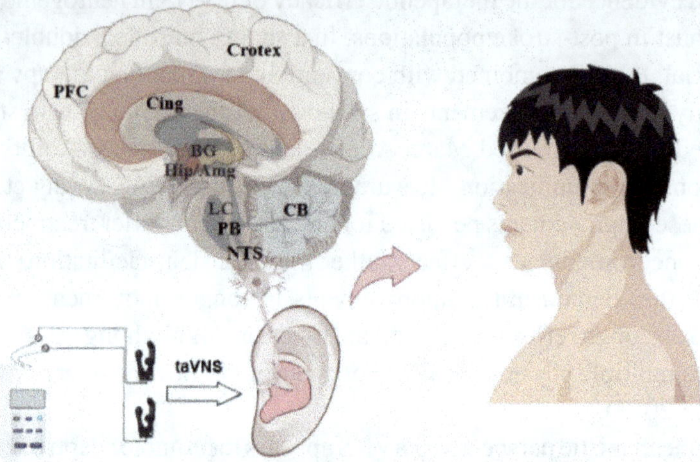

2.4. Transcranial Direct Current Stimulation

Transcranial direct current stimulation (tDCS) is a noninvasive brain stimulation technique that modulates cortical neuronal membrane potentials by applying low-intensity direct current via scalp electrodes (Cheng et al., 2022; Sasegbon et al., 2020; Stampanoni Bassi et al., 2025). Anodal stimulation increases cortical excitability by depolarizing the resting membrane potential, whereas cathodal stimulation induces a hyperpolarizing shift, resulting in an inhibitory effect (Sasegbon et al., 2020; Stampanoni Bassi et al., 2025).

tDCS has been shown to modulate the swallowing motor cortex and associated physiological functions in healthy individuals. Jefferson et al. (2009) provided early evidence that anodal tDCS applied to the swallowing motor cortex increases cortical excitability in the targeted hemisphere. Subsequent studies indicate that tDCS effects extend beyond modulation of cortical excitability. Notably, tDCS can reverse swallowing impairments induced by cortical inhibition in "virtual lesion" paradigms, supporting a restorative effect on disrupted swallowing networks (Vasant et al., 2014). Additionally, high-resolution pharyngeal manometry research by Doeltgen et al. (2018) demonstrated that anodal tDCS increases bolus transit through the upper esophageal sphincter, suggesting measurable effects on peripheral swallowing biomechanics.

Across multiple clinical studies involving individuals with post-stroke dysphagia, anodal tDCS protocols have yielded clinically meaningful improvements (Cheng et al., 2021; Sasegbon et al., 2020; Stampanoni Bassi et al., 2025). Kumar et al. (2011) found that a five-session course of 2-mA anodal tDCS produced significant gains in DOSS scores. Similarly, Shigematsu et al. (2013) observed that a 10-session anodal tDCS protocol administered during the acute post-stroke stage produced therapeutic effects lasting up to 1 month. In a large-sample RCT, Suntrup-Krueger et al. (2018) reported that anodal tDCS improved Fiberoptic Endoscopic Dysphagia Severity Scale (FEDSS) scores after acute stroke and enhanced swallowing network activity in the stimulated hemisphere. Collectively, these findings indicate that tDCS facilitates early cortical reorganization during both the acute and subacute phases of stroke recovery. Duan et al. (2025) recently conducted a randomized controlled study in individuals with hemispheric stroke, demonstrating that anodal tDCS significantly improved swallowing function and concurrently increased cortical activity as measured by EEG. These results provide robust evidence that the therapeutic impact of tDCS extends beyond behavioral improvement, producing measurable electrophysiological signatures of neural enhancement (Duan et al., 2025).

tDCS has also demonstrated therapeutic potential in neurogenic dysphagia beyond stroke. In multiple sclerosis, where swallowing impairment is relatively common, preliminary evidence is promising but limited. Cosentino et al. (2018) found that anodal tDCS applied to the swallowing motor cortex produced modest yet significant improvements in DOSS scores, with effects persisting for up to one month in a small uncontrolled sample. In a more rigorous sham-controlled RCT, Restivo et al. (2019) showed that a five-session anodal tDCS protocol significantly improved VFS-based swallowing outcomes in MS-related dysphagia.

The effectiveness of tDCS protocols varies considerably depending on electrode montage and current polarity. Prevailing clinical evidence indicates that unilateral contralesional anodal stimulation provides the most consistent therapeutic benefits (Cheng et al., 2021; Sasegbon et al., 2020). In contrast, bilateral stimulation protocols have produced mixed results. Some studies have reported favorable outcomes with bilateral approaches (e.g., Yuan et al., 2017), whereas others (Ahn et al., 2017; Pingue et al., 2018) found no significant advantage of bilateral stimulation over sham conditions.

tDCS is considered one of the most well-tolerated noninvasive brain stimulation techniques. Across more than 100 sham-controlled clinical trials involving both healthy individuals and clinical populations, no serious adverse events have been reported. Reported side effects are generally mild and transient, most commonly including scalp tingling, slight burning sensations, or mild headache, all of which can be minimized through proper skin and electrode preparation (Cheng et al., 2022; Sasegbon et al., 2020).

2.5. Repetitive Transcranial Magnetic Stimulation

Repetitive transcranial magnetic stimulation (rTMS) is a non-invasive neuromodulation technique that induces electrical currents in cortical neurons via rapidly changing magnetic fields, thereby modulating synaptic transmission and cortical excitability in a frequency-dependent manner (Sasegbon et al., 2020). Swallowing is not merely a brainstem-mediated reflex. Rather, it is a complex sensorimotor process that requires integrated activity across cortical, subcortical, and cerebellar networks. Following neurological insults such as stroke, these networks often show pronounced disruption and hemispheric imbalance, making cortical excitability a critical therapeutic target for restoring swallowing function. For this reason, rTMS has emerged as an increasingly important intervention capable of directly modulating the cortical mechanisms underlying dysphagia (Sasegbon et al., 2020; Yang et al., 2021).

The neurophysiological foundation of rTMS is closely tied to its frequency-dependent effects. Low-frequency stimulation ($\leq$1 Hz) exerts an inhibitory influence by reducing cortical excitability, whereas high-frequency stimulation ($\geq$1 Hz) enhances excitability by facilitating synaptic activity (Wen et al., 2022; Yang et al., 2021). Within this framework, two primary models have been proposed to explain how neurostimulation may promote recovery from post-stroke dysphagia (Sasegbon et al., 2020). The first model suggests that, in some patients, improvement is associated with increased recruitment of corticobulbar pathways within the intact hemisphere, indicating that this hemisphere may support swallowing through compensatory activation. (Sasegbon et al., 2020; Wen et al., 2022). The second model emphasizes the interhemispheric imbalance that arises after unilateral brain injury; stroke often disrupts the reciprocal inhibitory equilibrium between the hemispheres, leading the intact hemisphere to exert excessive inhibitory influence over the damaged side. Accordingly, rTMS can be directed either to reduce this maladaptive inhibition via low-frequency stimulation of the intact hemisphere or to enhance excitability in the lesioned hemisphere through high-frequency stimulation, with both approaches reflecting complementary neuroplasticity mechanisms (Peng et al., 2025; Sasegbon et al., 2020; Wen et al., 2022; Yang et al., 2021) (Figure 3).

Figure 3. Interhemispheric modulation with low- and high-frequency rTMS

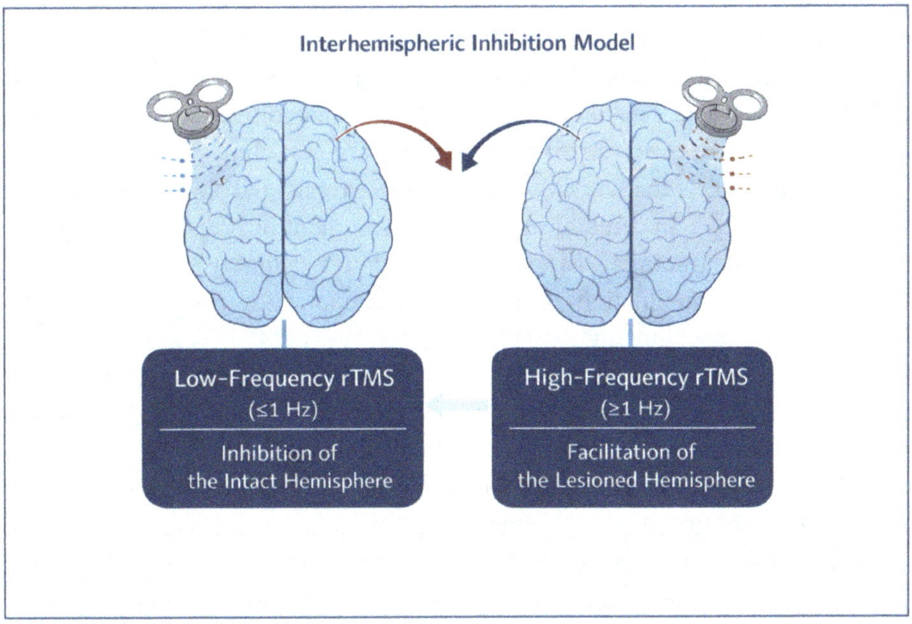

In addition to unilateral approaches, bilateral rTMS protocols have attracted attention as strategies for concurrently modulating both hemispheres. Existing studies report that this approach, which involves simultaneous modulation of both hemispheres, can improve swallowing safety, pharyngeal-phase function, and cortical excitability in some patients (Park et al., 2017; Zhang et al., 2019). Consistent with this overall trend, a recent meta-analysis (Peng et al., 2025) demonstrated that bilateral cerebral rTMS provides a more pronounced therapeutic benefit for post-stroke dysphagia compared with unilateral stimulation. These findings collectively suggest that bilateral stimulation may, in specific clinical profiles, provide broader or more effective neuromodulation than unilateral approaches. However, outcomes can still vary depending on lesion characteristics, stimulation parameters, and recovery stage (Peng et al., 2025; Sasegbon et al., 2020).

A notable development in recent years is the use of cerebellar rTMS as a therapeutic target in dysphagia rehabilitation. The cerebellum plays a central role in the temporal precision, coordination, and adaptive motor control required for effective swallowing, making it a biologically plausible site for neuromodulator intervention (Peng et al., 2025). Early experimental evidence provided foundational support for this approach. Jayasekeran et al. (2011) demonstrated that cerebellar stimulation can facilitate cortico-bulbar projections involved in swallowing, while Sasegbon et al. (2019) reported rapid increases in pharyngeal motor cortex excitability following cerebellar rTMS, further highlighting its capacity to modulate supramedullary components of the swallowing network. Further supporting this line of evidence, a meta-analysis by Liu et al. (2024) showed that cerebellar rTMS combined with traditional swallowing exercises produced significantly greater improvements in post-stroke dysphagia than exercises alone, suggesting an additive therapeutic benefit. More recently, Peng et al. (2025) provided the strongest clinical evidence to date, demonstrating that cerebellar rTMS can yield more robust and clinically meaningful therapeutic effects than cerebral rTMS in the treatment of post-stroke dysphagia. Collectively, these findings position the cerebellum as a highly effective and clinically relevant neuromodulation target within contemporary dysphagia rehabilitation.

Across the broader literature, the clinical benefits of rTMS have been consistently documented. Systematic reviews and meta-analyses report that rTMS improves swallowing function in patients with post-stroke dysphagia (Lin et al., 2025; Peng et al., 2025; Sasegbon et al., 2020; Stampanoni Bassi et al., 2025; Wen et al., 2022; Yang et al., 2021). Regarding safety, rTMS demonstrates a favorable tolerability profile across clinical studies. The most common mild, transient adverse events include headache and dizziness (Peng et al., 2025), and the risk of seizure remains extremely low (<0.03%) when established safety guidelines are followed (Cheng et al., 2022). Taken together, current evidence indicates that rTMS is a robust neuromodulation method capable of supporting the cortical and cerebellar reorganization required for swallowing recovery. Its ability to exert both inhibitory and excitatory effects, target either hemisphere, and modulate cerebellar circuits sets it apart from other neuromodulation techniques. However, as highlighted in the meta-analysis by Shen et al. (2024), the overall strength of the evidence is limited by methodological flaws and substantial heterogeneity across systematic reviews. The quality of the available evidence ranges from high to low, with most reported outcomes supported by only moderate-level evidence. Consequently, further rigorously designed, standardized, and comprehensive clinical studies are needed to more definitively establish the long-term efficacy and safety of repetitive transcranial magnetic stimulation for post-stroke dysphagia.

From a clinical standpoint, neuromodulation techniques should be implemented as adjunctive components of individualized, multimodal dysphagia rehabilitation programs rather than as standalone interventions. Clinical decision-making should integrate neuromodulation modality, stimulation parameters, and timing with patient-specific factors such as lesion characteristics, disease stage, cognitive status, and concurrent behavioral therapy to maximize functional outcomes and safety.

In conclusion, current evidence indicates that neuromodulation techniques have significant therapeutic potential for the rehabilitation of neurogenic dysphagia by targeting both peripheral and central components of the swallowing network. Peripheral interventions, such as PES and NMES, enhance afferent sensory drive and muscle activation, thereby strengthening brainstem–cortical integration through bottom-up mechanisms. In contrast, tDCS and rTMS directly modulate cortical and cerebellar excitability, supporting adaptive neuroplasticity via top-down pathways (see Tables 1 and 2). Despite these mechanistic differences, the literature consistently shows that neuromodulation can produce measurable neurophysiological improvements that translate into better swallowing safety, efficiency, and oral intake.

However, heterogeneity in stimulation parameters, patient characteristics, and outcome measures limits the comparability and generalizability of existing findings, and long-term effects remain insufficiently explored. Thus, rigorously designed, standardized multicenter trials are needed to clarify optimal protocols, identify patient-specific predictors of treatment response, and determine the durability of therapeutic gains. Even so, the growing evidence base positions neuromodulation as an increasingly valuable adjunct within individualized, multimodal rehabilitation programs for neurogenic dysphagia.

Table 1. Neuromodulation mechanisms in dysphagia rehabilitation.

Feature	rTMS (Central)	tDCS (Central)	NMES (Peripheral)	PES (Peripheral)	taVNS (Peripheral)
Delivery route	Scalp coil (non-invasive brain stimulation)	Scalp surface electrodes	Transcutaneous surface electrode pads	Intraluminal catheter positioned in the pharynx	Transcutaneous auricular stimulation (tragus / cymba conchae)
Primary target	Swallowing-related cortex and/or cerebellum	The swallowing motor cortex (pharyngeal motor cortex)	Swallowing-related muscles and motor axons	Pharyngeal sensory afferents (CN IX, CN X branches)	Auricular branch of the vagus nerve sensory afferents
Mechanism of action	Modulates synaptic plasticity and cortical excitability via magnetic pulses (frequency-dependent excitatory or inhibitory effects)	Alters neuronal firing threshold via weak direct current (anodal vs. cathodal polarity)	Depolarizes motor axons, inducing muscle contraction and strengthening with strong sensorimotor feedback	Dense sensory input activates the brainstem NTS and indirectly increases motor cortical excitability	Activates vagal afferent pathways via NTS and locus coeruleus, promoting ACh and NE release and facilitating global cortical plasticity
Focality	Relatively high cortical focality	Less focal; broader cortical engagement depending on montage	Less focal; current traverses skin and tissue layers	More focal; energy delivered directly to the pharyngeal mucosa	Peripheral nerve targeting with system-level neuromodulatory effects

Abbreviations: rTMS = repetitive transcranial magnetic stimulation; tDCS = transcranial direct current stimulation; NMES = neuromuscular electrical stimulation; PES = pharyngeal electrical stimulation; taVNS = transcutaneous auricular vagus nerve stimulation; NTS = nucleus tractus solitarius; ACh = acetylcholine; NE = norepinephrine.

Table 2. Evidence and clinical application of neuromodulation in dysphagia

Feature	rTMS (Central)	tDCS (Central)	NMES (Peripheral)	PES (Peripheral)	taVNS (Peripheral)
Evidence level in PSD	Highest efficacy for improving swallowing function (SUCRA[1] = **87.3%**)	Second-best for improving swallowing function (SUCRA = **75.3%**); second for QoL outcomes	Highest efficacy for improving quality of life (SUCRA = **79.3%**)	Strong evidence for increasing decannulation rates in severe dysphagia and tracheostomized patients	Accelerates recovery of swallowing function in acute stroke (e.g., MASA, PAS)
Clinical role	Direct modulation of cortical/cerebellar swallowing networks	Facilitates early cortical reorganization	Adjunct to behavioral therapy to enhance motor performance	Sensory-driven facilitation of brainstem–cortical integration	Peripheral–central hybrid neuromodulation paired with task-specific therapy
Key considerations	Equipment is bulky and costly (~**USD 35,000**); very low seizure risk (**<0.03%**)	Compact, portable, and relatively low cost (~**USD 1,500**); safe and well-tolerated	Considerable heterogeneity in protocols and parameters; typically combined with conventional therapy	Requires catheter placement; CE-approved for treatment of neurogenic dysphagia	Noninvasive; clinical improvements may persist ≥4 weeks post-treatment

Abbreviations: rTMS = repetitive transcranial magnetic stimulation; tDCS = transcranial direct current stimulation; NMES = neuromuscular electrical stimulation; PES = pharyngeal electrical stimulation; taVNS = transcutaneous auricular vagus nerve stimulation; NTS = nucleus tractus solitarius; PSD = post-stroke dysphagia; MASA = Mann Assessment of Swallowing Ability; PAS = Penetration–Aspiration Scale; QoL = quality of life.

3. THE USE OF SURFACE ELECTROMYOGRAPHY (sEMG) IN DYSPHAGIA MANAGEMENT

Early diagnosis and effective management of dysphagia are important for reducing patient morbidity and mortality (Kang et al., 2022; Selen Akıl et al., 2024). In this context, surface electromyography (sEMG) has an increasingly important role in the objective, non-invasive, and quantitative assessment of swallowing function. This subsection will address the purpose of sEMG applications and usage in dysphagia-related studies and its role in diagnostic evaluation and the rehabilitation process.

3.1. Purposes of sEMG Use in Dysphagia Literature

Swallowing requires the synchronized, sequential activation of oropharyngeal muscles during the act (Matsuo & Palmer, 2008). sEMG device records the electrical activity of the swallowing muscles via electrodes placed on the skin surface (Ye-Lin et al., 2022). sEMG is a useful method for examining muscle function because it records electrical signals that directly reflect muscle activation and contraction (Perlman, 2006).

The basic unit of muscle contraction is the motor unit. A motor unit consists of a motor neuron, the axon of the motor neuron, the neuromuscular junction, and the muscle fibers innervated by that specific motor neuron. A muscle fiber carries a constant membrane potential at rest. When a nerve impulse reaches the neuromuscular junction, acetylcholine is released, and the muscle fiber depolarizes. In this way, muscle contraction initiates, and depolarization observed during muscle contraction creates an electrical field. This is called the Motor Unit Action Potential (MUAP) (Perlman, 2006). sEMG is applied non-invasively from the skin surface. It is usually placed over the motor point of the muscle or muscle group to be evaluated. Therefore, the activations recorded with sEMG are not from a single motor unit but are the spatial and temporal sum of the action potentials of all muscle fibers near the electrode. The activation signal obtained with sEMG also consists of the sum of the MUAPs in the electrode's detection area (Perlman, 2006). The main purposes of sEMG in dysphagia studies are as follows:

3.1.1. Understanding Normal Swallowing Physiology

Studies have assessed swallowing patterns, muscle activation sequences, and intensities in healthy individuals to describe reference parameters of normal swallowing function (Crary et al., 2007; Monaco et al., 2008; Zhu et al., 2017). At the same time, sEMG has been used to evaluate dynamic characteristics, revealing temporal and spatial relationships among the muscles involved in swallowing (Zhu et al., 2017). According to the common findings of studies, although there is no single swallowing pattern in healthy individuals, the muscles that show the highest activation during swallowing are the suprahyoid muscles in the submental region. It has been reported that during swallowing, the suprahyoid muscles work in synergy with the infrahyoid and masticatory muscles, and that swallowing activations vary with factors such as bolus type, consistency, amount, and body position.

3.1.2. Screening and Diagnostic Tool

The usability of sEMG data has been investigated for the diagnosis of conditions such as neurogenic dysphagia and for differential diagnosis between oral and pharyngeal dysphagia (Vaiman & Nahlieli, 2009). Since neurogenic dysphagia is a common condition that can lead to serious complications, early diagnosis and management strategies are important (Ertekin, 2015; Panebianco et al., 2020). Neurophysiological assessment methods such as sEMG have been described as reliable, inexpensive, and easily applicable quantitative tests for detecting and monitoring both clinical and subclinical dysphagia (Ertekin, 2015). In this context, the "Dysphagia Limit" concept emerges as the most important diagnostic method. Patients suspected of having swallowing disorders can benefit from a simple diagnostic screening with sEMG before being referred for further evaluation

(Vaiman & Eviatar, 2009; Vaiman & Nahlieli, 2009). The dysphagia limit is a test derived from sEMG signals that helps quantify differences between normal and abnormal swallowing. Dysphagia limit refers to the maximum volume of liquid an individual can swallow in a single swallow. Individuals are asked to swallow 1, 3, 5, 10, 15, 20, and 30 ml of liquid in a single swallow. Piecemeal deglutition determines the dysphagia limit volume when more than one swallowing activation is observed. The normal dysphagia limit in healthy individuals is 20 ml (Ertekin et al., 1996). This testing method stands out as a reliable, cost-effective, and easy-to-administer quantitative assessment with the potential to detect and monitor both clinical and subclinical dysphagia (Ertekin, 2015; Ertekin et al., 1998).

3.1.3. Objective Monitoring of Treatment Effectiveness

With the widespread use of sEMG over the years, it has frequently been used to determine the effects of accepted rehabilitation practices, particularly on suprahyoid muscle activation, and to demonstrate treatment effectiveness (Chang et al., 2021; Sze et al., 2016; Wheeler-Hegland et al., 2008; White et al., 2008). It is also frequently used to objectively evaluate the effectiveness of newly developed therapeutic strategies, such as maneuvers and exercises (Cengiz et al., 2024; Park et al.,

2020; Yaşaroğlu et al., 2024). In particular, changes in muscle activation following rehabilitation provide valuable information regarding clinical significance.

3.1.4. Bolus Characterization

sEMG signals can exhibit different patterns depending on the characteristics of the ingested food or liquid. A recent study combined sEMG signals from the sternocleidomastoid muscle during swallowing with a motion-tracking sensor on the elbow that records eating and drinking movements (Hassan et al., 2024). According to the study's results, the daily intake and volume of liquids and solid foods were estimated with high accuracy. This offers hope for non-invasive monitoring of real-time eating and drinking events. It also indicates potential applicability in situations other than dysphagia, such as obesity and diabetes monitoring and management.

3.2. The role of sEMG in Assessment

sEMG provides several parameters for quantitative assessment of swallowing function, which provide important clues for diagnosing dysphagia. While non-instrumental assessment tools often yield subjective results, sEMG provides objective, detailed data (Ye-Lin et al., 2022).

3.2.1.Muscle Activation Patterns and Timing

sEMG provides precise information about the onset, duration, peak, and average values of swallowing muscle activation (Perlman, 2006; Suarez-Patiño et al., 2024). In patients with neurogenic oropharyngeal dysphagia, comparing muscle activation timing with the timing of bolus passage through anatomical structures may aid diagnosis when combined with instrumental assessment methods (Suarez-Patiño et al., 2024).

3.2.2. Signal Amplitude

Signal amplitude, which reflects the intensity of muscle activation, may indicate muscle weakness or insufficient activation. However, it should be remembered that although sEMG signals and the magnitude of activation are highly correlated with muscle strength, they do not represent actual muscle strength (Uysal, 2024). The greater the activation recorded during a therapeutic strategy, the more muscle from which the signal is collected is thought to be involved in that activity.

From a clinical decision-making perspective, sEMG findings can inform treatment selection by identifying specific impairments in muscle activation timing, coordination, or amplitude. Repeated sEMG measurements enable objective monitoring of therapeutic response over time and support outcome interpretation when combined with instrumental assessments such as VFSS or FEES. In this way, sEMG serves not only as a descriptive assessment tool but also as a clinically actionable measure guiding individualized dysphagia management.

3.3. The Role of sEMG in Rehabilitation and Therapeutic Applications

sEMG is used for both diagnostic and therapeutic purposes in dysphagia management. The use of it as a biofeedback, in particular, increases patient participation. sEMG biofeedback enables patients to instantly monitor the activity of the muscles involved in swallowing through visual or auditory feedback. This method stands out as one that supports motor learning, improves the effectiveness of swallowing therapy, and enhances swallowing skills (Bykova, 2024; Constantinescu & Garcia, 2024).

3.3.1. Guides Maneuvers and Exercises

sEMG biofeedback can increase muscle activity during swallowing therapy, which can improve maneuver or exercise performance (Archer et al., 2021; Benfield et al., 2019). sEMG biofeedback, applied by showing the patient their muscle activation during an effortful swallowing maneuver, has been shown to increase the effectiveness of the maneuver in geriatric patients (Archer et al., 2021). Also, it has been stated that patients find it easy to apply because their muscle activation increases during the maneuver, thereby increasing comprehensibility. In a study of patients with Parkinson's Disease, sEMG biofeedback applied during dry swallows and food-swallowing tasks resulted in significant improvements in patients' functional oral intake scores and residue status (Battel & Walshe, 2023). It has been shown that sEMG biofeedback applied after an acute stroke resulted in significant improvement in penetration and aspiration scores and dysphagia severity (Benfield et al., 2023).

3.3.2. Pediatric Applications

It has been stated that sEMG can be applied during swallowing therapy in pediatric populations (e.g., dysphagia-associated conditions such as cerebral palsy) (Bykova, 2024). Although sEMG is used for research purposes as an assessment tool, there are insufficient application examples regarding the potential of sEMG biofeedback in pediatric dysphagia management. As it is a potential tool for motor learning, there is a need for more sEMG biofeedback research (Bykova, 2024).

3.3.3. Evidence of Effectiveness

A systematic review and meta-analysis demonstrated that swallowing therapy supported by biofeedback significantly increased hyolaryngeal elevation in adults with dysphagia (Benfield et al., 2019). However, it has been stated that more research is needed to examine the marked improvement in broader clinical outcomes, such as functional oral intake or reduced dependence on tube feeding (Benfield et al., 2019). This indicates that biofeedback has mechanical effects, but its impact on clinical outcomes remains unclear.

3.4. Limitations of sEMG and Future Studies

The widespread use of sEMG in dysphagia studies involves methodological differences, including electrode placement, data-collection task, and normalization procedures. To interpret these differences in broader populations, standardized protocols need to be developed. Also, integrating sEMG biofeedback into game-based exercise methods designed using accelerometers could create an innovative treatment strategy aligned with motor learning principles, both in adult and pediatric populations with dysphagia.

Table 3 summarizes the clinical roles, evidence maturity, and practical considerations of the assessment-oriented technologies discussed in Sections 1 and 3. Across these innovations, evidence maturity varies. Some tools are currently feasible for clinician-supervised decision support (e.g., selected AI-assisted VFSS/FEES workflows and standardized sEMG protocols). In contrast, other approaches remain primarily investigational and should be used within structured implementation or research pathways (e.g., AI-based acoustic screening in unsupervised community settings).

Table 3. Assessment-oriented emerging technologies in dysphagia management.

Technology	Primary role	Clinical context	Evidence maturity	Key notes
AI-assisted VFSS/FEES analysis	Automated, objective interpretation	Instrumental assessment in clinical settings	Emerging	Decision support. Requires validation and clinician oversight
AI-based screening (signals/sounds)	Early screening and monitoring	Community, home, low-access settings	Emerging	Useful for triage; not a standalone diagnostic tool
sEMG assessment	Objective quantification of muscle activity	Screening, differential diagnosis, outcome tracking	Moderate	Protocol standardization needed

Building on this assessment framework, Table 4 synthesizes intervention-oriented technologies that support clinical decision-making across rehabilitation contexts. From a clinical decision-making perspective, intervention selection is typically guided by (i) impairment profile (sensory, motor, or cortical control), (ii) setting and available resources (home-based versus specialized center), and (iii) safety and monitoring requirements.

Table 4. Intervention-oriented emerging technologies in dysphagia management

Technology	Primary role	Typical application	Evidence maturity	Key notes
AI-enabled therapy / digital feedback	Personalized training and adherence	Home-based or hybrid rehabilitation	Emerging	Best for motivated patients with supervision
PES	Peripheral sensory neuromodulation	Post-stroke, ICU/tracheostomy patients	Moderate	Adjunct to behavioral therapy
NMES	Muscle activation and sensorimotor input	Multimodal swallowing therapy	Moderate	Parameter standardization required
taVNS	Vagal afferent neuromodulation	Post-stroke dysphagia (early evidence)	Emerging	Paired with task-specific therapy
tDCS	Cortical excitability modulation	Acute/subacute stroke rehabilitation	Moderate	Protocol fidelity essential
rTMS	Cortical/cerebellar neuromodulation	Specialized neurorehabilitation centers	Moderate	High resource requirements
sEMG biofeedback	Motor learning and performance monitoring	Exercise-based swallowing therapy	Emerging–Moderate	Functional outcome evidence evolving

4. DIGITAL TECHNOLOGIES IN DYSPHAGIA REHABILITATION

Digital technologies have emerged as a transformative force in dysphagia rehabilitation, offering personalized exercise delivery, remote monitoring, real-time feedback, and enhanced accessibility. Recent evidence demonstrates that digital health solutions lead to measurable improvements in swallowing physiology, functional performance, treatment adherence, and patient engagement (Hwang et al., 2025). Digital dysphagia interventions can be broadly categorized into three primary modalities: (1) mHealth-based home rehabilitation, (2) synchronous telepractice and remote supervision, and (3) game-based and sensor-driven biofeedback systems.

mHealth applications provide structured swallowing exercises, supported by video demonstrations and real-time feedback mechanisms. These programs have been shown to enhance swallowing physiology, improve performance, and increase quality of life while maintaining high patient adherence rates (Hwang et al., 2025). Consistent findings have been reported in tele-intervention studies among individuals with head and neck cancer, where home-based telerehabilitation improved swallowing safety, oral intake, nutritional status, and emotional well-being, while also demonstrating intense patient satisfaction and cost-effectiveness (Yang et al., 2023).

Telepractice-based dysphagia rehabilitation has become particularly critical in the post-pandemic era. Synchronous video-based therapy allows clinicians to supervise exercise execution, provide immediate feedback, offer educational support, and maintain motivational engagement. This model effectively overcomes geographic, mobility-related, and health-related barriers to care, enabling a more continuous and equitable rehabilitation process (Yang et al., 2023).

A rapidly expanding domain within digital rehabilitation involves *gamified and AI-enhanced biofeedback technologies*. These systems use surface electromyography, pressure sensors, accelerometers, or computer vision algorithms to convert physiological activity into interactive visual displays. Grounded in motor learning principles, such platforms increase patient motivation, support accurate skill acquisition, and provide objective performance tracking. A randomized controlled trial evaluating an AI-based video game intervention demonstrated significant improvements in swallowing function, oral intake, nutritional status, and quality of life in post-stroke patients, with markedly higher adherence and satisfaction compared with standard care (Zhang et al., 2025). These results align with broader evidence underscoring the essential role of biofeedback in facilitating motor control adaptations during swallowing rehabilitation (Huckabee et al., 2023).

Despite their promise, several challenges limit the widespread adoption of digital dysphagia technologies. Barriers include digital illiteracy, inequities in device and internet access, technical malfunctions, and the absence of standardized, evidence-based digital rehabilitation protocols (Hwang et al., 2025). In addition, AI-enabled and telehealth solutions require explicit attention to data privacy, informed consent, and secure storage of audiovisual health records, particularly when deployed outside hospital networks. Equity considerations are also critical, as technology-assisted care may widen disparities unless low-resource implementation pathways are actively incorporated. For future implementation, experts emphasize the need for adaptive exercise progression models, automated performance monitoring, and hybrid therapy structures that blend technological innovations with clinician oversight (Yang et al., 2023).

Taken together, current evidence positions digital technologies as powerful, complementary, and, in some cases, primary modalities in dysphagia rehabilitation. With continued advancements in artificial intelligence, sensor engineering, and immersive environments, dysphagia management is expected to evolve toward more personalized, continuous, accessible, and neurophysiologically targeted therapeutic paradigms (Duchac, 2025).

REFERENCES

Ahn, Y. H., Sohn, H. J., Park, J. S., Ahn, T. G., Shin, Y. B., Park, M., Ko, S. H., & Shin, Y. I. (2017). Effect of bihemispheric anodal transcranial direct current stimulation for dysphagia in chronic stroke patients: A randomized clinical trial. *Journal of Rehabilitation Medicine*, *49*(1), 30–35. DOI: 10.2340/16501977-2170 PMID: 27904911

Alfonsi, E., Bergamaschi, R., Cosentino, G., Ponzio, M., Montomoli, C., Restivo, D. A., Brighina, F., Ravaglia, S., Prunetti, P., Bertino, G., Benazzo, M., Fontana, D., & Moglia, A. (2013). Electrophysiological patterns of oropharyngeal swallowing in multiple sclerosis. *Clinical Neurophysiology*, *124*(8), 1638–1645. DOI: 10.1016/j.clinph.2013.03.003 PMID: 23601703

Alowais, S. A., Alghamdi, S. S., Alsuhebany, N., Alqahtani, T., Alshaya, A. I., Almohareb, S. N., Aldairem, A., Alrashed, M., Bin Saleh, K., Badreldin, H. A., Al Yami, M. S., Al Harbi, S., & Albekairy, A. M. (2023). Revolutionizing healthcare: The role of artificial intelligence in clinical practice. *BMC Medical Education*, *23*(1), 689. DOI: 10.1186/s12909-023-04698-z PMID: 37740191

Archer, S. K., Smith, C. H., & Newham, D. J. (2021). Surface Electromyographic Biofeedback and the Effortful Swallow Exercise for Stroke-Related Dysphagia and in Healthy Ageing. *Dysphagia*, *36*(2), 281–292. DOI: 10.1007/s00455-020-10129-8 PMID: 32445060

Badran, B. W., Dowdle, L. T., Mithoefer, O. J., LaBate, N. T., Coatsworth, J., Brown, J. C., DeVries, W. H., Austelle, C. W., McTeague, L. M., & George, M. S. (2018). Neurophysiologic effects of transcutaneous auricular vagus nerve stimulation (taVNS) via electrical stimulation of the tragus: A concurrent taVNS/fMRI study and review. *Brain Stimulation*, *11*(3), 492–500. DOI: 10.1016/j.brs.2017.12.009 PMID: 29361441

Bath, P. M., Scutt, P., Love, J., Clavé, P., Cohen, D., Dziewas, R., Iversen, H. K., Ledl, C., Ragab, S., Soda, H., Warusevitane, A., Woisard, V., & Hamdy, S. (2016). Pharyngeal Electrical Stimulation for Treatment of Dysphagia in Subacute Stroke: A Randomized Controlled Trial. *Stroke*, *47*(6), 1562–1570. DOI: 10.1161/STROKEAHA.115.012455 PMID: 27165955

Battel, I., & Walshe, M. (2023). An intensive neurorehabilitation programme with sEMG biofeedback to improve swallowing in idiopathic Parkinson's disease (IPD): A feasibility study. *International Journal of Language & Communication Disorders*, *58*(3), 813–825. DOI: 10.1111/1460-6984.12824 PMID: 36478035

Benfield, J. K., Everton, L. F., Bath, P. M., & England, T. J. (2019). Does Therapy With Biofeedback Improve Swallowing in Adults With Dysphagia? A Systematic Review and Meta-Analysis. *Archives of Physical Medicine and Rehabilitation*, *100*(3), 551–561. DOI: 10.1016/j.apmr.2018.04.031 PMID: 29859178

Benfield, J. K., Hedstrom, A., Everton, L. F., Bath, P. M., & England, T. J. (2023). Randomized controlled feasibility trial of swallow strength and skill training with surface electromyographic biofeedback in acute stroke patients with dysphagia. *Journal of Oral Rehabilitation*, *50*(6), 440–451. DOI: 10.1111/joor.13437 PMID: 36810785

Burdea, G., Kim, N., Polistico, K., Kadaru, A., Grampurohit, N., Roll, D., & Damiani, F. (2021). Assistive game controller for artificial intelligence-enhanced telerehabilitation post-stroke. *Assistive Technology*, *33*(3), 117–128. DOI: 10.1080/10400435.2019.1593260 PMID: 31180276

Bykova, K. M. (2024). Measurement of surface electromyography activity during swallowing in paediatrics: A scoping literature review. *European Journal of Pediatrics*, *183*(10), 4145–4157. PMID: 39037451

Carnaby-Mann, G. D., & Crary, M. A. (2007). Examining the evidence on neuromuscular electrical stimulation for swallowing: A meta-analysis. *Archives of Otolaryngology—Head & Neck Surgery*, *133*(6), 564–571. DOI: 10.1001/archotol.133.6.564 PMID: 17576907

Cengiz, E., Serel Arslan, S., Yaşaroğlu, Ö. F., Alıcı, R., Demir, N., Topçuoğlu, M. A., & Mutlu, A. (2024). Effects of the eccentric chin closure exercise on submental muscle activation, muscle strength, dysphagia limit, perceived exertion and pain in healthy volunteers: A prospective, randomized parallel group study. *PLoS One*, *19*(11), e0313995. DOI: 10.1371/journal.pone.0313995 PMID: 39570948

Chang, M. C., Park, S., Cho, J. Y., Lee, B. J., Hwang, J. M., Kim, K., & Park, D. (2021). Comparison of three different types of exercises for selective contractions of supra- and infrahyoid muscles. *Scientific Reports*, *11*(1), 7131. DOI: 10.1038/s41598-021-86502-w PMID: 33785793

Cheng, I., Hamad, A., Sasegbon, A., & Hamdy, S. (2022). Advances in the Treatment of Dysphagia in Neurological Disorders: A Review of Current Evidence and Future Considerations. *Neuropsychiatric Disease and Treatment*, *18*, 2251–2263. DOI: 10.2147/NDT.S371624 PMID: 36268265

Cheng, I., Sasegbon, A., & Hamdy, S. (2021). Effects of Neurostimulation on Post-stroke Dysphagia: A Synthesis of Current Evidence From Randomized Controlled Trials. *Neuromodulation*, *24*(8), 1388–1401. DOI: 10.1111/ner.13327 PMID: 33301231

Constantinescu, G., & Garcia, R. (2024). Surface Electromyography Biofeedback as an Adjuvant to Dysphagia Management: What It Is, What It Is Not, Why You Need It, and How to Get It. *Perspectives of the ASHA Special Interest Groups*, *9*(6), 1725–1736. DOI: 10.1044/2023_PERSP-23-0007

Cordella, C., Marte, M. J., Liu, H., & Kiran, S. (2025). An Introduction to Machine Learning for Speech-Language Pathologists: Concepts, Terminology, and Emerging Applications. *Perspectives of the ASHA Special Interest Groups*, *10*(2), 432–450. DOI: 10.1044/2024_persp-24-00037 PMID: 40786002

Cosentino, G., Gargano, R., Bonura, G., Realmuto, S., Tocco, E., Ragonese, P., Gangitano, M., Alfonsi, E., Fierro, B., Brighina, F., & Salemi, G. (2018). Anodal tDCS of the swallowing motor cortex for treatment of dysphagia in multiple sclerosis: A pilot open-label study. *Neurological Sciences*, *39*(8), 1471–1473. DOI: 10.1007/s10072-018-3443-x PMID: 29756180

Crary, M. A., Carnaby Mann, G. D., & Groher, M. E. (2007). Identification of swallowing events from sEMG Signals Obtained from Healthy Adults. *Dysphagia*, *22*(2), 94–99. DOI: 10.1007/s00455-006-9059-y PMID: 17294299

Doeltgen, S. H., Rigney, L., Cock, C., & Omari, T. (2018). Effects of cortical anodal transcranial direct current stimulation on swallowing biomechanics. *Neurogastroenterology and Motility*, *30*(11), e13434. DOI: 10.1111/nmo.13434 PMID: 30101445

Duan, G., Yuan, Y., Hua, H., Zhang, X., Liu, B., Li, Y., Zhao, J., Wang, Q., Wang, J., & Wu, D. (2025). Effect of transcranial direct current stimulation on swallowing improvement and cortical activity in hemispheric stroke patients: A randomized, controlled trial. *Scientific Reports*, *15*(1), 19586. DOI: 10.1038/s41598-025-04939-9 PMID: 40467882

Duchac, S. (2025). Navigating the Future of Dysphagia Management: From Advanced Innovations to Personalized Therapies. In *Innovations in Healthcare and Outcome Measurement: New Approaches for a Healthy Lifestyle* (pp. 199–211). Springer Nature Switzerland.

Dudik, J. M., Coyle, J. L., & Sejdić, E. (2015). Dysphagia Screening: Contributions of Cervical Auscultation Signals and Modern Signal-Processing Techniques. *IEEE Transactions on Human-Machine Systems*, *45*(4), 465–477. DOI: 10.1109/THMS.2015.2408615 PMID: 26213659

Dziewas, R., Stellato, R., van der Tweel, I., Walther, E., Werner, C. J., Braun, T., Citerio, G., Jandl, M., Friedrichs, M., Nötzel, K., Vosko, M. R., Mistry, S., Hamdy, S., McGowan, S., Warnecke, T., Zwittag, P., & Bath, P. M. (2018). Pharyngeal electrical stimulation for early decannulation in tracheotomised patients with neurogenic dysphagia after stroke (PHAST-TRAC): A prospective, single-blinded, randomised trial. *Lancet Neurology*, *17*(10), 849–859. PMID: 30170898

Ebdah, S., & Searl, J. (2024). Neuromuscular Electrical Stimulation for Dysphagia Treatment: Adoption, Perceived Barriers, and Clinical Practices. *American Journal of Speech-Language Pathology*, *33*(6), 2839–2854. DOI: 10.1044/2024_AJSLP-24-00175 PMID: 39265131

. Ertekin C. (2015). Electrophysiological Techniques to Evaluate Swallowing in Central and Peripheral Nervous System Disorders. Journal of clinical neurophysiology: official publication of the American Electroencephalographic Society, 32(4), 314–323. https://doi.org/DOI: 10.1097/WNP.0000000000000189

Ertekin, C., Aydoğdu, I., & Yüceyar, N. (1996). Piecemeal deglutition and dysphagia limit in normal subjects and in patients with swallowing disorders. *Journal of Neurology, Neurosurgery, and Psychiatry*, *61*(5), 491–496. DOI: 10.1136/jnnp.61.5.491 PMID: 8937344

Ertekin, C., Aydogdu, I., Yüceyar, N., Tarlaci, S., Kiylioglu, N., Pehlivan, M., & Celebi, G. (1998). Electrodiagnostic methods for neurogenic dysphagia. *Electroencephalography and Clinical Neurophysiology*, *109*(4), 331–340. DOI: 10.1016/s0924-980x(98)00027-7 PMID: 9751296

Frank, D. L., Khorshid, L., Kiffer, J. F., Moravec, C. S., & McKee, M. G. (2010). Biofeedback in medicine: Who, when, why and how? *Mental Health in Family Medicine*, *7*(2), 85–91. PMID: 22477926

Fraser, C., Power, M., Hamdy, S., Rothwell, J., Hobday, D., Hollander, I., Tyrell, P., Hobson, A., Williams, S., & Thompson, D. (2002). Driving plasticity in human adult motor cortex is associated with improved motor function after brain injury. *Neuron*, *34*(5), 831–840. DOI: 10.1016/s0896-6273(02)00705-5 PMID: 12062028

Gallano, G., Giglio, A., & Ferre, A. (2025). Artificial Intelligence in Speech-Language Pathology and Dysphagia: A Review From Latin American Perspective and Pilot Test of LLMs for Rehabilitation Planning. *Journal of Voice*. Advance online publication. DOI: 10.1016/j.jvoice.2025.04.010 PMID: 40312192

Gerges, A. N. H., Williams, E. E. R., Hillier, S., Uy, J., Hamilton, T., Chamberlain, S., & Hordacre, B. (2024). Clinical application of transcutaneous auricular vagus nerve stimulation: A scoping review. *Disability and Rehabilitation*, *46*(24), 5730–5760. DOI: 10.1080/09638288.2024.2313123 PMID: 38362860

Girardi, A. M., Cardell, E. A., & Bird, S. P. (2023). Artificial Intelligence in the Interpretation of Videofluoroscopic Swallow Studies: Implications and Advances for Speech–Language Pathologists. *Big Data and Cognitive Computing*, *7*(4), 178. DOI: 10.3390/bdcc7040178

Gugatschka, M., Egger, N. M., Haspl, K., Hortobagyi, D., Jauk, S., Feiner, M., & Kramer, D. (2024). Clinical evaluation of a machine learning-based dysphagia risk prediction tool. *European Archives of Oto-Rhino-Laryngology*, *281*(8), 4379–4384. DOI: 10.1007/s00405-024-08678-x PMID: 38743079

Gujrania, S., Long, D., & Magerko, B. (2019). Moving in Virtual Space: A Laban-inspired Framework for Procedural Animation. N Proceedings of the Experimental AI in Games Workshop (EXAG) at the 15th AAAI Conference on Artificial Intelligence and Interactive Digital Entertainment (AIIDE'19).

Hamdy, S., Rothwell, J. C., Aziz, Q., Singh, K. D., & Thompson, D. G. (1998). Long-term reorganization of human motor cortex driven by short-term sensory stimulation. *Nature Neuroscience*, *1*(1), 64–68. DOI: 10.1038/264 PMID: 10195111

Hassan, E. A., Khalifa, Y., & Morsy, A. A. (2024). sEMG-based automatic characterization of swallowed materials. *Biomedical Engineering Online*, *23*(1), 48. DOI: 10.1186/s12938-024-01241-z PMID: 38760808

Heo, S., Uhm, K. E., Yuk, D., Kwon, B. M., Yoo, B., Kim, J., & Lee, J. (2024). Deep learning approach for dysphagia detection by syllable-based speech analysis with daily conversations. *Scientific Reports*, *14*(1), 20270. DOI: 10.1038/s41598-024-70774-z PMID: 39217249

Huckabee, M. L., Mills, M., & Flynn, R.. (2023). The Evolution of Swallowing Rehabilitation and Emergence of Biofeedback Modalities. *Current Otorhinolaryngology Reports*, *11*, 144–153. DOI: 10.1007/s40136-023-00451-8

Hwang, N. K., Yoon, T. H., Chang, M. Y., & Park, J. S. (2025). Dysphagia Rehabilitation Using Digital Technology: A Scoping Review. *Journal of Evidence-Based Medicine*, *18*(1), e70009. DOI: 10.1111/jebm.70009 PMID: 40012116

Jayasekeran, V., Rothwell, J., & Hamdy, S. (2011). Non-invasive magnetic stimulation of the human cerebellum facilitates cortico-bulbar projections in the swallowing motor system. *Neurogastroenterology and Motility*, *23*(9), 831–e341. DOI: 10.1111/j.1365-2982.2011.01747.x PMID: 21838728

Jayasekeran, V., Singh, S., Tyrrell, P., Michou, E., Jefferson, S., Mistry, S., Gamble, E., Rothwell, J., Thompson, D., & Hamdy, S. (2010). Adjunctive functional pharyngeal electrical stimulation reverses swallowing disability after brain lesions. *Gastroenterology*, *138*(5), 1737–1746. DOI: 10.1053/j.gastro.2010.01.052 PMID: 20138037

Jefferson, S., Mistry, S., Michou, E., Singh, S., Rothwell, J. C., & Hamdy, S. (2009). Reversal of a virtual lesion in human pharyngeal motor cortex by high frequency contralesional brain stimulation. *Gastroenterology*, *137*(3), 841–849.e1. DOI: 10.1053/j.gastro.2009.04.056 PMID: 19427312

Jeong, C. W., Lee, C. S., Lim, D. W., Noh, S. H., Moon, H. K., Park, C., & Kim, M. S. (2024). The Development of an Artificial Intelligence Video Analysis-Based Web Application to Diagnose Oropharyngeal Dysphagia: A Pilot Study. *Brain Sciences*, *14*(6), 546. DOI: 10.3390/brainsci14060546 PMID: 38928546

Jeong, S. Y., Kim, J. M., Park, J. E., Baek, S. J., & Yang, S. N. (2023). Application of deep learning technology for temporal analysis of videofluoroscopic swallowing studies. *Scientific Reports*, *13*(1), 17522. DOI: 10.1038/s41598-023-44802-3 PMID: 37845272

Kang, Y. J., Arafa, H. M., Yoo, J.-Y., Kantarcigil, C., Kim, J.-T., Jeong, H., Yoo, S., Oh, S., Kim, J., & Wu, C. (2022). Soft skin-interfaced mechano-acoustic sensors for real-time monitoring and patient feedback on respiratory and swallowing biomechanics. *NPJ Digital Medicine*, *5*(1), 147. DOI: 10.1038/s41746-022-00691-w PMID: 36123384

Khalifa, Y., Donohue, C., Coyle, J. L., & Sejdic, E. (2023). Autonomous Swallow Segment Extraction Using Deep Learning in Neck-Sensor Vibratory Signals From Patients With Dysphagia. *IEEE Journal of Biomedical and Health Informatics*, *27*(2), 956–967. DOI: 10.1109/JBHI.2022.3224323 PMID: 36417738

Kim, J. M., Kim, M. S., Choi, S. Y., Lee, K., & Ryu, J. S. (2024). A deep learning approach to dysphagia-aspiration detecting algorithm through pre- and post-swallowing voice changes. *Frontiers in Bioengineering and Biotechnology*, *12*, 1433087. DOI: 10.3389/fbioe.2024.1433087 PMID: 39157445

Kim, J. M., Kim, M. S., Choi, S. Y., & Ryu, J. S. (2024). Prediction of dysphagia aspiration through machine learning-based analysis of patients' postprandial voices. *Journal of Neuroengineering and Rehabilitation*, *21*(1), 43. DOI: 10.1186/s12984-024-01329-6 PMID: 38555417

Koestenberger, M., Neuwersch, S., Hoefner, E., Breschan, C., Weissmann, H., Stettner, H., & Likar, R. (2020). A Pilot Study of Pharyngeal Electrical Stimulation for Orally Intubated ICU Patients with Dysphagia. *Neurocritical Care*, *32*(2), 532–538. DOI: 10.1007/s12028-019-00780-x PMID: 31313142

Koyama, Y., Ohmori, N., Momose, H., Kondo, E., Yamada, S. I., & Kurita, H. (2021). Detection of swallowing disorders using a multiple channel surface electromyography sheet: A preliminary study. *Journal of Dental Sciences*, *16*(1), 160–167. DOI: 10.1016/j.jds.2020.06.009 PMID: 33384793

Kumar, A., Shankar, A., Hollebeek, L. D., Behl, A., & Lim, W. M. (2025). Generative artificial intelligence (GenAI) revolution: A deep dive into GenAI adoption. *Journal of Business Research*, *189*, 115160.

Kumar, S., Wagner, C. W., Frayne, C., Zhu, L., Selim, M., Feng, W., & Schlaug, G. (2011). Noninvasive brain stimulation may improve stroke-related dysphagia: A pilot study. *Stroke*, *42*(4), 1035–1040. DOI: 10.1161/STROKEAHA.110.602128 PMID: 21441148

Kwak, S., Kim, J. K., Moon, J. S., Lee, G. W., Kim, S., & Chang, M. C. (2025). Deep learning-based video analysis for automatically detecting penetration and aspiration in videofluoroscopic swallowing study. *Scientific Reports*, *15*(1), 24296. DOI: 10.1038/s41598-025-10397-0 PMID: 40624237

Langmore, S. E. (1998). FEES: State of the Science. *Perspectives on Swallowing and Swallowing Disorders (Dysphagia)*, *7*(4), 8–10.

Lin, X., Li, H., Wu, X., & Huang, R. (2025). Effects of four non-invasive stimulations on swallowing function and quality of life of stroke patients-a network meta-analysis. *Frontiers in Human Neuroscience*, *19*, 1519660. DOI: 10.3389/fnhum.2025.1519660 PMID: 40183069

Liu, Y., Yin, S., Yang, X., Luo, S., Zhu, F., Zeng, Z., Hu, Q., Xu, L., & Yu, Q. (2024). Effects of Cerebellar Repetitive Transcranial Magnetic Stimulation in the Treatment of Post-Stroke Dysphagia: A Meta-Analysis and Systematic Review of Randomized Controlled Trials. *European Neurology*, *87*(2), 67–78. DOI: 10.1159/000538130 PMID: 38432194

Liu, Z., Cheng, J., Tan, C., Liu, H., & Han, D. (2024). Pharyngeal Cavity Electrical Stimulation-Assisted Swallowing for Post-stroke Dysphagia: A Systematic Review and Meta-analysis of Randomized Controlled Studies. *Dysphagia*, *39*(4), 541–551. DOI: 10.1007/s00455-023-10644-4 PMID: 38117313

Malandraki, G. A., Arkenberg, R. H., Mitchell, S. S., & Malandraki, J. B. (2021). Telehealth for Dysphagia Across the Life Span: Using Contemporary Evidence and Expertise to Guide Clinical Practice During and After COVID-19. *American Journal of Speech-Language Pathology*, *30*(2), 532–550. DOI: 10.1044/2020_AJSLP-20-00252 PMID: 33555933

Maleki Varnosfaderani, S., & Forouzanfar, M. (2024). The Role of AI in Hospitals and Clinics: Transforming Healthcare in the 21st Century. *Bioengineering (Basel, Switzerland)*, *11*(4), 337. DOI: 10.3390/bioengineering11040337 PMID: 38671759

Martin-Harris, B., & Jones, B. (2008). The videofluorographic swallowing study. *Physical Medicine and Rehabilitation Clinics of North America*, *19*(4), 769–785. DOI: 10.1016/j.pmr.2008.06.004 PMID: 18940640

Matsuo, K., & Palmer, J. B. (2008). Anatomy and physiology of feeding and swallowing: Normal and abnormal. *Physical Medicine and Rehabilitation Clinics of North America*, *19*(4), 691–707. DOI: 10.1016/j.pmr.2008.06.001 PMID: 18940636

Miller, S., Peters, K., & Ptok, M. (2022). Review of the effectiveness of neuromuscular electrical stimulation in the treatment of dysphagia - an update. German medical science: GMS e-journal, 20, Doc08. https://doi.org/DOI: 10.3205/000310

Monaco, A., Cattaneo, R., Spadaro, A., & Giannoni, M. (2008). Surface electromyography pattern of human swallowing. *BMC Oral Health*, *8*, 6. DOI: 10.1186/1472-6831-8-6 PMID: 18366770

Morinière, S., Boiron, M., Alison, D., Makris, P., & Beutter, P. (2008). Origin of the sound components during pharyngeal swallowing in normal subjects. *Dysphagia*, *23*(3), 267–273. DOI: 10.1007/s00455-007-9134-z PMID: 18071792

Nakamori, M., Ishikawa, R., Watanabe, T., Toko, M., Naito, H., Takahashi, T., Simizu, Y., Yamazaki, Y., & Maruyama, H. (2023). Swallowing sound evaluation using an electronic stethoscope and artificial intelligence analysis for patients with amyotrophic lateral sclerosis. *Frontiers in Neurology*, *14*, 1212024. DOI: 10.3389/fneur.2023.1212024 PMID: 37602264

. Panebianco, M., Marchese-Ragona, R., Masiero, S., & Restivo, D. A. (2020). Dysphagia in neurological diseases: a literature review. Neurological sciences: official journal of the Italian Neurological Society and of the Italian Society of Clinical Neurophysiology, 41(11), 3067–3073. https://doi.org/DOI: 10.1007/s10072-020-04495-2

Park, E., Kim, M. S., Chang, W. H., Oh, S. M., Kim, Y. K., Lee, A., & Kim, Y. H. (2017). Effects of Bilateral Repetitive Transcranial Magnetic Stimulation on Post-Stroke Dysphagia. *Brain Stimulation*, *10*(1), 75–82. DOI: 10.1016/j.brs.2016.08.005 PMID: 27593709

Park, J. S., Jung, Y. J., Kim, H. H., & Lee, G. (2020). A Novel Method Using Kinesiology Taping for the Activation of Suprahyoid Muscles in Healthy Adults: A Preliminary Research. *Dysphagia*, *35*(4), 636–642. DOI: 10.1007/s00455-019-10071-4 PMID: 31620860

Peng, X. M., Gong, C., Xiao, M. X., Chen, L. S., Li, Y., Chen, J., Wang, M. Y., & Luo, Y. (2025). Effect of repetitive transcranial magnetic stimulation with different stimulation parameters on post-stroke dysphagia: A systematic review and meta-analysis of randomized controlled trials. *Frontiers in Neurology*, *16*, 1586734. DOI: 10.3389/fneur.2025.1586734 PMID: 40474922

. Perlman, A. L. (2006). Electromyography in oral and pharyngeal motor disorders. GI Motility online.

Pikov, V. (2025). Electrical Stimulation of Cranial Nerves for Treating Dysphagia: A Critical Review. *Journal of Translational Gastroenterology*, *3*(4), 197–203. DOI: 10.14218/jtg.2025.00048

Pingue, V., Priori, A., Malovini, A., & Pistarini, C. (2018). Dual Transcranial Direct Current Stimulation for Poststroke Dysphagia: A Randomized Controlled Trial. *Neurorehabilitation and Neural Repair*, *32*(6-7), 635–644. DOI: 10.1177/1545968318782743 PMID: 29926772

Pisegna, J. M., Kaneoka, A., Pearson, W. G.Jr, Kumar, S., & Langmore, S. E. (2016). Effects of non-invasive brain stimulation on post-stroke dysphagia: A systematic review and meta-analysis of randomized controlled trials. *Clinical Neurophysiology*, *127*(1), 956–968. DOI: 10.1016/j.clinph.2015.04.069 PMID: 26070517

Prabhu, R., Kumaresan, A., Vishnuram, S., Suganthirababu, P., Srinivasan, V., Kumar, P., & Dhanusia, S. (2024). Effect of Vagal Nerve Stimulation on Swallowing in Subjects with Post Stroke Dysphagia. *Indian Journal of Physiotherapy and Occupational Therapy*, *18*. Advance online publication. DOI: 10.37506/6jf9m928

Vasant, D. H., Michou, E., O'Leary, N., Vail, A., Mistry, S., & Hamdy, S., & Greater Manchester Stroke Research Network. (2016). Pharyngeal electrical stimulation in dysphagia poststroke: A prospective, randomized single-blinded interventional study. *Neurorehabilitation and Neural Repair*, *30*(9), 866–875.

Restivo, D. A., Alfonsi, E., Casabona, A., Hamdy, S., Tassorelli, C., Panebianco, M., Marchese-Ragona, R., Quartarone, A., Centonze, D., Pavone, A., & Stampanoni Bassi, M. (2019). A pilot study on the efficacy of transcranial direct current stimulation applied to the pharyngeal motor cortex for dysphagia associated with brainstem involvement in multiple sclerosis. *Clinical Neurophysiology*, *130*(6), 1017–1024. DOI: 10.1016/j.clinph.2019.04.003 PMID: 31009904

Restivo, D. A., Casabona, A., Centonze, D., Marchese-Ragona, R., Maimone, D., & Pavone, A. (2013). Pharyngeal electrical stimulation for dysphagia associated with multiple sclerosis: A pilot study. *Brain Stimulation*, *6*(3), 418–423. DOI: 10.1016/j.brs.2012.09.001 PMID: 23040375

Restivo, D. A., Casabona, A., Centonze, D., Marchese-Ragona, R., Maimone, D., & Pavone, A. (2013). Pharyngeal electrical stimulation for dysphagia associated with multiple sclerosis: A pilot study. *Brain Stimulation*, *6*(3), 418–423. PMID: 23040375

Riebold, B., Seidl, R. O., & Schauer, T. (2024). Electromyography- and Bioimpedance-Based Detection of Swallow Onset for the Control of Dysphagia Treatment. *Sensors (Basel)*, *24*(20), 6525. DOI: 10.3390/s24206525 PMID: 39460005

Roldan-Vasco, S., Orozco-Duque, A., & Orozco-Arroyave, J. R. (2023). Swallowing disorders analysis using surface EMG biomarkers and classification models. *Digital Signal Processing*, *133*, 103815. DOI: 10.1016/j.dsp.2022.103815

Saab, R., Balachandar, A., Mahdi, H., Nashnoush, E., Perri, L. X., Waldron, A. L., Sadeghian, A., Rubenfeld, G., Crowley, M., Boulos, M. I., Murray, B. J., & Khosravani, H. (2023). Machine-learning assisted swallowing assessment: A deep learning-based quality improvement tool to screen for post-stroke dysphagia. *Frontiers in Neuroscience*, *17*, 1302132. DOI: 10.3389/fnins.2023.1302132 PMID: 38130696

Sanjeevi, G., Gopalakrishnan, U., Pathinarupothi, R. K., & Iyer, K. S. (2025). Artificial Intelligence in Videofluoroscopy Swallow Study Analysis: A Comprehensive Review. *Dysphagia*, *40*(5), 1035–1048. DOI: 10.1007/s00455-025-10812-8 PMID: 39961823

Sasegbon, A., Cheng, I., Zhang, M., & Hamdy, S. (2020). Advances in the Use of Neuromodulation for Neurogenic Dysphagia: Mechanisms and Therapeutic Application of Pharyngeal Electrical Stimulation, Transcranial Magnetic Stimulation, and Transcranial Direct Current Stimulation. *American Journal of Speech-Language Pathology, 29*(2S), 1044–1064. DOI: 10.1044/2020_AJSLP-19-00073 PMID: 32650660

Sasegbon, A., Watanabe, M., Simons, A., Michou, E., Vasant, D. H., Magara, J., Bath, P. M., Rothwell, J., Inoue, M., & Hamdy, S. (2019). Cerebellar repetitive transcranial magnetic stimulation restores pharyngeal brain activity and swallowing behaviour after disruption by a cortical virtual lesion. *The Journal of Physiology, 597*(9), 2533–2546. DOI: 10.1113/JP277545 PMID: 30907429

Sejdić, E., Khalifa, Y., Mahoney, A. S., & Coyle, J. L. (2020). Artificial intelligence and dysphagia: Novel solutions to old problems. *Arquivos de Gastroenterologia, 57*(04), 343–346. DOI: 10.1590/S0004-2803.202000000-66 PMID: 33331470

Sejdić, E., Malandraki, G. A., & Coyle, J. L. (2019). Computational deglutition: Signal and image processing methods to understand swallowing and associated disorders. *IEEE Signal Processing Magazine, 36*(1), 138–146. DOI: 10.1109/MSP.2018.2875863 PMID: 31631954

Selen Akıl, D., Bengisu, S., Sezer, E., Krespi, Y., & Topbaş, S. S. (2024). Reliability, validity and normative data of the timed water swallow test accompanied by sEMG. *European Archives of Oto-Rhino-Laryngology, 281*(11), 5885–5897. DOI: 10.1007/s00405-024-08884-7 PMID: 39107548

Shen, M., Zhang, L., Li, C., Wei, X., Li, Y., Wu, H., Zhang, X., Gao, S., Ma, Y., & Ma, Y. (2024). Repetitive transcranial magnetic stimulation as a therapy for post-stroke dysphagia: An overview of systematic reviews and meta-analysis. *Clinical Rehabilitation, 38*(10), 1289–1305. DOI: 10.1177/02692155241264757 PMID: 39053022

Shigematsu, T., Fujishima, I., & Ohno, K. (2013). Transcranial direct current stimulation improves swallowing function in stroke patients. *Neurorehabilitation and Neural Repair, 27*(4), 363–369. DOI: 10.1177/1545968312474116 PMID: 23392916

Silva, R. D. D., Almeida, S. B., Gonçalves, F. M., Zeigelboim, B. S., Stechman-Neto, J., Schroder, A. G. D., Nascimento, W. V., Santos, R. S., & Araujo, C. M. (2025). Artificial intelligence in the diagnosis and management of dysphagia: A scoping review. *CoDAS, 37*(4), e20240305. DOI: 10.1590/2317-1782/e20240305en PMID: 40767676

Simons, A., & Hamdy, S. (2017). The Use of Brain Stimulation in Dysphagia Management. *Dysphagia*, *32*(2), 209–215. DOI: 10.1007/s00455-017-9789-z PMID: 28353151

Stampanoni Bassi, M., Centonze, D., Gjikolaj, B., Alito, A., Tisano, A., Marchese-Ragona, R., & Restivo, D. A. (2025). Neurogenic Dysphagia: Peripheral and Central Neuromodulation. *Clinics and Practice*, *15*(9), 163. DOI: 10.3390/clinpract15090163 PMID: 41002778

. Suarez-Patiño, L. V., Roldan-Vasco, S., Suarez-Escudero, J. C., Orozco-Duque, A., & Perez-Giraldo, E. (2024). sEMG as complementary tool for VFSS: A synchronized study in patients with neurogenic oropharyngeal dysphagia. Journal of electromyography and kinesiology: official journal of the International Society of Electrophysiological Kinesiology, 78, 102913. https://doi.org/DOI: 10.1016/j.jelekin.2024.102913

Sun, J., Li, X., Zhou, Y., Liu, H., Ma, C., Hao, C., Liu, S., Zhao, J., Zhang, X., & Xiao, X. (2025). Clinical advances in transcutaneous auricular vagus nerve stimulation for post-stroke disorders: State of the art and future perspectives. *Frontiers in Neurology*, *16*, 1676727. DOI: 10.3389/fneur.2025.1676727 PMID: 41245869

Suntrup, S., Marian, T., Schröder, J. B., Suttrup, I., Muhle, P., Oelenberg, S., Hamacher, C., Minnerup, J., Warnecke, T., & Dziewas, R. (2015). Electrical pharyngeal stimulation for dysphagia treatment in tracheotomized stroke patients: A randomized controlled trial. *Intensive Care Medicine*, *41*(9), 1629–1637. DOI: 10.1007/s00134-015-3897-8 PMID: 26077087

Suntrup-Krueger, S., Ringmaier, C., Muhle, P., Wollbrink, A., Kemmling, A., Hanning, U., Claus, I., Warnecke, T., Teismann, I., Pantev, C., & Dziewas, R. (2018). Randomized trial of transcranial direct current stimulation for poststroke dysphagia. *Annals of Neurology*, *83*(2), 328–340. DOI: 10.1002/ana.25151 PMID: 29350775

Suzuki, K., Shimizu, Y., Ohshimo, S., Oue, K., Saeki, N., Sadamori, T., Tsutsumi, Y., Irifune, M., & Shime, N. (2022). Real-time assessment of swallowing sound using an electronic stethoscope and an artificial intelligence system. *Clinical and Experimental Dental Research*, *8*(1), 225–230. DOI: 10.1002/cre2.531 PMID: 35018714

Sze, W. P., Yoon, W. L., Escoffier, N., & Rickard Liow, S. J. (2016). Evaluating the Training Effects of Two Swallowing Rehabilitation Therapies Using Surface Electromyography—Chin Tuck Against Resistance (CTAR) Exercise and the Shaker Exercise. *Dysphagia*, *31*(2), 195–205. DOI: 10.1007/s00455-015-9678-2 PMID: 26837612

Uysal, Ö. (2024). A Letter to the Editor on "Effect of Visual Biofeedback Obtained Using the Iowa Oral Performance Instrument on the Suprahyoid Muscle Activation Level During Effortful Swallowing Maneuver". *Dysphagia*, *39*(6), 1218–1219. DOI: 10.1007/s00455-024-10698-y PMID: 38581479

Vaiman, M., & Eviatar, E. (2009). Surface electromyography as a screening method for evaluation of dysphagia and odynophagia. *Head & Face Medicine*, *5*, 9. DOI: 10.1186/1746-160X-5-9 PMID: 19232090

Vaiman, M., & Nahlieli, O. (2009). Oral vs. pharyngeal dysphagia: Surface electromyography randomized study. *BMC Ear, Nose, and Throat Disorders*, *9*, 3. DOI: 10.1186/1472-6815-9-3 PMID: 19460159

Vasant, D. H., Mistry, S., Michou, E., Jefferson, S., Rothwell, J. C., & Hamdy, S. (2014). Transcranial direct current stimulation reverses neurophysiological and behavioural effects of focal inhibition of human pharyngeal motor cortex on swallowing. *The Journal of Physiology*, *592*(4), 695–709. DOI: 10.1113/jphysiol.2013.263475 PMID: 24247983

Wang, Z., Xiao, Z., Shen, Q., Zhao, N., & Zhang, W. (2024). Neuromuscular Electrical Stimulation for Post-Stroke Dysphagia Treatment: A Systemic Evaluation and Meta-Analysis of Randomized Controlled Trials. *Dysphagia*, *39*(3), 424–432. DOI: 10.1007/s00455-023-10626-6 PMID: 37914887

Wen, X., Liu, Z., Zhong, L., Peng, Y., Wang, J., Liu, H., & Gong, X. (2022). The Effectiveness of Repetitive Transcranial Magnetic Stimulation for Post-stroke Dysphagia: A Systematic Review and Meta-Analysis. *Frontiers in Human Neuroscience*, *16*, 841781. DOI: 10.3389/fnhum.2022.841781 PMID: 35370584

Weng, W., Imaizumi, M., Murono, S., & Zhu, X. (2022). Expert-level aspiration and penetration detection during flexible endoscopic evaluation of swallowing with artificial intelligence-assisted diagnosis. *Scientific Reports*, *12*(1), 21689. DOI: 10.1038/s41598-022-25618-z PMID: 36522385

Wheeler-Hegland, K. M., Rosenbek, J. C., & Sapienza, C. M. (2008). Submental sEMG and hyoid movement during Mendelsohn maneuver, effortful swallow, and expiratory muscle strength training. *Journal of Speech, Language, and Hearing Research: JSLHR*, *51*(5), 1072–1087. DOI: 10.1044/1092-4388(2008/07-0016) PMID: 18728114

White, K. T., Easterling, C., Roberts, N., Wertsch, J., & Shaker, R. (2008). Fatigue analysis before and after shaker exercise: Physiologic tool for exercise design. *Dysphagia*, *23*(4), 385–391. DOI: 10.1007/s00455-008-9155-2 PMID: 18369673

Wong, D. W., Wang, J., Cheung, S. M., Lai, D. K., Chiu, A. T., Pu, D., Cheung, J. C., & Kwok, T. C. (2025). Current Technological Advances in Dysphagia Screening: Systematic Scoping Review. *Journal of Medical Internet Research*, *27*, e65551. DOI: 10.2196/65551 PMID: 40324167

Yang, W., Cao, X., Zhang, X., Wang, X., Li, X., & Huai, Y. (2021). The Effect of Repetitive Transcranial Magnetic Stimulation on Dysphagia After Stroke: A Systematic Review and Meta-Analysis. *Frontiers in Neuroscience*, *15*, 769848. DOI: 10.3389/fnins.2021.769848 PMID: 34867171

Yang, W., Du, Y., Chen, M., Li, S., Zhang, F., Yu, P., & Xu, X. (2023). Effectiveness of Home-Based Telerehabilitation Interventions for Dysphagia in Patients With Head and Neck Cancer: Systematic Review. *Journal of Medical Internet Research*, *25*, e47324. DOI: 10.2196/47324 PMID: 37682589

Yaşaroğlu, Ö. F., Serel Arslan, S., Cengiz, E., Alıcı, R., Demir, N., Oğuz, B., & Düger, T. (2024). Swallowing kinematics and submental muscles activation during a newly designed maneuver called Mouth Open Swallowing Maneuver: A comparative study. *PLoS One*, *19*(3), e0299845. DOI: 10.1371/journal.pone.0299845 PMID: 38527058

Ye-Lin, Y., Prats-Boluda, G., Galiano-Botella, M., Roldan-Vasco, S., Orozco-Duque, A., & Garcia-Casado, J. (2022). Directed Functional Coordination Analysis of Swallowing Muscles in Healthy and Dysphagic Subjects by Surface Electromyography. *Sensors (Basel)*, *22*(12), 4513. DOI: 10.3390/s22124513 PMID: 35746295

Yuan, Y., Wang, J., Wu, D., Huang, X., & Song, W. (2017). Effect of transcranial direct current stimulation on swallowing apraxia and cortical excitability in stroke patients. *Topics in Stroke Rehabilitation*, *24*(7), 503–509. DOI: 10.1080/10749357.2017.1322250 PMID: 28476095

Zhang, B., Wong, K. P., Liu, M., Hui, V., Guo, C., Liu, Z., Liu, Y., Xiao, Q., & Qin, J. (2025). Effect of artificial intelligence-based video-game system on dysphagia in patients with stroke: A randomized controlled trial. *Clinical Nutrition (Edinburgh, Lothian)*, *45*, 81–90. DOI: 10.1016/j.clnu.2024.12.022 PMID: 39765160

Zhang, C., Zheng, X., Lu, R., Yun, W., Yun, H., & Zhou, X. (2019). Repetitive transcranial magnetic stimulation in combination with neuromuscular electrical stimulation for treatment of post-stroke dysphagia. *The Journal of International Medical Research*, *47*(2), 662–672. DOI: 10.1177/0300060518807340 PMID: 30354918

Zhu, M., Yu, B., Yang, W., Jiang, Y., Lu, L., Huang, Z., Chen, S., & Li, G. (2017). Evaluation of normal swallowing functions by using dynamic high-density surface electromyography maps. *Biomedical Engineering Online*, *16*(1), 133. DOI: 10.1186/s12938-017-0424-x PMID: 29157238

1 SUCRA (Surface Under the Cumulative Ranking Curve) is a metric used in network meta-analyses to quantify the relative ranking of interventions. Higher SUCRA values indicate a greater probability that an intervention is among the most effective options.

Chapter 5
Dysphagia in Dementia: Clinical Findings, Assessment, and Management Approaches

Mümüne Merve Parlak
http://orcid.org/0000-0003-1827-4694
Ankara Yıldırım Beyazıt University, Turkey

Cansu Yıldırım
http://orcid.org/0000-0002-9957-3006
İzmir Bakırçay University, Turkey

ABSTRACT

Dysphagia is a frequent and clinically significant complication in individuals with dementia, contributing to malnutrition, aspiration pneumonia, and reduced quality of life. Its prevalence and clinical presentation vary according to dementia subtype, disease stage, and underlying neuropathology. This chapter provides an overview of dysphagia across major dementia types, including Alzheimer's disease, vascular dementia, frontotemporal dementia, and Lewy body dementia. Dementia-specific swallowing profiles are discussed with emphasis on sensory, motor, and cognitive mechanisms affecting swallowing safety and efficiency. Current assessment approaches are reviewed, highlighting the limitations of self-report measures in cognitively impaired populations and the importance of caregiver input, clinical bedside evaluations, and instrumental assessments. Evidence-based management strategies—including postural techniques, diet modification, behavioral and environmental interventions, rehabilitative exercises, and enteral feeding—are also addressed.

DOI: 10.4018/979-8-3373-6405-6.ch005

INTRODUCTION

Dementia is defined as a syndrome characterized by a decline in cognitive functions beyond what would be expected during normal aging and is generally progressive in nature (Organization, 2017, 2021). Dementia is not a single disease; rather, it is classified as a syndrome because it is characterized by a constellation of symptoms (Bayles & Tomoeda, 2007). It is a general term used to describe conditions that affect memory, other cognitive functions, and behavior, significantly reducing an individual's ability to perform activities of daily living (Organization, 2017). Current epidemiological data indicate that approximately 55 million people worldwide are living with dementia, with nearly 10 million new cases diagnosed each year (Better, 2023).

From an etiological perspective, dementia can be classified into two main categories: primary (degenerative) and secondary (non-degenerative) dementias. The most common degenerative types include Alzheimer's disease (AD), Frontotemporal Dementia (FTD), Dementia with Lewy Body Dementia (LBD), and Parkinson's disease dementia (Association, 2016; Prince et al., 2013; Selkoe, 2004). Non-degenerative dementia refers to cognitive impairment occurring during the course of psychiatric or neurological disorders. The most common causes of non-degenerative dementia include vascular dementia, vitamin deficiencies (e.g., vitamin B12, thiamine), hypothyroidism, chronic alcohol use, infections (e.g., HIV), and traumatic brain injury (Gale et al., 2018). The boundaries between different dementia types are often unclear, and multiple etiologies may coexist within the same individual (Organization, 2017).

Dysphagia, derived from the Greek words dys (difficulty) and phagia (eating), refers to difficulty in swallowing resulting from any disruption in the passage of food from the mouth to the stomach and is considered a symptom rather than a disease (Holt, 2004; Parlak et al., 2022; Sleisenger et al., 2010). Dysphagia may arise from motor, sensory, and behavioral impairments or a combination of these factors (Parlak, Altan, et al., 2022). The severity of dementia, along with cortical and/or subcortical lesions observed in these patients, may disrupt the neural control of swallowing and lead to dysphagia (Easterling & Robbins, 2008; Yıldırım, 2023).

Studies investigating the prevalence of dysphagia in dementia report highly variable results. Both the type and severity of dementia appear to influence dysphagia prevalence (Groher & Crary, 2015; Parlak, Babademez, et al., 2022; Parlak, Tokgöz, et al., 2022). Several studies have demonstrated that swallowing dysfunction worsens as dementia severity increases (Edahiro et al., 2012; Parlak, Babademez, et al., 2022; Wada et al., 2001). Dysphagia may emerge during the early stages of Alzheimer's disease (Humbert et al., 2010; Parlak, Babademez, et al., 2022), whereas it is more commonly observed in the later stages of other dementia types (Ikeda et al., 2002).

Dysphagia in advanced dementia has been extensively documented in the literature (Easterling & Robbins, 2008; Langmore, 2007). A systematic review by Alagiakrishnan, Bhanji, and Kurian (2013) reported that the prevalence of dysphagia across all dementia types ranges widely from 13% to 57% (Alagiakrishnan et al., 2013).

As dementia progresses, individuals typically exhibit a marked reduction in pharyngeal clearance and upper esophageal sphincter opening, frequently accompanied by penetration and/or aspiration events (De Stefano et al., 2020; Mira et al., 2022). These changes substantially increase the risk of serious health complications, underscoring the need for sensitive diagnostic and intervention strategies (Peranovic et al., 2025). However, dysphagia manifestations differ considerably across dementia subtypes (Parlak, Altan, et al., 2022; Yıldırım, 2023). Therefore, careful examination of swallowing characteristics specific to each dementia type is of critical clinical importance. This section reviews dysphagia characteristics, dementia-specific swallowing assessment, and intervention approaches across common dementia types based on current evidence.

1. DYSPHAGIA IN DIFFERENT TYPES OF DEMENTIA

Different types of dementia may present with distinct swallowing impairments. In Alzheimer's disease, dysphagia primarily affects sensory components of swallowing, often resulting in a prolonged oral phase. In contrast, vascular dementia predominantly affects motor aspects, leading to difficulties in mastication and bolus manipulation (Suh et al., 2009). Frontotemporal dementia may be associated with eating-related behavioral disturbances, such as hyperphagia and rapid eating (Ikeda et al., 2002). People with Lewy body dementia is particularly associated with impaired esophageal motility (Londos, Hanxsson, Hirsch, et al., 2013). Considering the sensory, motor, and cognitive changes associated with dementia that affect swallowing in varying ways and degrees, diverse and dementia-specific intervention approaches may be required.

1.1. Dysphagia in Alzheimer's Disease

Alzheimer's disease (AD) is a neurodegenerative disorder that affects multiple domains of cognition and typically presents with a gradual and progressive pattern of cognitive decline (Parlak, Bizpınar Munis, et al., 2025; Parlak et al., 2024; Parlak, Saylam, et al., 2023). Among all causes of dementia, AD represents the most prevalent form (Munis & Parlak, 2023; Parlak, Bizbinar, et al., 2023; Parlak & Köse, 2023). The initial clinical manifestation is most commonly episodic memory impairment, followed by progressive deterioration in other cognitive domains, including language, executive functions, and visuospatial abilities (Parlak & Köse, 2022; Ramirez-Gomez et al., 2017). In addition to memory deficits, aphasia, apraxia, and agnosia are also frequently observed clinical features of AD (Parlak, Altan, et al., 2022; Parlak & Köse, 2022).

Studies investigating dysphagia in AD generally involve relatively small sample sizes and employ methodologically similar approaches. The inclusion of age-matched control groups in some studies (Humbert et al., 2010; Priefer & Robbins, 1997) strengthens the interpretation that observed swallowing impairments are independent of normal age-related changes. Across studies, both oral and pharyngeal phase abnormalities have been shown to emerge in the early stages of the disease and to progressively worsen with increasing disease severity (Parlak, Altan, et al., 2022).

A prolonged oral phase has been consistently identified as a common feature across all stages of AD, whereas delayed swallow initiation typically becomes more pronounced during the moderate stage of the disease. As AD progresses, the severity of both oral and pharyngeal phase impairments increases, with pharyngeal phase dysfunctions substantially elevating the risk of aspiration (Humbert et al., 2010).

The study by Humbert and colleagues (2010) is particularly noteworthy for its use of functional magnetic resonance imaging (fMRI) to compare cortical activation patterns during swallowing in individuals with mild AD and age-matched healthy controls. Their findings demonstrated significantly reduced activation within the cortical swallowing network in the AD group, accompanied by diminished hyolaryngeal excursion and elevation (Humbert et al., 2010). Supporting evidence from additional studies has reported similar swallowing abnormalities. Suh, Kim, and Na (2009) identified oral residue, food accumulation in the sulcus, delayed oral transit, delayed initiation of the swallowing reflex, pharyngeal residue, and penetration of material into the laryngeal vestibule (Suh et al., 2009). Furthermore, Seçil et al. (2016), using submental/suprahyoid electromyography (SM-EMG), reported increased swallowing latency and a greater number of swallows required during sequential swallowing tasks (Seçil et al., 2016). Collectively, these findings indicate a substantial loss of functional reserve in swallowing that worsens with disease progression, yielding important implications for dysphagia assessment and management across all stages of AD.

Despite the growing body of literature, significant knowledge gaps remain due to small sample sizes, inconsistent use of age-matched control groups, and variability in the reporting of AD severity. Nevertheless, existing evidence consistently demonstrates that dysphagia symptoms emerge in the early stages of AD, progressively deteriorate over time, and exert a considerable impact on the health and well-being of individuals with Alzheimer's disease (Parlak, Altan, et al., 2022; Parlak, Babademez, et al., 2022).

1.2. Dysphagia in Vascular Dementia

Vascular Dementia (VaD) is characterized by damage to both gray and white matter of the brain resulting from vascular pathologies (Bayles & Tomoeda, 2007). Following Alzheimer's disease, VaD is considered the second most common type of dementia, accounting for approximately 20% of all dementia cases (Morgan & Mc Auley, 2024). Recurrent cerebrovascular insults lead to cumulative neural damage, and VaD is typically described as exhibiting a "staircase step'' pattern of cognitive decline, in which periods of relative stability follow sudden deteriorations (Bayles et al., 2018). Cognitive changes in VaD are difficult to predict and depend on the location and severity of vascular pathology; however, mood disturbances and behavioral changes are common clinical features (Smith, 2017). In addition, physical impairments such as balance and gait disturbances may frequently accompany the condition (Bayles et al., 2018).

The presentation of dysphagia in VaD has not been sufficiently investigated, and similar to the cognitive profile, its clinical characteristics are difficult to predict. Stach (2000) described oral phase impairments in VaD, including reduced swallowing speed, repetitive lingual movements, and delayed oral transit, as well as pharyngeal phase abnormalities such as delayed swallow initiation, reduced hyolaryngeal excursion, and incomplete closure of the laryngeal vestibule. However, the reliability of these observations is limited, as they were largely based on clinical hypotheses and the author's professional experience rather than objective instrumental assessment (Stach, 2000).

Using more robust methodological approaches, the study conducted by Suh and colleagues (2009) provided empirical support for several of Stach's observations. In a videofluoroscopic swallowing study (VFSS) involving 34 individuals with VaD, pharyngeal phase impairments such as delayed swallow initiation, reduced hyolaryngeal excursion, diminished epiglottic inversion, and pharyngeal residue were identified. Additionally, approximately two-fifths of the sample exhibited difficulties with mastication and bolus formation. More than half of the participants experienced laryngeal penetration, while slightly fewer than half aspirated, with 32% of aspiration events classified as silent aspiration (Suh et al., 2009). The authors suggested that the observed swallowing impairments were primarily related to motor dysfunction due to reduced pharyngeal movement. However, given the high incidence of silent aspiration and delayed swallow initiation, impairment of afferent sensory pathways represents a plausible alternative explanation (Suh et al., 2009).

Overall, the current literature is insufficient to draw definitive conclusions regarding the nature of dysphagia in VaD. Nevertheless, the underlying disease mechanisms suggest a high likelihood of swallowing impairment, indicating that individuals presenting with VaD should be prioritized for comprehensive clinical and instrumental dysphagia assessment within healthcare services (Stach, 2000; Suh et al., 2009).

1.3. Dysphagia in Frontotemporal Dementia

Frontotemporal Dementia (FTD) encompasses a spectrum of clinical syndromes characterized by degeneration of the frontal and temporal lobes, resulting in progressive impairments in executive functioning, behavior, language, and motor abilities (Olney et al., 2017). This syndrome is generally classified into two primary subtypes: the behavioral variant and the language variant. A less common subtype characterized predominantly by movement disorders has also been described. The behavioral variant typically presents with early symptoms such as impulsivity, apathy, disinhibition, and marked personality changes. In contrast, the language variant—commonly referred to as Primary Progressive Aphasia (PPA)—is characterized by initial impairments in speech and language. PPA is further subdivided into three variants: nonfluent/agrammatic, semantic, and logopenic (Marshall et al., 2018). FTD is also closely associated with other neurodegenerative conditions, including motor neuron disease, progressive supranuclear palsy, and corticobasal degeneration (Olney et al., 2017).

Compared to the more overt feeding and mealtime difficulties observed in FTD, dysphagia has received relatively limited research attention. Nevertheless, available evidence suggests that swallowing impairment represents a clinically relevant concern that warrants consideration. In a study conducted by Langmore and colleagues (2007), individuals with FTD and their caregivers were interviewed, and participants underwent Clinical Bedside Evaluations (CBE) and Fiberoptic Endoscopic Evaluation of Swallowing (FEES). While most individuals with FTD did not self-report swallowing difficulties, caregivers frequently described behavioral feeding problems and occasional choking episodes. FEES findings revealed premature spillage of the bolus into the pharynx during mastication, markedly delayed swallow initiation—often occurring when the bolus was located at the level of the valleculae or mid-pharynx—and post-swallow pharyngeal residue in approximately one-third of participants. Premature bolus spillage, delayed swallow initiation, and pharyngeal residue are all factors that substantially increase the risk of aspiration. The dysphagia characteristics identified in individuals with FTD in this study carry important clinical implications, underscoring the necessity of dysphagia management strategies and the routine use of objective swallowing assessments in this population (Langmore et al., 2007).

1.4. Dysphagia in Lewy Body Dementia (LBD) and Parkinson's Disease Dementia

In Lewy body dementia (LBD), cognitive impairment, extrapyramidal system involvement, and psychiatric symptoms may emerge either simultaneously or sequentially at different stages of the disease course (Kane et al., 2018). Following Alzheimer's disease, LBD is the second most common neurodegenerative dementia in individuals aged 65 years and older. The condition is characterized by a constellation of clinical features, including parkinsonism, fluctuating attention, visual hallucinations, and rapid eye movement (REM) sleep behavior disorder. LBD is considered an umbrella term that also encompasses Parkinson's disease dementia (PDD). Although LBD and PDD share overlapping pathological and clinical characteristics, they are typically differentiated by the temporal relationship between motor and cognitive symptoms. In LBD, cognitive symptoms usually precede or emerge within one year of the onset of motor symptoms, whereas in PDD, motor symptoms are the initial manifestation and cognitive decline develops at least one year after the onset of parkinsonism (Scholz et al., 2025). In LBD, cognitive deficits primarily affect visuospatial abilities, attention, and executive functions. Memory is often relatively preserved in the early stages but may decline as the disease progresses (Kane et al., 2018).

Research describing dysphagia in LBD is limited by small sample sizes and insufficient detail regarding dementia severity and swallowing phase involvement. Nevertheless, available evidence indicates that systematic swallowing assessment and dysphagia management are necessary in individuals with LBD. Retrospective analyses of VFSS records have demonstrated that LBD and PDD subtypes exhibit similar swallowing profiles, with pharyngeal residue observed in approximately 50% of cases and silent aspiration identified in 27% of individuals (Larsson et al., 2017).

Self-reported assessments of swallowing difficulties appear to lack adequate sensitivity in individuals with LBD. Yamamoto and colleagues (2010) reported silent aspiration in 55% of individuals with LBD, the majority of whom did not report any subjective swallowing difficulties. This finding suggests that reliance on low-sensitivity screening methods, such as self-report, may result in dysphagia being overlooked even at the stage of referral for objective instrumental assessment (VFSS or FEES) (Yamamoto et al., 2010). Supporting this observation, Londos and colleagues (2013) reported that despite minimal self-reported symptoms, a substantial proportion of individuals with LBD (88%) demonstrated pharyngeal phase impairments on VFSS, including delayed swallow initiation, pharyngeal residue, and penetration or aspiration. Follow-up data from the same study indicated that a considerable number of participants with dysphagia subsequently died, with pneumonia identified as the leading cause of death (Londos, Hanxsson, Hirsch, et al., 2013). These findings underscore the high likelihood that dysphagia in LBD may remain undetected in the absence of routine objective swallowing assessments, particularly given the elevated risk of silent aspiration, and highlight the potentially severe consequences for patient health outcomes.

Furthermore, in a study comparing individuals with PDD and LBD, the incidence of pneumonia within two years was significantly higher among patients with aspiration identified on VFSS in both groups, with the risk being more pronounced in the LBD group (Yamamoto et al., 2010). This evidence further supports the necessity of routine screening and comprehensive evaluation of pharyngeal phase dysphagia in individuals with LBD. Across these studies (Londos, Hanxsson, Hirsch, et al., 2013; Yamamoto et al., 2010), the consistent identification of pharyngeal phase impairments—particularly silent aspiration—suggests that dysphagia may be frequently overlooked in both LBD and PDD when objective swallowing assessments are not incorporated into routine clinical practice. Given the well-established association between silent aspiration and the development of aspiration pneumonia, these findings carry critical clinical implications for the health, survival, and quality of life of individuals with LBD.

2. DYSPHAGIA ASSESSMENT IN INDIVIDUALS WITH DEMENTIA

Swallowing is a complex process involving multiple anatomical structures and physiological mechanisms and requires a comprehensive evaluation of all contributing factors and underlying causes to ensure safe and adequate nutrition. The primary goals of dysphagia assessment include the identification of swallowing impairment, localization of the affected anatomical region, and the development of appropriate treatment strategies. However, standard swallowing assessments are often challenging to administer in individuals with dementia and typically necessitate multidisciplinary, comprehensive evaluations to accurately reflect daily swallowing function. Evidence regarding the clinical assessment, intervention, and medical management of dysphagia in individuals with dementia remains limited (Parlak, Altan, et al., 2022).

2.1. Anamnesis

During history taking, individuals with dementia may provide inaccurate or incomplete information about their condition due to cognitive impairment. Therefore, in the clinical assessment of dysphagia in individuals with dementia, detailed information should be obtained not only from the patient but also from family members or caregivers who spend substantial time with the individual (Parlak, Altan, et al., 2022). When obtaining anamnesis, clinicians should inquire about dysphagia-related symptoms as well as associated and potential risk factors. Patients and caregivers may lack awareness of dysphagia symptoms; thus, the use of guided and targeted questions may facilitate more accurate information gathering. For example, individuals in the early stages of dementia frequently report complaints of xerostomia related to reduced salivary secretion, while often remaining unaware of underlying swallowing difficulties (Ekberg, 2012). Accordingly, anamnesis should not be limited to overt dysphagia symptoms but should also encompass questions addressing related factors and risk indicators. Table 1 presents example questions that may be used during anamnesis in clinical cases involving individuals with dementia, along with the rationale for each question.

Table 1. Anamnesis Questions Used in Dysphagia Assessment of Individuals with Dementia

Question	Rationale / Explanation
When was the diagnosis of dementia made?	Important for determining disease duration and progression
What stage of dementia is the patient in?	Aspiration risk increases with disease severity
Are there any comorbid conditions (neurological/psychiatric)?	Parkinson's disease, MS, ALS, depression, etc.
What medications is the patient currently using?	Sedatives and antipsychotics may contribute to dysphagia
Has there been any weight change?	Indicator of malnutrition risk
Is the patient able to feed themselves?	Functional independence
How is the patient's appetite?	Reduced appetite may indicate dysphagia or depression
What is the current mode of nutrition? (oral, gastrostomy, etc.)	History of enteral feeding
Are there specific food preferences?	Texture and consistency preferences
Is there any difficulty with chewing?	Assessment of the oral phase
Is there a history of recurrent pneumonia?	Indicator of silent aspiration
Does the patient experience frequent fever?	Suspicion of aspiration pneumonia
Is there a change in voice quality after meals?	Wet or gurgly voice suggests aspiration
Is there coughing, choking, throat clearing, or a sensation of food sticking during or after eating?	Suspicion of aspiration or penetration
Does food or liquid regurgitate through the nose during or after swallowing?	Nasal regurgitation

continued on following page

Table 1. Continued

Question	Rationale / Explanation
Has a swallowing assessment been performed previously?	Clinical or instrumental evaluation
Has the patient received swallowing therapy before?	Response to previous intervention
Have any diet texture modifications been implemented?	IDDSI levels
How long does a typical meal take?	Prolonged duration may indicate oral phase impairment
Does the patient experience fatigue during meals?	Muscle weakness
What are the number and portion size of meals?	Nutritional pattern
Is there difficulty with saliva control?	Drooling or saliva pooling
Are there difficulties with tongue movements?	Oral preparatory phase
Is there a history of COPD, asthma, or other respiratory disease?	Swallowing–breathing coordination
Is a tracheostomy present?	Alters swallowing risk
Is hoarseness present?	Laryngeal closure insufficiency
Are there symptoms of reflux?	LPR/GERD increases aspiration risk
Is there belching or regurgitation after oral intake?	Esophageal phase involvement
How are attention and monitoring abilities?	Swallowing safety
Is the patient able to understand commands?	Therapy compliance
Is caregiver support available?	Safety of feeding at home

2.2. Dysphagia Screening Tools in Dementia

Various screening tools have been developed to identify individuals who are at risk for dysphagia. Reliance solely on patient self-report to determine the presence and severity of dysphagia may compromise diagnostic accuracy, particularly in populations with cognitive impairment such as individuals with dementia (Leonard, 2023). Accordingly, recent studies suggest that clinician-administered screening tools may yield more effective results in individuals with dementia, given the reduced self-awareness associated with cognitive decline (Parlak, İnceoğlu, et al., 2025). For example, the Eating Assessment Tool (EAT-10) is a ten-item dysphagia screening questionnaire based on patient self-report and is widely used in both clinical practice and research settings (Arslan et al., 2017; Demir et al., 2016). However, Parlak and colleagues (2025) examined the agreement between EAT-10 scores obtained from individuals with AD and their caregivers, and compared both sets of EAT-10 results with findings from FEES. Their results demonstrated low agreement between EAT-10 and FEES outcomes, particularly in the identification of aspiration, regardless of whether the information was obtained from the individual with AD or from the caregiver (Parlak, İnceoğlu, et al., 2025).

In a systematic review and meta-analysis conducted by Doan and colleagues (2022), oropharyngeal dysphagia screening tests were evaluated in adults aged 60 years and older across various settings, including community-dwelling populations, nursing homes, and hospital environments. Among the 32 studies meeting the inclusion criteria, the most frequently used screening tools were the Standardized Swallowing Assessment (SSA), the Volume–Viscosity Swallow Test (V-VST), the Gugging Swallowing Screen (GUSS), and the EAT-10. While EAT-10 is questionnaire-based, GUSS and V-VST involve water swallow or multiple-consistency swallow tests, and SSA comprises a more comprehensive clinical assessment. Regardless of the care setting, the highest prevalence of oropharyngeal dysphagia was identified using SSA, whereas the lowest prevalence was detected using EAT-10. The authors emphasized that the risk of underestimating or overlooking oropharyngeal dysphagia is strongly influenced by the choice of screening tool (Doan et al., 2022).

Individuals with dementia are particularly vulnerable to clinical deterioration in hospital settings, as unfamiliar environments often exacerbate confusion. Changes in mealtime routines and food types may further aggravate feeding and swallowing difficulties. Consequently, the assessment of eating and nutritional behaviors may provide valuable insight into the overall clinical status of individuals with dementia. The Edinburgh Feeding Evaluation in Dementia Questionnaire (EdFED-Q) is a valid and reliable observational tool designed to identify feeding and eating difficulties and to determine the level of assistance required (Watson, 1994). However, EdFED-Q is primarily a feeding and nutrition assessment instrument, and its diagnostic accuracy for dysphagia has not been evaluated against instrumental swallowing assessments in validity and reliability studies.

In recent years, novel screening tools such as the Rastreamento de Disfagia Orofaríngea em Idosos (RaDI) and the Dysphagia Screening Tool for Geriatric Patients (DSTG) have been developed for older adults with swallowing disorders (Magalhães Junior et al., 2022; Thiem et al., 2023). Nevertheless, these tools have not yet been widely disseminated or sufficiently validated. Recent literature consistently emphasizes the need to develop new dysphagia screening instruments tailored specifically to individuals with dementia—and even to specific dementia subtypes—that do not rely on cognitive function and can be completed either by caregivers or by clinicians (Parlak, İnceoğlu, et al., 2025).

2.3. Clinical Swallowing Assessment in Dementia

Clinical swallowing assessment is performed to identify most patients at risk for dysphagia at an early stage and to evaluate the effectiveness and safety of swallowing. Patients in whom dysphagia is suspected during clinical assessment should undergo more comprehensive evaluations to prevent potential complications. Although clinical swallowing assessment provides detailed information about the oral phase of swallowing, it cannot yield definitive data regarding the timing of swallow initiation or the integrity of the pharyngeal swallow (Boccardi et al., 2016; O'Rourke et al., 2014).

The Clinical Bedside Swallowing Screening (CBSS) is used to screen for potential swallowing problems and to determine the appropriateness of instrumental assessment. During CBSS, the clinician observes how the patient places a liquid or solid bolus into the mouth, how effectively the bolus is contained during the oral phase, the time required to manipulate or chew the bolus, and the overall duration from oral preparation to swallow initiation. CBSS protocols are designed to address individual patient needs, including feeding history, medical diagnosis, and mental status. These protocols range from observing a single 3-ounce water swallow to assessing the chewing of solid boluses such as cookies (Logemann, 1998). CBSS serves as an important early screening tool for dysphagia and aspiration risk. However, due to its variable sensitivity (42–92%) and specificity (59–91%), careful selection of protocol components is required (Ramsey et al., 2003). CBSS should be considered complementary to instrumental assessment and should not be used as a stand-alone diagnostic tool, as it does not allow clinicians to identify the physiological mechanisms underlying dysphagia. Furthermore, CBSS does not permit direct observation of the physiological processes necessary for safe bolus transport and airway protection. Although patients may cough or exhibit changes in voice quality following trial swallows, bedside screening alone cannot determine the physiological cause of coughing or voice alterations (Easterling & Robbins, 2008).

The Water Swallow Test is one of the most traditional and widely used tools for dysphagia screening in hospitals, community settings, and nursing homes (Rofes et al., 2014). This test is simple, low-cost, and well suited for use in primary healthcare settings. However, in older adults, degenerative changes in the tissues of the oral cavity, pharynx, and esophagus may reduce sensitivity to aspiration, thereby increasing the risk of missed diagnoses due to silent aspiration (Nakashima et al., 2018). In a study by Parlak et al. (2022), which employed both the 10 mL water swallow test and EAT-10, findings from the water swallow test were reported to be more consistent with FEES results than those obtained from EAT-10. Nevertheless, sensitivity and specificity values were not reported in this study (Parlak, Altan, et al., 2022).

V-VST has been recommended by the European Geriatric Medicine Society as a preferred screening tool for dysphagia in older adults (Baijens, Clavé, et al., 2016). The V-VST requires the preparation of boluses with three different viscosities (thin liquid, nectar-thick, and pudding-thick) and three different volumes (5 mL, 10 mL, and 20 mL), resulting in nine test combinations. The test is easy to administer and can be completed in approximately 8.7 ± 2.7 minutes in older adults, demonstrating high clinical efficiency (Michel et al., 2018). However, it should be noted that validation studies specifically tailored to individuals with dementia are lacking. During administration of these screening tools, individuals with dementia may experience difficulty due to behavioral and psychological symptoms associated with the disease (Parlak, İnceoğlu, et al., 2025). In individuals with dementia, further research is required to determine which of the currently available standardized, valid, and reliable swallowing assessments is most functional and which demonstrates the highest diagnostic performance in this population. Alternatively, there is a clear need for the development of new clinical dysphagia assessment protocols or tools tailored to the clinical characteristics of different dementia subtypes.

2.4. Instrumental Assessment Methods

Following clinical observation and examination, instrumental assessment may be required in patients with suspected dysphagia to confirm the diagnosis and/or to guide treatment planning. Findings obtained from instrumental swallowing assessments contribute to understanding the pathophysiology of swallowing disorders and to evaluating the natural course of the disease as well as the response to treatment. When selecting an instrumental assessment method, indications and contraindications such as the patient's cognitive–linguistic status and overall medical condition should be carefully considered. As described in the literature, instrumental swallowing assessments include VFSS, FEES, ultrasound, and manometry (Langmore, 2003). According to current position statements of the European Society for Swallowing Disorders (ESSD), patients who exhibit dysphagia or impaired airway protection during clinical evaluation should undergo an instrumental assessment such as VFSS or FEES (Baijens, Clavé, et al., 2016).

FEES allows direct visualization of the pharynx and larynx and their functions during and after swallowing. FEES can identify findings such as vallecular and pyriform sinus residue, premature spillage or uncontrolled bolus flow, penetration, aspiration, and piecemeal deglutition. In addition, FEES is well tolerated, easy to administer, repeatable, and can be performed at the bedside by the clinician (Baijens, Clavé, et al., 2016). It is widely recognized as a reliable bedside diagnostic tool for the assessment of swallowing disorders in geriatric populations (Peranovic et al., 2025). Langmore et al. (2007) reported a case series evaluating swallowing function using FEES in individuals with FTD. While only 4 of the 21 caregivers (21.05%) reported swallowing difficulties, instrumental assessment revealed moderate swallowing abnormalities in 12 of the 21 patients (57.14%). The authors interpreted these findings as reflecting deficits in cortical and subcortical pathways connected to the brainstem swallowing center (Langmore et al., 2007). Recent studies in AD have also demonstrated the widespread use of FEES (Parlak, Babademez, et al., 2022; Parlak, İnceoğlu, et al., 2025). Peronovic et al. (2025) provided insights into the prevalence and characteristics of various dysphagia pathologies across different dementia types using FEES. In their study, bolus residue in the vallecula and pyriform sinuses was detected in nearly all individuals with dementia (96%). The authors emphasized that this high prevalence exceeded rates reported in prospective age-matched cohorts and suggested that dementia-specific neurodegenerative changes, in addition to age-related sensory loss, contribute to residue formation (Labeit et al., 2022; Peranovic et al., 2025).

Clinical experience plays a critical role in the interpretation of FEES recordings. In the national literature, Yıldırım (2025), within the scope of a doctoral dissertation, aims to develop a deep learning–based artificial intelligence model using FEES videos obtained from both healthy individuals and individuals with various types of dementia. The proposed model is intended to be trained to automatically detect findings such as residue, penetration, and aspiration on FEES images. The integration of standardized scales into the model and the evaluation of thin liquids, purees, and solid consistencies are also planned. Successful implementation of this approach may enable FEES images to be interpreted more easily and independently of the clinician's training and experience, thereby facilitating rapid and effective therapy planning.

The primary aims of VFSS are to assess swallowing safety and efficiency, to characterize swallowing disorders based on VFSS findings, and to support treatment selection and outcome evaluation. To minimize interpretation errors, VFSS recordings should be reviewed in a darkened room. VFSS should be performed in the lateral projection, and images should include the lips, oral cavity, pharynx, cervical spine, and esophagus, preferably with dentures in place (Baijens, Clave, et al., 2016). Studies evaluating individuals with dementia using VFSS have reported higher dysphagia prevalence rates compared to those identified using other diagnostic tools (Affoo et al., 2013; Humbert et al., 2010). Londos et al. (2013) investigated the prevalence of swallowing disorders in LBD and PDD using VFSS. In their study, 82 individuals with LBD or PDD enrolled in a clinical follow-up program were questioned about dysphagia symptoms, and those reporting symptoms underwent VFSS examination. The authors reported pathological VFSS findings—predominantly of pharyngeal origin—in nearly all individuals with LBD or PDD who exhibited subjective dysphagia symptoms (Londos, Hanxsson, Alm Hirsch, et al., 2013).

In addition, noninvasive and easily applicable electrophysiological instrumental swallowing assessments are available (Gürgör et al., 2013). Mild to moderate, and even in some cases severe, cognitive impairment does not constitute a barrier to electrophysiological evaluation (Aydogdu et al., 2015). Seçil et al. (2016) investigated electrophysiological swallowing parameters across all stages of Alzheimer's disease. Their results demonstrated dysphagia in 30 of 40 individuals with AD (75%). The authors concluded that electrophysiological features of dysphagia are present even in the early stages of AD, that cortical involvement and the severity of cognitive impairment may exacerbate swallowing difficulties, and that subclinical signs of dysphagia may be observed even in individuals with mild to moderate AD (Seçil et al., 2016).

2.5. Current Assessment Approaches

Instrumental assessments such as VFSS and FEES require specialized equipment and skilled technical personnel; moreover, their application may be challenging in some individuals with dementia due to communication and cognitive impairments (Parlak, Altan, et al., 2022). Although instrumental methods are essential for accurate diagnosis, their dependence on specialized equipment, trained personnel, and time limits their widespread use in routine clinical practice. This situation highlights the need for assessment methods that are valid, reliable, and practical. Recent advances in artificial intelligence (AI) offer a promising solution in this regard (Imaizumi et al., 2024; Wong et al., 2025). Within the scope of TÜBİTAK 1001 projects, Parlak et al. (2025) aim to develop a novel artificial intelligence–based model grounded in speech and voice analysis to objectively assess the presence and severity of dysphagia in individuals with AD. The project proposes a standardized assessment protocol encompassing swallowing tasks with different consistencies (water, yogurt, biscuit) and volumes, and aims to provide a reliable clinical tool capable of reflecting FEES findings through speech and voice signals. If successfully implemented, this approach may enable the identification of the presence, localization, and severity of dysphagia in individuals with AD using speech analysis alone across different consistencies and bolus volumes. This assessment approach, which is simple, practical, and does not impose cognitive demands on the individual, may facilitate not only early dysphagia evaluation in individuals with dementia but also frequent reassessments over time. Such repeated evaluations would allow clearer monitoring of therapeutic outcomes and disease progression, thereby supporting more timely and individualized dysphagia management.

3. DYSPHAGIA INTERVENTION APPROACHES IN DEMENTIA

The primary goals of dysphagia management in individuals with dementia include ensuring adequate nutrition, protecting the airway, preventing aspiration pneumonia, and maintaining quality of life (Forster et al., 2011; Sato et al., 2014). Regardless of the dementia subtype, dysphagia intervention should be individualized, with patient comfort, safety, and respect for human dignity placed at the center of care. Within this framework, intervention strategies span a broad spectrum, ranging from simple environmental modifications to dietary adjustments, physical and behavioral therapies, and, as a last resort, enteral feeding (Priefer & Robbins, 1997). However, evidence regarding the effectiveness of dysphagia interventions in individuals with dementia remains limited, and the feasibility of most strategies is directly related to the severity of cognitive impairment (Boccardi et al., 2016).

When planning interventions for individuals with dementia, multiple factors beyond dysphagia must be considered, including comorbid conditions, cognitive and physical capacities, and the age and abilities of caregivers (Chan et al., 2024). Recent meta-analyses and systematic reviews suggest that various dysphagia treatment approaches may potentially improve swallowing function in individuals with dementia; however, treatment effectiveness remains highly dependent on individual clinical profiles. Existing studies are characterized by low levels of evidence, a lack of randomized controlled trials, and substantial methodological heterogeneity. Consequently, future research emphasizing homogeneous sample populations and long-term follow-up through well-designed randomized controlled trials is needed to draw more definitive conclusions regarding the effectiveness of dysphagia interventions in dementia (Hu et al., 2024; Tong et al., 2025).

3.1. Positioning and Postural Modifications

For safe swallowing, it is essential that the patient assumes an upright and symmetrical seated posture. This position optimizes the oropharyngeal pathway, facilitates bolus flow, and reduces the risk of aspiration (Forster et al., 2011). Therefore, patients should be encouraged and assisted to sit upright during meals. For individuals who are fed in bed, elevating the head of the bed to at least 60–90 degrees is recommended to facilitate bolus transit and enhance swallowing safety (Carr et al., 2010).

Figure 1. Positional recommendations for eating (Adapted from Carr et al,2010)

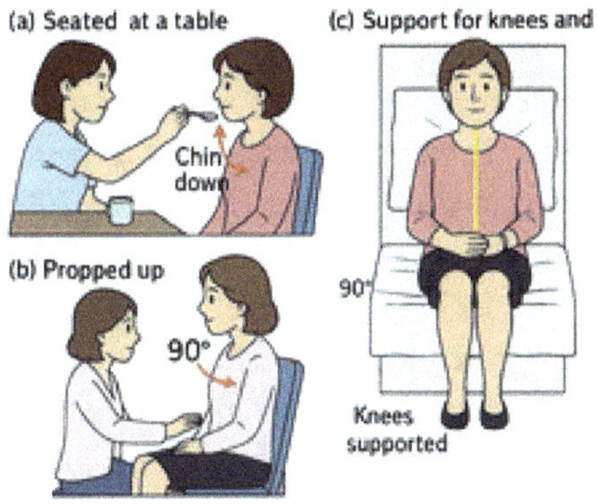

Postural modifications—such as the chin-tuck maneuver, head rotation, and lateral flexion—may alter bolus speed and flow direction and contribute to airway protection (Groher, 2015). The selection of an appropriate postural strategy should be tailored to the individual patient's swallowing profile. However, particularly in individuals with moderate to advanced dementia, cognitive impairment, memory deficits, and reduced cooperation may limit the clinical effectiveness of these techniques, as they may be forgotten or inconsistently applied during each swallow (Bautmans et al., 2008; Robbins et al., 2008). In individuals with dementia, the presence of a caregiver during meals—providing verbal cues and reminders for each eating behavior—may facilitate adherence to postural strategies. Similarly, the use of external memory aids, such as visual or video cues during meals, may support recall of required positional adjustments and enhance compliance with swallowing strategies.

Benigas and Bourgeois (2016) investigated whether Spaced Retrieval (SR), when combined with an external memory aid, is an effective technique for teaching compensatory swallowing strategies to individuals with dementia. In their study, SR paired with a visual external memory strategy was implemented to teach compensatory behaviors (e.g., chin tuck, alternating liquids and solids) to five nursing home residents with mild to moderate dementia and concomitant dysphagia. Following intervention, functional improvement was observed in learning two to three compensatory swallowing behaviors for each participant. However, the authors noted that participants consumed meals in a quiet and controlled environment, and therefore the generalizability of these gains to typical mealtime settings and the long-term effectiveness of the intervention remain uncertain (Benigas & Bourgeois, 2016).

3.2. Dietary and Food Modifications

Dietary interventions are among the most common and evidence-based approaches in dysphagia management. Texture modification has been shown to significantly reduce the risk of aspiration and penetration (Ney et al., 2009). In particular, nectar-thick and honey-thick liquids are associated with lower aspiration rates compared with thin liquids. In the study by Logemann et al. (2008), most patients with dementia aspirated thin liquids even when using the chin-tuck posture; therefore, avoidance of thin liquids was recommended. In the same study, patient preference favored the chin-tuck posture most frequently, followed by nectar-thick liquids. Individuals with advanced-stage dementia demonstrated the lowest level of effectiveness across all interventions (Logemann et al., 2008). In contrast, Robbins et al. (2008) compared chin-tuck posture and thickened liquids and found no significant difference in pneumonia incidence after three months of follow-up. While increasing liquid viscosity may reduce aspiration risk in the short term in individuals with dementia, it should be noted that long-term use may lead to complications related to nutrition, respiratory health, and hydration (Flynn et al., 2018; Robbins et al., 2008).

Regarding solid foods, mashed textures or small, soft bite-sized foods are generally preferred. In addition, sensory stimuli such as taste, temperature, aroma, and viscosity may contribute to earlier triggering of the swallowing reflex. Given that diminished taste perception is common in individuals with dementia, the use of more flavorful, sour, or sweet foods may enhance the meaningfulness and enjoyment of eating (Aliani et al., 2013; Behrman et al., 2014). Importantly, dietary modification should also support nutritional status; therefore, it should be planned in conjunction with nutritional supplementation when necessary, and caregivers should be clearly educated regarding liquid viscosity levels and texture recommendations (Parlak, Altan, et al., 2022).

3.3. Oral Hygiene and Airway Protection

Poor oral hygiene is a common issue in individuals with dementia and represents a significant risk factor for pneumonia. Systematic reviews have demonstrated that regular mechanical oral care (e.g., tooth brushing and tongue cleaning) reduces respiratory tract infections and pneumonia-related mortality (Fernández & Clavé, 2013). Oral hygiene remains essential even in individuals receiving enteral nutrition or those who are edentulous, as colonized saliva can still be aspirated into the lungs in the absence of oral feeding. However, due to cognitive impairment, individuals with dementia often have limited cooperation with oral care procedures. In such cases, caregivers should provide support using strategies such as verbal cueing, visual prompts, and the establishment of consistent routines to facilitate adherence to oral hygiene practices (Bomfim et al., 2013; Park et al., 2013).

3.4. Swallowing Exercises

Swallowing function is closely related to the strength and coordination of the tongue, lips, jaw, hyolaryngeal structures, and head–neck range of motion. Accordingly, active exercise programs aim to enhance muscular strength and coordination (Burkhead et al., 2007; Kays & Robbins, 2006). Techniques such as the Mendelsohn maneuver, the Shaker exercise, and Expiratory Muscle Strength Training (EMST) have been shown to be effective in strengthening the swallowing reflex. Rehabilitation approaches based on these exercises appear to influence both neural and behavioral plasticity (Burkhead et al., 2007; Kays & Robbins, 2006). Resistance exercises targeting the tongue and oropharyngeal muscles have also demonstrated effectiveness in older adults with dysphagia (Lazarus, 2006; Robbins et al., 2007). Nevertheless, learning and maintaining these exercises in individuals with dementia is challenging due to cognitive and behavioral limitations. Significant uncertainty remains regarding the feasibility of teaching and implementing swallowing exercises in this population. Therefore, adapted, simplified, and visually supported exercise protocols should be developed for individuals with dementia (Parlak, Altan, et al., 2022; Tong et al., 2025). For example, video modeling may enhance the learning effectiveness of exercise programs in individuals with dementia (Sura et al., 2012).

Ye et al. (2024), conducted a multicenter randomized controlled trial investigating the effects of oropharyngeal muscle training in individuals with AD and dysphagia. The intervention group received a video-based, systematic, progressive swallowing exercise program targeting routine dysphagia management, delivered once daily, five days per week for four weeks (Figure 2). The control group received routine dysphagia care, including dietary and postural management and health education regarding swallowing dysfunction. Based on water swallowing tests and standardized swallowing assessments, the intervention group demonstrated significantly greater improvements in swallowing function, independence level, and nutritional status compared with the control group. Although the authors acknowledged that rehabilitation interventions may be challenging for individuals living with AD due to cognitive decline, they emphasized the importance of active participation in therapy, as participants showed meaningful improvements in swallowing function through learning and practicing swallowing muscle exercises (Wu et al., 2022; Ye et al., 2024).

Figure 2. Stepwise swallowing exercise training protocol proposed by Ye et al. (2024) and Wu et al. (2022)

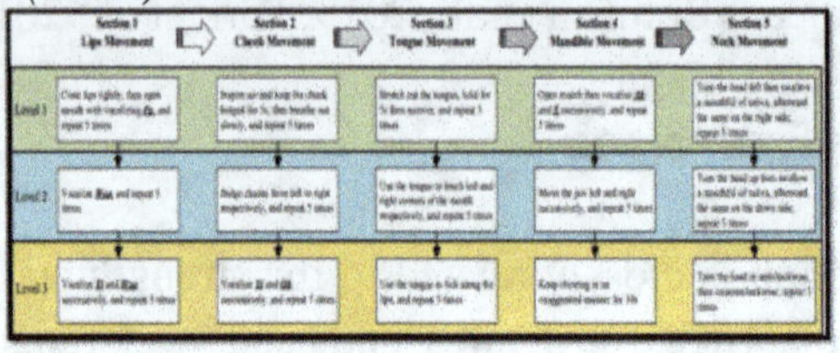

In their meta-analysis, Tong et al. (2025) demonstrated that swallowing exercise training exhibited superior intervention effects compared with various other treatment approaches. The authors reported that a 4–6-week swallowing exercise program yielded optimal outcomes in individuals with early-stage dementia and dysphagia. While multiple dysphagia intervention strategies were shown to effectively improve swallowing function in patients with dementia-related dysphagia, the findings indicated that structured swallowing exercise training delivered over a 4–6-week period may represent the most effective approach. Subgroup analyses based on dysphagia severity revealed that interventions were more effective in individuals at the mild stage compared with those at moderate to advanced stages. The authors emphasized that early interventions, implemented before swallowing function becomes severely impaired, are likely to be more beneficial when initiated during the early phases of the disease trajectory. Furthermore, Tong et al. (2025) highlighted that emerging technologies—such as video games, virtual reality, and artificial intelligence—may be integrated with swallowing muscle strengthening exercises in future research to simultaneously enhance both swallowing and cognitive functions. Based on the results of their meta-analysis, the authors proposed a structured clinical pathway outlining the effectiveness and cost considerations of different dysphagia interventions for individuals with dementia, as illustrated in Figure 3 (Tong et al., 2025).

Figure 3. Effect size and cost-effectiveness framework of dysphagia interventions in dementia based on the meta-analysis by Tong et al. (2025).

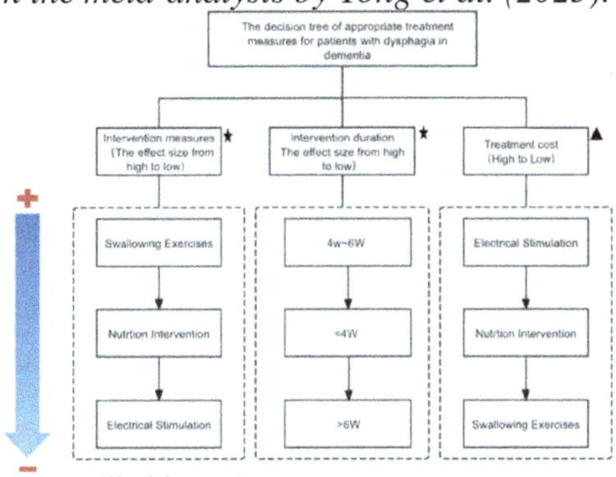

3.5. Cervical Mobilization

Cervical mobilization techniques may contribute to improvements in swallowing function by enhancing strength and range of motion in the head and neck musculature, which play a critical role in swallowing. Based on this rationale, a randomized controlled study investigated the effects of cervical spine mobilization in individuals with advanced AD presenting with dysphagia. In this study, mobilization was administered three times per week, on alternate days, with each session lasting approximately 20 minutes. Participants were seated comfortably with their head supported against the therapist's chest, while the therapist stabilized the patient's head using the arm and hand. Gentle mobilization of the head and cervical spine was performed to align the head in a neutral position over the shoulders. All mobilization techniques were applied within the patient's available range of motion and discontinued if muscle guarding or discomfort occurred. After one week of intervention, significant improvements were reported in single-swallow capacity and overall swallowing function. Nevertheless, the evidence supporting cervical mobilization in dysphagia management among individuals with dementia remains at a pilot level, and further large-scale randomized controlled trials are required to establish its efficacy (Bautmans et al., 2008).

3.6. Behavioral and Environmental Interventions

In individuals with dementia, eating is not only a physiological activity but also an emotional and social experience. Therefore, the mealtime environment should be carefully structured. Recommended strategies include (Lin et al., 2010; Whear et al., 2014):

- Providing a calm, quiet, and well-lit environment,
- Maintaining consistency by having the same caregivers serve meals using the same routine,
- Delivering simple, repetitive verbal instructions (e.g., "Pick up the fork," "Open your mouth"),
- Interpreting behaviors such as head turning, food holding in the mouth, or spitting not as pathological symptoms but as forms of communication

Sensory preparation before meals—such as allowing the individual to smell the food or visually inspect the plate—may help trigger the swallowing reflex. Some studies have demonstrated that the use of calming background music during meals can reduce anxiety and shorten mealtime duration (Whear et al., 2014).

Caregivers play a crucial role in supporting individuals with dementia by monitoring nutritional intake, providing verbal, visual, and/or physical assistance during eating and swallowing, and implementing and following up on prescribed intervention programs (Yıldırım, 2023). Accordingly, caregivers should receive education regarding signs of aspiration, safe swallowing techniques, oral hygiene practices, and appropriate scheduling of mealtimes. Table 2 presents practical recommendations that may be provided to caregivers to support safe and effective feeding in individuals with dementia (Yıldırım, 2023).

Table 2. Recommendations for Caregivers of Individuals with Dementia During Mealtime

Domain	Caregiver Recommendations
Mealtime Environment	• Eating utensils should be reserved exclusively for mealtimes to reinforce routine and contextual cues. • Mealtimes should be scheduled during periods of the day when the individual is most alert and stable. • If distressing, environmental distractions (e.g., background noise, unnecessary objects) should be minimized or eliminated. • Individuals with dementia may require rest breaks during meals; pauses should be permitted as needed. • Pleasant and supportive conversation should be maintained during meals. • Calming music tailored to the individual's preferences may be provided. • Meals should not be rushed; sufficient time should be allowed for completion. • Verbal and non-verbal communication should be maintained throughout the meal.
Meal Planning and Scheduling	• A structured and predictable meal schedule should be established and consistently followed.
Food Presentation and Access	• Food items or containers may be placed directly into the individual's hand to facilitate initiation of self-feeding. • Foods should be prepared in appropriate portion sizes and textures consistent with the individual's swallowing abilities.
Support for Self-Feeding	• Self-feeding should be encouraged, initiated, and gently guided when necessary. • Assistance should be provided to prompt mouth opening when required.
Chewing and Swallowing Facilitation	• Verbal cues may be used to remind and encourage chewing when necessary. • Swallowing should be gently prompted using verbal encouragement. • If required, verbal instructions and manual cues may be provided to encourage tongue use for clearing oral residue after swallowing.

3.7. Enteral Nutrition

Enteral feeding methods, including nasogastric (NG) tube feeding and percutaneous endoscopic gastrostomy (PEG), are generally implemented following acute aspiration pneumonia or severe malnutrition. However, in individuals with advanced dementia, tube feeding does not prolong survival, reduce aspiration risk, or improve quality of life (Alagiakrishnan et al., 2013; Kuo et al., 2009). Studies comparing feeding modalities in individuals with dementia and dysphagia have demonstrated that NG tube feeding is associated with a higher incidence of aspiration pneumonia compared with oral feeding (Cintra et al., 2014; Yuen et al., 2022), while PEG feeding has been shown to result in a higher aspiration pneumonia incidence compared with total caregiver-assisted feeding (Masaki & Kawamoto, 2019). The 2023 guidelines of the European Society for Clinical Nutrition and Metabolism (ESPEN) explicitly emphasize that tube feeding is not recommended in this population (Volkert et al.,

2015). Instead, individualized oral approaches such as hand feeding represent a more ethical and clinically appropriate alternative, preserving eating pleasure, social interaction, and human dignity in individuals with dementia (Parlak, Altan, et al., 2022).

3.8. Multidisciplinary Approach

A multidisciplinary team includes healthcare professionals, caregivers, and the individual with dementia. The selection and combined use of one or more intervention options should be determined through shared decision-making by the multidisciplinary team, taking into account the preferences and needs of both the individual with dementia and their family members (Chan et al., 2024; Tong et al., 2025).

Arahata et al. (2017) conducted a comprehensive intervention program monitoring the clinical course of eating and swallowing disorders in 90 individuals with dementia. Using a multidisciplinary approach involving physicians, dentists, pharmacists, nurses, speech and language therapists, physiotherapists, occupational therapists, dietitians, and certified care workers, the team performed detailed assessments to clarify etiologies and implemented individualized therapeutic interventions. The study demonstrated that comprehensive evaluation of physical, cognitive, chewing, swallowing, and sensory functions—using the most appropriate assessment procedures for each individual—facilitated accurate determination of reversibility. Detailed etiological identification contributed to improvements in functional eating status, enhanced independence, and improved survival without reliance on artificial nutrition (Arahata et al., 2017).

3.9. Neuromodulation and Other Techniques

Tang et al. (2017) divided 103 individuals with Alzheimer's disease and dysphagia into two groups. The control group received swallowing function training only, whereas the intervention group received swallowing rehabilitation training combined with neuromuscular electrical stimulation (NMES) and electromyographic (EMG) biofeedback therapy. After 12 weeks of treatment, swallowing function was assessed using a water swallowing test, and the incidence and course of aspiration pneumonia were recorded. Although no significant difference was observed between groups in Mini Nutritional Assessment scores, the intervention group demonstrated greater improvements in swallowing function, better nutritional status, and a lower frequency and shorter duration of aspiration pneumonia. These findings suggest that combining swallowing rehabilitation with NMES and EMG biofeedback may enhance swallowing function and significantly reduce adverse outcomes (Tang et al., 2017).

Electrical stimulation used for rehabilitation purposes includes therapeutic electrical stimulation to increase muscle strength, functional electrical stimulation to facilitate compensatory muscle contractions, and transcutaneous electrical nerve stimulation (TENS) for analgesia. These modalities primarily target nerves and muscles, and many TENS procedures employ low-frequency stimulation. In dysphagia rehabilitation, low-frequency electrical stimulation is commonly applied to enhance cervical muscle strength. However, because TENS cannot effectively stimulate deep anatomical structures, interferential current stimulation has been developed to overcome this limitation. Hara et al. (2020) investigated the effects of interferential current transcutaneous electrical sensory stimulation (IFC-TESS) on swallowing function in individuals with chronic dysphagia and dementia for whom active training is difficult. IFC-TESS was administered twice daily, five days per week, for three weeks. The upper electrodes were placed directly below the mandibular angle, and the lower electrodes were positioned along the anterior border of the sternocleidomastoid muscle at the level of the thyroid cartilage (Figure 4). Their findings indicated that cervical IFC-TESS improved the cough reflex and increased oral caloric intake in nursing home residents with dementia and dysphagia. The authors concluded that IFC-TESS may be a feasible intervention for individuals with dementia who are unable to participate in active rehabilitation approaches (Hara et al., 2021).

Figure 4. Electrode placement for IFC-TESS (Hara et al., 2020)

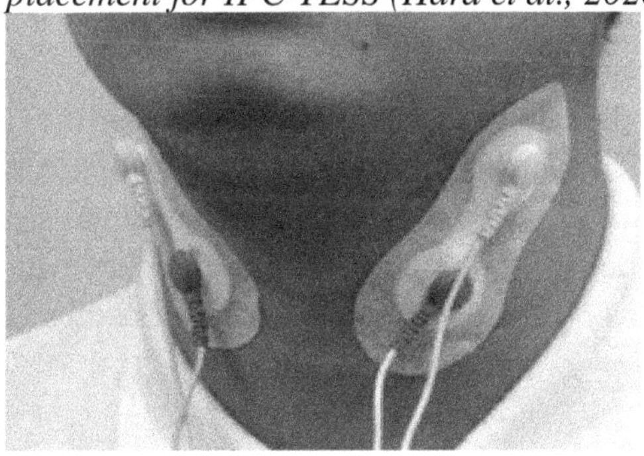

For individuals with moderate to severe dysphagia, advanced interventions targeting central swallowing dysfunction—such as transcranial magnetic stimulation or transcranial electrical stimulation —may be required (Liu et al., 2024; Marchina et al., 2021). However, to date, no studies have reported the use of neuromodulation techniques specifically to improve swallowing function in individuals with dementia.

Therefore, future research employing high-quality randomized controlled trials is necessary to explore the efficacy and safety of these approaches in this population.

CONCLUSION

The clinical profiles of individuals with dementia vary according to dementia subtype and individual characteristics. The features of dysphagia in individuals with dementia may change throughout the course of the disease; therefore, their needs and challenges can also evolve over time. Regular reassessments are essential to monitor changes in dysphagia profiles and to evaluate the effectiveness of interventions in this population. However, there is a notable lack of dementia-specific clinical dysphagia screening and assessment tools, and instrumental evaluations may also be challenging to implement in this group. Further research is required to address these assessment-related limitations.

Dysphagia intervention in individuals with dementia requires an individualized, multidimensional, and dynamic approach. Interventions should be planned according to the stage and etiology of dementia and delivered within a multidisciplinary team framework. Dysphagia management in dementia should not be limited to restoring physiological swallowing function; rather, it should adopt a holistic approach that also addresses emotional, behavioral, and social needs. Intervention plans should be personalized and multidimensional, taking into account the individual's cognitive level, behavioral profile, motivation for eating, and caregiving environment.

Among evidence-based interventions, texture-modified diets, meticulous oral hygiene, behavioral support, and adaptive environmental modifications emerge as key components. Swallowing exercises and postural maneuvers may be beneficial, particularly when implemented over a 4–6 week period in the early stages of dementia. Enteral feeding, when considered within a quality-of-life framework, should be regarded as a last resort. Finally, dysphagia management in dementia is likely to be more effective when delivered through a multidisciplinary team involving healthcare professionals, caregivers, and the individual with dementia.

REFERENCES

Affoo, R. H., Foley, N., Rosenbek, J., Kevin Shoemaker, J., & Martin, R. E. (2013). Swallowing dysfunction and autonomic nervous system dysfunction in Alzheimer's disease: A scoping review of the evidence. *Journal of the American Geriatrics Society*, *61*(12), 2203–2213. PMID: 24329892

Alagiakrishnan, K., Bhanji, R. A., & Kurian, M. (2013). Evaluation and management of oropharyngeal dysphagia in different types of dementia: A systematic review. *Archives of Gerontology and Geriatrics*, *56*(1), 1–9. PMID: 22608838

Aliani, M., Udenigwe, C. C., Girgih, A. T., Pownall, T. L., Bugera, J. L., & Eskin, M. N. (2013). Aroma and taste perceptions with Alzheimer disease and stroke. *Critical Reviews in Food Science and Nutrition*, *53*(7), 760–769. PMID: 23638935

Arahata, M., Oura, M., Tomiyama, Y., Morikawa, N., Fujii, H., Minani, S., & Shimizu, Y. (2017). A comprehensive intervention following the clinical pathway of eating and swallowing disorder in the elderly with dementia: Historically controlled study. *BMC Geriatrics*, *17*(1), 146. PMID: 28705163

Arslan, S. S., Demir, N., Kılınç, H. E., & Karaduman, A. A. (2017). The ability of the Eating Assessment Tool-10 to detect aspiration in patients with neurological disorders. *Journal of Neurogastroenterology and Motility*, *23*(4), 550. PMID: 28545185

Association, A. s. (2016). 2016 Alzheimer's disease facts and figures. *Alzheimer's & dementia*, *12*(4), 459-509.

Aydogdu, I., Kiylioglu, N., Tarlaci, S., Tanriverdi, Z., Alpaydin, S., Acarer, A., & Secil, Y. (2015). Diagnostic value of "dysphagia limit" for neurogenic dysphagia: 17 years of experience in 1278 adults. *Clinical Neurophysiology*, *126*(3), 634–643. PMID: 25088732

Baijens, L. W., Clave, P., Cras, P., Ekberg, O., Forster, A., Kolb, G. F., & Ortega, O. (2016). European Society for Swallowing Disorders–European Union Geriatric Medicine Society white paper: Oropharyngeal dysphagia as a geriatric syndrome. *Clinical Interventions in Aging*, *11*, 1403. PMID: 27785002

Baijens, L. W., Clavé, P., Cras, P., Ekberg, O., Forster, A., Kolb, G. F., & Ortega, O. (2016). European Society for Swallowing Disorders–European Union Geriatric Medicine Society white paper: Oropharyngeal dysphagia as a geriatric syndrome. *Clinical Interventions in Aging*, *11*, 1403. PMID: 27785002

Bautmans, I., Demarteau, J., Cruts, B., Lemper, J.-C., & Mets, T. (2008). Dysphagia in elderly nursing home residents with severe cognitive impairment can be attenuated by cervical spine mobilization. *Journal of Rehabilitation Medicine*, *40*(9), 755–760. PMID: 18843429

Bayles, K., McCullough, K., & Tomoeda, C. K. (2018). *Cognitive-communication disorders of MCI and dementia: Definition, assessment, and clinical management.* Plural Publishing.

Bayles, K., & Tomoeda, C. (2007). *Assessment of Cognitive-Communication Disorders of Dementia. Cognitive-Communication Disorders of Dementia.* Plural Publishing.

Bayles, K. A., & Tomoeda, C. K. (2007). *Cognitive-communication disorders of dementia*. Plural Publishing.

Behrman, S., Chouliaras, L., & Ebmeier, K. P. (2014). Considering the senses in the diagnosis and management of dementia. *Maturitas*, *77*(4), 305–310. PMID: 24495787

Benigas, J. E., & Bourgeois, M. (2016). Using spaced retrieval with external aids to improve use of compensatory strategies during eating for persons with dementia. *American Journal of Speech-Language Pathology*, *25*(3), 321–334. PMID: 27538017

Better, M. A. (2023). Alzheimer's disease facts and figures. *Alzheimer's & Dementia*, *19*(4), 1598–1695. PMID: 36918389

Boccardi, V., Ruggiero, C., Patriti, A., & Marano, L. (2016). Diagnostic assessment and management of dysphagia in patients with Alzheimer's disease. *Journal of Alzheimer's Disease*, *50*(4), 947–955. PMID: 26836016

Bomfim, F., Chiari, B. M., & Roque, F. P. (2013). Factors associated to suggestive signs of oropharyngeal dysphagia in institutionalized elderly women. *CEP*, *57035*, 130. PMID: 24408245

Burkhead, L. M., Sapienza, C. M., & Rosenbek, J. C. (2007). Strength-training exercise in dysphagia rehabilitation: Principles, procedures, and directions for future research. *Dysphagia*, *22*(3), 251–265. PMID: 17457549

Carr, M., McKeown, L., & MacEntee, M. I. (2010). Oral health, dysphagia, and aspiration pneumonia. *Oral Healthcare and the Frail Elder: A Clinical Perspective*, 111-125.

Chan, C. T. W., Wu, T. Y., & Cheng, I. (2024). A systematic review on dysphagia treatments for persons living with dementia. *European Geriatric Medicine*, *15*(6), 1573–1585. PMID: 39612080

Cintra, M., De Rezende, N., De Moraes, E., Cunha, L., & da Gama Torres, H. (2014). A comparison of survival, pneumonia, and hospitalization in patients with advanced dementia and dysphagia receiving either oral or enteral nutrition. *The Journal of Nutrition, Health & Aging*, *18*(10), 894–899. PMID: 25470805

De Stefano, A., Di Giovanni, P., Kulamarva, G., Gennachi, S., Di Fonzo, F., Sallustio, V., & Dispenza, F. (2020). Oropharyngeal dysphagia in elderly population suffering from mild cognitive impairment and mild dementia: Understanding the link. *American Journal of Otolaryngology*, *41*(4), 102501. PMID: 32409161

Demir, N., Arslan, S. S., İnal, Ö., & Karaduman, A. A. (2016). Reliability and validity of the Turkish Eating Assessment Tool (T-EAT-10). *Dysphagia*, *31*(5), 644–649. PMID: 27405421

Doan, T.-N., Ho, W.-C., Wang, L.-H., Chang, F.-C., Nhu, N. T., & Chou, L.-W. (2022). Prevalence and methods for assessment of oropharyngeal dysphagia in older adults: A systematic review and meta-analysis. *Journal of Clinical Medicine*, *11*(9), 2605. PMID: 35566731

Easterling, C. S., & Robbins, E. (2008). Dementia and dysphagia. *Geriatric Nursing*, *29*(4), 275–285. PMID: 18694703

Edahiro, A., Hirano, H., Yamada, R., Chiba, Y., Watanabe, Y., Tonogi, M., & Yamane, G. y. (2012). Factors affecting independence in eating among elderly with Alzheimer's disease. *Geriatrics & Gerontology International*, *12*(3), 481–490. PMID: 22233202

Ekberg, O. (2012). *Dysphagia: Diagnosis and treatment.* Springer Science & Business Media.

Fernández, O. O., & Clavé, P. (2013). Oral hygiene, aspiration, and aspiration pneumonia: From pathophysiology to therapeutic strategies. *Current Physical Medicine and Rehabilitation Reports*, *1*(4), 292–295.

Flynn, E., Smith, C. H., Walsh, C. D., & Walshe, M. (2018). Modifying the consistency of food and fluids for swallowing difficulties in dementia. *Cochrane Database of Systematic Reviews*, 9. PMID: 30251253

Forster, A., Samaras, N., Gold, G., & Samaras, D. (2011). Oropharyngeal dysphagia in older adults: A review. *European Geriatric Medicine*, *2*(6), 356–362.

Gale, S. A., Acar, D., & Daffner, K. R. (2018). William J. Mullally, MD, Neurology Series Editor.

Groher, M. E. (2015). Issues and Challenges in Managing Patients with Dementia and Dysphagia. , *30*(2), 61-67.

Groher, M. E., & Crary, M. A. (2015). *Dysphagia: clinical management in adults and children*. Elsevier Health Sciences.

Gürgör, N., Arıcı, Ş., Incesu, T. K., Seçil, Y., Tokuçoğlu, F., & Ertekin, C. (2013). An electrophysiological study of the sequential water swallowing. *Journal of Electromyography and Kinesiology*, *23*(3), 619–626. PMID: 23466271

Hara, Y., Nakane, A., Tohara, H., Kubota, K., Nakagawa, K., Hara, K., & Minakuchi, S. (2021). Cervical interferential current transcutaneous electrical sensory stimulation for patients with dysphagia and dementia in nursing homes. *Clinical Interventions in Aging*, •••, 2431–2437. PMID: 33456308

Holt, P. (2004). Management and evaluation of dysphagia. *Supplement to Annals of Long-Term Care*, 2-7.

Hu, X., Ma, Y.-n., Karako, K., Tang, W., Song, P., & Xia, Y. (2024). Comprehensive assessment and treatment strategies for dysphagia in the elderly population: Current status and prospects. *Bioscience Trends*, *18*(2), 116–126. PMID: 38658363

Humbert, I. A., McLaren, D. G., Kosmatka, K., Fitzgerald, M., Johnson, S., Porcaro, E., & Robbins, J. (2010). Early deficits in cortical control of swallowing in Alzheimer's disease. *Journal of Alzheimer's Disease*, *19*(4), 1185–1197. PMID: 20308785

Ikeda, M., Brown, J., Holland, A. J., Fukuhara, R., & Hodges, J. (2002). Changes in appetite, food preference, and eating habits in frontotemporal dementia and Alzheimer's disease. *Journal of Neurology, Neurosurgery, and Psychiatry*, *73*(4), 371–376. PMID: 12235302

Imaizumi, M., Weng, W., Zhu, X., & Murono, S. (2024). Effectiveness of FEES with artificial intelligence-assisted computer-aided diagnosis. *Auris, Nasus, Larynx*, *51*(2), 251–258. PMID: 37980257

Kane, J. P., Surendranathan, A., Bentley, A., Barker, S. A., Taylor, J.-P., Thomas, A. J., & McKeith, I. G. (2018). Clinical prevalence of Lewy body dementia. *Alzheimer's Research & Therapy*, *10*(1), 19. PMID: 29448953

Kays, S., & Robbins, J. A. (2006). Effects of sensorimotor exercise on swallowing outcomes relative to age and age-related disease. Seminars in speech and language, Kuo, S., Rhodes, R. L., Mitchell, S. L., Mor, V., & Teno, J. M. (2009). Natural history of feeding-tube use in nursing home residents with advanced dementia. *Journal of the American Medical Directors Association*, *10*(4), 264–270.

Labeit, B., Ahring, S., Boehmer, M., Sporns, P., Sauer, S., Claus, I., & Warnecke, T. (2022). Comparison of simultaneous swallowing endoscopy and videofluoroscopy in neurogenic dysphagia. *Journal of the American Medical Directors Association, 23*(8), 1360–1366. PMID: 34678269

Langmore, S. E. (2003). Evaluation of oropharyngeal dysphagia: Which diagnostic tool is superior? *Current Opinion in Otolaryngology & Head & Neck Surgery, 11*(6), 485–489. PMID: 14631184

Langmore, S. E., Olney, R. K., Lomen-Hoerth, C., & Miller, B. L. (2007). Dysphagia in patients with frontotemporal lobar dementia. *Archives of Neurology, 64*(1), 58–62. PMID: 17210809

Larsson, V., Torisson, G., Bülow, M., & Londos, E. (2017). Effects of carbonated liquid on swallowing dysfunction in dementia with Lewy bodies and Parkinson's disease dementia. *Clinical Interventions in Aging*, •••, 1215–1222. PMID: 28848329

Lazarus, C. (2006). Tongue strength and exercise in healthy individuals and in head and neck cancer patients. Seminars in speech and language, Leonard, R. (2023). Dysphagia and dementia: A 'double dilemma'. *Current Opinion in Otolaryngology & Head & Neck Surgery, 31*(6), 357–361.

Lin, L. C., Watson, R., & Wu, S. C. (2010). What is associated with low food intake in older people with dementia? *Journal of Clinical Nursing, 19*(1-2), 53–59. PMID: 20500244

Liu, Y., Yin, S., Yang, X., Luo, S., Zhu, F., Zeng, Z., & Yu, Q. (2024). Effects of cerebellar repetitive transcranial magnetic stimulation in the treatment of post-stroke dysphagia: A meta-analysis and systematic review of randomized controlled trials. *European Neurology, 87*(2), 67–78. PMID: 38432194

Logemann, J. A. (1998). The evaluation and treatment of swallowing disorders. *Current Opinion in Otolaryngology & Head & Neck Surgery, 6*(6), 395–400.

Logemann, J. A., Gensler, G., Robbins, J., Lindblad, A. S., Brandt, D., Hind, J. A.,… Gramigna, G. D. (2008). A randomized study of three interventions for aspiration of thin liquids in patients with dementia or Parkinson's disease.

Londos, E., Hanxsson, O., Alm Hirsch, I., Janneskog, A., Bülow, M., & Palmqvist, S. (2013). Dysphagia in Lewy body dementia-a clinical observational study of swallowing function by videofluoroscopic examination. *BMC Neurology, 13*(1), 140. PMID: 24099488

Londos, E., Hanxsson, O., Hirsch, I. A., Janneskog, A., Bülow, M., & Palmqvist, S. (2013). Dysphagia in Lewy body dementia-a clinical observational study of swallowing function by videofluoroscopic examination. *BMC Neurology*, *13*(1), 140. PMID: 24099488

Magalhães, H. V.Junior, Pernambuco, L. A., Cavalcanti, R. V. A., Silva, R. G. d., Lima, K. C., & Ferreira, M. A. F. (2022). Accuracy of an epidemiological oropharyngeal dysphagia screening for older adults. *Gerodontology*, *39*(4), 418–424. PMID: 34913514

Marchina, S., Pisegna, J. M., Massaro, J. M., Langmore, S. E., McVey, C., Wang, J., & Kumar, S. (2021). Transcranial direct current stimulation for post-stroke dysphagia: A systematic review and meta-analysis of randomized controlled trials. *Journal of Neurology*, *268*(1), 293–304. PMID: 32797300

Marshall, C. R., Hardy, C. J., Volkmer, A., Russell, L. L., Bond, R. L., Fletcher, P. D., & Rossor, M. N. (2018). Primary progressive aphasia: A clinical approach. *Journal of Neurology*, *265*(6), 1474–1490. PMID: 29392464

Masaki, S., & Kawamoto, T. (2019). Comparison of long-term outcomes between enteral nutrition via gastrostomy and total parenteral nutrition in older persons with dysphagia: A propensity-matched cohort study. *PLoS One*, *14*(10), e0217120. PMID: 31577813

Michel, A., Vérin, E., Gbaguidi, X., Druesne, L., Roca, F., & Chassagne, P. (2018). Oropharyngeal dysphagia in community-dwelling older patients with dementia: Prevalence and relationship with geriatric parameters. *Journal of the American Medical Directors Association*, *19*(9), 770–774. PMID: 29861192

Mira, A., Gonçalves, R., & Rodrigues, I. T. (2022). Dysphagia in Alzheimer's disease: A systematic review. *Dementia & Neuropsychologia*, *16*(3), 261–269. PMID: 36619845

Morgan, A. E., & Mc Auley, M. T. (2024). Vascular dementia: From pathobiology to emerging perspectives. *Ageing Research Reviews*, *96*, 102278. PMID: 38513772

Munis, Ö. B., & Parlak, M. M. (2023). Validity and reliability of the Turkish version of the Holden Communication Scale. *Brain and Behavior*, •••, 3223. PMID: 37587848

Nakashima, T., Maeda, K., Tahira, K., Taniguchi, K., Mori, K., Kiyomiya, H., & Akagi, J. (2018). Silent aspiration predicts mortality in older adults with aspiration pneumonia admitted to acute hospitals. *Geriatrics & Gerontology International*, *18*(6), 828–832. PMID: 29388314

Ney, D. M., Weiss, J. M., Kind, A. J., & Robbins, J. (2009). Senescent swallowing: Impact, strategies, and interventions. *Nutrition in Clinical Practice*, *24*(3), 395–413. PMID: 19483069

O'Rourke, F., Vickers, K., Upton, C., & Chan, D. (2014). Swallowing and oropharyngeal dysphagia. *Clinical Medicine*, *14*(2), 196–199. PMID: 24715134

Olney, N. T., Spina, S., & Miller, B. L. (2017). Frontotemporal dementia. *Neurologic Clinics*, *35*(2), 339. PMID: 28410663

Organization, W. H. (2017). Global action plan on the public health response to dementia 2017–2025.

Organization, W. H. (2021). Rise, respond, recover: renewing progress on women's, children's and adolescents' health in the era of COVID-19.

Park, Y.-H., Han, H.-R., Oh, B.-M., Lee, J., Park, J.-a., Yu, S. J., & Chang, H. (2013). Prevalence and associated factors of dysphagia in nursing home residents. *Geriatric Nursing*, *34*(3), 212–217. PMID: 23528180

Parlak, M. M., Altan, E., & Saylam, G. (2022). Dysphagia in Individuals with Dementia. *Journal of Ear Nose Throat and Head Neck Surgery*(30(2)), 88-96. https://doi.org/DOI: DOI: 10.24179/kbbbbc.2021-86783

Parlak, M. M., Babademez, M. A., Tokgöz, S. A., Bizpınar, Ö., & Saylam, G. (2022). Evaluation of Swallowing Function according to the Stage of Alzheimer's Disease. *Folia Phoniatrica et Logopaedica*, *74*(3), 186–194. PMID: 34469898

Parlak, M. M., Bizbinar, Ö., & Köse, A. (2023). The Effect of Holistic Therapy in Alzheimer's Disease. *Alternative Therapies in Health and Medicine*, •••, AT7591. PMID: 36689358

Parlak, M. M., Bizpinar, Ö., & Saylam, G. (2022). Dysphagia in patients in acute period of ischemic stroke: What is the relationship of dysphagia with infarct localization, cognition, malnutrition, and independence level? *Neurology Asia*, *27*(1), 63–71.

Parlak, M. M., Bizpınar Munis, Ö., Köse, A., Yıldırım, C., & Ülker, C. A. (2025). The Turkish validity and reliability of Addenbrooke's Cognitive Examination III. *International Journal of Language & Communication Disorders*, *60*(1), e13147. PMID: 39698920

Parlak, M. M., İnceoğlu, P., Tokgöz, S. A., Munis, Ö. B., & Saylam, G. (2025). Use of EAT-10 in Individuals with Alzheimer's Disease: Who Should be the Source of Information? *Dysphagia*, *40*(3), 668–679. PMID: 39466385

Parlak, M. M., & Köse, A. (2022). Cognitive Communication Disorders in Alzheimer's Disease. In Akkaya, R., & Akkaya, B. (Eds.), *Current Debates on Health Sciences 4* (pp. 239–250). Bilgin Kültür Sanat Yayınları., https://www.bidgecongress.org/wp-content/uploads/2023/02/Current-Debates-in-Health-Sciences-4-13.pdf

Parlak, M. M., & Köse, A. (2023). Investigation of the knowledge, experiences, and opinions of Speech and Language Pathologists on assessments and therapies for cognitive communication disorders in people with Alzheimer's disease-A cross-sectional survey in Turkey. *Hacettepe University Faculty of Health Sciences Journal*, *10*(1), 45–57.

Parlak, M. M., Köse, A., Güç, M., & Munis, Ö. B. (2024). Development of mobile compatible software for cognitive–communication disorder in individuals with Alzheimer's disease. *International Journal of Language & Communication Disorders*, *59*(1), 234–254. PMID: 37528064

Parlak, M. M., Saylam, G., Babademez, M. A., Munis, Ö. B., & Tokgöz, S. A. (2023). Voice analysis results in individuals with Alzheimer's disease: How do age and cognitive status affect voice parameters? *Brain and Behavior*, *13*(11), e3271. PMID: 37794703

Parlak, M. M., Tokgöz, S. A., Bizpinar, Ö., Saylam, G., & Köse, A. (2022). Investigation of cognition, nutrition, independence and swallowing difficulty, relationship with quality of life, and effect levels in elderly people with Alzheimer's disease living with their families. *Neurology Asia*, *27*(3), 701–708.

Peranovic, S., Pourhassan, M., Labeit, B., Muhle, P., Suntrup-Krueger, S., Warnecke, T., & Lueg, G. (2025). Endoscopic characterization of oropharyngeal dysphagia in patients with dementia. *Frontiers in Aging*, *6*, 1535137. PMID: 40642379

Priefer, B. A., & Robbins, J. (1997). Eating changes in mild-stage Alzheimer's disease: A pilot study. *Dysphagia*, *12*(4), 212–221. PMID: 9294942

Prince, M., Bryce, R., Albanese, E., Wimo, A., Ribeiro, W., & Ferri, C. P. (2013). The global prevalence of dementia: a systematic review and metaanalysis. *Alzheimer's & dementia, 9*(1), 63-75. e62.

Ramirez-Gomez, L., Zheng, L., Reed, B., Kramer, J., Mungas, D., Zarow, C., & Chui, H. (2017). Neuropsychological profiles differentiate Alzheimer disease from subcortical ischemic vascular dementia in an autopsy-defined cohort. *Dementia and Geriatric Cognitive Disorders*, *44*(1-2), 1–11. PMID: 28595184

Ramsey, D. J., Smithard, D. G., & Kalra, L. (2003). Early assessments of dysphagia and aspiration risk in acute stroke patients. *Stroke*, *34*(5), 1252–1257. PMID: 12677020

Robbins, J., Gensler, G., Hind, J., Logemann, J. A., Lindblad, A. S., Brandt, D., & Lundy, D. (2008). Comparison of 2 Interventions for Liquid Aspiration on Pneumonia IncidenceA Randomized TrialRandomized Trial of 2 Interventions for Aspiration. *Annals of Internal Medicine*, *148*(7), 509–518. PMID: 18378947

Robbins, J., Kays, S. A., Gangnon, R. E., Hind, J. A., Hewitt, A. L., Gentry, L. R., & Taylor, A. J. (2007). The effects of lingual exercise in stroke patients with dysphagia. *Archives of Physical Medicine and Rehabilitation*, *88*(2), 150–158. PMID: 17270511

Rofes, L., Arreola, V., Mukherjee, R., & Clave, P. (2014). Sensitivity and specificity of the Eating Assessment Tool and the Volume-Viscosity Swallow Test for clinical evaluation of oropharyngeal dysphagia. *Neurogastroenterology and Motility*, *26*(9), 1256–1265. PMID: 24909661

Sato, E., Hirano, H., Watanabe, Y., Edahiro, A., Sato, K., Yamane, G., & Katakura, A. (2014). Detecting signs of dysphagia in patients with Alzheimer's disease with oral feeding in daily life. *Geriatrics & Gerontology International*, *14*(3), 549–555. PMID: 23992204

Scholz, S. W., Okubadejo, N. U., Prakash, P., Liddelow, S. A., Ryten, M., & Halliday, G. M. (2025). Advances in the genetics and pathology of Lewy body dementia. *Lancet Neurology*, *24*(12), 1026–1037. PMID: 41240918

Seçil, Y., Arıcı, Ş., İncesu, T. K., Gürgör, N., Beckmann, Y., & Ertekin, C. (2016). Dysphagia in Alzheimer's disease. *Neurophysiologie Clinique. Clinical Neurophysiology*, *46*(3), 171–178. PMID: 26924307

Selkoe, D. J. (2004). Cell biology of protein misfolding: The examples of Alzheimer's and Parkinson's diseases. *Nature Cell Biology*, *6*(11), 1054–1061. PMID: 15516999

Sleisenger, M. H., Feldman, M., Friedman, L. S., & Brandt, L. J. (2010). *Sleisenger and Fordtran's gastrointestinal and liver disease: pathophysiology, diagnosis, management/Gastrointestinal and liver disease*. Saunders/Elsevier.

Smith, E. E. (2017). Clinical presentations and epidemiology of vascular dementia. *Clinical Science*, *131*(11), 1059–1068. PMID: 28515342

Stach, C. B. (2000). Vascular dementia and dysphagia. *Topics in Stroke Rehabilitation*, *7*(3), 1–10.

Suh, M. K., Kim, H., & Na, D. L. (2009). Dysphagia in patients with dementia: Alzheimer versus vascular. *Alzheimer Disease and Associated Disorders*, *23*(2), 178–184. PMID: 19474573

Sura, L., Madhavan, A., Carnaby, G., & Crary, M. A. (2012). Dysphagia in the elderly: Management and nutritional considerations. *Clinical Interventions in Aging*, 7, 287. PMID: 22956864

Tang, J. A., Salapatas, A. M., Bonzelaar, L. B., & Friedman, M. (2017). Long-term incidence of velopharyngeal insufficiency and other sequelae following uvulopalatopharyngoplasty. *Otolaryngology - Head and Neck Surgery*, *156*(4), 606–610. PMID: 28116979

Thiem, U., Jäger, M., Stege, H., & Wirth, R. (2023). Diagnostic accuracy of the 'Dysphagia Screening Tool for Geriatric Patients' (DSTG) compared to Flexible Endoscopic Evaluation of Swallowing (FEES) for assessing dysphagia in hospitalized geriatric patients–a diagnostic study. *BMC Geriatrics*, *23*(1), 856. PMID: 38097922

Tong, L., Chen, L., Xiao, P., Zhang, Y., Cao, Q., & Zhu, W. (2025). Treatment of Dysphagia in Patients with Dementia: A Systematic Review and Meta-Analysis. *Dysphagia*, •••, 1–13. PMID: 40622605

Volkert, D., Chourdakis, M., Faxen-Irving, G., Frühwald, T., Landi, F., Suominen, M. H., & Schneider, S. M. (2015). ESPEN guidelines on nutrition in dementia. *Clinical Nutrition (Edinburgh, Lothian)*, *34*(6), 1052–1073. PMID: 26522922

Wada, H., Nakajoh, K., Satoh-Nakagawa, T., Suzuki, T., Ohrui, T., Arai, H., & Sasaki, H. (2001). Risk factors of aspiration pneumonia in Alzheimer's disease patients. *Gerontology*, *47*(5), 271–276. PMID: 11490146

Watson, R. (1994). Measuring feeding difficulty in patients with dementia: Replication and validation of the EdFED Scale# 1. *Journal of Advanced Nursing*, *19*(5), 850–855. PMID: 8056912

Whear, R., Abbott, R., Thompson-Coon, J., Bethel, A., Rogers, M., Hemsley, A., & Stein, K. (2014). Effectiveness of mealtime interventions on behavior symptoms of people with dementia living in care homes: A systematic review. *Journal of the American Medical Directors Association*, *15*(3), 185–193. PMID: 24405641

Wong, D. W.-C., Wang, J., Cheung, S. M.-Y., Lai, D. K.-H., Chiu, A. T.-S., Pu, D., & Kwok, T. C.-Y. (2025). Current Technological Advances in Dysphagia Screening: Systematic Scoping Review. *Journal of Medical Internet Research*, *27*, e65551. PMID: 40324167

Wu, C., Zhang, K., Ye, J., Huang, X., Yang, H., Yuan, L., & Guo, J. (2022). Evaluating the effectiveness of stepwise swallowing training on dysphagia in patients with Alzheimer's disease: Study protocol for a randomized controlled trial. *Trials, 23*(1), 490. PMID: 35698162

Yamamoto, T., Kobayashi, Y., & Murata, M. (2010). Risk of pneumonia onset and discontinuation of oral intake following videofluorography in patients with Lewy body disease. *Parkinsonism & Related Disorders, 16*(8), 503–506. PMID: 20584622

Ye, J., Wu, C., Chen, J., Wang, H., Pan, Y., Huang, X., & Wang, W. (2024). Effectiveness of nurse-delivered stepwise swallowing training on dysphagia in patients with Alzheimer's disease: A multi-center randomized controlled trial. *International Journal of Nursing Studies, 150*, 104649. PMID: 38070229

Yıldırım, C. S. A., Merve (2023). *Demansı Olan Bireylerde Görülen Yutma Bozuklukları*. Ankara Nobel Tıp Kitabevleri.

Yuen, J. K., Luk, J. K., Chan, T.-C., Shea, Y.-F., Chu, S. T., Bernacki, R.,…Chan, F. H. (2022). Reduced pneumonia risk in advanced dementia patients on careful hand feeding compared with nasogastric tube feeding. *Journal of the American Medical Directors Association, 23*(9), 1541-1547. e1542.

Chapter 6
Dysphagia in Head and Neck Cancers

Eren Balo
http://orcid.org/0000-0002-4215-0192
Anadolu University, Turkey

Batuhan Ökte
Anadolu University, Turkey

ABSTRACT

Head and neck cancers comprise malignant tumors that arise in various sites, including the oral cavity, pharynx, larynx, nasal cavity, paranasal sinuses, and salivary glands. Surgical treatments for head and neck cancer can cause dysphagia and aspiration by compromising both anatomical and neurological functions. The type and severity of the resulting swallowing disorders depend on the tumor location, the extent of resection, and the reconstruction method used. Reconstruction involves repairing tissues removed during surgery with flaps, grafts, or prostheses, while aiming to preserve functional integrity. The risk of dysphagia after oral and/or oropharyngeal surgery is especially linked to resection of the tongue and related structures. A systematic assessment of dysphagia is essential to ensure safe swallowing in patients undergoing head and neck cancer treatment. This section will outline the factors that influence swallowing function and lead to dysphagia in head and neck cancer patients

1. HEAD AND NECK CANCERS

Worldwide, cancer is the second leading cause of death among non-communicable diseases after cardiovascular diseases and is characterized by uncontrolled cell

DOI: 10.4018/979-8-3373-6405-6.ch006

growth primarily caused by damage to cellular DNA. This growth process results in hyperplasia and abnormal tissue formation, leading to the development of malignant tumors. Cancer cells can spread from the primary site to distant organs through the bloodstream or lymphatic system, forming metastases. When looking at the global causes of head and neck cancers, tobacco products and heavy alcohol use remain the most significant risk factors (Figure 1). However, there has been a notable rise in HPV-related oropharyngeal cancers, especially in developed countries. Additionally, factors like poor oral hygiene, consumption of processed foods and foods high in nitrosamines, and exposure to environmental and occupational irritants also play important roles in developing head and neck cancer (Sung et al., 2021).

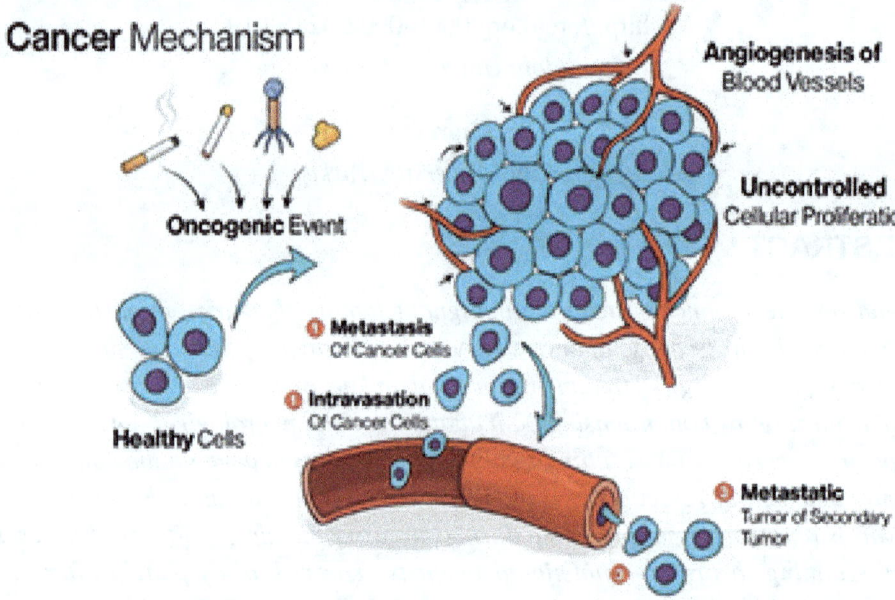

. Although the clinical presentation of the disease usually involves tumor formation, not all tumors are malignant (cancerous). The diagnostic process is based on the subjective complaints (symptoms) reported by the patient and the objective signs (findings) observed by the physician. Although it varies depending on the type and location of the cancer, unexplained weight loss, fever, and persistent fatigue are considered general warning signs(Rositch, 2020). More specific symptoms for the head and neck region include non-healing sores, white patches in the mouth, difficulty swallowing (dysphagia), hoarseness, abnormal bleeding, and skin changes. Additionally, pain and chronic fatigue, which develop due to tumor growth or treatments, are among the most common issues faced by patients and can diminish their quality of life.

One of the most damaging physiological effects of cancer is significant weight loss and malnutrition, which also weaken patients' immune systems. Between 30% and 50% of head and neck cancer patients are already malnourished at diagnosis and have lost 5-10% of their initial body weight(Hunter et al., 2020). This weight loss results not only from reduced food intake but also from increased metabolic energy demands caused by the tumor and impaired nutrient absorption. The patient's inadequate nutrition despite higher caloric needs creates a vicious cycle called 'cachexia.' This condition, worsened by anorexia, nausea, and constipation, delays wound healing and raises the risk of infection, negatively impacting the treatment process.

Signs and symptoms associated with cancer can occur in many patients, not just those with head and neck cancer. General warning signs include unexplained weight loss, fever, fatigue, pain, and skin changes. Specific symptoms might involve changes in bowel or bladder function, persistent sores, white patches or spots in the mouth or on the tongue, unusual bleeding or discharge, lumps or thickening anywhere in the body, indigestion or difficulty swallowing, recent changes in skin features like warts or moles, and ongoing coughing or hoarseness. A key feature of cancer-related fatigue is feeling exhausted, tired, or worn out despite enough sleep. People may find it hard to have the energy for daily tasks; they might also have trouble focusing, thinking clearly, or remembering. Fatigue often pairs with negative emotions, restlessness, impatience, and low motivation. Behavioral signs such as less interest in daily activities, neglecting personal care, or spending more time in bed or sleeping may also be seen. Malnutrition can lead to serious risks like higher chances of infection and a weakened immune system. Poor nutrition can cause respiratory failure, slow wound healing, and skin damage. In extreme cases, severe malnutrition could even be fatal.

In the Tumor, Node, Metastasis (TNM) classification of oropharyngeal cancer, the primary tumor size is defined in increasing levels from T1 to T4, with T1 indicating a tumor smaller than 2 cm, T2 between 2–4 cm, T3 larger than 4 cm, and T4 indicating invasion of adjacent structures. Lymph node involvement is graded from N0 to N3; N1 indicates a single ipsilateral lymph node metastasis smaller than 3 cm, N2 indicates more extensive or multiple lymph node involvement, and N3 indicates a metastatic lymph node larger than 6 cm. The presence of distant metastasis is assessed as M0 (absent) and M1 (present). When staging is performed according to these TNM characteristics, early-stage disease is limited to Tis or T1 tumors, whereas T2 lesions correspond to Stage II, and larger or lymph node-positive tumors correspond to Stage III. Invasion of adjacent structures or advanced lymph node involvement is classified as Stage IVA and IVB, while the presence of distant metastasis defines the disease as Stage IVC. This system provides a basic framework for determining the extent of the disease based on tumor size, lymph node spread, and metastasis status, and for guiding treatment planning(Amin & Edge, 2017).

2. DYSPHAGIA IN HEAD AND NECK CANCERS

Swallowing is a complex process divided into three main phases: oral, pharyngeal, and esophageal; it requires a brief pause in breathing and precise neuromuscular coordination of the upper aerodigestive tract. An adult swallows approximately 600 times per day, averaging 35 times per hour while awake and 6 times per hour while asleep(Kronenberger & Meyers, 1994).

Normal swallowing is a complex neuromuscular process involving sequential voluntary and involuntary movements and consists of three main phases (Figure 2): oral, pharyngeal, and esophageal (Leonard & Kendall, 2019). The oral phase is entirely under voluntary control and is divided into two sub-phases: oral preparation and oral transfer. During the oral preparation phase, food is brought to an appropriate consistency through chewing; lip closure, buccal muscle tone, rotational movements of the jaw, and lateralization of the tongue play critical roles in bolus formation. The intrinsic and extrinsic muscles of the tongue bring the bolus together and form a consistent structure. During the oral phase proper, the tongue pushes the bolus upward and backward along the hard palate into the oropharynx. The propulsive force of the tongue's midline and the closure of the lateral edges against the alveolar ridges enable the controlled transition of the bolus to the pharyngeal phase. This phase is completed in approximately 1–1.5 seconds in healthy individuals, and the pharyngeal swallowing reflex is triggered when the bolus reaches the pharynx.

The pharyngeal phase is the most critical stage of swallowing in terms of airway protection and is completely involuntary. During this phase, breathing stops briefly, the soft palate rises to prevent nasopharyngeal leakage, and the larynx moves upward and anteriorly, contributing to airway closure. The closure of the vocal folds, along with the epiglottis and aryepiglottic structures, effectively protects the airway. At the same time, the root of the tongue moves strongly backward, pushing the bolus toward the pharynx, and the pharyngeal constrictor muscles contract sequentially to allow the bolus to move downward. The upper esophageal sphincter (UES) opens with the movement of the larynx and neural relaxation mechanisms. This phase lasts approximately 1 second and is minimally affected by age, gender, or changes in consistency.

The esophageal phase is an entirely autonomous process and ensures the transport of the bolus from the UES to the stomach. The bolus advances through the esophagus in approximately 8–10 seconds with a primary peristaltic wave; if this wave is insufficient, secondary peristaltic waves associated with bolus distension are activated. The upper third of the esophagus consists of striated muscle, while the lower two-thirds consist of smooth muscle and are controlled by the vagus nerve and the myenteric nervous system. The lower esophageal sphincter (LES) reflexively relaxes as the bolus approaches and then provides a tonic closure after passage is complete, preventing reflux. Thus, the act of swallowing is safely completed.

Figure 2. (McKean et al., 2017)

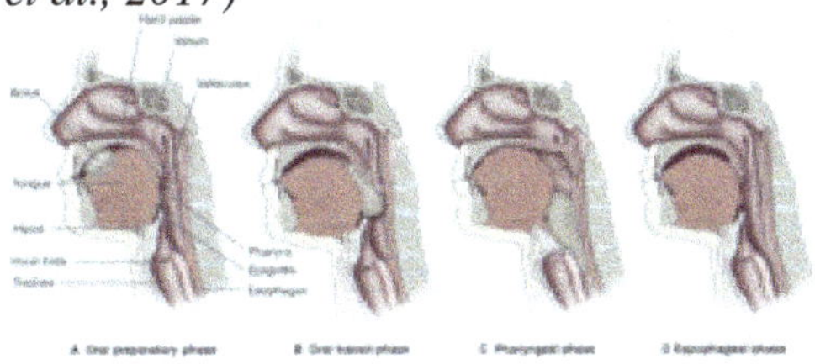

Dysphagia is a symptom originating from the Greek words *dys* (difficulty) and *phagein* (to eat), indicating a delay in the passage of solid or liquid food from the oral cavity to the stomach(Amitrano, 2024; WHO, 2004). Patients with head and neck cancer may experience dysphagia due to both the tumor itself and the treatments administered. Although there has been an increase in the use of organ-preserving treatment approaches in recent years, it cannot be said that these methods always provide functional preservation (Gillespie et al., 2004) .

Dysphagia and aspiration are among the potentially serious complications of head and neck cancer treatment. Any condition that restricts the opening of the upper esophageal sphincter can lead to material building up and leaking into the airway. As a result, aspiration can occur due to dysphagia. Normally, aspiration can be prevented by a robust cough reflex; however, the true rate of "silent aspiration" remains unknown.

The causes of aspiration can be divided into three groups: pre-swallowing, during swallowing, and post-swallowing. Pre-swallowing aspiration is associated with decreased oromotor control or delayed/absent swallowing reflex. Aspiration during swallowing may occur as a result of decreased laryngeal closure, inadequate epiglottic inversion, or decreased laryngeal elevation. Post-swallowing aspiration may develop due to decreased pharyngeal peristalsis, cricopharyngeal sphincter dysfunction, inadequate laryngeal elevation, or structural anomalies. The risk of aspiration is higher in patients undergoing chemotherapy and radiotherapy; moreover, aspiration may be challenging to detect in these patients as laryngeal sensory loss may also be present.

3. SURGICAL INTERVENTIONS AND DYSPHAGIA

Although chemoradiotherapy is currently favored as the primary treatment for many oropharyngeal, hypopharyngeal, and laryngeal cancers, surgery remains the mainstay of treatment for oral cavity, oral tongue, and selected early-stage laryngeal tumors, as well as for salvage cases following treatment failure. Postoperatively, oral intake is typically withheld for 1–2 weeks to allow adequate wound healing. The timing of swallowing assessment and resumption of oral feeding should be individualized, taking into account surgical healing, local edema, fistula formation, comorbid medical conditions, and the patient's overall clinical and psychological status. Although substantial spontaneous recovery of swallowing function is uncommon, many patients develop compensatory strategies over time, highlighting the critical role of long-term swallowing rehabilitation after surgery (Lester & Yang, 2015).

The type and extent of surgical intervention are among the primary determinants of which phases and mechanisms of swallowing will be affected. Surgeries for oral cavity cancers predominantly impair the oral phase of swallowing and bolus control, whereas resections involving the pharyngeal and laryngeal levels more profoundly affect the pharyngeal phase, airway protection, and aspiration risk.

Resection of lip tumors primarily affects oral sphincter competence, with functional outcomes determined by defect size, sensory preservation, and structural support. While resections involving up to half of the lower lip can often be closed primarily with minimal functional impairment, larger defects frequently require reconstructive techniques and may result in microstomia, compromising bolus intake. Sensory loss due to mental nerve injury further impairs oral competence, increasing the risk of anterior bolus loss and drooling during mastication (Chen, 2019; Howard et al., 2021; Ihara et al., 2022).

Impairment of mastication and swallowing is common following surgical procedures involving the oral cavity, mandible, and tongue, with the severity of dysfunction closely related to the type and extent of resection. Mandibulectomy, particularly segmental resections without reconstruction, may lead to marked deterioration in chewing and swallowing function, whereas mandibular reconstruction is generally associated with more limited functional deficits. Glossectomy and tongue resections have the greatest impact on swallowing function and are commonly associated with delayed swallow initiation, prolonged oral preparatory time, impaired oral-to-pharyngeal bolus transfer, premature bolus spillage due to sensory loss, reduced bolus control, and increased oral and pharyngeal residue. These impairments primarily result from reduced oral competence and insufficient intraoral pressure generation for effective bolus propulsion. Involvement of the floor of the mouth further restricts anterior–posterior tongue mobility and stabilization, leading to additional difficulties in bolus preparation and propulsion (Pauloski et al., 1995). Moreover, resection or dysfunction of the suprahyoid musculature compromises hyoid–laryngeal elevation and limits opening of the pharyngoesophageal segment, substantially increasing dysphagia severity and, in extreme cases, precluding safe swallowing (Lazarus, 2000). Tethering of the tongue to the floor of the mouth reduces contact with the posterior pharyngeal wall, resulting in weak pharyngeal constriction, increased pharyngeal residue, and an elevated risk of aspiration. Sensory and motor deficits due to lingual or hypoglossal nerve involvement may further exacerbate swallowing impairment (Sharma et al., 2022). Despite these deficits, preservation of the larynx often allows maintenance of oral intake with appropriate dietary modifications. Nasal regurgitation and pharyngeal residue are also frequently observed following oropharyngeal and tonsillar resections, reflecting direct disruption of the pharyngeal phase of swallowing.

Defects in the floor of the mouth directly affect a patient's swallowing ability. Performing closure in a way that pulls the tongue forward or using local flaps that reduce tongue volume can worsen existing movement restrictions. Therefore, surgeons should avoid techniques that might cause the tongue to be pulled forward during reconstruction. Pulling the tongue forward makes backward movement difficult and prevents contact with the posterior pharyngeal wall. When contact cannot be made, pharyngeal constriction weakens, leading to residual food in the pharynx and a risk of aspiration. Conversely, a large regional flap placed in the defect may push the tongue too far back, disrupting normal bolus control. For the tongue to deliver the bolus to the pharynx, it must make sequential contact along the palate from front to back; disrupting this mechanism significantly reduces swallowing efficiency. To transfer the bolus to the pharynx, the tongue must make successive contacts with the palate in the anterior-posterior direction(Hirano et al., 1992).

The degree of impairment is related to the location and extent of the resection(Logemann et al., 1994). Surgical removal of 50% or more of the tongue base (≥50% tongue base resection) has emerged as the strongest risk factor for the development of postoperative dysphagia. In patients with oral cavity and oropharyngeal cancer, resection at this level is associated with a significant impairment of swallowing function in both the short and long term. Since the tongue base plays a fundamental role in propelling the bolus into the oropharynx and initiating the swallowing reflex, removal of more than half of the tongue base leads to decreased pharyngeal pressure, increased oral and vallecular residue, and an elevated risk of aspiration(Zhang et al., 2025).

Loss of tongue volume following tongue cancer resection is a major determinant of dysphagia severity, affecting both the oral and pharyngeal phases of swallowing. Anterior tongue resections primarily impair bolus manipulation and oral propulsion, particularly when palatal contact cannot be adequately achieved. In contrast, posterior tongue resections compromise the generation of pharyngeal driving pressure, resulting in weak pharyngeal constriction, increased vallecular and pharyngeal residue, and an elevated risk of aspiration on instrumental swallowing assessment(McConnel & O'Connor, 1994). These deficits reflect the tongue's central role in bolus formation, propulsion, and pharyngeal clearance and highlight the importance of preserving tongue volume and mobility during surgical planning and reconstruction. With the development of transoral robotic surgery (TORS), this method has gained popularity in the treatment of small tongue root tumors. Robotic arms are inserted through the mouth, allowing for better visualization of the surgical site and removal of the tumor using two robotic arms. Such defects are usually left to secondary healing, and it is thought that patients may have better swallowing function than those treated with chemoradiotherapy. However, most studies in these patients have focused on patients' subjective perceptions of swallowing and gastrostomy tube use rates rather than on modified barium swallow studies. It has been reported that patients receiving adjuvant therapy, such as additional radiotherapy, have a higher need for gastrostomy tubes in the short term(Hutcheson et al., 2015).

Since tumors involving the floor of the mouth, anterior region of the tongue, or lateral pharyngeal wall often spread to the mandible, resection of part of the mandible may be necessary to ensure safe surgical margins. This can result in sensory loss in the lower lip and lower teeth due to involvement of the alveolar and mental nerves that run within the mandible. Resection of mandibular segments can also cause malocclusion by disrupting jaw alignment. Anterior mandibular resections can lead to the "Andy Gump" deformity, which results in a significant loss of jaw contour and severely reduces oral competence. Following mandibular resections, the loss of the attachment points of the hyoid elevator muscles also reduces hyoid elevation, preventing adequate opening of the pharyngoesophageal sphincter.

Hard palate defects lead to the formation of oro-nasal fistulas. The fistula increases the volume of the oral cavity to that of the nasal cavity, turning what should be a closed structure into an open cavity. As a result, during bolus preparation, food or liquids can easily escape into the nasal cavity. The tongue is often insufficient to retrieve material that enters the nasal cavity, making bolus manipulation more difficult. The hard palate provides a stable surface necessary for the tongue to push the bolus toward the pharynx; therefore, pressure generation and bolus transfer are significantly impaired in defects involving the palate. Closing hard palate defects with obturator prostheses usually greatly improves dysphagia.

Soft palate defects disrupt the dual sphincter function of the palate. During the oral phase, the soft palate is relaxed and rests on the root of the tongue, separating the oral and pharyngeal cavities. During the pharyngeal phase, the soft palate elevates, separating the nasopharynx from the oropharynx. Tissue loss or limited mobility disrupts both functions and causes pressure leakage and bolus material to escape into unintended areas. Soft palate reconstruction is technically challenging.

Most existing techniques cannot recreate the original muscle structure of the palate, and mobility is limited. Tissue volume can usually be restored with local flaps. Prosthetic obturators can help bring limited-mobility palatal tissue into a more functional swallowing position, but this often comes at the cost of restricted nasal breathing (Barata et al., 2013).

Surgical resections in cases like tonsillar fossa cancer, which involve removing part of the pharyngeal walls, can weaken the wall and cause serious disruptions in swallowing. The pharynx normally acts as a reservoir, creating resistance against the backward movement of the tongue root, which helps generate the pressure needed for the bolus to pass through the pharyngoesophageal sphincter. Additionally, the sequential contraction of the pharyngeal muscles helps clear the bolus from this space. Postoperative separation (dehiscence) in muscle tissue can lead to diverticulum formation and residue remaining after swallowing. Especially in surgeries involving the posterior pharyngeal wall, there is a risk of tethering the pharynx to the prevertebral fascia. Although pharyngeal elevation is not considered critical for swallowing, it has been linked to weak pharyngeal constriction and severe dysphagia in dynamic videofluoroscopic studies. From a reconstruction standpoint, primary closure offers the best functional outcome if the defect size allows. However, when large, immobile (adynamic) flaps are necessary, dysphagia can worsen due to muscle tone loss in the flap area or obstruction caused by the flap's own mass (Zafereo et al., 2010).

The larynx consists of three anatomical regions: supraglottic, glottic, and subglottic. Subglottic tumors are rare and most often extend into the glottic region (Groher & Crary, 2016). Supraglottic tumors carry a higher risk of metastasis to the neck lymph nodes due to a more extensive lymphatic network. Tumors in the supraglottic and glottic regions often cause early changes in voice and swallowing functions, so patients seek treatment early and can be treated with limited surgical interventions (e.g., laser surgery) (Preuss et al., 2009). However, as tumor size increases or there is spread to surrounding tissues, more extensive resections are required, necessitating partial or total laryngectomy.

Partial laryngectomy is an organ-preserving surgical method preferred in cases of unilateral or supraglottic laryngeal carcinoma, with cure rates comparable to those of total laryngectomy in appropriately selected patients. Although this approach offers significant advantages, such as preservation of voice and avoidance of a permanent tracheostomy, it differs from total laryngectomy, which completely separates the respiratory and digestive tracts. It entails a challenging rehabilitation process requiring the patient to relearn aspiration-free swallowing with altered laryngeal anatomy. There are three main types of partial laryngectomy: supraglottic laryngectomy, hemilaryngectomy, and supracricoid laryngectomy. In supraglottic laryngectomy, the epiglottis, pre-epiglottic area, and false vocal cords are removed.

However, preserving the true vocal folds confers an advantage in phonation; the risk of aspiration increases with loss of supraglottic protective mechanisms. Supraglottic laryngectomy is a surgical procedure that involves the removal of the epiglottis, ar-iepiglottic folds, false vocal folds, and often one or both superior laryngeal nerves; however, the true vocal cords, arytenoid cartilages, tongue base, and hyoid bone are preserved12. It can be performed using an open, endoscopic, or more recent technique, the transoral robotic approach. The loss of supraglottic structures predisposes to aspiration by eliminating mechanisms critical for protecting the laryngeal inlet; this is usually attributed to inadequate closure of the laryngeal inlet, accumulation of secretions in the pharynx, or dysfunction of the upper esophageal sphincter. Hyoid-laryngeal elevation and approximation of the tongue base to the laryngeal inlet during swallowing constitute important compensatory mechanisms; therefore, hyoid or tongue base resection markedly worsens functional outcomes (Mendelsohn et al., 2013; Weinstein et al., 2007).

Clinically, supraglottic laryngectomy is applicable only to young patients with adequate pulmonary reserve who are expected to tolerate postoperative aspiration. In traditional open surgery, most patients regain oral intake within 1–3 months, whereas in more extensive resections, oral intake begins later. In a small group of patients, swallowing function does not improve, and total laryngectomy may be necessary to prevent aspiration. Supraglottic laryngectomy performed with endoscopic laser has been reported to yield better swallowing outcomes compared to the open technique; the transoral robotic approach has not been reported in the literature to result in long-term feeding tube dependency.

In hemilaryngectomy, the epiglottis is preserved, while the unilateral vocal cord and aryepiglottic fold are excised; this can lead to asymmetric airway closure. Traditional supraglottic laryngectomy, performed for tumors involving supraglottic structures, involves resection of structures above the hyoid bone and repair of the defect by suturing the remaining tissues to the root of the tongue. However, loss of the pre-epiglottic area and false vocal cords weakens airway protection during swallowing and significantly increases the risk of aspiration pneumonia. For this reason, some surgeons have previously recommended anterior suspension of the larynx to the mandible as an additional protective strategy. Today, however, endoscopic supraglottic laser resection has come to the fore in appropriate cases where the tumor has not spread to the pre-epiglottic area. In this transoral technique, the hyoid bone, thyrohyoid membrane, and muscles connecting the larynx to the hyoid bone are preserved; thus, the anterior movement of the larynx during swallowing is not impaired. Preserving anatomical integrity in this manner allows the endoscopic method to yield better swallowing outcomes compared to traditional open surgery.

Vertical partial laryngectomies are surgical procedures used to remove early-stage glottic tumors confined to the vocal folds, accessed through a window opened in the thyroid cartilage. This technique includes different subtypes such as laryngofissure cordectomy, vertical hemilaryngectomy, frontolateral, and anterior-frontal laryngectomy. All vertical procedures involve resection of the glottic, supraglottic, and subglottic structures in the vertical plane. Postoperatively, patients generally experience short-term difficulty swallowing; however, the intact laryngeal structures on the contralateral side are seen to assume a compensatory role over time. The decrease in laryngeal closure causes difficulty, especially in fluid intake; however, in most cases, the vocal fold on the intact side crosses the midline within a few weeks and supports closure.

Laryngofissure cordectomy involves limited removal of the vocal fold and adjacent thyroid cartilage and is preferred for early tumors that do not show anterior-posterior commissure or subglottic spread; today, it has mostly been replaced by endoscopic cordectomy. Vertical hemilaryngectomy is performed when the tumor is located on a single vocal fold, and the affected vocal fold is removed along with the adjacent thyroid cartilage. In cases where cricoid cartilage involvement is limited, it can be preserved after debridement. However, because this procedure entails resection of approximately half of the larynx, swallowing function may be significantly affected.

Anterior-frontal laryngectomy is performed only for tumors smaller than 1 cm located at the anterior commissure and involves removing the front third of both vocal folds along with the commissure. Frontolateral laryngectomy is preferred for bilateral vocal fold tumors, provided there is no fixation; while the larger side undergoes complete resection, the opposite side is partially preserved and re-sutured to the thyroid cartilage. The extended form, called extended frontolateral laryngectomy, involves additional resection inferiorly in cases of vocal protrusion metastasis. Since this approach results in significant tissue loss from both vocal folds, recovering swallowing function can take a long time and requires intensive rehabilitation.

Supracricoid Laryngectomy (SCL) is a conservative surgical technique in which the entire thyroid cartilage and the true and false vocal cords are resected, but at least one arytenoid cartilage is left for functional preservation(Chawla & Carney, 2009). SCL involves two different reconstruction techniques depending on the condition of the epiglottis and the pre-epiglottic space: (1) In glottic carcinomas, the epiglottis, hyoid bone, and tongue root are sutured to the cricoid cartilage to perform cricohyoidomysopalatopharyngopexy (CHEP). (2) In supraglottic and transglottic carcinomas, resection of the epiglottis and pre-epiglottic space is required, and the cricoid cartilage is suspended directly to the hyoid bone and tongue root, performing Cricohyoidopexy (CHP) (Flint, 2021; Ganly et al., 2009). Overall, the current literature shows that despite high rates of early dysphagia after partial laryngectomy, most patients achieve a good level of functional swallowing ability over time, but results are heterogeneous due to the lack of a standard evaluation protocol (Lips et al., 2015).

Dysphagia developing after partial laryngectomy is closely related not only to the surgical technique but also to the functional integrity of the preserved and resected anatomical structures. Therefore, speech-language pathologists (SLPs) should assess patients in the postoperative period based on risk, according to the type of surgery and extent of resection. Since the risk of aspiration is high in patients after supraglottic and supracricoid laryngectomy, early objective swallowing assessments (VFSS or FEES) are recommended to determine the functional profile. Considering that preservation of hyoid-laryngeal elevation and tongue-base-laryngeal contact is critical for swallowing safety, rehabilitation programs should include exercises targeting these structures (e.g., Mendelsohn maneuver, effortful swallow, tongue-base strengthening exercises). Furthermore, individualization of compensatory strategies (chin-down, bolus modification, postural adaptations) based on anatomical changes developing after surgery and supporting functional adaptations with long-term follow-up should be considered a fundamental approach in regaining oral intake and reducing the risk of aspiration(Alicandri–Ciufelli et al., 2013a; Rademaker et al., 1993).

During the postoperative period, a temporary tracheostomy is performed to secure the airway, and a nasogastric (NG) tube is placed for feeding; however, swallowing therapy is usually delayed until the 10th to 14th day, when these tubes are removed, because the NG tube prevents closure of the soft palate and causes discomfort. Despite suspension of the larynx to the tongue root during surgical repair, resection of the external muscles that move the larynx during swallowing (suprahyoid muscles in supraglottic type, infrahyoid muscles in hemilaryngectomy) causes the larynx to remain in a lower position in the neck (laryngeal ptosis) (Wang et al., 2014). This situation prevents the larynx from rising sufficiently below the root of the tongue during the pharyngeal phase of swallowing and weakens protection. In addition, damage to the superior laryngeal nerve creates sensory loss in the hypopharynx, increasing the risk of aspiration.

The literature indicates that arytenoid cartilage resection is associated with the strongest statistical correlation with postoperative dysphagia, primarily due to the presence of an unclosed posterior glottal opening. McConnel and colleagues' manofluorographic analyses explain the mechanism leading to aspiration in these patients with three main abnormalities: Inability to elevate sufficiently during swallowing due to the low resting position of the larynx, aspiration of uncleared residue at the laryngeal inlet due to impaired contact between the tongue and larynx, and delayed triggering of the laryngeal elevation reflex. This combination of physiological deficiencies constitutes the fundamental causes of dysphagia seen after arytenoid resection(Mcconnel et al., 1994).

Partial laryngectomy significantly alters the anatomy of the upper aerodigestive tract, causing permanent effects on swallowing and voice functions; however, studies comprehensively examining the functional outcomes of these surgeries are quite limited in the literature. Current publications generally focus on a single surgical technique, do not compare different types of partial laryngectomy, and do not sufficiently evaluate the anatomical factors that affect functional outcomes. Due to similar survival rates achieved with radiotherapy and chemotherapy, swallowing and voice outcomes after partial laryngectomy have become increasingly important (Alicandri–Ciufelli et al., 2013b).

Significant anatomical changes in phonation and swallowing function occur after partial laryngectomy, and outcomes vary with the surgical technique employed, the formation of the neoglottic structure, a history of radiotherapy, and other patient-specific factors. In supracricoid laryngectomies, voice production relies on the tongue base, epiglottis, and 1–2 arytenoid units forming a new sphincter structure, whereas in supraglottic laryngectomies, phonatory outcomes are significantly better due to the preservation of the vocal folds. Preserving one or both arytenoids has not been shown to have a significant effect on voice quality; however, radiotherapy has been shown to increase the fundamental frequency and thus have adverse effects on phonation. No significant effect of arytenoid number or neoglottis type on swallowing function has been identified; however, radiotherapy has been shown to significantly worsen dysphagia scores, aspiration risk, and MDADI outcomes. Age and time since surgery generally did not have a significant effect on phonation and swallowing, although there are conflicting findings in the literature suggesting that aspiration risk may increase with advanced age. Overall, radiotherapy was a significant negative predictor, while no major differences in swallowing were observed between different types of partial laryngectomy.

Total laryngectomy is a radical surgical procedure involving the removal of the epiglottis, thyroid and cricoid cartilages, hyoid bone, true and false vocal folds, ary-epiglottic folds, pyriform fossa, the initial ring of the trachea, the entire larynx, and part of the tongue root. If part of the pharynx is also removed along with the larynx, the operation is called a *pharyngolaryngectomy*32. Today, total laryngectomy is no longer the first-line treatment option; rather, it is preferred in advanced-stage tumors that invade cartilage, spread outside the larynx, or threaten the safety of the airway. After surgery, patients may experience significant functional impairments, including loss of nasal function, reduced cough effectiveness, changes in pulmonary function, loss of voice, and varying degrees of difficulty swallowing. Although the risk of aspiration is quite low due to the complete separation of the trachea and esophagus, dysphagia can develop after total laryngectomy through various mechanisms. These mechanisms include abnormal pharyngeal muscle contraction patterns, failure of the upper esophageal sphincter to open, decreased mobility of the tongue base, formation of a structure called a “pseudoeptglottis” between the tongue base and scar tissue, and accumulation of food in this area. In addition, resection of the hyoid bone may make it difficult to move the bolus anterior-posteriorly during chewing.

Narrowing of the pharynx or esophagus slows bolus transit, whereas pouches in the esophagus can lead to food retention in these areas. Considering all these functional effects, swallowing and voice production emerge as the two most important parameters determining quality of life for most patients who have undergone total laryngectomy(Arenaz Búa et al., 2018).

Physiologically, with the loss of the larynx, the laryngeal elevation mechanism that opens the pharyngoesophageal sphincter is also lost. Therefore, patients become dependent on the pressure applied by the root of the tongue to the pharyngeal walls and the "tongue pumping" movement to push the bolus down; thus, severe dysphagia is inevitable in cases involving tongue root resection. Although the risk of aspiration is eliminated after surgery because the airway and digestive system are completely separated, this does not mean that swallowing difficulties do not occur. Studies have reported that 72% of patients experience difficulty swallowing, 86% require liquid support to swallow solid foods, and many are forced to modify their diet (especially avoiding meat) (Maclean et al., 2009).

The hyoid bone and laryngeal elevation are fundamental mechanisms for protecting the airway and preventing aspiration during swallowing. The effects of tracheostomy on swallowing function, however, involve multiple factors that cannot be explained solely by a direct cause-and-effect relationship. It is accepted that dysphagia and aspiration findings observed in individuals with tracheostomy are often related to the individual's underlying disease, general clinical condition, and accompanying medical factors rather than the presence of the tracheostomy tube. In particular, disease severity, respiratory failure, sedative medication use, advanced age, and existing comorbidities can negatively affect swallowing function. However, tracheostomy can affect swallowing safety through indirect mechanisms such as decreased subglottic air pressure, weakened laryngeal and pharyngeal sensory feedback, and decreased cough effectiveness. Furthermore, impairments in smell and taste can negatively affect nutritional performance by reducing the desire and motivation for oral intake. Therefore, the assessment and management of swallowing function in individuals with tracheostomy requires a comprehensive and individualized clinical approach, independent of the presence of a tracheostomy(Kang et al., 2012; Terk et al., 2007).

The management of dysphagia resulting from surgical interventions depends largely on the type and extent of the surgical procedure performed. Rehabilitation approaches generally involve the use of compensatory strategies, dietary modifications, and joint range of motion and strengthening exercises. The primary goal of intervention is to ensure safe and effective swallowing with the least possible restriction and adaptation. In this regard, it is recommended that strategies that patients can maintain in social settings and that mimic more natural eating behaviors be preferred when appropriate. Indeed, it has been reported that compensatory maneuvers can eliminate aspiration in up to 81% of patients after head and neck surgery (Heijnen et al., 2016)

Ensuring adequate closure of the pharynx during swallowing and maintaining this closure until swallowing is complete is critical for airway safety. The cough reflex that occurs before inspiration contributes to the clearance of residual material remaining at the laryngeal inlet. The supraglottic swallowing maneuver narrows the laryngeal vestibule entrance by bringing the tongue base closer to the laryngeal inlet, further enhancing airway protection. Strategies that increase the narrowing of the laryngeal vestibule entrance are often needed after surgeries focused at the glottic level. For this purpose, chin tuck and effortful swallow maneuvers are frequently used. Turning the head toward the affected side can improve swallowing safety by increasing the degree of glottic closure. In patients who have undergone total laryngectomy, the main problem is bolus clearance due to the absence of pharyngeal propulsion. In these individuals, the liquid wash strategy is often beneficial, especially when applied with increased effort. After partial laryngeal resection, patients can generally tolerate thicker consistencies better, while after total laryngectomy, thinner consistencies are easier to clear.

Therapeutic exercises that may be beneficial after laryngeal surgery include effortful swallow, Mendelsohn maneuver, effortful pitch glide, supraglottic and super-supraglottic swallowing maneuvers, Shaker exercise, and laryngeal adduction exercises. Direct exercises targeting range of motion and strengthening generally require the surgeon's approval and are usually initiated approximately two weeks after surgery in most patients. This period allows sufficient time for tissue healing; however, in patients who have undergone complex reconstruction or whose healing is delayed, the initiation of exercises may be postponed to a later date. Exercise programs should target preserved muscle groups to increase the safety and effectiveness of swallowing. Swallowing therapy also involves a gradual progression from the least challenging diet to the most challenging diet, accompanied by appropriate strategies. However, it should be noted that patients often undergo complex resections involving multiple anatomical regions and frequently receive combined treatments (e.g., salvage surgery after chemoradiotherapy). Therefore, individualized and often combined rehabilitation strategies are required to ensure safe and effective swallowing function(Suiter & Gosa, 2019; Tsou et al., 2025; Zhang et al., 2022)

4. EFFECT OF RADIOTHERAPY/CHEMORADIOTHERAPY ON SWALLOWING FUNCTION

The pathophysiological changes that occur in the upper aerodigestive system after radiation exposure and lead to dysphagia are not fully understood, and there is limited information available. The fundamental difference between normal trauma-related wound healing and radiation damage is that radiation causes repeated damage at regular intervals. This repeated effect disrupts cellular regulatory processes, leading to tissue homeostasis disruption in tumor and epithelial cells. The direct and indirect effects of radiation alter oxidative stress and signaling pathways at the cellular and molecular levels.

Radiation-induced early changes primarily occur in the epidermis and oral–pharyngeal mucosa, and the inflammatory response develops within hours to weeks after exposure. Increased cell membrane permeability and histamine release lead to epithelial cell loss, resulting in mucositis, xerostomia, erythema, and soft tissue edema. These acute effects negatively impact swallowing function, particularly in the oral and pharyngeal phases, through pain, sensory changes, and anatomical narrowing. Acute radiation effects are mostly temporary and usually subside within 3–6 months. However, there is no direct correlation between the severity of acute symptoms and the fibrosis and chronic dysphagia that develop in the late phase. Indeed, while some patients may develop significant fibrotic changes and persistent swallowing disorders in the late phase despite mild acute findings, some patients with severe mucositis may experience minimal functional limitations in the long term (Eisbruch et al., 2002). The edema during the acute phase narrows anatomical spaces like the vallecula and piriform sinuses, which normally guide the esophagus, causing the bolus to shift toward the airway and increasing the risk of aspiration, which is common during this time. This edema typically subsides within 3 months of completing treatment.

The severity of radiation toxicity depends on factors such as total dose, dose per fraction, irradiated tissue volume, and dose intensity, as the tissue's capacity for self-renewal is related to these factors(Trotti et al., 2003). Acute inflammation begins in the submucosa minutes after radiation exposure, and certain proinflammatory cytokines and chemokines are released. This increases vascular permeability, leading to neutrophil and macrophage accumulation. Although most patients can partially maintain their swallowing function during radiotherapy, significant dysphagia generally results from a combination of multiple factors, such as decreased tongue root retraction, inadequate epiglottic retroflexion, decreased laryngeal elevation, prolonged pharyngeal transit time, and coordination disorder in the swallowing muscles. Pain associated with oral mucositis adversely affects the oral phase, and smoking, oral hygiene, nutritional status, and infections can further exacerbate this condition. Dependence on gastrostomy or nasogastric tube feeding due to decreased oral intake during radiotherapy leads to “disuse atrophy” and fibrotic changes in the swallowing muscles in the long term; this condition creates a fibroatrophic process characterized by the gradual replacement of muscle fibers with fibrotic tissue and decreased range of motion. Therefore, long-term tube dependence is considered an important precursor to late-onset dysphagia (Gómez et al., 2025; Roe et al., 2010).

In oropharyngeal tumors of the head and neck region, particularly tumors of the tongue base, tonsils, posterior pharyngeal wall, and soft palate, chemoradiotherapy protocols consisting of concurrent chemotherapy and radiotherapy have been preferred as the primary treatment approach in recent years. Similarly, hypopharyngeal tumors and laryngeal tumors without cartilage invasion are also mostly treated with this method. However, although designed as an organ-preserving approach, dysphagia persists as a common and persistent problem after chemoradiotherapy. According to SEER data, dysphagia occurs in approximately 64% of patients receiving this treatment, and it has been reported that swallowing-related quality of life scores are significantly reduced in patients with tongue base and tonsil cancer. The literature shows that even if patients report returning to a normal diet, objective assessments reveal a significant level of dysphagia.

One of the most critical components of dysphagia after chemoradiotherapy is aspiration(Xu et al., 2015). In a study by Langerman et al. (2007), the aspiration rate was reported to be 69%; 75% of these patients were unaware that they had silent aspiration(Langerman et al., 2007; Nguyen et al., 2004). Furthermore, some studies have shown that silent aspiration can persist for up to 5 years after diagnosis. These findings suggest that sensory changes following chemoradiotherapy may impair patients' perception of the severity of their swallowing disorders. Furthermore, increasing age, tumor location in the larynx or hypopharynx, and tumor size are among the clinical factors that increase the risk of persistent dysphagia after treatment. The dose of radiation therapy and the targeted anatomical regions play a critical role in the development of dysphagia. Various studies have shown that high radiation doses to the upper constrictor muscles, supraglottic region, or larynx significantly worsen dysphagia Intensity-modulated radiation therapy (IMRT) is a modern radiotherapy technique designed to spare normal tissues by allowing precise modulation of radiation dose distribution. In head and neck cancers, IMRT theoretically reduces radiation exposure to critical swallowing-related structures, particularly the pharyngeal constrictor muscles. However, clinical evidence indicates that this dosimetric advantage does not consistently translate into meaningful reductions in dysphagia rates. In a cohort of 83 patients treated with IMRT, one year after treatment, 22% remained dependent on gastrostomy feeding, 45% demonstrated aspiration on instrumental assessment, and 20% developed severe pharyngoesophageal strictures. (Caudell et al., 2010). Although some recent studies have reported reduced acute toxicity and lower PEG dependence with IMRT, late-stage dysphagia rates appear comparable to those observed with conventional radiotherapy, suggesting that radiation-induced fibrosis, sensory impairment, and disuse-related muscular atrophy continue to play a major role in long-term swallowing dysfunction (Al-Mamgani et al., 2014). The three- to six-month period after treatment is when dysphagia becomes most pronounced. During this period, patients report a marked deterioration in their swallowing function, and objective examinations show that the aspiration rate can reach up to 69%. Nevertheless, this period is a window of recovery during which patients are encouraged to increase their oral intake. Therefore, careful clinical monitoring and evaluation of the effectiveness of swallowing strategies are essential in reducing the risk of aspiration (Langendijk et al., 2008).

In summary, it is crucial for speech-language pathologists (SLPs) working with individuals with dysphagia to ensure the accessibility of post-treatment services in order to help these individuals adapt to the sequelae of their primary disease and maintain their lives at the highest possible level of functionality . These services must address not only physical needs but also emotional and psychosocial needs. In a qualitative study examining speech therapists' experiences in dysphagia management, it was shown that caregivers often did not feel adequately prepared for their roles; clinicians emphasized the importance of timely and adequate training and support for caregivers (Nund et al., 2014). Similarly, Krisciunas and colleagues reported that there is no standardized rehabilitation protocol for head and neck cancer (HNC) patients in the field of speech therapy and that evidence strongly supporting a particular approach is limited(Krisciunas et al., 2012).

Dysphagia rehabilitation in head and neck cancers should be individualized according to the underlying mechanism of the swallowing disorder, the tumor location, and the treatment modality used. Physiological changes such as decreased tongue mobility, weak pharyngeal thrust, limited laryngeal elevation, and impaired bolus clearance are frequently observed in the postoperative period following surgery, radiotherapy, and chemotherapy. Therefore, rehabilitation programs should not be limited to compensatory strategies; they should include a structured and targeted approach that incorporates active swallowing exercises(Heijnen et al., 2016).

Exercises used in dysphagia rehabilitation generally aim to increase tongue strength and range of motion, support pharyngeal muscle activity, and improve laryngeal elevation. Tongue exercises (anterior–posterior and lateral range of motion exercises and resistive tongue thrust exercises) are particularly effective in bolus formation during the oral phase and bolus propulsion into the pharynx. The Masako (tongue-hold) maneuver and effortful swallow are frequently used in patients with tongue root weakness or insufficient posterior bolus propulsion to increase pharyngeal wall contact and bolus clearance. Exercises aimed at improving laryngeal elevation and upper esophageal sphincter (UES) opening play a critical role in reducing the risk of aspiration. The Mendelsohn maneuver aims to increase cricopharyngeal opening by prolonging laryngeal elevation during swallowing, while the Shaker exercise and its modified versions support UES opening by strengthening the suprahyoid muscles. Additionally, effortful pitch glide and laryngeal adduction exercises can be incorporated into the rehabilitation program to improve glottic closure and airway protection(Hutcheson et al., 2013).

In the early postoperative period or in patients at high risk of aspiration, compensatory maneuvers constitute an important component of rehabilitation. Postural strategies such as chin tuck, head rotation, or head tilt can reduce the risk of aspiration by allowing the bolus to travel more safely. However, it should be emphasized that these strategies are not permanent solutions; they are supportive approaches used until functional improvement is achieved. The long-term goal is to restore safe and effective swallowing function with as little adaptation as possible. The rehabilitation process often progresses in conjunction with dietary modifications. Patients typically begin oral intake with consistencies considered safer (e.g., purees or thick liquids) and gradually progress to more challenging consistencies with appropriate exercises and strategies. During this process, it is recommended to regularly monitor functional gains using patient-reported scales, oral intake levels, and instrumental assessments (VFSS/FEES) when necessary. In conclusion, dysphagia rehabilitation in head and neck cancers should be approached as a dynamic and long-term process that combines the right exercises, appropriate strategies, and multidisciplinary clinical management(Suiter & Gosa, 2019).

5. ASSESSMENT OF DYSPHAGIA IN HEAD AND NECK CANCERS

Current data in the literature indicate that pre-treatment swallowing function in patients with head and neck cancer is an important predictor of dysphagia that may develop after treatment. Therefore, assessments performed before treatment begins are critical both as a reference point for comparing treatment effects and for predicting long-term functional loss (Denaro et al., 2013; Murphy & Gilbert, 2009). Even if patients have not yet undergone treatment, they may exhibit severe symptoms such as pain, aspiration, trismus, and weight loss due to the tumor disrupting the anatomical structure, invading nerves, or affecting mucosal surfaces. Managing this complex picture requires the collaboration of a multidisciplinary team consisting of surgeons, speech-language pathologists, oncologists, and dietitians. This interdisciplinary team should follow a protocol that begins with a clinical swallowing assessment and is supplemented with instrumental methods, such as videofluoroscopic swallowing study (MBS), fiberoptic endoscopic evaluation of swallowing (FEES), to minimize the risk of aspiration and to provide patient education before treatment. These assessments, performed before and after surgery, radiotherapy, or chemoradiotherapy, establish a reference point for the patient's anatomical and functional status. Particularly in laryngeal and hypopharyngeal tumors, it should be remembered that dysphagia and aspiration may develop depending on the size and location of the tumor even before treatment begins. The literature supports that prophylactic exercises started before treatment reduce dependence on a gastrostomy tube by improving tongue root contact and epiglottis mobility; conversely, it emphasizes that oral intake deficiency lasting longer than two weeks increases the risk of dysphagia after treatment.

Clinical Swallowing Evaluation (CSE), the first step in the evaluation process, begins with taking the patient's history, examining the tumor's location, size, and histopathological characteristics, and evaluating the planned treatment modalities. During this consultation, triggering symptoms such as coughing during swallowing, a 'wet' sound, a feeling of choking, food getting stuck, prolonged eating times, or unexplained weight loss should be inquired about. The presence of any of these symptoms requires the patient to be referred to a speech-language pathologist (SLP) immediately. The clinical examination phase of CSE involves assessing oral motor function, cranial nerves, the integrity of intraoral structures, saliva management, phonation, and respiratory coordination. Subsequently, water swallowing tests or trials with different consistencies are performed to determine the aspiration risk and the general profile of swallowing physiology. This assessment both establishes a functional baseline prior to treatment and reveals the level of the patient's existing dysphagia before starting the treatment process. The pre-treatment assessment is also the most appropriate time to initiate the patient on preventive swallowing exercises, known as pretreatment swallowing exercises. The literature indicates that these exercises reduce the severity of post-treatment dysphagia by maintaining the range of motion of the swallowing muscles; furthermore, maintaining oral intake (even at a minimal level) is important in reducing long-term G-tube dependence. Therefore, it is critically important for the SLP to train the patient in appropriate exercises and to coordinate with the treatment team. CSE results are supported by instrumental assessments (videofluoroscopic swallowing study—MBS, fiberoptic endoscopic evaluation of swallowing—FEES) when necessary. These tests provide a detailed analysis of swallowing physiology and help determine appropriate swallowing strategies. Considering the functional changes that the applied treatment (surgery, radiotherapy, or chemoradiotherapy) may cause, the assessment should be repeated both before and after treatment. In conclusion, clinical swallowing assessment is an indispensable component of head and neck cancer management, as it helps reduce the risk of aspiration, maintain adequate nutrition and hydration, and ensure the patient is better prepared for treatment. This comprehensive approach has a significant impact on patients' quality of life, both during the acute treatment period and during long-term rehabilitation.

Instrumental assessments are considered the gold standard in swallowing assessment because they objectively examine oropharyngeal swallowing physiology and bolus movement and can predict adverse health outcomes such as pneumonia and malnutrition. Identifying aspiration risk and silent swallowing disorders in patients with advanced head and neck cancer optimizes treatment by enabling speech and language therapists to implement appropriate compensatory maneuvers and dietary modifications. Therefore, pre-treatment instrumental assessment can influence both the rehabilitation approach and oncological decisions aimed at improving the patient's post-treatment functionality and quality of life. Videofluoroscopic swallowing study (VFSS) and flexible endoscopic evaluation of swallowing are complementary methods; VFSS remains the gold standard for detailed assessment of the anatomical and physiological causes of swallowing, aspiration risk, and oral and pharyngeal transit times. FEES, on the other hand, allows direct visualization of pharyngeal structures using a flexible endoscope inserted through the nasal route; it does not provide information about the oral phase but offers significant advantages, such as bedside applicability and the absence of radiation. In addition to instrumental assessments, patient-reported outcome (PRO) scales provide a complementary perspective on understanding the impact of physiological impairments on daily life and quality of life; however, PRO results often show inconsistencies with objective measurements and therefore do not fully reflect actual swallowing competence. Therefore, a multidimensional assessment approach that incorporates objective-instrumental findings, patient reports, and clinician evaluations enables a more accurate definition of dysphagia and a more comprehensive understanding of its symptoms.

In the assessment of dysphagia in head and neck cancers, screening and self-assessment scales, in addition to instrumental examinations, constitute one of the fundamental components of clinical management. Among the tests used for screening purposes, the Water Swallow Test (WST), the Yale Swallow Protocol, and bedside clinical assessments enable the early identification of patients at risk of aspiration. However, as the sensitivity of these tests may be limited, patient-reported outcome measures (PROMs), which reveal the patient's perceived swallowing difficulty and functional impairment, are of great importance. The most commonly used self-assessment scales for head and neck cancers include the MD Anderson Dysphagia Inventory (MDADI), Eating Assessment Tool-10 (EAT-10), Functional Oral Intake Scale (FOIS), and Swallowing Quality of Life Questionnaire (SWAL-QOL). The MDADI, in particular, is widely used in clinical and research settings because it was developed specifically for head and neck cancers and includes physical, functional, and emotional subscales. The EAT-10 is preferred for dysphagia screening and monitoring treatment response due to its short and practical structure. However, it is known that self-report scales alone may not fully reflect physiological abnormalities and may be inadequate, especially in the presence of silent aspiration. Therefore, current approaches recommend that dysphagia assessment in head and neck cancer patients be addressed using a multidimensional assessment model that combines clinical screening tests, self-assessment scales, and instrumental methods .

6. THE IMPACT OF DYSPHAGIA ON QUALITY OF LIFE

The long-term effects of head and neck cancer treatment greatly influence patients' health-related quality of life. When several treatment options with similar oncological outcomes are available, the functional outcomes of these treatments are crucial to decision-making, particularly with respect to swallowing function. It is well established that combining surgery and radiotherapy with primary chemoradiotherapy in laryngeal cancers yields comparable survival outcomes; however, the impact of these two approaches on swallowing performance differentially shapes long-term quality of life.

Studies conducted on patients undergoing chemoradiotherapy show a significant decline in all parameters related to quality of life during and immediately after treatment(Lotempio et al., 2005). Although recovery begins approximately six months later with the reduction of acute toxicities, specific assessments of swallowing function reveal a marked deterioration three months after treatment and only limited improvement even at 12 months(Wilson et al., 2011). This finding suggests that chemoradiotherapy may have lasting effects on swallowing physiology. Studies examining long-term swallowing function after chemoradiotherapy indicate that aspiration persists even years after treatment. For example, significant aspiration and silent aspiration were detected in a significant proportion of patients with five-year or longer survival; these conditions have been reported to be associated with a marked decline in quality-of-life domains such as chewing, swallowing, and dietary normality(Campbell et al., 2004). Another study conducted on a larger patient group revealed that less than half of the treated individuals assessed their eating functions as normal or close to normal, demonstrating that dysphagia can be persistent in the long term (Funk, 2012). Some studies examining the relationship between swallowing function and quality of life have shown that there is no strong correlation between objective swallowing measurements and patients' self-reports (Kendall et al., 2014). This finding suggests that patients may perceive their swallowing performance as better than the physiological reality and that relying solely on subjective assessments may be insufficient for clinical decision-making. Studies comparing quality of life by treatment type indicate that speech is the primary source of dissatisfaction among patients undergoing total laryngectomy, as this surgery causes voice loss and significantly affects long-term communication skills. In contrast, patients treated with chemoradiotherapy, an organ-preserving approach, largely preserve their speech function but report a marked decline in quality of life in chewing and swallowing functions due to side effects of the treatment, such as mucosal toxicity, fibrosis, and sensory loss. This contrast highlights the need to carefully evaluate not only oncological outcomes but also long-term functional outcomes when selecting treatment.

REFERENCES

Al-Mamgani, A., van Rooij, P. H., Mehilal, R., Verduijn, G. M., Tans, L., & Kwa, S. L. S. (2014). Radiotherapy for T1a glottic cancer: The influence of smoking cessation and fractionation schedule of radiotherapy. *European Archives of Oto-Rhino-Laryngology, 271*(1), 125–132. DOI: 10.1007/s00405-013-2608-8 PMID: 23797970

Alicandri–Ciufelli, M., Piccinini, A., Grammatica, A., Chiesi, A., Bergamini, G., Luppi, M. P., Nizzoli, F., Ghidini, A., Tassi, S., & Presutti, L. (2013a). Voice and swallowing after partial laryngectomy: Factors influencing outcome. *Head & Neck, 35*(2), 214–219. DOI: 10.1002/hed.22946 PMID: 22307985

Alicandri–Ciufelli, M., Piccinini, A., Grammatica, A., Chiesi, A., Bergamini, G., Luppi, M. P., Nizzoli, F., Ghidini, A., Tassi, S., & Presutti, L. (2013b). Voice and swallowing after partial laryngectomy: Factors influencing outcome. *Head & Neck, 35*(2), 214–219. DOI: 10.1002/hed.22946 PMID: 22307985

Amin, M. B., & Edge, S. B. (2017). *AJCC cancer staging manual* (8th ed.). Springer.

Amitrano, A. (2024). Dysphagia in Adulthood and the Geriatric Age. In *Dysphagia and Nutrition* (pp. 13–34). Springer Nature Switzerland., DOI: 10.1007/978-3-031-77449-2_2

Arenaz Búa, B., Pendleton, H., Westin, U., & Rydell, R. (2018). Voice and swallowing after total laryngectomy. *Acta Oto-Laryngologica, 138*(2), 170–174. DOI: 10.1080/00016489.2017.1384056 PMID: 28978261

Barata, L. F., de Carvalho, G. B., Carrara-de Angelis, E., de Faria, J. C. M., & Kowalski, L. P. (2013). Swallowing, speech and quality of life in patients undergoing resection of soft palate. *European Archives of Oto-Rhino-Laryngology, 270*(1), 305–312. DOI: 10.1007/s00405-012-2006-7 PMID: 22526573

Campbell, B. H., Spinelli, K., Marbella, A. M., Myers, K. B., Kuhn, J. C., & Layde, P. M. (2004). Aspiration, Weight Loss, and Quality of Life in Head and Neck Cancer Survivors. *Archives of Otolaryngology—Head & Neck Surgery, 130*(9), 1100. DOI: 10.1001/archotol.130.9.1100 PMID: 15381598

Caudell, J. J., Schaner, P. E., Desmond, R. A., Meredith, R. F., Spencer, S. A., & Bonner, J. A. (2010). Dosimetric Factors Associated With Long-Term Dysphagia After Definitive Radiotherapy for Squamous Cell Carcinoma of the Head and Neck. *International Journal of Radiation Oncology*Biology*Physics, 76*(2), 403–409. https://doi.org/DOI: 10.1016/j.ijrobp.2009.02.017

Chawla, S., & Carney, A. S. (2009). Organ preservation surgery for laryngeal cancer. *Head & Neck Oncology*, *1*(1), 12. DOI: 10.1186/1758-3284-1-12 PMID: 19442314

Chen, S.-C. (2019). Oral Dysfunction in Patients With Head and Neck Cancer: A Systematic Review. *The Journal of Nursing Research*, *27*(6), e58. DOI: 10.1097/jnr.0000000000000363 PMID: 31688276

Denaro, N., Merlano, M. C., & Russi, E. G. (2013). Dysphagia in Head and Neck Cancer Patients: Pretreatment Evaluation, Predictive Factors, and Assessment during Radio-Chemotherapy, Recommendations. *Clinical and Experimental Otorhinolaryngology*, *6*(3), 117. DOI: 10.3342/ceo.2013.6.3.117 PMID: 24069513

Eisbruch, A., Lyden, T., Bradford, C. R., Dawson, L. A., Haxer, M. J., Miller, A. E., Teknos, T. N., Chepeha, D. B., Hogikyan, N. D., Terrell, J. E., & Wolf, G. T. (2002). Objective assessment of swallowing dysfunction and aspiration after radiation concurrent with chemotherapy for head-and-neck cancer. *International Journal of Radiation Oncology*Biology*Physics*, *53*(1), 23–28. https://doi.org/DOI: 10.1016/S0360-3016(02)02712-8

Flint, P. W. (2021). *Cummings otolaryngology : head and neck surgery*. Elsevier.

Funk, G. F. (2012). Long-term Health-Related Quality of Life in Survivors of Head and Neck Cancer. *Archives of Otolaryngology—Head & Neck Surgery*, *138*(2), 123. DOI: 10.1001/archoto.2011.234 PMID: 22248560

Ganly, I., Patel, S. G., Matsuo, J., Singh, B., Kraus, D. H., Boyle, J., Wong, R., Shaha, A. R., & Shah, J. P. (2009). Analysis of postoperative complications of open partial laryngectomy. *Head & Neck*, *31*(3), 338–345. DOI: 10.1002/hed.20975 PMID: 19073010

Gillespie, M. B., Brodsky, M. B., Day, T. A., Lee, F., & Martin-Harris, B. (2004). Swallowing-Related Quality of Life After Head and Neck Cancer Treatment. *The Laryngoscope*, *114*(8), 1362–1367. DOI: 10.1097/00005537-200408000-00008 PMID: 15280708

Gómez, Á., García-Chabur, M. A., Peñaranda, D., Gómez-Mendoza, A., & Forero, J. C. (2025). Chemotherapy/Radiotherapy-Induced Dysphagia in Head and Neck Tumors: A Challenge for Otolaryngologists in Low- to Middle-Income Countries. *Dysphagia*, *40*(3), 515–527. DOI: 10.1007/s00455-024-10756-5 PMID: 39317843

Groher, M. E., & Crary, M. A. (2016). *Dysphagia : clinical management in adults and children*. Elsevier.

Heijnen, B. J., Speyer, R., Kertscher, B., Cordier, R., Koetsenruijter, K. W. J., Swan, K., & Bogaardt, H. (2016). Dysphagia, Speech, Voice, and Trismus following Radiotherapy and/or Chemotherapy in Patients with Head and Neck Carcinoma: Review of the Literature. *BioMed Research International*, *2016*, 1–24. DOI: 10.1155/2016/6086894 PMID: 27722170

Hirano, M., Matsuoka, H., Kuroiwa, Y., Sato, K., Tanaka, S., & Yoshida, T. (1992). Dysphagia following Various Degrees of Surgical Resection for Oral Cancer. *The Annals of Otology, Rhinology, and Laryngology*, *101*(2), 138–141. DOI: 10.1177/000348949210100206 PMID: 1739258

Howard, A., Agrawal, N., & Gooi, Z. (2021). Lip and Oral Cavity Squamous Cell Carcinoma. *Hematology/Oncology Clinics of North America*, *35*(5), 895–911. DOI: 10.1016/j.hoc.2021.05.003 PMID: 34274176

Hunter, M., Kellett, J., Toohey, K., D'Cunha, N. M., Isbel, S., & Naumovski, N. (2020). Toxicities Caused by Head and Neck Cancer Treatments and Their Influence on the Development of Malnutrition: Review of the Literature. *European Journal of Investigation in Health, Psychology and Education*, *10*(4), 935–949. DOI: 10.3390/ejihpe10040066 PMID: 34542427

Hutcheson, K. A., Bhayani, M. K., Beadle, B. M., Gold, K. A., Shinn, E. H., Lai, S. Y., & Lewin, J. (2013). Eat and Exercise During Radiotherapy or Chemoradiotherapy for Pharyngeal Cancers. *JAMA Otolaryngology-Head & Neck Surgery*, *139*(11), 1127. DOI: 10.1001/jamaoto.2013.4715 PMID: 24051544

Hutcheson, K. A., Holsinger, F. C., Kupferman, M. E., & Lewin, J. S. (2015). Functional outcomes after TORS for oropharyngeal cancer: A systematic review. *European Archives of Oto-Rhino-Laryngology*, *272*(2), 463–471. DOI: 10.1007/s00405-014-2985-7 PMID: 24643851

Ihara, Y., Kato, H., Tashimo, Y., Iizumi, Y., Fukunishi, Y., Sato, H., Shimane, T., & Takahashi, K. (2022). Changes in oral function, swallowing function, and quality of life in patients with head and neck cancer: A prospective cohort study. *BMC Oral Health*, *22*(1), 293. DOI: 10.1186/s12903-022-02329-5 PMID: 35843950

Kang, J. Y., Choi, K. H., Yun, G. J., Kim, M. Y., & Ryu, J. S. (2012). Does Removal of Tracheostomy Affect Dysphagia? A Kinematic Analysis. *Dysphagia*, *27*(4), 498–503. DOI: 10.1007/s00455-012-9396-y PMID: 22327860

Kendall, K. A., Kosek, S. R., & Tanner, K. (2014). Quality-of-life scores compared to objective measures of swallowing after oropharyngeal chemoradiation. *The Laryngoscope*, *124*(3), 682–687. DOI: 10.1002/lary.24344 PMID: 23929736

Krisciunas, G. P., Sokoloff, W., Stepas, K., & Langmore, S. E. (2012). Survey of Usual Practice: Dysphagia Therapy in Head and Neck Cancer Patients. *Dysphagia*, *27*(4), 538–549. DOI: 10.1007/s00455-012-9404-2 PMID: 22456699

Kronenberger, M. B., & Meyers, A. D. (1994). Dysphagia following head and neck cancer surgery. *Dysphagia*, *9*(4), 236–244. DOI: 10.1007/BF00301917 PMID: 7805423

Langendijk, J. A., Doornaert, P., Verdonck-de Leeuw, I. M., Leemans, C. R., Aaronson, N. K., & Slotman, B. J. (2008). Impact of Late Treatment-Related Toxicity on Quality of Life Among Patients With Head and Neck Cancer Treated With Radiotherapy. *Journal of Clinical Oncology*, *26*(22), 3770–3776. DOI: 10.1200/JCO.2007.14.6647 PMID: 18669465

Langerman, A., MacCracken, E., Kasza, K., Haraf, D. J., Vokes, E. E., & Stenson, K. M. (2007). Aspiration in Chemoradiated Patients With Head and Neck Cancer. *Archives of Otolaryngology—Head & Neck Surgery*, *133*(12), 1289. DOI: 10.1001/archotol.133.12.1289 PMID: 18086974

Lazarus, C. L. (2000). Management of Swallowing Disorders in Head and Neck Cancer Patients: Optimal Patterns of Care. *Seminars in Speech and Language, Volume 21*(Number 4), 0293–0310. https://doi.org/DOI: 10.1055/s-2000-8383

Lester, S., & Yang, W.-Y. (2015). Principles and management of head and neck cancer. *Surgery (Oxford)*, *33*(12), 620–626. DOI: 10.1016/j.mpsur.2015.09.007

Lips, M., Speyer, R., Zumach, A., Kross, K. W., & Kremer, B. (2015). Supracricoid laryngectomy and dysphagia: A systematic literature review. *The Laryngoscope*, *125*(9), 2143–2156. DOI: 10.1002/lary.25341 PMID: 26013745

Logemann, J. A., Rademaker, A. W., Pauloski, B. R., & Kahrilas, P. J. (1994). Effects of postural change on aspiration in head and neck surgical patients. *Otolaryngology - Head and Neck Surgery*, *110*(2), 222–227. DOI: 10.1177/019459989411000212 PMID: 8108157

Lotempio, M. M., Wang, K. H., Sadeghi, A., Delacure, M. D., Juillard, G. F., & Wang, M. B. (2005). Comparison of quality of life outcomes in laryngeal cancer patients following chemoradiation vs. total laryngectomy. *Otolaryngology - Head and Neck Surgery*, *132*(6), 948–953. DOI: 10.1016/j.otohns.2004.12.014 PMID: 15944570

Maclean, J., Cotton, S., & Perry, A. (2009). Post-Laryngectomy: It's Hard to Swallow. *Dysphagia*, *24*(2), 172–179. DOI: 10.1007/s00455-008-9189-5 PMID: 18784911

McConnel, F. M., & O'Connor, A. (1994). Dysphagia secondary to head and neck cancer surgery. *Acta Oto-Rhino-Laryngologica Belgica*, *48*(2), 165–170. PMID: 8209679

Mcconnel, F. M. S., Logemann, J. A., Rademaker, A. W., Pauloski, B. R., Baker, S. R., Lewin, J., Shedd, D., Heiser, M. A., Cardinale, S., Collins, S., Graner, D., Cook, B. S., Milianti, F., & Baker, T. (1994). Surgical variables affecting postoperative swallowing efficiency in oral cancer patients: A pilot study. *The Laryngoscope*, *104*(1), 87–90. DOI: 10.1288/00005537-199401000-00015 PMID: 8295463

McKean, S. C. ., Ross, J. J. ., Dressler, D. D.., & Scheurer, D. (2017). *Principles and practice of hospital medicine*. McGraw-Hill Education.

Mendelsohn, A. H., Remacle, M., Van Der Vorst, S., Bachy, V., & Lawson, G. (2013). Outcomes following transoral robotic surgery: Supraglottic laryngectomy. *The Laryngoscope*, *123*(1), 208–214. DOI: 10.1002/lary.23621 PMID: 23008093

Murphy, B. A., & Gilbert, J. (2009). Dysphagia in Head and Neck Cancer Patients Treated With Radiation: Assessment, Sequelae, and Rehabilitation. *Seminars in Radiation Oncology*, *19*(1), 35–42. DOI: 10.1016/j.semradonc.2008.09.007 PMID: 19028344

Nguyen, N. P., Moltz, C. C., Frank, C., Vos, P., Smith, H. J., Karlsson, U., Dutta, S., Midyett, F. A., Barloon, J., & Sallah, S. (2004). Dysphagia following chemoradiation for locally advanced head and neck cancer. *Annals of Oncology : Official Journal of the European Society for Medical Oncology*, *15*(3), 383–388. DOI: 10.1093/annonc/mdh101 PMID: 14998839

Nund, R. L., Ward, E. C., Scarinci, N. A., Cartmill, B., Kuipers, P., & Porceddu, S. V. (2014). Carers' Experiences of Dysphagia in People Treated for Head and Neck Cancer: A Qualitative Study. *Dysphagia*, *29*(4), 450–458. DOI: 10.1007/s00455-014-9527-8 PMID: 24844768

Pauloski, B. R., Logemann, J. A., Fox, J. C., & Colangelo, L. A. (1995). Biomechanical Analysis of the Pharyngeal Swallow in Postsurgical Patients With Anterior Tongue and Floor of Mouth Resection and Distal Flap Reconstruction. *Journal of Speech, Language, and Hearing Research: JSLHR*, *38*(1), 110–123. DOI: 10.1044/jshr.3801.110 PMID: 7731203

Preuss, S. F., Cramer, K., Klussmann, J. P., Eckel, H. E., & Guntinas-Lichius, O. (2009). Transoral laser surgery for laryngeal cancer: Outcome, complications and prognostic factors in 275 patients. [EJSO]. *European Journal of Surgical Oncology*, *35*(3), 235–240. DOI: 10.1016/j.ejso.2008.01.012 PMID: 18281184

Rademaker, A. W., Logemann, J. A., Pauloski, B. R., Bowman, J. B., Lazarus, C. L., Sisson, G. A., Milianti, F. J., Graner, D., Cook, B. S., Collins, S. L., Stein, D. W., Beery, Q. C., Johnson, J. T., & Baker, T. M. (1993). Recovery of postoperative swallowing in patients undergoing partial laryngectomy. *Head & Neck*, *15*(4), 325–334. DOI: 10.1002/hed.2880150410 PMID: 8360055

Roe, J. W. G., Carding, P. N., Dwivedi, R. C., Kazi, R. A., Rhys-Evans, P. H., Harrington, K. J., & Nutting, C. M. (2010). Swallowing outcomes following Intensity Modulated Radiation Therapy (IMRT) for head & neck cancer – A systematic review. *Oral Oncology*, *46*(10), 727–733. DOI: 10.1016/j.oraloncology.2010.07.012 PMID: 20850370

Rositch, A. F. (2020). Global burden of cancer attributable to infections: The critical role of implementation science. *The Lancet. Global Health*, *8*(2), e153–e154. DOI: 10.1016/S2214-109X(20)30001-2 PMID: 31981543

Sharma, B. K., Contrera, K. J., Jia, X., Fleming, C., Lorenz, R. R., Koyfman, S. A., Mahomva, C., Arianpour, K., Burkey, B. B., Fritz, M., Ku, J. A., Lamarre, E. D., Scharpf, J., & Prendes, B. L. (2022). Outcomes After Oral Cavity and Oropharyngeal Salvage Surgery. *The Laryngoscope*, *132*(10), 1984–1992. DOI: 10.1002/lary.30070 PMID: 35191537

Suiter, D. M., & Gosa, M. M. (2019). *Assessing and treating dysphagia : a lifespan perspective*. Thieme.

Sung, H., Ferlay, J., Siegel, R. L., Laversanne, M., Soerjomataram, I., Jemal, A., & Bray, F. (2021). Global Cancer Statistics 2020: GLOBOCAN Estimates of Incidence and Mortality Worldwide for 36 Cancers in 185 Countries. *CA: a Cancer Journal for Clinicians*, *71*(3), 209–249. DOI: 10.3322/caac.21660 PMID: 33538338

Terk, A. R., Leder, S. B., & Burrell, M. I. (2007). Hyoid Bone and Laryngeal Movement Dependent Upon Presence of a Tracheotomy Tube. *Dysphagia*, *22*(2), 89–93. DOI: 10.1007/s00455-006-9057-0 PMID: 17287926

Trotti, A., Bellm, L. A., Epstein, J. B., Frame, D., Fuchs, H. J., Gwede, C. K., Komaroff, E., Nalysnyk, L., & Zilberberg, M. D. (2003). Mucositis incidence, severity and associated outcomes in patients with head and neck cancer receiving radiotherapy with or without chemotherapy: A systematic literature review. *Radiotherapy and Oncology : Journal of the European Society for Therapeutic Radiology and Oncology*, *66*(3), 253–262. DOI: 10.1016/S0167-8140(02)00404-8 PMID: 12742264

Tsou, Y.-A., Meng, N.-H., Chang, W.-D., & Hua, C.-H. (2025). Does swallow rehabilitation improve recovery of swallow function after treatment for advanced head and neck cancer. *Scientific Reports*, *15*(1), 8300. DOI: 10.1038/s41598-025-87877-w PMID: 40064906

Wang, J., Liu, M., Liu, C., Ye, Y., & Huang, G. (2014). Percutaneous endoscopic gastrostomy versus nasogastric tube feeding for patients with head and neck cancer: A systematic review. *Journal of Radiation Research*, *55*(3), 559–567. DOI: 10.1093/jrr/rrt144 PMID: 24453356

Weinstein, G. S., O'Malley, B. W., Snyder, W., & Hockstein, N. G. (2007). Transoral Robotic Surgery: Supraglottic Partial Laryngectomy. *The Annals of Otology, Rhinology, and Laryngology*, *116*(1), 19–23. DOI: 10.1177/000348940711600104 PMID: 17305273

WHO. (2004). *International statistical classification of diseases and related health problems*. World Health Organization.

Wilson, J. A., Carding, P. N., & Patterson, J. M. (2011). Dysphagia after Nonsurgical Head and Neck Cancer Treatment. *Otolaryngology - Head and Neck Surgery*, *145*(5), 767–771. DOI: 10.1177/0194599811414506 PMID: 21746839

Xu, B., Boero, I. J., Hwang, L., Le, Q., Moiseenko, V., Sanghvi, P. R., Cohen, E. E. W., Mell, L. K., & Murphy, J. D. (2015). Aspiration pneumonia after concurrent chemoradiotherapy for head and neck cancer. *Cancer*, *121*(8), 1303–1311. DOI: 10.1002/cncr.29207 PMID: 25537836

Zafereo, M. E., Weber, R. S., Lewin, J. S., Roberts, D. B., & Hanasono, M. M. (2010). Complications and functional outcomes following complex oropharyngeal reconstruction. *Head & Neck*, *32*(8), 1003–1011. DOI: 10.1002/hed.21290 PMID: 19953614

Zhang, J., Li, Q., Wu, H.-Y., & Yang, Y. (2022). A Systematic Review of Swallowing Training Measures for Postoperative Oral Cancer Patients. *Dysphagia*, *37*(6), 1839–1850. DOI: 10.1007/s00455-022-10445-1 PMID: 35435477

Zhang, J., Zhu, Y.-K., Wan, Y.-F., Wu, H.-Y., Yang, C., Li, X.-K., Tan, L.-B., & Yang, Y. (2025). Risk Factors for Postoperative Dysphagia in Patients with Oral Cavity and Oropharyngeal Cancer: A Systematic Review and Meta-analysis. *Dysphagia*. Advance online publication. DOI: 10.1007/s00455-025-10854-y PMID: 40542856

Chapter 7
Post-Stroke Dysphagia

Pooja Vijay Shevale
http://orcid.org/0009-0001-6075-6497
National Centre for Ageing, AIIMS, New Delhi, India

Anshu Tikariha
http://orcid.org/0009-0007-9064-7324
Datta Meghe Institute of Higher Education and Research, Wardha, India

ABSTRACT

Post-stroke dysphagia is a common, serious complication increasing risks of aspiration pneumonia, malnutrition, and mortality. This chapter covers swallowing neurophysiology, epidemiology, acute and chronic phases, quality of life impact, and prognosis. It details bedside and instrumental screening, evidence-based compensatory and rehabilitative interventions, and emerging neuromodulatory therapies. The role of a multidisciplinary team in optimizing recovery and preventing complications is highlighted, illustrated through a case study.

A. INTRODUCTION

Dysphagia is a well-known problem that frequently develops 50%–80% of the time following a stroke. A bad prognosis or even mortality can result from post-stroke dysphagia (PSD), which frequently causes major consequences such pneumonia and starvation. PSD causes these adverse physical and psychological impairments to patients, which becomes a challenge for both patients and physicians. (Wang et al., 2025)

When dysphagia makes it impossible to share meals with loved ones, it not only raises morbidity and mortality following a stroke but also has a major negative impact on quality of life. Early diagnosis and treatment of swallowing difficulties

DOI: 10.4018/979-8-3373-6405-6.ch007

can promote quick reintegration into society and prevent the emergence of secondary issues. Over half of stroke survivors experience dysphagia. Thankfully, only 11–13% of these patients are still dysphagic after six months, and most of them regain the ability to swallow within seven days. (González-Fernández et al., 2013) Eighty percent of patients with persistent dysphagia needed different enteral feeding methods, according to one study. (Broadley et al., 2003)

B. NEUROPHYSIOLOGICAL FOUNDATION OF SWALLOWING

The coordinated contraction and inhibition of the muscles around the mouth, as well as at the tongue, larynx, pharynx, and oesophagus on both sides, is a complicated sensorimotor activity that occurs during swallowing. Many of the striated muscles innervated by the cranial nerves (CN) are sequentially excited and/or inhibited to carry out the bolus passage from the mouth to the stomach during a swallow, involving various levels of the central nervous system from the cerebral cortex to the medulla oblongata. (Ertekin & Aydogdu, 2004)

The mouth cavity, pharynx, and larynx are the three morphologically and functionally distinct upper aerodigestive tract structures that must work together to swallow. Food and liquid can be moved into the stomach without going via the respiratory system thanks to these structures, which function as a hydrodynamic pump with valves. The oral, pharyngeal, and esophageal phases of swallowing are separated by the placement of the food bolus inside the swallowing mechanism. The pharyngeal and esophageal stages of deglutition follow the voluntary oral phase, which is the first stage. (Ertekin & Aydogdu, 2004)

Figure 1. Phases of Swallowing

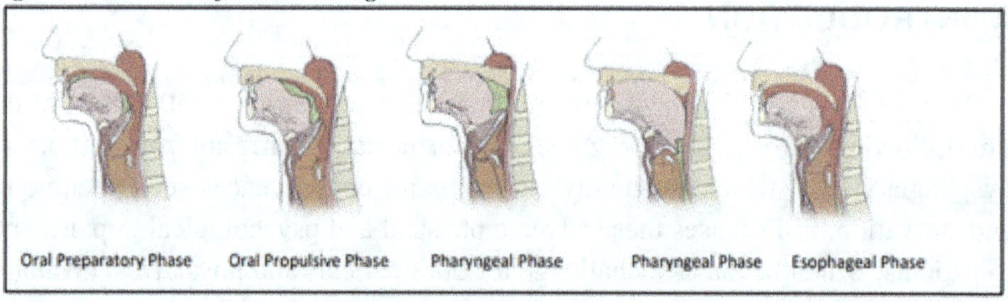

It is now convenient to say that there are three phases to swallowing: oral, pharyngeal, and esophageal. However, the swallow has also been divided into two parts: the esophageal and buccopharyngeal (or oropharyngeal) stages. The three stages of swallowing are likely connected by their innervation patterns: the oesophagus phase is primarily controlled by the somatic and autonomic neural systems, the pharyngeal phase is thought to be a reflex response, and the oral phase is frequently seen as voluntary. In addition to the pharyngeal and laryngeal muscles, the oral cavity's tongue and suprahyoid muscles are also involved in the pharyngeal phase of deglutition. The involuntary swallows are actively caused by the periorbital muscles. The oropharyngeal phase (also known as the buccopharyngeal phase) and the succeeding esophageal phase comprise the actual motor activities of swallowing. The entire oropharyngeal swallowing sequence lasts between 0.6 and 1.0 seconds, and it is extremely consistent across all mammals studied, including humans (Gordon et al., 1987). The oesophagus phase of swallowing is slower and simpler than the oropharyngeal phase, which is remarkably intricate and quick. It is made up of a peristaltic wave of smooth and striated muscular contraction that travels to the stomach. In a cognisant individual, the entire esophageal phase may last longer than ten seconds.

Table 1. Anatomy of the oropharangeal and oesophageal stages of swallowing

Table 1. Anatomy of the oropharyngeal and oesophageal stages of swallowing

Muscle groups		Individual muscles	Main function in swallowing
Jaw	Jaw closing muscles	Masseter	Mastication and food processing
		Temporalis	
		Medial pterygoid	
	Jaw opening muscles	Digastric	
		Mylohyoid	
		Suprahyoid	
		Lateral pterygoid	
Lips and cheek		Orbicularis oris	Containment of the food bolus in the oral cavity during the oral stage
		Risorius	
		Lip elevators	
		Lip depressors	
		Buccinator	
Tongue	Intrinsic muscles	Vertical	Manipulation of the food bolus in the oral cavity to enable processing and propulsion during the oral stage
		Transverse	
		Superior longitudinal	
		Inferior longitudinal	
	Extrinsic muscles	Genioglossus	
		Styloglossus	
		Hyoglossus	
		Palatoglossus	
Soft palate		Levator veli palatine	Elevation of the soft palate during the pharyngeal stage to seal the entrance from the oral to the nasal cavity
		Tensor veli palatine	
		Palatoglossus	
		Palatopharyngeus	
		Musculus uvulae	
Larynx	Intrinsic laryngeal muscles	Lateral cricoarytenoid	Control of the opening to the laryngeal inlet
		Transverse and oblique arytenoid	
		Aryepiglotticus	
		Thyroepiglotticus	
Pharynx		Anterior digastric	Constriction of the pharyngeal wall and elevation of the pharynx and larynx during the pharyngeal stage
		Geniohyoid	
		Stylohyoid	
		Styloglossus	
	External circular muscles of pharyngeal wall	Superior, middle, and inferior constrictors	
		Palatoglossus	
	Internal longitudinal muscles of pharyngeal wall	Palatopharyngeus	
		Stylopharyngeus	
		Salpingopharyngeus	
Oesophagus	Upper oesophageal sphincter	Cricopharyngeus	Relaxation of the upper oesophageal sphincter allows passage of the bolus from the pharynx to the oesophagus
			Propulsion of the bolus towards the stomach through peristaltic waves during the oesophageal stage
		Thyropharyngeus	
	Oesophagus	Internal circular muscle	
		External longitudinal muscle	

1. Oral Phase of Swallowing

The oral phase of swallowing is mostly voluntary and varies greatly in length based on the human's flavour, environment, hunger, motivation, and consciousness. The maxillary branch of the trigeminal nerve, the glossopharyngeal nerve, and the vagus nerve, particularly its superior laryngeal branch, are thought to contain the afferent fibres that initiate swallowing. Peripheral regions such the dorsum of the tongue, the epiglottis, the pillar of the fauces, and the pharyngeal walls are innervated by these nerves. All of the afferent fibres that initiate or facilitate swallowing at the brain stem level converge in the solitary tract and terminate in the nucleus tractus solitarius (NTS). As a result, the primary afferent central structure is the NTS.

In addition to receiving the primary sensory fibres from the laryngeal and oro-pharangeal regions, homologous regions of the NTS receive cortical descending signals. The area of the cortex that assists the onset of swallowing receives some of the sensory inputs that cause swallowing. The threshold to elicit swallowing may be lowered by descending signals from the swallowing- related brain regions during recurrent swallowing. In humans, however, swallowing start or triggering is likely more complicated and may rely more on areas above the brainstem. The kind of bolus, single or continuous swallows, and voluntary or reflexively triggered swallowing may all have an impact. The initiation of deliberately induced swallows in humans appears to be modulated by certain circumstances. These are the sub-mental/suprahyoid muscles at the floor of the mouth (V and XII CN), the bolus in the mouth (food or saliva), and the corticobulbar drive to the tongue muscles (XII CN). The amount of saliva that accumulates in the mouth during non-REM sleep and in between meals may induce the spontaneous swallows, which most likely do not require cerebral driving but may include communication with the cortex and subcortical regions. Without a doubt, the oral cavity, tongue, and pharyngeal mechanoreceptors, chemoreceptors, and thermoreceptors give crucial information for bolus recognition. Swallows have been suggested to be triggered by sensory inputs from the oropharangeal region, particularly the tonsillar pillara, base of the tongue, and oropharangeal mucosa (IX and X CN).

Water infusion into the valleculae does not cause a swallow until the liquid reaches the pyriform sinuses and aryepiglottic folds, according to the majority of human research, including investigations of continuous eating or drinking. However, if the bolus touches the top third of the epiglottis rather than just the valleculae and pyriform sinuses at the throat, a swallow may start sooner. It is clear that prepared food typically builds up gradually on the posterior surface of the tongue in healthy human individuals, and this solid food reaches the valleculae before the swallow begins. In order for sensory impulses to trigger the pharyngeal reflex swallow, the mucosa around the larynx and in the hypopharynx must remain intact. Therefore, depending on the type of bolus, the start of the swallow can be anticipated from the posterior region of the oral cavity to the hypopharynx. The oral and pharyngeal stages happen sequentially in a small volume swallow (1-2 ml), like saliva, and there is no oral preparation. The oral and pharyngeal phases, on the other hand, overlap and happen concurrently when consuming a big volume liquid bolus. The bolus's size modifies the time of each stage of the swallow but has no effect on the order of events during oropharyngeal swallowing. The pharyngeal transit time, laryngeal closure, and elevation all increase with bolus size (1–20 ml). Normal persons often split a 20 ml volume of water into two or more parts. Piecemeal deglutition is the term for this. Individuals who suffer from neurogenic dysphagia must split the bolus into two or more swallows, each of which must be less than 20 millilitres of drinking water. Once swallowing is started, the cascade of sequential muscle activation does not fundamentally change from the perioral muscles downward, even though the location, timing, and density of the oropharyngeal sensory input may differ from bolus to bolus and from normal subjects to patients with sensory impairment. The central pattern generator (CPG) for human swallowing is supported by this line of data.

2. Pharyngeal Phase of Swallowing

The pharynx and oral cavity are physically distinct but functionally connected parts of the head and neck, as was previously mentioned. Feeding, chewing, swallowing, speaking, and breathing are examples of complicated motor responses that include these two areas. The oral and pharyngeal phases are closely linked from the point of swallowing, and it is frequently difficult to distinguish between them. Because of their close relationship, we frequently refer to oropharynx and oropharyngeal swallowing. When the movement of the bolus from the oral cavity to the pharyngeal spaces triggers the swallowing reflex or response, the following physiological events occur in rapid overlapping

All of the events until the esophageal phase are mainly controlled by the CPG of the brain stem. These events are as follows:

A number of "reflex" events, such as the palate closing the velopharyngeal isthmus, the suprahyoid/submental muscles elevating and suspending the larynx, and the laryngeal muscles of the vocal folds and epiglottis closing the larynx, protect the nasal, laryngeal, and tracheal airways. Because it helps close the vestibulae and relocate the larynx anterosuperiorly beneath the base of the tongue, laryngeal elevation is an essential part of airway protection. Every swallow occurs between late inspiration and late expiration, and the pharyngeal phase of swallowing always includes an apneic phase. Because of the CPG, airway protection is crucial. In accordance with the urgent demand, the laryngeal closure is additionally supported by the orolaryngopharyngeal protective reflexes.

To force the bolus past the pharynx and into the oesophagus, the tongue thrusts posteriorly (XII CN). Any leftover material is cleared into the oesophagus by a series of waves of contraction of the pharyngeal constrictor muscles (X CN). Thus, the tongue's posterior movement provides the primary propulsive force acting on the bolus. Although it helps future pharyngeal clearance in conjunction with a significant shortening of the pharynx, the pharyngeal contraction appears to be minor in relation to bolus propulsion.

The bolus is transported into the oesophagus by the relaxation and opening of the upper esophageal sphincter (UES). The striated cricopharyngeus muscle, which contracts tonically, is the main component of the UES. This muscle relaxes and opens during swallowing, and the contraction of the suprahyoid/submental muscle groups pulls on the sphincter anteriorly. The UES then closes until the subsequent swallow once the pharyngeal phase of swallowing is finished. The CP sphincter muscle's tonic EMG activity stops and the UES opens at the same time during a swallow. Since there is a connection and correlation between the laryngeal relocation time and the opening of the UES, the mechanism governing the opening and relaxation of the CP muscle of the UES is under neurological control rather than biomechanical factors. (Ertekin & Aydogdu, 2004). A summary of both phases is depicted in Table 1.

C. NEUROPHYSIOLOGY OF SWALLOWING

To understand the pathophysiology of PSD, it is important to appreciate the intricacies of the neurological basis for swallowing. Much of the basic knowledge concerning the neural control of swallowing has traditionally come from studies on anaesthetised or awake mammals using direct electrical stimulation of the brain and extracellular or intracellular recordings of neuronal activity. These studies collectively showed that swallowing can be elicited through stimulating peripheral nerves, the brainstem, and various cortical and sub-cortical structures.

1. Brainstem

The command centre for swallowing is thought to be the brainstem. It receives afferent inputs from the cerebral cortex and peripheral nerves, integrates and interprets the data, and produces efferent motor impulses to carry out the swallowing motor sequence. Swallowing neurones, comprising motor neurones and interneurones, are found in the medulla oblongata, which is at the base of the brainstem, according to research based on microelectrode recordings in animals. The swallowing central pattern generator (CPG), a complex unit made up of these neurones, is in charge of creating and controlling the swallowing motor sequence.

The CPG's neurones are divided into two groups: the ventral swallowing group (VSG), which is found in the ventrolateral medulla, and the dorsal swallowing group (DSG), which is found in the nucleus tractus solitarii and the nearby reticular formation. The generator interneurones that make up the DSG are responsible for initiating and sequencing motor actions. Prior to swallowing motor events, these neurones show a pattern of discharges. This discharge activity ceases if there are no swallowing events, but it increases when swallowing is started, creating a swallowing discharge pattern. This firing pattern implies that these neurones are in charge of programming and initiating swallowing-related motor activities. The VSG, on the other hand, consists of switching interneurones and functions as a relay unit in which DSG neurones activate neurones, which subsequently transmit signals to motor neurones in motor nuclei that innervate the muscles in the oesophagus and oropharynx. These motor neurones can be found in the dorsal motor nucleus of the vagus, the nucleus ambiguus, and the trigeminal (V), facial (VII), and hypoglossal (XII) motor nuclei.

2. Cerebral Cortex and Subcortical Structures

Swallowing can be made rhythmically by stimulating the anterolateral areas of the primary motor cortex, indicating the involvement of cortical input in swallowing. The peripheral muscles that correspond to the stimulated cortical region receive a volley of action potentials when the motor cortex is activated. Surface EMG electrodes can then detect the impulses from the muscles, known as motor evoked potentials (MEPs). Eliciting MEPs is a potent method to study neurophysiological processes because different characteristics of MEPs represent various facets and the integrity of neural circuits. Primary motor cortex, primary somatosensory cortex, insula, cingulate cortex, supplementary motor area, pre-motor cortex, auditory cortex, inferior frontal gyrus, parietooccipital and prefrontal cortex, operculum, putamen, thalamus, global pallidus, internal capsule, corpus callosum, basal ganglia, caudate, pons and mid-brain, inferior parietal lobule, and the cerebellum are among them.

Swallowing is initiated and carried out by the primary motor cortex. It is believed that during swallowing, afferent information is processed by the main somatosensory cortex. During swallowing, sensory information is crucial because it gives the system feedback to modify muscle motions based on the characteristics and condition of the bolus. During sensory stimulation and swallowing in MRI investigations, the somatosensory and primary motor cortices are frequently seen to be active concurrently. Taste information and mechanical sensory information from vagal and spinal afferents are processed by the insula and frontal operculum, which are thought to be the main taste centres. The commencement of swallowing may be attributed to the insula, a main integrative area for voluntary swallowing. The processing of visceral discomfort, higher cognitive level processing, and swallowing focus may all be mediated by the anterior cingulate cortex. Moreover, the swallowing network's functional loop includes the basal ganglia. They may be in charge of controlling different motor functions during swallowing because of their responsibilities in the selection of suitable motor programs.

3. Cerebellum

Similar to how it fine-tunes limb motions, the cerebellum, a motor modulatory organ, is thought to fine-tune the muscle contractions that take place during swallowing. Although the brainstem is the only structure involved in swallowing, the cerebellum aids in modulating the central neuronal regulation of swallowing. When considered collectively, the physiology of regular swallowing is extremely intricate, including dynamic interactions between the nervous system's afferent and efferent circuits. The brainstem, cerebellum, subcortical regions, and cerebral cortex are all essential for controlling swallowing. Therefore, it should come as no surprise that impairment to these tissues after a neurological injury (such as a stroke) might cause dysphagia by interfering with regular swallowing (Ertekin & Aydogdu, 2004).

D. EPIDEMIOLOGY AND RISK FACTORS OF POST-STROKE DYSPHAGIA

1. Prevalence

Post-stroke dysphagia was seen in 46.6% of cases overall. The diagnosing method has the biggest impact on prevalence. Risk variables for post-stroke dysphagia included hypertension, a history of stroke, atrial fibrillation, patient age, and the severity of the stroke. Patients with PSD are two to four times more likely than those without PSD to experience aphasia, dysarthria, respiratory tract infections, and pneumonitis. (Wang et al., 2025)

The prevalence of poststroke dysphagia was originally reported by Rosemary in 2005. (Martino R,et al., 2005) Numerous researchers have carried out comparable studies,(Meng et al., 2020) (Banda et al., 2022) (Chang et al., 2022) and their findings showed that improving PSD screening can result in a threefold decreased risk of stroke-associated pneumonia (SAP).(Hinchey et al., 2005) Nevertheless, none of this research thoroughly examined the variables affecting PSD occurrence from a variety of angles.

The data included in this integrated study of PSD prevalence in epidemiology studies was published between 2000 and 2022. Compared to the rate of 42% among acute stroke patients in 2022, the total prevalence of PSD is 38.69% (Banda KJ.et al.,2022) The prevalence of PSD is influenced by a number of factors, including temporal, geographical, demographic, and stroke-related factors. (Finestone et al., 1995)

Dysphagia is most common in South America and least common in Oceania, according to the spatial distribution.

The incidence rates vary across different study years, regions, situations, evaluation instruments, and personnel. The highest rates of dysphagia are found in patients in rehabilitation facilities, which is a clear sign that people in need of rehabilitation typically have more severe stroke consequences, which is correlated with the severity of their disease. Prevalence rates are also influenced by the experience level of screening staff, with more experienced workers generally reporting higher PSD instances. (Wen et al., 2025)

2. Risk Factors

A higher percentage of those with dysphagia had a history of dementia, hypertension, coronary artery disease, congestive heart failure, and previous stroke. Risk factors were excessive cholesterol, alcohol use, current cigarette smoking status, and a history of transient ischemic attacks.

Dysphagia and heart problems make recovery more challenging and frequently result in worse outcomes. However, it is challenging to ascertain whether there is a causative association between these cardiac diseases and swallowing deficits or whether these conditions made patients more vulnerable to developing dysphagia following stroke simply because these individuals are more medically impaired.

Additional risk variables for dysphagia following a stroke were being older, Black, having a hemorrhagic stroke (as opposed to an infarct), having a right hemisphere stroke, and having a higher NIHSS score at presentation. Patients with a history of elevated cholesterol, a lower prestroke mRS, and any WMD shown on clinical imaging were factors linked to a lower risk. Black people experience more severe strokes than White people, according to previously published statistics. (Krekeler et al., 2024)

Figure 2. Geographical representation of prevalence of post stroke dysphagia

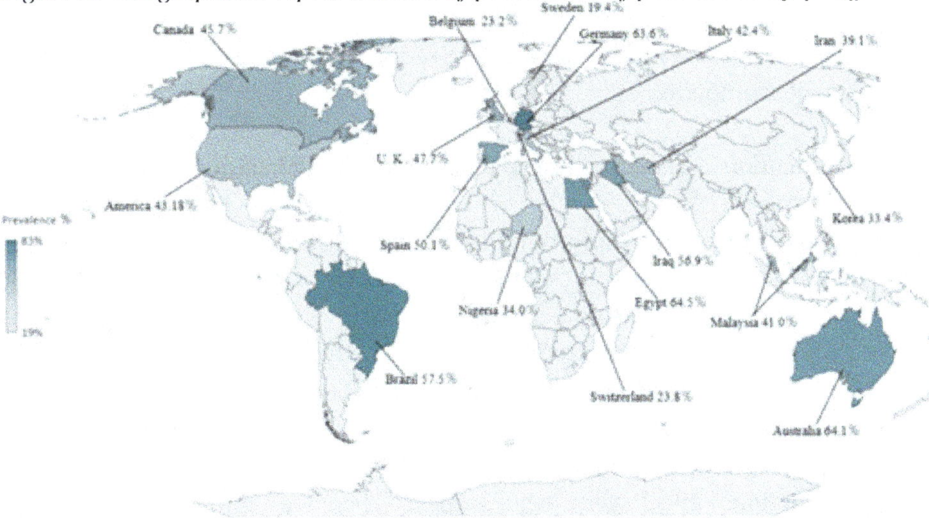

E. DYSPHAGIA IN ACUTE STROKE VERSUS CHRONIC STROKE

While chronic dysphagia is linked to ongoing difficulties, long-term dependency, increased mortality rates, and a much lower quality of life, acute dysphagia following a stroke is frequently a transient condition with a high chance of significant improvement.

1. **Outcomes of Acute Dysphagia:** The majority of stroke victims have acute dysphagia during the initial days or weeks. Most of these people experience a quick and spontaneous improvement in their ability to swallow during the first week or two.
2. **Complications:** Even when they do occur, the difficulties are frequently treatable with early intervention (e.g., diet change, positioning procedures, tube feeding if severe).
3. **Recovery:** A speech-language pathologist's early, focused intervention can greatly lower the chance of problems and hasten the return to a regular diet.
4. **Prognosis:** Although many patients still make a full recovery, dysphagia during the acute period is a sign of the severity of the stroke and is linked to worse short-term outcomes.

2. Outcomes of Chronic Dysphagia

The prognosis is more difficult for the 8–13% of stroke survivors who still have dysphagia at six months.

i. **Complications:** There is always a chance of major health problems. Among them are:
   a. **Recurrent aspiration pneumonia:** The most dreaded consequence, frequently brought on by "silent aspiration" (food or liquid getting into the airway without causing a cough).
   b. **Malnutrition and dehydration:** Frequently caused by insufficient oral intake or dependence on thickened liquids or altered diets.
   c. **Increased mortality:** Higher long-term mortality is independently predicted with severe, persistent dysphagia.
   d. **Functional and Psychosocial Impact:** There are significant psychosocial repercussions linked to persistent dysphagia.

ii. **Increased dependency:** A greater chance of needing long-term institutionalised care (such as a nursing home) or assistance with everyday tasks.

iii. **Reduced quality of life:** Many patients claim that eating is no longer pleasurable, which can result in despair, anxiety, and social isolation.

iv. **Employment issues:** Patients of working age who have persistent dysphagia are much less likely to return to work. (Smithard, et al., 2007) (Karisik et al., 2025) (Khedr et al.,2021)

F. DYSPHAGIA SCREENING

Before problems like pneumonia, dehydration, malnutrition, or airway obstruction arise, dysphagia screening can identify the likelihood of aspiration (overt or silent). A number of these tests are utilised for both screening and bedside evaluations. The majority of tools evaluate a water swallowing trial and/or a few clinical characteristics. (González-Fernández et al., 2013). If any two of the following are true, the screening is deemed successful: 1) abnormal gagging, 2) dysarthria, 3) abnormal volitional coughing, 5) coughing after swallowing, or 6) voice changes following swallowing. (Daniels et al., 1997). The only screening instrument that evaluates pharyngeal feeling is the Toronto Bedside Swallowing Screening Test (TOR-BSST©). (Broadley et al., 2003)

Bours et al. (2009) suggested a water swallowing test in conjunction with pulse oximetry with end points of coughing, dysphonia, and choking as a way to screen patients for aspiration and dysphagia in a systematic review of bedside screening tests. The Modified Mann Assessment of Swallowing Ability (MMASA) has been suggested by Antonios et al. (2010) as a physician-specific screening tool for dysphagia. (Gordon et al., 1987) According to their initial results, the MMASA is a valid and reliable screening tool for dysphagia in stroke survivors. (Finestone et al., 1995)

1. Clinical Bedside Assessments

For the purposes of screening and/or evaluation, a number of clinical or bedside swallowing assessments have been described. While some of these techniques assess swallowing abilities using a combined approach, others employ clinical markers or indicators, such as abnormalities of speech or voice (e.g., dysarthria, dysphonia, vocal alteration), sensitivity of the gag reflex, or volitional cough strength. A water-swallowing test to assess voice change or coughing after swallowing may or may not be part of these techniques.

2. Clinical Assessment of Bulbar Muscle Function

a. **Gag reflex:** When the velum or posterior pharyngeal wall elevates unilaterally or bilaterally in response to tactile stimulation, this is referred to as a normal gag reflex response; when the reaction is decreased or absent, it is referred to as an abnormal gag reflex. (b) The patient's response to a voluntary cough command is known as the voluntary cough response; an aberrant cough reflex is taken into consideration when there is no response, a vocalised cough, or a weaker cough. (González-Fernández et al., 2013) (Wang et al., 2025)
b. **Water swallowing test (WST):** In order to determine if dysphagia was present or not, WST asked the patient to swallow 30 milliliters of water at room temperature as usual. They then tracked how many times the patient swallowed and whether they choked. If the patient can swallow everything at once without coughing, choking, or changing the quality of their speech within five seconds, it is deemed affirmative. For two days in a row, the test was administered twice. (González-Fernández et al., 2013) (Wang et al., 2025)

When an abnormal water swallowing test is combined with an abnormal gag reflex and volitional cough response, dysphagia is diagnosed.

3. Dysphagia Outcome Severity Scale (DOSS)

A straightforward, user-friendly seven-level scale designed to assess the degree of dysphagia and suggest the degree of feeding dependence. Level 1 mounts to severe dysphasia because the patient cannot tolerate per oral intake. Level 2 mounts to moderate-severe dysphagia as maximal help with partial per oral intake only, where the patient can safely tolerate at least one consistency with maximum precautions. Level 3 dysphagia is characterised by complete supervision and restrictions on two or more meal consistencies. Level 4 progresses to mild-to-moderate dysphagia when one or two consistencies are limited and intermittent supervision is required. Level 5 progresses to mild dysphagia, requiring one diet consistency restriction and remote supervision. Level 6 mount to swallowing within functional limits/ modified independence. Level 7 refers to swallowing that is normal in all situations. (González-Fernández et al., 2013) (Wang et al., 2025)

i. **Gugging Swallowing Screen (GUSS):** The only dysphagia screening instrument that tests swallowing function using several consistencies is the Gugging Swallowing Screen (GUSS). Because individuals with dysphagia are more likely to aspirate liquids than semi-solids, this is a significant component in acute stroke-related dysphagia. The test's objective is to evaluate the degree of aspiration risk and, if required, make suggestions for dietary changes. Even minor indicators of silent aspiration, such as drooling, delayed swallowing, and vocal changes, can be detected by the GUSS. A straightforward swallow test is the first part of the bedside GUSS exam. Next comes a direct swallowing test with three subtests: the Semisolid Swallowing Trial, the Liquid Swallowing Trial and Solid Swallowing Trial. In the semisolid swallowing trial, participants swallow a pudding-like concoction made by combining 1/3 to 1/2 teaspoon of distilled water with instant food thickener, then five more 1/2 teaspoons. Aqua bi is swallowed in different volumes during the liquid swallowing trial: 3 ml, 5 ml, 10 ml, 20 ml, and 50 ml. Lastly, a tiny piece of dry bread is used as the bolus in the solid swallowing trial. Every ten seconds, this trial is repeated five times (Trapl et al., 2007). It was discovered that the GUSS has 69% specificity and 100% sensitivity in predicting aspiration risk (Ekberg et al., 2002)
ii. **Swallowing Provocation Test (SPT):** A less common two-stage screening test called the swallowing provocation test (SPT) uses a tiny nasal catheter with an internal diameter of 0.5 mm to inject a bolus of 0.4 mL and then 2.0 mL of distilled water to the suprapharynx in order to induce an involuntary swallow (Finestone et al., 1995) (Smithard et al., 1996). Next, a stopwatch is used to quantify the latent time between the water injection and the start of swallowing, which is determined by visual observation of the distinctive laryngeal movement. The activation of the swallowing reflex following the water injection determines whether the responses to the SPT are considered normal or abnormal. A cut-off point in seconds is utilised to distinguish between a normal and pathological swallow. (González-Fernández et al., 2013) (Wang et al., 2025)

iii. **Toronto Bedside Swallowing Screening Test (TOR-BSST):** Patients who are at risk for dysphagia after a stroke can be identified using the Toronto Bedside Swallowing Screening Test (TOR-BSST©), a screening tool given at the bedside by qualified screeners. Five things make up the TOR-BSST©: baseline voice quality, tongue movement, cup sip, 50mL water test, and final evaluation of vocal quality. In an effort to generate dysphagia screening results with high sensitivity and negative predictive value between the acute and rehabilitation periods following a stroke, this screening method integrates independent indicators with strong predictive values. The TOR-BSST was reported to have a sensitivity of 91.3% and a negative predictive value of 93.3% in acute settings and 89.5% in rehabilitative settings.

4. Instrumental Methods Used in the Detection of Dysphagia/Aspiration

i. **Videofluoroscopic Modified Barium Swallow (VMBS) Examination:** Videofluoroscopic Modified Barium Swallow (VMBS) examination is often considered the "gold standard" for confirming the diagnosis. A speech-language pathologist and a radiologist work together to conduct a VMBS study that examines the oral preparation, oral, and pharyngeal phases of swallowing as depicted in Table 2. The patient must have sufficient cognitive and physical skills in order to be assessed. The person is seated in a chair designed to resemble a typical lunchtime position. Common radio-opaque materials tested include bread, cookies, custard, and thin and thick liquids impregnated with barium. Different features of oral, laryngeal, and pharyngeal involvement are shown by the radiography examination (Table 2) (Bach et al., 1989) After the VMBS examination, a chest x-ray may be obtained to document any aspirated barium into the tracheobronchial tree. The VMBS evaluation may reveal the mechanism causing the swallowing problem in addition to identifying the presence and degree of aspiration. Aspiration is most frequently caused by reduced laryngeal closure, pharyngeal paresis, or a functional disturbance in the pharyngeal phase of swallowing. If the patient is obviously struggling to stay properly hydrated and nourished, if frequent choking during meals is a worry, or if the patient has repeated respiratory infections, a VMBS study is recommended. Other hazards, such as depression, immunocompromised lung disease, cognition, recurrent stroke, and depression, must also be considered (Sasegbon et al., 2025)

Table 2. Radiological Evaluation during VMBS (Ertekin & Aydogdu, 2004)

Oral Phase • Lips: Closure • Tongue: Anterior and posterior motion with consonants; motion and coordination during transport, and manipulation of bolus • Soft palate: Evaluation and retraction with consonants • Jaw: Motion • Oral: Pocketing
Pharyngeal Phase • Swallow: Delay, absence • Peristalsis: Residue in valleculae, pyriform sinuses nasopharyngeal regurgitation
Laryngeal Function • Elevation of larynx • Penetration into laryngeal vestibule • Aspiration • Cough: Presence, delay, effectiveness • Vocal cord function
Post-Exam Chest X-Ray • Chronic changes • Presence of barium in valleculae, pyriform sinuses, tracheobroncheal tree, lungs

ii. **Fiberoptic Endoscopic Evaluation of Swallowing (FEES):** When there are restrictions, fiberoptic endoscopic assessment of swallowing (FEES) frequently supplements the VFSS. When performed by an otolaryngologist and/or speech pathologist alone, FEES is a safe and well-tolerated treatment. When evaluating aspiration, pharyngeal residue, and delayed swallow beginning, FEES is just as sensitive as VFSS. Flexible endoscopy is used in the FEES examination to assess the presence and control of oropharyngeal secretions, swallowing various solid and liquid consistencies, and static and dynamic pharyngeal architecture. The length of the transition, signs of aspiration and penetration, the number of swallows required to remove the bolus, and the degree of airway closure are all recorded during swallowing. The scope is moved transnasally along the nose's floor until it reaches the base of the uvula or the tip of the epiglottis. This makes it possible to see the endolarynx, pyriform sinus, lateral and posterior pharyngeal walls, and tongue base. (Sasegbon et al., 2025)

iii. **Pharyngeal Manometry:** Pharyngoesophageal manometry is used to study intra-bolus pressures, pharyngeal peristalsis integrity, and the physiological functions of the upper esophageal sphincter. The gold standard for assessing esophageal motor function is esophageal manometry. It is only used when endoscopy, videoflurography, or history have not been able to identify a motor issue or provide a diagnosis, and it is not the main diagnostic method for dysphagia in stroke. A gastroenterologist typically does manometry, which is recommended in cases of solid meal dysphagia linked to regurgitation and weight loss. (Sasegbon et al., 2025)

iv. **Pulse Oximetry:** Based on the idea that aspirating food into the airway causes bronchospasm or airway blockage, which lowers oxygen saturation, pulse oximetry has been proposed as a technique for detecting aspiration. This method is simple to obtain, non-invasive, and requires minimal patient cooperation. However, it is still unclear if oxygen desaturation can predict aspiration, and the accuracy of pulse oximetry in identifying aspiration has not been demonstrated. (Sasegbon et al., 2025)

v. **Ultrasonography:** A potential new technique for evaluating dysphagia following a stroke is ultrasound. Compared to the conventional VFSS and FEES, it is believed to provide a more useful bedside method for assessing swallowing function. As an alternative, this approach may provide further data to support these instrumental methods or other bedside evaluations. Both the oral and pharyngeal phases of swallowing can be captured by ultrasonography

G. EVIDENCE BASED RESEARCH

Both compensatory and rehabilitative methods are used in dysphagia therapy. While rehabilitative methods aim to enhance swallowing physiology and increase swallow safety and tolerance of the least restrictive diet, compensatory tactics are employed to lessen dysphagia symptoms without changing the physiology.

Certain techniques can both alleviate acute dysphagia symptoms and improve swallowing physiology over time, making them both compensatory and rehabilitative in nature (Table 3).

In dysphagia rehabilitation, a number of methods are frequently used. The Mendelsohn manoeuvre, supraglottic and super-supraglottic swallow, effortful swallow, tongue hold exercises, thermal-tactile stimulation, tongue strengthening exercises, and the Shaker exercise are examples of traditional therapy methods. (Broadley et al., 2003) (Wang et al., 2025)

Table 3. Behavioral Treatment Approaches (González-Fernández M. et al., 2008)

Compensatory	Both	Rehabilitative
• Postural adjustments • Altering bolus characteristics (consistency, viscosity, volume of bolus, temperature, taste) • Increase volitional control	• Effortful swallow • Mendelsohn maneuver • Supraglottic Safety Swallow & Super Supraglottic Safety Swallow (breath hold) • Increase sensory input	• Tongue hold exercise • Shaker exercise (head-raise) • Lingual exercise/ resistance training • LSVT • EMST • NMES

LSVT, Lee Silverman Voice Therapy; EMST, Expiratory Muscle Strength Training; NMES, Neuromuscular Electrical Stimulation*

Table 4. Dysphagia Therapeutic Techniques (Bahia MM, et.al. 2020) (C. Lazarus 2013)

Treatment Technique	Effect on Swallow Function
Effortful Swallow	Improves base of tongue retraction during the swallow and improves clearance of the bolus from the vallecula.
Mendelsohn Maneuver	Increases extent and duration of laryngeal elevation and thereby enhancing during and width of cricopharyngeal opening
Shaker Exercise (Head lift exercise)	Indicated for patients with reduced extent or duration of cricopharyngeal opening resulting in pyriform sinus residue
Supraglottic Safety Swallow	Breath hold closes vocal folds prior to swallow initiation and clears possible residue from the laryngeal vestibule
Super-Supraglottic Safety Swallow	Increase chance of true vocal fold and false vocal fold closure by bearing down
Tongue Hold Exercise	Improves contact between the base of tongue and posterior pharyngeal wall

Rehabilitative Exercises

For patients with acute brain injuries to successfully recover, dysphagia must be carefully managed. Three different kinds of rehabilitation programs have been reported for stroke patients with dysphagia, depending on the swallowing function condition upon admission: 1) not feeding; 2) feeding and facilitation; and 3) progressive feeding. Developing self-sufficiency in eating abilities is one of the objectives of dysphagia treatment. People with dysphagia who are fed by someone else are reported to be 20 times more likely to get pneumonia than those who can feed themselves. In order to prepare very low-level patients for later feeding, the non-feeding program was created as a stimulation program.

i. **Oral Motor Exercises:** Various oral motor activities, as summarized in Table 4, such as range-of-motion exercises for the tongue and pharyngeal structures, are presented with individuals who have developed a swallowing issue. The purpose of these exercises is to enhance swallowing muscle coordination, strength, mobility, and awareness. Exercises that support tongue elevation and lateralisation may be used to help enhance oral transit. Here, in an attempt to enhance speaking and swallowing, the patient could be encouraged to carry out extremely specialised tongue exercises. Additionally, patients may be asked to engage in bolus control exercises (which teach the patient how to control or manipulate objects placed in the mouth) and tongue resistance exercises (which involve pressing the tongue against a tongue blade or popsicle stick for one second).
ii. **Range of Motion Exercises:** The person is instructed to bear down while holding their breath while seated during range-of-motion exercises. It is not advised for people with uncontrolled blood pressure to perform this activity. It is advised to perform this workout for five minutes five to ten times a day.
iii. **Vocal Fold Adduction Exercises:** The goal of vocal fold adduction exercises is to lower the risk of aspiration and enhance vocal quality. People are instructed to speak clearly while bearing down and pressing one hand against a chair. This is carried out five times. After then, the person is requested to make the sound "ah" five times. Once more, it is advised to perform these exercises five to ten times a day for five minutes, three times in a row. People may be requested to pull up on the seat of a chair while seated and prolong phonation if, after a week, there is no discernible improvement in swallowing. For people whose vocal folds do not fully close, this exercise is advised.
iv. **Strengthening Exercises:** Swallowing function may be enhanced by exercises that strengthen the neck and throat muscles. However, in order to apply this therapeutic approach, patients must be able to physically do the necessary motions without becoming hurt. The Shaker Exercise: Patients are instructed to elevate their heads high enough to see their toes while lying flat on the floor or in bed. The patient rests for one minute after holding this position for a minute. Three repetitions of the workout are performed. The patient next looks at their toes, raises their head, and then lowers it. This head-up, head-down pattern is repeated thirty times. For six weeks, it is advised to perform the Shaker exercise three times a day. It has been demonstrated that this exercise can somewhat improve hyolaryngeal mobility.
v. **Chin Tuck Against Resistance:** The chin tuck against resistance exercise is an alternate method of strengthening the suprahyoid muscles. Participants must take two steps in this process: 1) Squeezing a rubber ball with the chin tucked in for ten seconds (isometric); 2) Squeezing a rubber ball with the chin as hard as

possible ten times in a row (isokinetic). The chin tuck produced higher maximal surface electromyography as compared to the Shaker exercises, according to a preliminary investigation that used healthy participants to assess the prospective efficacy of this technique against strength exercise in populations with dysphagia. However, the authors noted that clinical trials are required to ascertain the efficacy of exercising suprahyoid muscles for dysphagia (Broadley et al., 2003)

vi. **Swallow Maneuvers**: Patients may have more difficulty swallowing during the initial phase of recovery than they do during subsequent rehabilitation. If swallowing problems are not addressed and treated in the early stages, there may be problems adhering to the suggested diets and potential setbacks due to aspiration pneumonia. In general, this may make it more difficult for the patient to engage in official rehabilitation. Eating too rapidly, taking big bites, cognitive deficits, and impaired swallowing sensitivity are all common causes of post-ABI swallowing issues. Four manoeuvres can help with swallowing difficulties, but they need the patient to pay attention, follow instructions, and be able to put in the necessary physical effort.

vii. **Supraglottic Swallow:** This technique is intended to eliminate residue after swallowing and to shut the airway at the level of the real vocal folds both before and during the swallow. People are instructed to hold their breath while swallowing and to cough right away. In an attempt to treat impaired or delayed vocal fold closure or delayed pharyngeal swallow, this technique promotes closure of the actual vocal cords. The purpose of this maneuver's cough phase is to expel any residue or items from the laryngeal vestibule.

viii. **Super-Supraglottic Swallow:** This technique tries to eliminate residue after the swallow is finished, enhances pressure generation, and closes the airway entry both before and during the swallow. The patient completes the following steps during this manoeuvre: 1) inhale deeply; 2) hold the breath while bearing down firmly; 3) swallow forcefully while holding this breath; 4) cough and clear your throat right away after the swallow; and 5) swallow again.

ix. **Effortful Swallow:** The goal of an effortful swallow is to increase the tongue base's posterior movement. This method is urging the person to squeeze firmly with all of the swallowing muscles (neck and throat muscles) when they swallow.

x. **Mendelsohn Maneuver:** Reduced laryngeal movement and swallow discoordination are the goals of this technique. Increasing the degree and duration of laryngeal elevation, which lengthens and widens the cricopharyngeal aperture, improves swallowing performance. Patients are usually instructed to hold their larynx (also known as Adam's apple) raised for two to three seconds before finishing the swallow.

xi. **Thermal-tactile Stimulation:** Thermal stimulation, also known as thermal-tactile stimulation, was created to encourage people with neurological impairments to swallow. A cold laryngeal mirror is applied to the base of the facial arches while the patient opens their mouth as part of the thermal-tactile stimulation technique. The mirror is stroked up and down five times while it is in contact with the arch. Contact will be made on the normal (uninjured) side of the mouth for patients who have experienced trauma. The goal is to increase the sensitivity for swallowing through the central nervous system, even when pharyngeal swallow may not be initiated at the moment of stimulation. It is envisaged that the pharyngeal swallow will occur more rapidly once a patient tries to swallow. (Sasegbon et al., 2025)

xii. **Postural Techniques:** In order to improve pharyngeal clearance and/or lower the risk of aspiration, physically shifting the patient's head, neck, and/or body may help modify the direction of the bolus flow. Table 5 lists five positions that have been demonstrated to help people enhance their ability to swallow. It may be difficult to get a patient to use any one of these strategies if they have severe cognitive impairments following an injury. Patients with oral and pharyngeal deficits have been advised to regularly do the following: take controlled bites or sips, alternate solids and liquids, take several swallows, clear or remove food that has pocketed in the mouth, and stay upright for 30 minutes after a meal to lower the risk of aspiration.

Table 5. Five Postures to Improve Swallowing Function

Chin Down Posture	• Helpful for those who have tongue base retraction issues; • Mechanism of change widens the valleculae, allowing the valleculae to contain the bolus in event of pharyngeal delay.
Chin Up Posture	• Helpful for those who have oral tongue propulsion problems; • Aids in gaining adequate lingual pressure to drive the food or liquid out of the mouth and into the pharynx.
Head Turn (left or right)	• Involves rotating the head to the side that is damaged; • Bolus is then directed through the "normal" safe side.
Head Tilt (left or right)	• Head is tilted toward the stronger side, to promote the flow of food and liquid through that side.
Lying Down	• Effective in those with posterior pharyngeal wall contraction or reduced laryngeal elevation with resulting residue and subsequent aspiration after swallowing. • Residual or pooling of food or liquid in the pharynx is less able to enter the airway as gravity pulls the bolus towards the posterior pharyngeal wall and in more easily moved through to the esophagus

H. ADJUNCTIVE AND TECHNOLOGY-ASSISTED THERAPIES

Several devices have now been shown to produce promising results in improving swallowing through neuromodulation.

1. Pharyngeal Electrical Stimulation (PES)

It is a technique that stimulates the peripheral sensory component of the swallowing pathway, further modulating neuronal activities in the higher swallowing centre. Electrodes are placed in contact with the mucosa of the pharynx, which is introduced using a catheter either transnasally or transorally.

On stimulation, a neuropeptide substance P is released. The body typically produces substance P in response to the passage of food, and its decreased level is associated with swallowing problems. Additionally, stimulation induces neuroplasticity by activating the bulbar cranial nerves, pathways in the medulla, and the primary sensory cortex. (Sasegbon et al., 2025)

2. Neuromuscular Electrical Stimulation (NMES)

Electrical stimulation helps in muscle strengthening and sensorimotor recovery. It also works peripherally on the neuromuscular system, reinforcing damaged oropharyngeal musculature by using surface electrodes that trigger muscle contraction by depolarising nerve fibres in neck muscles.

Electrodes are either placed in the suprahyoid or infrahyoid muscles. Since contractions of these muscles can pull the hyoid bone and larynx down, this placement is sometimes used as resistive training, in which patients are asked to perform swallowing actions, such as effortful swallowing, during stimulation. Although studies have reported favourable clinical outcomes, further research is warranted to gain a better understanding of the underlying mechanisms of NMES and the effects of different stimulation parameters on swallowing neurophysiology. (Alamer et al., 2020; Sasegbon et al., 2025; Wang et al., 2023)

3. Repetitive Transcranial Magnetic Stimulation (rTMS)

It is a noninvasive technique that uses magnetic pulses to induce neuroplasticity. High-frequency impulses (≥1 Hz) increase neuronal activity, while low-frequency impulses (<1 Hz) inhibit it. Therefore, while HF-rTMS promotes the excitability of the stroke-affected hemisphere, LF-rTMS is intended to inhibit the cortical excitability of the healthy hemisphere. Long-term depression (LTD) and long-term potentiation (LTP), which alter synaptic plasticity, are the main explanations underlying the effect of rTMS.

Although the most effective stimulation sites have not been conclusively determined, some studies suggest that stimulation of both hemispheres may lead to better swallowing outcomes. In most studies, the oesophageal cortex, mylohyoid and pharyngeal areas were targeted. (Khedr & Abo-Elfetoh, 2010; Sasegbon et al., 2025; Yang et al., 2021)

4. Transcranial Direct Current Stimulation (tDCS)

A continuous, comparatively low-intensity direct current is applied to particular cortical regions via transcranial direct current stimulation (tDCS). It affects synaptic activity and neuronal connectivity by altering the resting membrane potential of neurons. Typically, a signal generator is connected to two saline-soaked sponge electrodes, one serving as the active electrode and the other as the reference electrode. The reference electrode is typically positioned on the opposite side of the active electrode, which is placed over the targeted cortical region (such as the primary motor cortex). Current moves between the two electrodes in the brain once the signal generator is turned on.

The electrodes can be placed ipsilesionally, contralesionally, or bilaterally, depending on the stimulation approach. In studies on swallowing recovery, they are often positioned over the orofacial sensorimotor cortex. According to preliminary data, compensatory reorganization in the contralesional hemisphere is associated with recovery from post-stroke dysphagia. It has been suggested that functional remodelling of the swallowing-related cortex in the contralesional hemisphere is necessary for the recovery of swallowing function following a unilateral stroke.

In dysphagia research, a new bimodal balance-recovery model has been presented more recently that leads to interhemispheric balance and functional recovery. (Ahn et al., 2017; Duan et al., 2025; Sasegbon et al., 2025)

5. Transcutaneous Auricular Vagus Nerve Stimulation

Transcutaneous auricular vagus nerve stimulation (taVNS) modulates central pathways related to neuroplasticity, anti-inflammatory processes, angiogenesis, and blood–brain barrier protection by focusing on the auricular branch of the vagus nerve. This offers a comprehensive strategy for stroke recovery. TaVNS is believed to have neuroprotective effects through several mechanisms. Most notably, it directly affects pharyngeal and laryngeal muscle function by activating specific brainstem nuclei that are part of the central pattern generator for swallowing.

Clinical evidence suggests that taVNS enhances laryngeal sensory feedback and motor control, thereby improving soft palate function, cough reflex, and swallowing ability. It has also demonstrated potential advantages in promoting cognitive recovery and mitigating post-stroke complications, such as sleep disturbances. Nevertheless, it remains unclear exactly how taVNS controls salivation, especially in relation to the central pattern generator's activation. (Sun et al., 2025)

I. MULTIDISCIPLINARY REHABILITATION TEAM

For an optimal rehabilitation, synergistic supervision of a multidisciplinary team is required. This team is composed of:

1. *Neurologist/Physician*- oversees neurological deficit and medical management.
2. *Speech and Language Therapists*- Specialist professionals are primarily responsible for dysphagia screening and assessment, diagnosis and management. They supervise instrumental swallowing assessments, such as videofluoroscopic swallowing studies (VFSS) or fiberoptic endoscopic evaluations of swallowing (FEES). Based on findings, SLPs implement evidence-based interventions and systematically monitor therapeutic progress. When communication disorders co-occur with dysphagia, SLPs also assess and treat them. (Dilworth, 2008; Saitoh et al., 2018)
3. *Nurses*- They perform a critical role in the early detection of dysphagia, specifically in acute care, when nurses maintain continuous bedside presence with direct contact with patients. They supervise and ensure safe feeding practices. (Ferreira et al., 2023)
4. *Dietician and Nutritionist*- Dysphagia directly influences the nutritional level of the patient. These specialists help manage malnutrition and dehydration. Dietitians are trained to assess, interpret and monitor nutritional status (e.g., based on anthropometric, biochemical and dietary data); to develop the nutritional care plan, including texture modification; to monitor and evaluate the effectiveness of the nutrition care plan for the management of dysphagia; to identify the need for nutritional supplements and/or assistive devices; to recognize when nutrition support is indicated; and to develop enteral and parental nutrition support regimes. (Dietitians Of Canada, 2015)
5. *Physiotherapist:* They contribute to improving other neurological deficits along with targeting muscle and motor control of swallowing using evidence-based

swallowing exercises, postural control and other neuromodulation techniques. (Khalil et al., 2025; Saitoh et al., 2018)

6. *Psychologist-* They significantly address the psychological burden using interventions such as cognitive behavioural therapy (CBT), supportive psychotherapy and counselling. (Lei et al., 2025) Recent evidence highlights that post-stroke dysphagia affects the psychological function and is an independent predictor for post-stroke depression and anxiety. (Karisik et al., 2025)

J. IMPACT ON QUALITY OF LIFE

The impact of dysphagia goes beyond just a swallowing dysfunction; it affects all domains of quality of life, influencing social and psychological areas. Usually, it is underrecognized, which affects the overall rehabilitation of a person. Among all phases, particularly the pharyngeal-phase dysphagia has a negative impact on the physical, emotional and social quality of stroke survivors. When compared with oral feeding, tube-dependent patients face an additional burden and experience sleep disturbances, as indicated by lower Swallowing Quality of Life (SWAL-QOL) scores. (Kim et al., 2020)

1. **Social impacts:** Patient suffering from dysphagia knowingly or unknowingly prefers to avoid social gatherings and eating with others, leading to a psychological impact on them. Patients have demonstrated a need for a relative or healthcare professional to facilitate a positive mealtime experience. Lack of choice and control, as well as social engagement, can lead to a negative experience. Often, food modifications or tube feeding result in the patient's isolation. (Farri & Accornero, n.d.; Smith et al., 2024)
2. **Psychological impacts:** Evidence proves a clear association between post-stroke dysphagia and psychological symptoms of depression, and to a lesser extent, anxiety. Apart from isolation and lack of confidence, there is a pathophysiology affecting neuronal connections. (Karisik et al., 2025)

K. PROGNOSIS

1. **Trajectory of stroke recovery:** Six months after a stroke, recovery increases to 95% from 13.53% in the first week. After the damage, the affected cell dies within the first 7 days, followed by the secretion of pro-inflammatory factors within (Smithard et al., 1996) days. Consequently, neural repair and regeneration, known as neuroplasticity, start within hours and peak in the subacute stage

known as the "critical time window", which then continues leading to recovery. With supportive rehabilitation, neuroplasticity further strengthens recovery. (Ballester et al., 2019; Jin et al., 2025)

2. **Stroke severity-** In several studies, it has been documented that elevated NIHSS is correlated with severe dysphagia. Greater neurological deficits resulted in a higher NIH Stroke Scale score (NIHSS), which is associated with poorer recovery of swallowing. (3) NIHSS score 1 (González-Fernández et al., 2013) was a risk factor for poor prognosis of swallowing function after stroke. (Jin et al., 2025)
3. **Lesion location-** In terms of the location of strokes, lesions in the carotid circulation were more common, particularly in left-sided strokes. Involvement of the anterior circulation can lead to lesions affecting the insular cortex, frontal operculum, and basal ganglia that are crucial for the neural control of swallowing.

Additionally, recent research highlights the significance of the intact, unaffected hemisphere in predicting swallowing recovery, especially the contralateral frontal operculum. On the other hand, recovery outcomes for patients with bilateral strokes only reach roughly one-third of those seen in people with unilateral strokes, suggesting that bilateral strokes are a negative factor for swallowing function recovery. (Jin et al., 2025)

4. **Age-** Ageing is linked to sarcopenia, cerebral atrophy, and a decline in neural function, all of which can impair swallowing by interfering with the oral and pharyngeal phases. In the elderly, patients typically exhibit lower, less coordinated swallowing motions, reduced sensory feedback, and diminished strength in the muscles involved in deglutition. Consequently, advanced age (70 years) is often linked to a poorer prognosis for swallowing recovery after stroke. (Jin et al., 2025)
5. **BMI-** In the early phases following a stroke, a low body mass index (BMI) is also thought to be a predictor of poor recovery of total oral intake. Sarcopenia and general physical frailty are frequently seen in people with a BMI below 18.5. It has been demonstrated that sarcopenia, in particular, decreases tongue pressure and pharyngeal muscle strength, which can exacerbate dysphagia. Additionally, patients with low BMI are more likely to experience nutritional deficiencies during the course of the disease, which exacerbates their swallowing function. Malnutrition is closely linked to swallowing difficulties. (Jin et al., 2025)
6. **Comorbidities-** The swallowing function recovery of patients with post-stroke dysphagia who required tracheal intubation was around one-fifth compared to those patients who were not intubated. On the other hand, the recovery rate in patients with aspiration was approximately one-fifth that of those without

aspiration. Therefore, both tracheal intubation and aspiration are negative predictors for swallowing recovery. Tracheal intubation can disrupt the typical structure and function of the respiratory tract, potentially causing mechanical injury to the larynx and vocal cords or leading to local ulcers and granulomas. Constant mechanical stimulation can also irritate the laryngeal mucosa, leading to swelling, pain, and reduced mobility. These changes make it harder for the larynx to function normally, which can slow down the recovery of swallowing after a stroke. The natural synchronization of breathing and swallowing may also be disrupted by tracheal intubation. By interfering with normal vocal cord closure and laryngeal elevation during swallowing, this disruption may compromise airway protection mechanisms. Food passage becomes less efficient as a result, and the risk of aspiration rises. Recurrent aspiration can result in aspiration pneumonia, retarding recovery. (Félix et al., 2025; Jin et al., 2025)

L. CASE STUDY

The role of the multidisciplinary team can be easily understood through a study by Zheng et. al. In this study, (Ertekin & Aydogdu, 2004) acute stroke patients with dysphagia were divided into 2 groups: one group received a conventional rehabilitation program. In contrast, the other group received individualized rehabilitation interventions from a multidisciplinary team, comprising a neurologist, a language therapist, a psychologist, a qualified primary nurse, and two associate nurses.

To aid in treatment planning, the neurologist conducted specialized neurological exams and thorough systemic assessments. To evaluate mental health, offer counselling, and assist in lowering anxiety and depression—factors known to affect adherence to rehabilitation—the psychologist collaborated closely with patients and their families. The language therapist focused on creating customized eating and swallowing training regimens, offering guidance on specific safety measures, and promoting collaboration between patients and their caregivers during their recovery.

The nursing staff played a crucial role in implementing the prescribed oral and non-oral feeding plans, maintaining oral hygiene, and providing support for daily swallowing training. The pharyngeal and laryngeal muscles were the focus of exercises performed twice a day, each lasting about half an hour. The attending physician or nurse selected the most suitable diet type, feeding position, and mealtime schedule for each patient based on their individual swallowing assessment.

The nursing staff played a crucial role in implementing the prescribed oral and non-oral feeding plans, maintaining oral hygiene, and providing support for daily swallowing training. The pharyngeal and laryngeal muscles were the focus of exercises performed twice a day, each lasting about half an hour. The attending physician or nurse selected the most suitable diet type, feeding position, and mealtime schedule for each patient based on their individual swallowing assessment.

In contrast to traditional rehabilitation methods, the study showed that individualized rehabilitation interventions administered by a coordinated multidisciplinary team produced noticeably better therapeutic outcomes in patients with acute post-stroke dysphagia. This study highlights the importance of an integrated, patient-centred team approach in maximizing recovery and improving quality of life. (Zheng et al., 2014)

REFERENCES

Antonios, N., Carnaby-Mann, G., & Crary, M., (2010). Analysis of a physician tool for evaluating dysphagia on an inpatient stroke unit: The modified Mann Assessment of Swallowing Ability. *Journal of Stroke and Cerebrovascular Diseases, 19*(1), 49–57. DOI: 10.1016/j.jstrokecerebrovasdis.2009.03.007

Bach, D. B., Pouget, S., & Belle, K., (1989). An integrated team approach to the management of patients with oropharyngeal dysphagia. *Journal of Allied Health, 18*(5), 459–468.

Banda, K. J., Chu, H., & Kang, X. L., (2022). Prevalence of dysphagia and risk of pneumonia and mortality in acute stroke patients: A meta-analysis. *BMC Geriatrics, 22*(1), 420. DOI: 10.1186/s12877-022-02960-5

Bours, G. J., Speyer, R., Lemmens, J., Limburg, M., & de Wit, R. (2009). Bedside screening tests vs. videofluoroscopy or fibreoptic endoscopic evaluation of swallowing to detect dysphagia in patients with neurological disorders: Systematic review. *Journal of Advanced Nursing, 65*(3), 477–493. DOI: 10.1111/j.1365-2648.2008.04915.x

Broadley, S., Croser, D., & Cottrell, J., (2003). Predictors of prolonged dysphagia following acute stroke. *Journal of Clinical Neuroscience, 10*(3), 300–305. DOI: 10.1016/s0967-5868(03)00022-5

Chang, M. C., Choo, Y. J., & Seo, K. C., (2022). The relationship between dysphagia and pneumonia in acute stroke patients: A systematic review and meta-analysis. *Frontiers in Neurology, 13*, 834240. DOI: 10.3389/fneur.2022.834240

Daniels, S. K., McAdam, C. P., Brailey, K., & Foundas, A. L. (1997). Clinical assessment of swallowing and prediction of dysphagia severity. *American Journal of Speech-Language Pathology, 6*(1), 17–24.

Ekberg, O., Hamdy, S., Woisard, V., Wuttge-Hannig, A., & Ortega, P. (2002). Social and psychological burden of dysphagia: Its impact on diagnosis and treatment. *Dysphagia, 17*(2), 139–146. DOI: 10.1007/s00455-001-0113-5

Ertekin, C., & Aydogdu, I. (2004). Neurology of swallowing. *Clinical Neurophysiology, 114*(11), 2226–2244. DOI: 10.1016/S1388-2457(03)00237-2

Finestone, H. M., Greene-Finestone, L. S., Wilson, E. S., & Teasell, R. W. (1995). Malnutrition in stroke patients on the rehabilitation service and at follow-up: Prevalence and predictors. *Archives of Physical Medicine and Rehabilitation, 76*(4), 310–316. DOI: 10.1016/s0003-9993(95)80655-5

González-Fernández, M., Ottenstein, L., Atanelov, L., & Christian, A. B. (2013). Dysphagia after stroke: An overview. *Current Physical Medicine and Rehabilitation Reports*, *1*(3), 187–196. DOI: 10.1007/s40141-013-0017-y

González-Fernández, M., Ottenstein, L., Atanelov, L., & Christian, A. B. (2013). Dysphagia after stroke: An overview. *Current Physical Medicine and Rehabilitation Reports*, *1*(3), 187–196. DOI: 10.1007/s40141-013-0017-y

Gordon, C., Hewer, R. L., & Wade, D. T. (1987). Dysphagia in acute stroke. *British Medical Journal*, *295*(6595), 411–414. DOI: 10.1136/bmj.295.6595.411

Hinchey, J. A., Shephard, T., & Furie, K., (2005). Formal dysphagia screening protocols prevent pneumonia. *Stroke*, *36*(9), 1972–1976. DOI: 10.1161/01.STR.0000177529.86868.8d

Karisik, A., Moelgg, K., & Buergi, L., (2025). Impact of dysphagia on early psychosocial consequences after acute ischemic stroke. *Journal of the Neurological Sciences*, *476*, 123624. DOI: 10.1016/j.jns.2025.123624

Khedr, E. M., Abbass, M. A., & Soliman, R. K., (2021). Post-stroke dysphagia: Frequency, risk factors, and topographic representation: Hospital-based study. *The Egyptian Journal of Neurology, Psychiatry and Neurosurgery*, *57*, 23. DOI: 10.1186/s41983-021-00281-9

Krekeler, B. N., Schieve, H. J. P., & Khoury, J., (2024). Health factors associated with development and severity of poststroke dysphagia: An epidemiological investigation. *Journal of the American Heart Association*, *13*(7), e033922. DOI: 10.1161/jaha.123.033922

Martino, R., Foley, N., & Bhogal, S., (2005). Dysphagia after stroke: Incidence, diagnosis, and pulmonary complications. *Stroke*, *36*(12), 2756–2763. DOI: 10.1161/01.STR.0000190056.76543.eb

Meng, P. P., Zhang, S. C., & Han, C., (2020). The occurrence rate of swallowing disorders after stroke patients in Asia: A PRISMA-compliant systematic review and meta-analysis. *Journal of Stroke and Cerebrovascular Diseases*, *29*(10), 105113. DOI: 10.1016/j.jstrokecerebrovasdis.2020.105113

Sasegbon, A., Cheng, I., & Hamdy, S. (2025). The neurorehabilitation of post-stroke dysphagia: Physiology and pathophysiology. *The Journal of Physiology*, *603*(2), 617–634. DOI: 10.1113/JP285564

Smithard, D. G., O'Neill, P. A., Parks, C., & Morris, J. (1996). Complications and outcome after acute stroke. Does dysphagia matter? *Stroke*, *27*(7), 1200–1204. DOI: 10.1161/01.str.27.7.1200

Smithard, D. G., Smeeton, N. C., & Wolfe, C. D. A. (2007). Long-term outcome after stroke: Does dysphagia matter? *Age and Ageing*, *36*(1), 90–94. DOI: 10.1093/ageing/afl149

Trapl, M., Enderle, P., & Nowotny, M., (2007). Dysphagia bedside screening for acute-stroke patients: The Gugging Swallowing Screen. *Stroke*, *38*(11), 2948–2952. DOI: 10.1161/strokeaha.107.483933

Wang, Z., Shi, R., & Moreira, P. (2025). Post-stroke dysphagia: Identifying the evidence missing. *Frontiers in Medicine*, *12*, 1494645. DOI: 10.3389/fmed.2025.1494645

Wen, X., Fan, B., & Zhan, J., (2025). Integrated analysis of the prevalence and influencing factors of poststroke dysphagia. *European Journal of Medical Research*, *30*(1), 27. DOI: 10.1186/s40001-024-02263-y

Chapter 8
A Comprehensive Overview of Dysphagia in Parkinson's Disease: Clinical Findings, Assessment, and Treatment Approaches

Merve Sapmaz Atalar
http://orcid.org/0000-0003-2556-1026
Hamidiye Faculty of Health Sciences, University of Health Sciences, Turkey

Özlem Oğuz
http://orcid.org/0000-0001-7590-0028
Faculty of Health Sciences, Üsküdar University, Turkey

ABSTRACT

Parkinson's disease (PD) is the second most common neurodegenerative disorder. Dysphagia, one of the symptoms, is one of the most important complications that seriously reduces the quality of life of individuals with PD (IwPD) and can lead to morbidity and mortality such as malnutrition, dehydration, and aspiration pneumonia. The neural mechanism of dysphagia is related to dopamine deficiency, as well as alpha-synuclein accumulation and decreased substance P concentration. This condition manifests itself as impaired swallowing function in the all phases. Assessment includes case history, medical history, self-assessment tools, physical examination. Fiberoptic endoscopic evaluation of swallowing and videofluoroscopic swallowing study are critical instrumental methods. Treatment options include swallowing therapy, treatment optimization, medical treatments and neuromodulation

DOI: 10.4018/979-8-3373-6405-6.ch008

applications. Finally, there is a need for advanced research evaluating long-term treatment efficacy using evidence-based, standardized, and cost-effective clinical assessment tools for dysphagia specific to PD.

INTRODUCTION

This section of the book offers a comprehensive overview of Parkinson's disease (PD). As a slowly progressive neurodegenerative condition, PD is among the most frequently diagnosed disorders worldwide and is often accompanied by motor, cognitive, communication, and swallowing impairments. These multifaceted difficulties emphasize the need for multidisciplinary intervention. Dysphagia is particularly common in individuals with PD (IwPD) and can result in malnutrition, reduced fluid intake and aspiration pneumonia, the leading cause of mortality in this population. Accordingly, this section provides detailed guidance on the diagnosis, assessment and treatment of dysphagia in PD. The proposed assessment protocol and described therapeutic approaches aim to support speech and language therapists, who play a central role in multidisciplinary care. Accordingly, the following sections will explore this critical issue in depth under the headings *"Definition, Neural Mechanism, Etiology, Prevalence and Clinical Features of Parkinson's Disease ", "Prevalence, Pathophysiology and Clinical Findings of Dysphagia in Parkinson's Disease," "Assessment of Dysphagia in Parkinson's Disease"* and *"Treatment of Dysphagia in Parkinson's Disease."*

DEFINITION, NEURAL MECHANISM, ETIOLOGY, PREVALENCE AND CLINICAL FEATURES OF PARKINSON'S DISEASE

Parkinson's disease (PD) is a slowly progressive neurodegenerative disorder characterized by the progressive loss of dopaminergic neurons in the substantia nigra (Freed, 2020; Kalia & Lang, 2015). Multiple neuroanatomical areas are affected in PD (Kalia & Lang, 2015). The neural mechanisms of PD include the loss of dopamine-secreting neurons in the substantia nigra pars compacta, Lewy body pathology and alpha-synuclein aggregation (Jellinger, 2019; Morris et al., 2024; Simon et al., 2020).

Although the exact cause of PD is unknown, it has been suggested that it stems from a combination of environmental and genetic factors (Kalia & Lang, 2015). A range of environmental factors has been associated with elevated PD risk including prolonged exposure to toxic chemicals, previous head trauma, rural residence, agricultural work, β-blocker use and consumption of well water (Goldman, 2014;

Noyce et al., 2012). These findings point to the role of both lifestyle and ecological conditions in modulating susceptibility to the disease. Genetic influences have also been implicated in PD etiology. For instance, individuals with a positive family history of PD or tremors show increased likelihood of developing the disorder, emphasizing the contribution of hereditary components (Noyce et al., 2012). The first gene identified in association with PD was SNCA which encodes the α-synuclein protein and plays a central role in the formation of Lewy bodies, a hallmark of the disease (Kalia & Lang, 2015; Polymeropoulos et al., 1997). Additional genes such as LRRK2 and parkin represent some of the most common autosomal dominant and recessive inherited causes of PD while mutations in GBA have emerged as the most prevalent genetic risk factor overall (Corti et al., 2011; Sidransky & Lopez, 2012). Beyond environmental and genetic determinants, demographic factors also may shape disease vulnerability. Age has consistently been identified as the strongest predictor of PD development with prevalence markedly increasing in older populations (Kalia & Lang, 2015; Pringsheim et al., 2014). Moreover, gender and ethnicity have also been identified as risk factors for PD, with a higher incidence in males than in females (de Lau & Breteler, 2006; Van Den Eeden et al., 2003). Collectively, these findings highlight the multifactorial nature of PD and the importance of considering both biological and contextual risk factors in understanding its onset and progression.

Parkinson's disease is recognized as the most common movement disorder and the second most prevalent neurodegenerative condition after Alzheimer's disease (Sun et al., 2024). Recent epidemiological evidence underscores its growing public health impact. According to Global Burden of Disease (GBD) data, the age-standardized prevalence of PD has increased globally from 1990 to 2021. Furthermore, the study results reported that the prevalence of PD was 138.63 per 100,000 people (Li et al., 2025). A systematic review and meta-analysis study indicated that PD prevalence has been on the rise between 1980 and 2023. The study also reported that the global PD prevalence is 1.51 per 1,000 (Zhu et al., 2024).

Clinically, PD is characterized by a constellation of both motor and non-motor symptoms, reflecting its heterogeneous and progressive nature (Bloem et al., 2021). Core motor symptoms typically include resting tremors, rigidity, bradykinesia and postural instability; features that remain central to diagnosis and disease monitoring (Kalia & Lang, 2015). In addition to these symptoms such as dysarthria, dysphagia, gait disturbance, and micrographia further contribute to functional impairment and daily activity limitations (Kalia & Lang, 2015; Moustafa et al., 2016). The non-motor symptoms of PD are also important. Non-motor symptoms include cognitive impairment, smell disorders, psychiatric symptoms, fatigue, autonomic dysfunction, sleep disorders, and pain (Kalia & Lang, 2015). Motor and non-motor symptoms negatively affect the quality of life of IwPD (Lacy et al., 2022; Liu et al., 2015). As such, a comprehensive understanding of the broad clinical spectrum of PD is essential for effective management, timely intervention, and improved long-term outcomes.

Dysphagia constitutes a major component of the adverse effects experienced by IwPD and is recognized as a symptom with serious clinical consequences, including increased morbidity and mortality (Simons, 2017). Given its profound impact on health outcomes, nutritional status and overall quality of life, dysphagia warrants dedicated and detailed examination within the broader symptomatology of PD. Accordingly, the following sections will explore this critical symptom. These sections aim to provide a comprehensive overview of the mechanisms, identification and management of dysphagia in IwPD, thereby emphasizing its central role in clinical care and therapeutic planning.

DYSPHAGIA IN PARKINSON'S DISEASE, DYSPHAGIA PREVALENCE, PATHOPHYSIOLOGY AND CLINICAL FINDINGS

Dysphagia is a commonly observed symptom in IwPD, frequently highlighted in research and increasingly emphasized in clinical practice. As early as the original description of the disease, James Parkinson identified dysphagia as a characteristic feature in this population (Parkinson, 2002). This symptom exerts a substantial psychosocial and physiological burden on affected individuals, contributing to malnutrition, reduced fluid intake and aspiration pneumonia which is one of the most common causes of mortality in IwPD (Akbar et al., 2015; Morgante et al., 2000; Paul et al., 2019; Plowman-Prine et al., 2009; Suttrup & Warnecke, 2016). In addition to these complications, dysphagia has been associated with longer hospital stays, repeated hospitalizations, increased medication consumption, higher healthcare costs, and mortality (Di Luca et al., 2021; Makaroff et al., 2011; Simons, 2017). Furthermore, its impact extends to psychosocial well-being, negatively affecting the quality of life of both IwPD and their caregivers (Perry et al., 2022; Plowman-Prine et al., 2009). Given these substantial consequences, early identification of dysphagia and comprehensive assessment procedures are considered essential components of effective intervention in PD.

The reported prevalence of dysphagia in IwPD varies widely across studies largely due to differences in assessment approaches and diagnostic criteria. A systematic review found prevalence rates ranging from 11% to 81% (Takizawa et al., 2016), reflecting the heterogeneity observed in the literature. More recently, a meta-analysis that included studies using both subjective and objective evaluation methods estimated a dysphagia prevalence of 50.4% in IwPD (Aghaz et al., 2024). Another meta-analysis further demonstrated the importance of assessment modality: the prevalence reached 82% when objective swallowing evaluations were used compared with 35% based on subjective reports (Kalf et al., 2012). These consistently high rates demonstrate the strong association between PD and dysphagia and highlight the need for accurate screening and diagnostic tools.

High prevalence rates indicate a strong association between PD and dysphagia. However, the underlying mechanisms of dysphagia, which is frequently observed in IwPD, are not fully understood. The pathophysiology of dysphagia seen in PD is thought to be caused by a decrease in dopamine in the substantia nigra affecting the supramedullary swallowing system (Leopold & Daniels, 2010; Suttrup & Warnecke, 2016). Impaired basal ganglia-thalamic-supplementary cortical circuits may affect voluntary swallowing in PD, leading to orally related dysphagia (Leopold & Daniels, 2010). The pathology of Lewy bodies in non-dopaminergic brain regions and the accumulation of alpha-synuclein in peripheral nerves innervating the pharyngeal muscles may also be associated with dysphagia in PD (Kwon & Lee, 2019). It has been suggested that another pathophysiological factor associated with dysphagia in this disease may be a decrease in the concentration of substance P in saliva (Suttrup & Warnecke, 2016). As a result, impairment of protective reflexes such as coughing and swallowing and subsequent silent aspiration may occur (Ebihara et al., 2003; Suttrup & Warnecke, 2016; Troche et al., 2014a).

Individuals with PD experience impaired swallowing function from the early stages (Sung et al., 2010; Umay et al., 2019). This impairment manifests in all phases of swallowing: oral, pharyngeal, and esophageal (Potulska et al., 2003). Associated with tremor, bradykinesia, and rigidity, problems with bolus formation and propulsion in the oral phase of swallowing, chewing difficulties, impaired tongue movement and pressure formation, and prolonged oral transit time occur. Consequently, these problems lead to fragmented swallowing, residue, and premature spillage (Fukuoka et al., 2019; Kwon & Lee, 2019; Nagaya et al., 1998; Patel et al., 2020; Simons, 2017). In the pharyngeal phase, delayed initiation of pharyngeal swallowing, prolonged pharyngeal transit time, problems with upper esophageal sphincter (UES) opening and duration, decreased hyo-laryngeal elevation, delayed laryngeal closure, decreased pharyngeal contraction and tongue base retraction, and sensory problems. This leads to residue in the vallecula and pyriform sinuses and airway safety issues (e.g., penetration, aspiration) (Curtis et al., 2020a; Ellerston et al., 2016; Ertekin et al., 2002; Kwon & Lee, 2019; Nagaya et al., 1998; Patel et al., 2020; Simons, 2017). In the esophageal phase, there is prolongation of the phase duration, esophageal spasm, abnormal contractions, and lower esophageal abnormalities (Castell et al., 2001; Potulska et al., 2003). The clinical findings of IwPD are summarized in Table 1.

Table 1. Clinical Findings Related to Dysphagia in Individuals with Parkinson's Disease

Swallowing Phase	Clinical Findings
Oral Phase	• Repetitive pumping motion of the tongue • Difficulty pushing food toward the back of the mouth with the tongue • Piecemeal deglutition • Drooling • Residue • Premature spillage
Pharyngeal Phase	• Delayed swallowing reflex • Prolonged pharyngeal transit time • Decreased hyolaryngeal elevation • Delayed laryngeal closure • Decreased tongue base retraction • Decreased pharyngeal contraction • Impaired with UES opening • Residue in the vallecula and/or pyriform sinus • Penetration aspiration • Silent aspiration • Decreased laryngeal and pharyngeal sensitivity • Decreased swallowing frequency
Esophageal Phase	• Impaired esophageal peristalsis • Prolongation of the phase • Lower esophageal sphincter problem • Spasm

Clinical findings play an essential role in diagnosing dysphagia and several clinical parameters may further assist in estimating dysphagia risk in this population. Clinical predictors of PD-related dysphagia include a Hoehn & Yahr score greater than 3, weight loss or a body mass index below 20 kg/m^2, drooling, dementia, dysarthria, disease duration exceeding 10 years and the presence of depression (Cereda et al., 2014; Coelho et al., 2010; Han et al., 2011; Lam et al., 2007; Perez-Lloret et al., 2012; Simons, 2017). These predictors show the multifactorial nature of swallowing impairment and the importance of considering both motor and non-motor features when evaluating dysphagia risk in IwPD.

Understanding the prevalence of dysphagia in IwPD, its underlying mechanisms, potential complications, associated clinical findings and predictive factors is crucial. Such comprehensive knowledge is thought to guide healthcare professionals in the early stages of assessment and treatment planning, enabling timely intervention and more effective management strategies.

ASSESSMENT OF DYSPHAGIA IN PARKINSON'S DISEASE

Individuals with PD may experience impaired self-perception of dysphagia symptoms; a challenge that can significantly hinder timely diagnosis and treatment (Pflug et al., 2018). When individuals are not fully aware of or cannot accurately interpret their swallowing difficulties, symptoms may go unreported, resulting in dysphagia being overlooked during routine neurological examinations. This under-recognition increases the likelihood that comprehensive assessment and appropriate intervention will be delayed. Given these risks, it becomes clear that dysphagia must be systematically assessed from the early stages of PD, using appropriate, sensitive and validated tools tailored to the needs of this population (Simons, 2017).

The assessment and management of dysphagia in PD require a multidisciplinary and coordinated clinical approach, as the disorder affects multiple physiological systems and may interact with both motor and non-motor symptoms. This multidisciplinary team typically includes a speech and language therapist, neurologist, otorhinolaryngologist, radiologist, gastroenterologist, physiatrist, nurse, dietitian, physical therapist and occupational therapist. Each of them contributes essential expertise to the evaluation and treatment process (Atalar & Genç, 2022; Umemoto & Furuya, 2020). In clinical practice, neurologists play a key role in identifying early signs of dysphagia during routine examinations and should promptly refer suspected cases to a SLT for detailed analysis. Broader PD assessment tools such as the *Non-Motor Symptoms Questionnaire (NMSQuest)* and the *Movement Disorder Society Unified Parkinson's Disease Rating Scale (MDS-UPDRS)* also include swallowing-related items that allow clinicians to capture dysphagia indicators within general PD evaluations (Chaudhuri et al., 2006; Goetz et al., 2008). To ensure ongoing monitoring, it is recommended that dysphagia-related symptoms be screened during the initial neurological evaluation with reassessments performed at least annually, especially as the disease progresses (Cosentino et al., 2022).

A wide range of clinical and instrumental assessment methods are available for evaluating dysphagia in IwPD. A comprehensive clinical swallowing assessment should include a detailed case history (e.g., demographic information, medical history) followed by a structured physical examination targeting swallowing-related functions such as oral-motor performance, voluntary cough strength, laryngeal elevation and swallowing trials using different consistencies. In addition, the assessment tools used in clinical evaluation also provide important information for clinicians (Groher & Crary, 2016).

Despite the clinical and academic importance of self-assessment tools used in clinical swallowing assessments, the number of valid and reliable self-assessment tools specifically developed for IwPD remains limited (Simons, 2017). Self-assessment tools specifically developed to assess dysphagia in IwPD include the

Swallowing Disorder Questionnaire (SDQ), the Radboud Oral Motor Inventory for Parkinson's Disease (ROMP), the Munich Dysphagia Test–Parkinson's Disease (MDT-PD) and the Sialorrhea Clinical Scale for PD (SCS-PD) (Kalf et al., 2011a; Manor et al., 2007; Perez Lloret et al., 2007; Simons et al., 2014). Each tool offers a unique contribution to screening and clinical decision-making. For instance, the SDQ supports early detection of dysphagia symptoms and is recommended for use in everyday clinical settings (Manor et al., 2007). The ROMP provides a broader functional perspective by assessing dysarthria, drooling and dysphagia across functional, activity and participation domains in both IwPD and individuals with atypical parkinsonism (Kalf et al., 2011a). MDT-PD has been shown to be effective not only for early identification of dysphagia and aspiration risk but also for the grading of dysphagia severity, making it a valuable screening tool (Simons et al., 2014). The SCS-PD, on the other hand, focuses on the multidimensional impact of drooling (sialorrhea), documenting its effects on daily activity and social functioning (Perez Lloret et al., 2007).

In addition to these PD-specific instruments, several widely used dysphagia tools can also be applied to IwPD. The Eating Assessment Tool (EAT-10) is a commonly used self-report measure covering both swallowing function and swallowing-related quality of life, it is applicable across diverse patient groups (Belafsky et al., 2008; Printza & Triaridis, 2022). Notably, the EAT-10 has demonstrated sensitivity in detecting the risk of penetration and aspiration in individuals with early- and mid-stage PD supporting its use as an effective preliminary screening tool (Ponsoni et al., 2024). Meanwhile, the Swallowing Quality of Life (SWAL-QOL) scale, although not developed specifically for PD, is frequently employed in PD research to assess disease-related changes in swallowing-related quality of life (Bengisu et al., 2024; Carneiro et al., 2014; McHorney et al., 2000; Plowman-Prine et al., 2009; Zimmerman et al., 2022).

Among bedside screening tools, the 50 ml water swallow test is commonly used but demonstrates limitations in detecting severe dysphagia in IwPD (Lam et al., 2007). In contrast, electrophysiological evaluations provide more detailed insight: a study involving electromyography (EMG) during water swallowing trials revealed that the swallowing volume of IwPD was often less than 20 ml, highlighting the challenges these individuals face even with small liquid volumes (Potulska et al., 2003). To improve clinical screening accuracy, Dutch speech and language therapy guidelines recommend including both observation of spontaneous drinking behaviors and structured water swallow tests that estimate maximum swallowing volume or swallowing speed (Kalf et al., 2011b).

To further support clinical evaluation in IwPD, the Swallowing Clinical Assessment Score in Parkinson's Disease (SCAS-PD) was developed as a standardized tool for detecting oral and pharyngeal swallowing impairments through controlled swallowing tasks (Branco et al., 2019; Loureiro et al., 2013). Additionally, the Functional Oral Intake Scale (FOIS) provides information on functional oral intake patterns and is widely applied in PD literature and international consensus studies (Bengisu et al., 2024; Cosentino et al., 2022; Crary et al., 2005; Luchesi et al., 2015). Because clinical evaluation alone may fail to detect critical findings such as residue, penetration or aspiration, studies emphasize the necessity of instrumental assessment following clinical examination (Simons, 2017).

Fiberoptic endoscopic evaluation of swallowing (FEES) and videofluoroscopic swallowing study (VFSS) are commonly used instrumental methods in dysphagia assessment. FEES and VFSS enable visualization of structures related to swallowing, measurement of changes in swallowing physiology, and detection of dysphagia, and are also used in IwPD (Rudisch et al., 2023). Swallowing efficiency (residue), particularly the presence and severity of residue, can be assessed using metrics such as the Bolus Clearance Ratio (BCR), Visual Analysis of Swallowing Efficiency and Safety (VASES) and the Yale Pharyngeal Residue Severity Rating Scale (YPRSRS). Swallowing safety, including penetration and aspiration, is typically rated using the Penetration-Aspiration Scale (PAS) and VASES (Curtis et al., 2022; Leonard, 2017; Neubauer et al., 2015; Rosenbek et al., 1996). The Dynamic Imaging Grade of Swallowing Toxicity (DIGEST) provides an integrated evaluation of overall pharyngeal swallowing function by combining safety and efficiency ratings (Hutcheson et al., 2017). In studies involving IwPD undergoing FEES or VFSS, BCR, PAS, VASES, YPRSRS and DIGEST-FEES have been routinely employed to evaluate swallowing safety and efficiency (Curtis et al., 2020b, 2022; Doruk et al., 2023; Labeit et al., 2024; Macedo et al., 2025).

Finally, outside FEES and VFSS, several additional methods have been used to evaluate swallowing physiology in IwPD. These include manometry for assessing pharyngoesophageal function, surface electromyography (sEMG) to measure swallowing muscle activity, the Iowa Oral Performance Instrument (IOPI) to quantify tongue pressure and ultrasonography to evaluate muscle thickness (Pitts et al., 2019; Sung et al., 2010; Ws Coriolano et al., 2012). Together, these approaches provide a multifaceted understanding of dysphagia in PD. The dysphagia assessment procedure in PD is summarized in Table 2.

Table 2. Dysphagia Assessment Procedure for Individuals with Parkinson's Disease

Neurological Examination **- Non-Motor Symptoms Questionnaire (NMSQuest)** **- The Movement Disorder Society Unified Parkinson's Disease Rating Scale (MDS-UPDRS)** **- Hoehn&Yahr Score**
Clinical Swallowing Assessment - Case History • Demographic information - Medical History • Diagnosis, comorbidities • Duration of illness • Medications used • Medication times • Surgeries history • Dysphagia history - Self-Assessment Tools • Swallowing Disturbance Questionnaire (SDQ) • Radboud Oral Motor Inventory for Parkinson's Disease (ROMP) • Sialorrhea Clinical Scale for PD (SCS-PD) • Munich Dysphagia Test-Parkinson's Disease (MDT-PD) • Eating Assessment Tool (EAT-10) • Swallowing Quality of Life (SWAL-QOL) -Physical Assessment • Clinical observation • Oral-motor assessment • Observation of voluntary coughing • Observation of laryngeal elevation • Swallowing trials using different consistencies
Instrumental Swallowing Assessment - Instrumental Tools • Videofluoroscopic Swallow Studies (VFSS) • Flexible Endoscopic Evaluations of Swallowing (FEES) • Surface Electromyography (sEMG) • Iowa Oral Performance Instrument (IOPI) • Manometry - Scales • Bolus Clearance Ratio (BCR) • Visual Analysis of Swallowing Efficiency and Safety (VASES) • Yale Pharyngeal Residue Severity Rating Scale (YPRSRS) • Penetration–Aspiration Scale (PAS) • Dynamic Imaging Grade of Swallowing Toxicity for Flexible Endoscopic Evaluation of Swallowing (DIGEST-FEES)

The above paragraphs provide an overview of the assessment process for dysphagia in PD. Building upon this foundation, it is important to emphasize that contemporary clinical practice increasingly recommends evaluating dysphagia within the broader conceptual framework of the International Classification of Functioning, Disability and Health (ICF). This framework offers a holistic and integrative perspective on health conditions and has been highlighted as a guiding model for dysphagia assessment (ASHA, 2004; Threats, 2007). In this context, the individual's body structures/functions, activities/participation, environmental and personal factors are considered (WHO, 2013). Within this approach, clinicians are encouraged not only to document physiological swallowing impairments but also to consider the full spectrum of factors influencing an individual's functioning and overall well-being. In accordance with the ICF model, assessment should encompass the individual's body structures and body functions, which in the context of dysphagia include the integrity and efficiency of oral, pharyngeal and esophageal mechanisms, neuromuscular control, sensory and motor functions and the presence of any disease-related structural changes. At the same time, attention must be directed to the person's activities and participation, acknowledging that dysphagia may hinder a range of activities such as safe eating and drinking, social dining or attending community events. Additionally, the ICF framework emphasizes the role of environmental factors which may either facilitate or hinder functional outcomes. For IwPD, environmental considerations may include the availability of caregiver support, access to dysphagia services, dietary modifications, mealtime adaptations and broader healthcare resources. Likewise, personal factors such as motivation and coping strategies should also be examined, as they affect both the presentation of dysphagia and the individual's capacity to engage in treatment (Threats, 2007).

Conducting dysphagia assessment within the ICF framework not only assists in the identification and grading of swallowing impairment but also enables clinicians to understand how dysphagia influences multiple dimensions of the lives of IwPD. This includes its impact on health-related quality of life, daily functioning and social participation as well as the emotional consequences of living with dysphagia. Furthermore, such an integrative assessment approach plays a critical role in guiding personalized treatment planning.

Overall, applying the ICF framework ensures that dysphagia assessment in PD moves beyond isolated physiological observations toward a comprehensive, person-centered and functionally oriented understanding. This perspective supports informed clinical decision-making and enhances the potential for meaningful improvements in swallowing function, independence and overall quality of life.

TREATMENT OF DYSPHAGIA IN PARKINSON'S DISEASE

All phases of swallowing are affected in PD although the specific physiological abnormalities observed in each phase may vary substantially across individuals. This variability highlights the heterogeneous nature of dysphagia in PD and shows the need for individualized assessment and treatment planning. The onset of dysphagia often has profound consequences for health and well-being, as it may lead to dehydration, malnutrition and aspiration pneumonia. These complications do not only endanger physiological stability but also significantly diminish quality of life

(Di Luca et al., 2021; Plowman-Prine et al., 2009). Given these risks, it becomes essential that intervention planning be grounded in a thorough and accurate evaluation of swallowing function.

Intervention decisions should be informed by holistic consideration of both clinical and instrumental assessment results. These complementary data sources help clinicians form a complete understanding of the physiological, functional and psychosocial facets of dysphagia. Importantly, once dysphagia is identified, the intervention process should begin promptly to reduce the risk of complications (Schindler et al., 2021). Instrumental assessment results, for example, may help delineate which phase(s) of swallowing are physiologically impaired, allowing clinicians to target specific biomechanical deficits. Meanwhile, clinical assessment findings often shed light on the broader psychosocial effects of dysphagia including changes in emotional well-being, social participation and daily routines. Collectively, these insights support the development of a personalized treatment plan which is widely recognized as the most effective approach for IwPD.

A variety of approaches are currently used for dysphagia intervention in PD and these approaches are increasingly supported by expert consensus. In a major consensus study on dysphagia treatment in PD, a range of evidence-informed management options were identified including *swallowing therapy, optimization of PD treatments, medical interventions* and *neuromodulation techniques* (Schindler et al., 2021). Together, these modalities reflect the multifaceted nature of dysphagia and the necessity of combining strategies to address both functional swallowing impairments and disease-related influences on eating and drinking.

In PD, *swallowing therapy* is performed by SLTs and plays an important role in the intervention process, as it does in other processes. In PD, the aims of swallowing therapy may include improving swallowing physiology, ensuring airway protection and supporting safe and sufficient nutrition, hydration and oral hygiene. Swallowing therapy generally involves both compensatory and rehabilitative methods. *Compensatory approaches* such as postural adjustments (e.g., chin tuck) and dietary modifications (e.g., nectar- or honey-thickened liquids) often provide short-term functional benefits although research has suggested that their long-term effects require further investigation (Logemann et al., 2008). Importantly, the chin tuck position has also been associated with reduced risk of choking (Kalf et al., 2011b). Additionally, an intervention program incorporating modifications to the feeding environment, postural adjustments, adjusted mealtime duration and proper oral hygiene has been shown to improve swallowing-related quality of life in IwPD (Ayres et al., 2016). Based on instrumental examination findings, the risk of pulmonary complications and dehydration as well as the preferences of patients and caregivers, compensatory strategies should be recommended in a targeted manner (Logemann et al., 2008; Schindler et al., 2021). *Rehabilitative approaches* aim to modify the underlying physiology of swallowing. These include exercises targeting the orofacial, laryngeal, pharyngeal, and respiratory muscles, swallowing maneuvers, and biofeedback-based therapies (Gandhi et al., 2022). For IwPD, effortful swallowing has often been recommended to improve pharyngeal clearance and reduce residue (Kalf et al., 2011b). The long-term effects of a therapy program combining compensatory and rehabilitative approaches have documented meaningful improvements in IwPD even over extended follow-up periods (Luchesi et al., 2015). Another study combining compensatory and rehabilitation approaches have also reported improvements in swallowing in IwPD (Argolo et al., 2013). Another rehabilitative approach that has received attention is the Lee Silverman Voice Treatment (LSVT) traditionally used for voice therapy. Research has reported positive effects of LSVT on swallowing function (El Sharkawi et al., 2002; Miles et al., 2017). However, because LSVT does not directly target swallowing physiology, consensus recommendations advise that it not be regarded as a primary dysphagia intervention (Schindler et al., 2021). Additionally, the effectiveness of expiratory muscle strength training (EMST) on swallowing function in IwPD has been studied and EMST may contribute to improving dysphagia outcomes in PD (Pitts et al., 2009; Troche et al., 2010, 2014b). Other rehabilitative approaches reported in the literature include Video-Assisted Swallowing Therapy (VAST), surface EMG biofeedback and IOPI biofeedback. While these methods have yielded positive preliminary results, further research is required to determine their long-term effectiveness in IwPD (Athukorala et al., 2014; Gandhi et al., 2023; Manor et al., 2013; Suttrup & Warnecke, 2016).

Another essential component of dysphagia management involves *optimizing PD-related treatments.* The effect of pharmacological treatments in dysphagia intervention is controversial. The consensus highlights several strategies in its recommendations for optimizing PD-related treatments in dysphagia treatment: (1) testing individuals in both "ON" and "OFF" states to evaluate how dopaminergic treatment affects swallowing; (2) optimizing dopaminergic treatments for individuals experiencing dysphagia; (3) encouraging individuals to eat during their best ON periods and (4) carefully monitoring swallowing function in individuals who have undergone Deep Brain Stimulation (DBS) including periodic reassessment and timely intervention should be performed when necessary (Schindler et al., 2021). In clinical practice, IwPD are commonly advised to take antiparkinsonian medications approximately 30 minutes before meals (Cereda et al., 2010). When dysphagia interferes with pill intake, modification strategies include taking tablets with a large amount of water or, if this is not feasible, mixing them into a spoonful of apple puree (Kalf et al., 2011b).

More targeted *medical interventions* have been used to treat swallowing impairments in addition to behavioral and medical optimization strategies. Among these, botulinum toxin (BT) injections have been applied to improve relaxation of the UES during swallowing, while injection laryngoplasty has been used to enhance glottic closure by medializing the vocal folds (Alfonsi et al., 2017; Howell et al., 2019). Consensus guidelines indicate that BT injection may be considered when UES dysfunction is identified as the primary physiological issue; however, current evidence remains insufficient to support injection laryngoplasty as a treatment for dysphagia in PD (Schindler et al., 2021).

Emerging treatment options include *neuromodulation techniques* such as transcranial direct current stimulation (tDCS) and repetitive transcranial magnetic stimulation (rTMS). Early studies have reported beneficial effects of these methods on swallowing function (Dashtelei et al., 2024; Khedr et al., 2019). Despite these promising findings, small sample sizes or methodological limitations indicate that further research is needed. The effects of DBS on swallowing function are controversial, and more studies investigating combinations of DBS and swallowing therapy are needed (Büyükönder & Parlak, 2025; Gandhi et al., 2022). It has been concluded that there is insufficient evidence to support the use of neuromodulation techniques in consensus (Schindler et al., 2021).

Finally, nutritional management is a critical component of dysphagia treatment in PD. Consensus recommendations state that *percutaneous endoscopic gastrostomy (PEG)* should be considered in cases where involuntary weight loss occurs (≥10% in three months) and/or when serious aspiration risk is accompanied by inadequate oral intake for more than four weeks. Additional guidance indicates that oral hygiene interventions should continue after PEG if oral intake remains safe based on clinical and instrumental findings. Nasogastric tube feeding may be used when dysphagia is considered reversible, while PEG placement is generally not recommended for IwPD who also have dementia (Schindler et al., 2021). Treatment methods for dysphagia in PD are listed in Table 3.

Table 3. Therapeutic Approaches for Dysphagia in Individuals with Parkinson's Disease

Swallowing Therapy (Compensatory and Rehabilitative Methods)
The method to be selected should be determined based on clinical and instrumental evaluation results. - Postural Adjustment • Head-neck postural adjustment • Body posture adjustment - Adjustment of Nutritional Conditions • Adjustment of food/drink size and speed • Taking pills with apple sauce when needed • Informing about the swallowing process with visual materials • Eliminating distractions - Diet Modifications - Thermal Tactile Stimulation - Oral Motor Exercises - Swallowing Maneuvers - Exercises for Respiratory, Laryngeal, Pharyngeal Muscles - Biofeedback-based therapies • Iowa Oral Performance Instrument (IOPI) • Surface Electromyography (sEMG) • Video-Assisted Swallowing Therapy (VAST) - Expiratory muscle strength training (EMST) - Lee Silverman Voice Treatment (LSVT)

CONCLUSION

This section of the book offers a thorough analysis of dysphagia and associated problems in PD, emphasizing its high prevalence, early onset, and significant effects on function, health, and quality of life. Significant morbidity and death are linked to dysphagia in IwPD, underscoring the importance of prompt diagnosis and tailored treatment. Clinicians can assess swallowing physiology in addition to functional, psychosocial, and environmental factors through comprehensive assessment that integrates clinical and instrumental methods and is guided by the ICF framework. This supports accurate diagnosis and focused intervention.

The significance of interdisciplinary cooperation is further highlighted by a wide range of therapeutic choices, such as swallowing therapy, medicinal interventions, neuromodulation approaches, and optimization of PD-specific treatments.

There are still a number of significant research gaps in the area of dysphagia linked to PD. Further investigation is required to clarify the pathophysiological mechanisms underlying dysphagia in IwPD to develop standardized, practical and cost-effective clinical assessment tools tailored to this population, and to conduct studies examining the evidence-based and long-term efficacy of different treatment approaches. It is anticipated that advancing these study areas would improve clinical treatment, aid in the creation of evidence-based guidelines, and eventually give IwPD and their caregivers more hope and better results (Atalar & Genç, 2022).

KEY POINTS

- Dysphagia is highly prevalent in IwPD and may appear from the early stages of the disease. Malnutrition, dehydration, aspiration pneumonia, extended and recurrent hospital stays, and higher healthcare expenses are all linked to it, which has an impact on the quality of life for both IwPD and their caregivers.
- The pathophysiology of dysphagia in PD involves dopaminergic deficiency and disruption of supramedullary swallowing control, basal ganglia-cortical circuits dysfunction, Lewy body pathology, alpha-synuclein accumulation and decreased substance P.
- Dysphagia in PD can affect all phases of swallowing. Oral phase impairments (e.g., repetitive pumping motion of the tongue, prolonged oral transit, piecemeal deglutition) contribute to residue and premature spillage. Pharyngeal phase deficits (e.g., delayed swallow initiation, reduced hyolaryngeal elevation, impaired UES opening, reduced pharyngeal contraction and tongue base retraction, sensory impairment) lead to vallecular and pyriform sinus residue, penetration and aspiration. Esophageal phase abnormalities include impaired peristalsis, spasms and lower esophageal sphincter dysfunction. Clinical predictors of PD-related dysphagia include higher Hoehn & Yahr stages, weight loss, drooling, dementia, dysarthria, longer disease duration and depression.
- Assessment of dysphagia in PD should begin early and follow a multidisciplinary, structured pathway including neurological examination and detailed clinical swallowing assessment. Case history, medical history, self-assessment instruments, and physical examination (e.g., oral motor assessment, swallowing trials) are all part of the clinical swallowing assessment process. PD-dysphagia specific such as SDQ, ROMP, MDT-PD help to capture symptoms, functional impact and swallowing-related quality of life.
- Instrumental assessment methods, particularly FEES and VFSS, are essential. Scales such as BCR, VASES, YPRSRS, PAS and DIGEST-FEES provide outcome measures for research and clinical decision-making in IwPD. Additional tools including manometry, surface EMG, IOPI and ultrasonography contributing to a more detailed understanding of dysphagia mechanisms and treatment effects in PD.
- Dysphagia management in PD is individualized and based on integrated clinical and instrumental findings. Swallowing therapy delivered by SLTs

includes compensatory strategies (e.g., postural adjustments, diet modifications, environmental adaptations) and rehabilitative approaches (e.g., oral motor, respiratory and laryngeal-pharyngeal exercises, swallowing maneuvers, and biofeedback-based therapies such as using sEMG, IOPI and VAST). Evidence suggests potential benefits of LSVT and EMST interventions for swallowing in PD although the strength of evidence varies and long-term effects require further study.

- Current data with neuromodulation techniques (tDCS, rTMS) are limited and larger and methodologically robust trials are needed.
- Treatment optimization, it is recommended that IwPD be tested during both on/off states to assess the effect of dopaminergic treatment on swallowing function and that patients eat their meals preferably during their best "ON" periods. From a nutritional perspective, PEG placement must balance nutritional needs, safety, disease progression and cognitive status.

REFERENCES

Aghaz, A., Ghelichi, L., Shahriyari, A., Noori, S., & Banari, A. (2024). The prevalence of dysphagia in Parkinson's disease: a systematic review and meta-analysis. *Journal of Iranian Medical Council*.

Akbar, U., Dham, B., He, Y., Hack, N., Wu, S., Troche, M., Tighe, P., Nelson, E., Friedman, J. H., & Okun, M. S. (2015). Incidence and mortality trends of aspiration pneumonia in Parkinson's disease in the United States, 1979-2010. *Parkinsonism & Related Disorders*, *21*(9), 1082–1086. DOI: 10.1016/j.parkreldis.2015.06.020

Alfonsi, E., Restivo, D. A., Cosentino, G., De Icco, R., Bertino, G., Schindler, A., Todisco, M., Fresia, M., Cortese, A., Prunetti, P., Ramusino, M. C., Moglia, A., Sandrini, G., & Tassorelli, C. (2017). Botulinum toxin is effective in the management of neurogenic dysphagia. Clinical-electrophysiological findings and tips on safety in different neurological disorders. *Frontiers in Pharmacology*, *8*, 80. DOI: 10.3389/fphar.2017.00080

American Speech-Language-Hearing Association. (2004). Preferred practice patterns for the profession of speech-language pathology. Available at: h ttp://www.asha.org/docs/html/PP2004-00191. html. Accessed November 22, 2025

Argolo, N., Sampaio, M., Pinho, P., Melo, A., & Nóbrega, A. C. (2013). Do swallowing exercises improve swallowing dynamic and quality of life in Parkinson's disease? *NeuroRehabilitation*, *32*(4), 949–955. DOI: 10.3233/NRE-130918

Atalar, M. S., & Genç, G. (2022). Parkinson hastalığında yutma bozukluklarına yaklaşım. *Muğla Sıtkı Koçman Üniversitesi Tıp Dergisi*, *9*(2), 189–203.

Athukorala, R. P., Jones, R. D., Sella, O., & Huckabee, M. L. (2014). Skill training for swallowing rehabilitation in patients with Parkinson's disease. *Archives of Physical Medicine and Rehabilitation*, *95*(7), 1374–1382. DOI: 10.1016/j.apmr.2014.03.001

Ayres, A., Jotz, G. P., Rieder, C. R., Schuh, A. F., & Olchik, M. R. (2016). The Impact of Dysphagia Therapy on Quality of Life in Patients with Parkinson's Disease as Measured by the Swallowing Quality of Life Questionnaire (SWALQOL). *International Archives of Otorhinolaryngology*, *20*(3), 202–206. DOI: 10.1055/s-0036-1582450

Belafsky, P. C., Mouadeb, D. A., Rees, C. J., Pryor, J. C., Postma, G. N., Allen, J., & Leonard, R. J. (2008). Validity and reliability of the Eating Assessment Tool (EAT-10). *The Annals of Otology, Rhinology, and Laryngology*, *117*(12), 919–924. DOI: 10.1177/000348940811701210

Bengisu, S., Savaş, M., Aygün, D., Beğen, S. K., Altıntaş, T., & Manay, B. (2024). Impact of Parkinson's disease-related dysphagia severity on quality of life: Comparison between self-reports and videofluoroscopic swallowing study results. *The Turkish Journal of Ear Nose and Throat, 34*(3), 84–91.

Bloem, B. R., Okun, M. S., & Klein, C. (2021). Parkinson's disease. *Lancet, 397*(10291), 2284–2303.

Branco, L. L., Trentin, S., Augustin Schwanke, C. H., Gomes, I., & Loureiro, F. (2019). The Swallowing Clinical Assessment Score in Parkinson's Disease (SCAS-PD) is a valid and low-cost tool for evaluation of dysphagia: A gold-standard comparison study. *Journal of Aging Research, 7984635*. Advance online publication. DOI: 10.1155/2019/7984635

Büyükönder, G., & Parlak, M. M. (2025). Deep brain stimulation in swallowing disorders in individuals with Parkinson's disease: a narrative review. *Sensory Neuroscience*, e70012.

Carneiro, D., das Graças Wanderley de Sales Coriolano, M., Belo, L. R., de Marcos Rabelo, A. R., Asano, A. G., & Lins, O. G. (2014). Quality of life related to swallowing in Parkinson's disease. *Dysphagia, 29*(5), 578–582. DOI: 10.1007/s00455-014-9548-3

Castell, J. A., Johnston, B. T., Colcher, A., Li, Q., Gideon, R. M., & Castell, D. O. (2001). Manometric abnormalities of the esophagus in patients with Parkinson's disease. *Neurogastroenterology and Motility, 13*(4), 361–364. DOI: 10.1046/j.1365-2982.2001.00275.x

Cereda, E., Barichella, M., Pedrolli, C., & Pezzoli, G. (2010). Low-protein and protein-redistribution diets for Parkinson's disease patients with motor fluctuations: A systematic review. *Movement Disorders, 25*(13), 2021–2034. DOI: 10.1002/mds.23226

Cereda, E., Cilia, R., Klersy, C., Canesi, M., Zecchinelli, A. L., Mariani, C. B., Tesei, S., Sacilotto, G., Meucci, N., Zini, M., Isaias, I. U., Cassani, E., Goldwurm, S., Barichella, M., & Pezzoli, G. (2014). Swallowing disturbances in Parkinson's disease: A multivariate analysis of contributing factors. *Parkinsonism & Related Disorders, 20*(12), 1382–1387. DOI: 10.1016/j.parkreldis.2014.09.031

Chaudhuri, K. R., Martinez-Martin, P., Schapira, A. H., Stocchi, F., Sethi, K., Odin, P., Brown, R. G., Koller, W., Barone, P., MacPhee, G., Kelly, L., Rabey, M., MacMahon, D., Thomas, S., Ondo, W., Rye, D., Forbes, A., Tluk, S., Dhawan, V., & Olanow, C. W. (2006). International multicenter pilot study of the first comprehensive self-completed nonmotor symptoms questionnaire for Parkinson's disease: The NMSQuest study. *Movement Disorders*, *21*(7), 916–923. DOI: 10.1002/mds.20844

Coelho, M., Marti, M. J., Tolosa, E., Ferreira, J. J., Valldeoriola, F., Rosa, M., & Sampaio, C. (2010). Late-stage Parkinson's disease: The Barcelona and Lisbon cohort. *Journal of Neurology*, *257*(9), 1524–1532. DOI: 10.1007/s00415-010-5566-8

Corti, O., Lesage, S., & Brice, A. (2011). What genetics tells us about the causes and mechanisms of Parkinson's disease. *Physiological Reviews*, *91*(4), 1161–1218. DOI: 10.1152/physrev.00022.2010

Cosentino, G., Avenali, M., Schindler, A., Pizzorni, N., Montomoli, C., Abbruzzese, G., Antonini, A., Barbiera, F., Benazzo, M., Benarroch, E. E., Bertino, G., Cereda, E., Clavè, P., Cortelli, P., Eleopra, R., Ferrari, C., Hamdy, S., Huckabee, M. L., Lopiano, L., & Alfonsi, E. (2022). A multinational consensus on dysphagia in Parkinson's disease: Screening, diagnosis and prognostic value. *Journal of Neurology*, *269*(3), 1335–1352. DOI: 10.1007/s00415-021-10739-8

Crary, M. A., Mann, G. D., & Groher, M. E. (2005). Initial psychometric assessment of a functional oral intake scale for dysphagia in stroke patients. *Archives of Physical Medicine and Rehabilitation*, *86*(8), 1516–1520. DOI: 10.1016/j.apmr.2004.11.049

Curtis, J. A., Borders, J. C., Perry, S. E., Dakin, A. E., Seikaly, Z. N., & Troche, M. S. (2022). Visual Analysis of Swallowing Efficiency and Safety (VASES): A standardized approach to rating pharyngeal residue, penetration, and aspiration during fees. *Dysphagia*, *37*(2), 417–435. DOI: 10.1007/s00455-021-10293-5

Curtis, J. A., Molfenter, S., & Troche, M. S. (2020b). Predictors of residue and airway invasion in Parkinson's disease. *Dysphagia*, *35*(2), 220–230. DOI: 10.1007/s00455-019-10014-z

Curtis, J. A., Molfenter, S. M., & Troche, M. S. (2020a). Pharyngeal area changes in Parkinson's disease and its effect on swallowing safety, efficiency, and kinematics. *Dysphagia*, *35*(2), 389–398. DOI: 10.1007/s00455-019-10052-7

Dashtelei, A. A., Nitsche, M. A., Salehinejad, M. A., Habibi, A. H., Bakhtyiari, J., & Khatoonabadi, A. R. (2024). Adjunctive transcranial direct current stimulation to improve swallowing functions in Parkinson's disease. *EXCLI Journal*, *23*, 95.

de Lau, L. M., & Breteler, M. M. (2006). Epidemiology of Parkinson's disease. *Lancet Neurology*, *5*(6), 525–535. DOI: 10.1016/S1474-4422(06)70471-9

Di Luca, D. G., McArthur, E. W., Willis, A., Martino, R., & Marras, C. (2021). Clinical and economic outcomes associated with dysphagia in hospitalized patients with Parkinson's Disease. *Journal of Parkinson's Disease*, *11*(4), 1965–1971. DOI: 10.3233/JPD-212798

Doruk, C., Çaytemel, B., Şahin, E., Kara, H., Samancı, B., Abay, S. N., Bilgiç, B., Hanağası, H., Başaran, B., Enver, N., & Rameau, A. (2023). Evaluation of post-swallow residue with visual analysis of swallowing efficiency and safety in patients with idiopathic Parkinson's Disease. *Ear, Nose, and Throat Journal, 1455613231210976*. Advance online publication. DOI: 10.1177/01455613231210976

Ebihara, S., Saito, H., Kanda, A., Nakajoh, M., Takahashi, H., Arai, H., & Sasaki, H. (2003). Impaired efficacy of cough in patients with Parkinson disease. *Chest*, *124*(3), 1009–1015. DOI: 10.1378/chest.124.3.1009

El Sharkawi, A., Ramig, L., Logemann, J. A., Pauloski, B. R., Rademaker, A. W., Smith, C. H., Pawlas, A., Baum, S., & Werner, C. (2002). Swallowing and voice effects of Lee Silverman Voice Treatment (LSVT): A pilot study. *Journal of Neurology, Neurosurgery, and Psychiatry*, *72*(1), 31–36. DOI: 10.1136/jnnp.72.1.31

Ellerston, J. K., Heller, A. C., Houtz, D. R., & Kendall, K. A. (2016). Quantitative measures of swallowing deficits in patients with Parkinson's disease. *The Annals of Otology, Rhinology, and Laryngology*, *125*(5), 385–392. DOI: 10.1177/0003489415617774

Ertekin, C., Tarlaci, S., Aydogdu, I., Kiylioglu, N., Yuceyar, N., Turman, A. B., Secil, Y., & Esmeli, F. (2002). Electrophysiological evaluation of pharyngeal phase of swallowing in patients with Parkinson's disease. *Movement Disorders*, *17*(5), 942–949. DOI: 10.1002/mds.10240

Freed, D. B. (2020). Hypokinetic dysarthria. In *Motor speech disorders: Diagnosis and treatment* (3rd ed., p. 208). Plural Publishing.

Fukuoka, T., Ono, T., Hori, K., Wada, Y., Uchiyama, Y., Kasama, S., Yoshikawa, H., & Domen, K. (2019). Tongue pressure measurement and videofluoroscopic study of swallowing in patients with Parkinson's disease. *Dysphagia*, *34*(1), 80–88. DOI: 10.1007/s00455-018-9916-5

Gandhi, P., Peladeau-Pigeon, M., Simmons, M., & Steele, C. M. (2023). Exploring the efficacy of the effortful swallow maneuver for improving swallowing in people with Parkinson disease-a pilot study. *Archives of Rehabilitation Research and Clinical Translation*, *5*(3), 100276. DOI: 10.1016/j.arrct.2023.100276

Gandhi, P., & Steele, C. M. (2022). Effectiveness of interventions for dysphagia in Parkinson disease: A systematic review. *American Journal of Speech-Language Pathology*, *31*(1), 463–485. DOI: 10.1044/2021_AJSLP-21-00145

Goetz, C. G., Tilley, B. C., Shaftman, S. R., Stebbins, G. T., Fahn, S., Martinez-Martin, P., Poewe, W., Sampaio, C., Stern, M. B., Dodel, R., Dubois, B., Holloway, R., Jankovic, J., Kulisevsky, J., Lang, A. E., Lees, A., Leurgans, S., LeWitt, P. A., & Nyenhuis, D.Movement Disorder Society UPDRS Revision Task Force. (2008). Movement Disorder Society-sponsored revision of the Unified Parkinson's Disease Rating Scale (MDS-UPDRS): Scale presentation and clinimetric testing results. *Movement Disorders*, *23*(15), 2129–2170. DOI: 10.1002/mds.22340

Goldman, S. M. (2014). Environmental toxins and Parkinson's disease. *Annual Review of Pharmacology and Toxicology*, *54*, 141–164. DOI: 10.1146/annurev-pharmtox-011613-135937

Groher, M. E., & Crary, M. A. (2016). *Dysphagia: Clinical management in adults and children* (2nd ed.). Elsevier.

Han, M., Ohnishi, H., Nonaka, M., Yamauchi, R., Hozuki, T., Hayashi, T., & Mori, M. (2011). Relationship between dysphagia and depressive states in patients with Parkinson's disease. *Parkinsonism & Related Disorders*, *17*(6), 437–439.

Howell, R. J., Webster, H., Kissela, E., Gustin, R., Kaval, F., Klaben, B., & Khosla, S. (2019). Dysphagia in Parkinson's disease improves with vocal augmentation. *Dysphagia*, *34*(6), 862–868. DOI: 10.1007/s00455-019-09982-z

Hutcheson, K. A., Barrow, M. P., Barringer, D. A., Knott, J. K., Lin, H. Y., Weber, R. S., Fuller, C. D., Lai, S. Y., Alvarez, C. P., Raut, J., Lazarus, C. L., May, A., Patterson, J., Roe, J. W., Starmer, H. M., & Lewin, J. S. (2017). Dynamic Imaging Grade of Swallowing Toxicity (DIGEST): Scale development and validation. *Cancer*, *123*(1), 62–70. DOI: 10.1002/cncr.30283

Jellinger K. A. (2019). Is Braak staging valid for all types of Parkinson's disease? *Journal of Neural Transmission (Vienna, Austria: 1996)*, *126*(4), 423–431. https://doi.org/DOI: 10.1007/s00702-018-1898-9

Kalf, H., de Swart, B., Bonnier-Baars, M., Kanters, J., Hofman, M., Kocken, J., & Munneke, M. (2011b). *Guidelines for speech-language therapy in Parkinson's disease*. ParkinsonNet/NPF.

Kalf, J. G., Borm, G. F., de Swart, B. J., Bloem, B. R., Zwarts, M. J., & Munneke, M. (2011a). Reproducibility and validity of patient-rated assessment of speech, swallowing, and saliva control in Parkinson's disease. *Archives of Physical Medicine and Rehabilitation, 92*(7), 1152–1158. DOI: 10.1016/j.apmr.2011.02.011

Kalf, J. G., de Swart, B. J., Bloem, B. R., & Munneke, M. (2012). Prevalence of oropharyngeal dysphagia in Parkinson's disease: A meta-analysis. *Parkinsonism & Related Disorders, 18*(4), 311–315. DOI: 10.1016/j.parkreldis.2011.11.006

Kalia, L. V., & Lang, A. E. (2015). Parkinson's disease. *Lancet, 386*(9996), 896–912.

Khedr, E. M., Mohamed, K. O., Soliman, R. K., Hassan, A. M. M., & Rothwell, J. C. (2019). The effect of high-frequency repetitive transcranial magnetic stimulation on advancing Parkinson's disease with dysphagia: Double blind randomized clinical trial. *Neurorehabilitation and Neural Repair, 33*(6), 442–452. DOI: 10.1177/1545968319847968

Kwon, M., & Lee, J. H. (2019). Oro-pharyngeal dysphagia in Parkinson's disease and related movement disorders. *Journal of Movement Disorders, 12*(3), 152–160. DOI: 10.14802/jmd.19048

Labeit, B., Lapa, S., Muhle, P., Suntrup-Krueger, S., Claus, I., Gandor, F., Ahring, S., Oelenberg, S., Dziewas, R., & Warnecke, T. (2024). Validation of the DIGEST-FEES as a global outcome measure for pharyngeal dysphagia in Parkinson's disease. *Dysphagia, 39*(4), 697–704. DOI: 10.1007/s00455-023-10650-6

Lacy, B., Piotrowski, H. J., Dewey, R. B.Jr, & Husain, M. M. (2022). Severity of depressive and motor symptoms impacts quality of life in Parkinson's disease patients at an academic movement clinic: A cross-sectional study. *Clinical Parkinsonism & Related Disorders, 8*, 100180. DOI: 10.1016/j.prdoa.2022.100180

Lam, K., Kwai Yi Lam, F., Kwong Lau, K., Kay Chan, Y., Yee Ling Kan, E., Woo, J., & Ko, A. (2007). Simple clinical tests may predict severe oropharyngeal dysphagia in Parkinson's disease. *Movement Disorders, 22*(5), 640–644.

Leonard, R. (2017). Two methods for quantifying pharyngeal residue on fluoroscopic swallow studies: Reliability assessment. *Annals of Otolaryngology and Rhinology, 4*(3), 1168.

Leopold, N. A., & Daniels, S. K. (2010). Supranuclear control of swallowing. *Dysphagia, 25*(3), 250–257. DOI: 10.1007/s00455-009-9249-5

Li, M., Ye, X., Huang, Z., Ye, L., & Chen, C. (2025). Global burden of Parkinson's disease from 1990 to 2021: A population-based study. *BMJ Open*, *15*(4), e095610. DOI: 10.1136/bmjopen-2024-095610

Liu, W. M., Lin, R. J., Yu, R. L., Tai, C. H., Lin, C. H., & Wu, R. M. (2015). The impact of nonmotor symptoms on quality of life in patients with Parkinson's disease in Taiwan. *Neuropsychiatric Disease and Treatment*, *11*, 2865–2873. DOI: 10.2147/NDT.S88968

Logemann, J. A., Gensler, G., Robbins, J., Lindblad, A. S., Brandt, D., Hind, J. A., Kosek, S., Dikeman, K., Kazandjian, M., Gramigna, G. D., Lundy, D., McGarvey-Toler, S., & Miller Gardner, P. J. (2008). A randomized study of three interventions for aspiration of thin liquids in patients with dementia or Parkinson's disease. *Journal of Speech, Language, and Hearing Research: JSLHR*, *51*(1), 173–183. DOI: 10.1044/1092-4388(2008/013)

Loureiro, F., Nóbrega, A. C., Sampaio, M., Argolo, N., Dalbem, A., Melo, A., & Gomes, I. (2013). A Swallowing Clinical Assessment Score (SCAS) to evaluate outpatients with Parkinson's disease. *PAJAR-Pan-American Journal of Aging Research*, *1*(1), 16–19.

Luchesi, K. F., Kitamura, S., & Mourão, L. F. (2015). Dysphagia progression and swallowing management in Parkinson's disease: An observational study. *Brazilian Journal of Otorhinolaryngology*, *81*(1), 24–30. DOI: 10.1016/j.bjorl.2014.09.006

Macedo, A. K. P. D., Araújo, R. C. P. D., Godoy, C. M. D. A., & Magalhães, H. (2025). Relationship between orofacial mobility and severity of pharyngeal residues in oropharyngeal dysphagia in individuals with PD. *Audiology - Communication Research*, *30*, e3028.

Makaroff, L., Gunn, A., Gervasoni, C., & Richy, F. (2011). Gastrointestinal disorders in Parkinson's disease: Prevalence and health outcomes in a US claims database. *Journal of Parkinson's Disease*, *1*(1), 65–74. DOI: 10.3233/JPD-2011-001

Manor, Y., Giladi, N., Cohen, A., Fliss, D. M., & Cohen, J. T. (2007). Validation of a swallowing disturbance questionnaire for detecting dysphagia in patients with Parkinson's disease. *Movement Disorders*, *22*(13), 1917–1921. DOI: 10.1002/mds.21625

Manor, Y., Mootanah, R., Freud, D., Giladi, N., & Cohen, J. T. (2013). Video-assisted swallowing therapy for patients with Parkinson's disease. *Parkinsonism & Related Disorders*, *19*(2), 207–211. DOI: 10.1016/j.parkreldis.2012.10.004

McHorney, C. A., Bricker, D. E., Kramer, A. E., Rosenbek, J. C., Robbins, J., Chignell, K. A., Logemann, J. A., & Clarke, C. (2000). The SWAL-QOL outcomes tool for oropharyngeal dysphagia in adults: I. Conceptual foundation and item development. *Dysphagia*, *15*(3), 115–121. DOI: 10.1007/s004550010012

Miles, A., Jardine, M., Johnston, F., de Lisle, M., Friary, P., & Allen, J. (2017). Effect of Lee Silverman Voice Treatment (LSVT LOUD®) on swallowing and cough in Parkinson's disease: A pilot study. *Journal of the Neurological Sciences*, *383*, 180–187. DOI: 10.1016/j.jns.2017.11.015

Morgante, L., Salemi, G., Meneghini, F., Di Rosa, A. E., Epifanio, A., Grigoletto, F., Ragonese, P., Patti, F., Reggio, A., Di Perri, R., & Savettieri, G. (2000). Parkinson disease survival: A population-based study. *Archives of Neurology*, *57*(4), 507–512. DOI: 10.1001/archneur.57.4.507

Morris, H. R., Spillantini, M. G., Sue, C. M., & Williams-Gray, C. H. (2024). The pathogenesis of Parkinson's disease. *Lancet*, *403*(10423), 293–304. DOI: 10.1016/S0140-6736(23)01478-2

Moustafa, A. A., Chakravarthy, S., Phillips, J. R., Gupta, A., Keri, S., Polner, B., Frank, M. J., & Jahanshahi, M. (2016). Motor symptoms in Parkinson's disease: A unified framework. *Neuroscience and Biobehavioral Reviews*, *68*, 727–740. DOI: 10.1016/j.neubiorev.2016.07.010

Nagaya, M., Kachi, T., Yamada, T., & Igata, A. (1998). Videofluorographic study of swallowing in Parkinson's disease. *Dysphagia*, *13*(2), 95–100. DOI: 10.1007/PL00009562

Neubauer, P. D., Rademaker, A. W., & Leder, S. B. (2015). The Yale Pharyngeal Residue Severity Rating Scale: An anatomically defined and image-based tool. *Dysphagia*, *30*(5), 521–528. DOI: 10.1007/s00455-015-9631-4

Noyce, A. J., Bestwick, J. P., Silveira-Moriyama, L., Hawkes, C. H., Giovannoni, G., Lees, A. J., & Schrag, A. (2012). Meta-analysis of early nonmotor features and risk factors for Parkinson disease. *Annals of Neurology*, *72*(6), 893–901. DOI: 10.1002/ana.23687

Parkinson, J. (2002). An essay on the shaking palsy. *The Journal of Neuropsychiatry and Clinical Neurosciences*, *14*(2), 223–236.

Patel, B., Legacy, J., Hegland, K. W., Okun, M. S., & Herndon, N. E. (2020). A comprehensive review of the diagnosis and treatment of Parkinson's disease dysphagia and aspiration. *Expert Review of Gastroenterology & Hepatology*, *14*(6), 411–424. DOI: 10.1080/17474124.2020.1769475

Paul, B. S., Singh, T., Paul, G., Jain, D., Singh, G., Kaushal, S., & Chhina, R. S. (2019). Prevalence of malnutrition in Parkinson's disease and correlation with gastrointestinal symptoms. *Annals of Indian Academy of Neurology*, *22*(4), 447–452. DOI: 10.4103/aian.AIAN_349_18

Perez-Lloret, S., Nègre-Pagès, L., Ojero-Senard, A., Damier, P., Destée, A., Tison, F., Merello, M., & Rascol, O.COPARK Study Group. (2012). Oro-buccal symptoms (dysphagia, dysarthria, and sialorrhea) in patients with Parkinson's disease: Preliminary analysis from the French COPARK cohort. *European Journal of Neurology*, *19*(1), 28–37. DOI: 10.1111/j.1468-1331.2011.03402.x

Perez Lloret, S., Pirán Arce, G., Rossi, M., Caivano Nemet, M. L., Salsamendi, P., & Merello, M. (2007). Validation of a new scale for the evaluation of sialorrhea in patients with Parkinson's disease. *Movement Disorders*, *22*(1), 107–111. DOI: 10.1002/mds.21152

Perry, S. E., Borders, J. C., Dakin, A. E., & Troche, M. S. (2022). Characterizing quality of life in caregivers of people with Parkinson's disease and dysphagia. *Dysphagia*, *37*(3), 523–532. DOI: 10.1007/s00455-021-10299-z

Pflug, C., Bihler, M., Emich, K., Niessen, A., Nienstedt, J. C., Flügel, T., Koseki, J. C., Plaetke, R., Hidding, U., Gerloff, C., & Buhmann, C. (2018). Critical dysphagia is common in Parkinson disease and occurs even in early stages: A prospective cohort study. *Dysphagia*, *33*(1), 41–50. DOI: 10.1007/s00455-017-9831-1

Pitts, L. L., Kanadet, R. M., Hamilton, V. K., Crimmins, S. K., & Cherney, L. R. (2019). Lingual pressure dysfunction contributes to reduced swallowing-related quality of life in Parkinson's Disease. *Journal of Speech, Language, and Hearing Research: JSLHR*, *62*(8), 2671–2679. DOI: 10.1044/2019_JSLHR-S-18-0366

Pitts, T., Bolser, D., Rosenbek, J., Troche, M., Okun, M. S., & Sapienza, C. (2009). Impact of expiratory muscle strength training on voluntary cough and swallow function in Parkinson disease. *Chest*, *135*(5), 1301–1308. DOI: 10.1378/chest.08-1389

Plowman-Prine, E. K., Sapienza, C. M., Okun, M. S., Pollock, S. L., Jacobson, C., Wu, S. S., & Rosenbek, J. C. (2009). The relationship between quality of life and swallowing in Parkinson's disease. *Movement Disorders: Disorders: Official Journal of the Movement Disorder Society*, *24*(9), 1352–1358. DOI: 10.1002/mds.22617

Polymeropoulos, M. H., Lavedan, C., Leroy, E., Ide, S. E., Dehejia, A., Dutra, A., Pike, B., Root, H., Rubenstein, J., Boyer, R., Stenroos, E. S., Chandrasekharappa, S., Athanassiadou, A., Papapetropoulos, T., Johnson, W. G., Lazzarini, A. M., Duvoisin, R. C., Di Iorio, G., Golbe, L. I., & Nussbaum, R. L. (1997). Mutation in the alpha-synuclein gene identified in families with Parkinson's disease. *Science*, *276*(5321), 2045–2047. DOI: 10.1126/science.276.5321.2045

Ponsoni, A., Costa, F. P., Soares, V. N., Santos, C. G. S., & Mourão, L. F. (2024). Sensitivity and specificity of the EAT-10 and SDQ-DP in identifying the risk of dysphagia in Parkinson's disease. Sensibilidade e especificidade do EAT-10 e SDQ-DP na identificação do risco de disfagia na doença de Parkinson. *Arquivos de Neuro-Psiquiatria*, *82*(2), 1–8. DOI: 10.1055/s-0044-1779055

Potulska, A., Friedman, A., Królicki, L., & Spychala, A. (2003). Swallowing disorders in Parkinson's disease. *Parkinsonism & Related Disorders*, *9*(6), 349–353. DOI: 10.1016/s1353-8020(03)00045-2

Pringsheim, T., Jette, N., Frolkis, A., & Steeves, T. D. (2014). The prevalence of Parkinson's disease: A systematic review and meta-analysis. *Movement Disorders*, *29*(13), 1583–1590. DOI: 10.1002/mds.25945

Printza, A., & Triaridis, S. (2022). Is the ability of the Eating Assessment Tool (EAT-10) to screen for aspiration in patients with dysphagia depending on the patients' disease?. *European Archives of Oto-Rhino-Laryngology: Official Journal of The European Federation of Oto-Rhino-Laryngological Societies (EUFOS): Affiliated with the German Society for Oto-Rhino-Laryngology - Head - and Neck Surgery*, *279*(7), 3745–3746. https://doi.org/DOI: 10.1007/s00405-021-06661-4

Rosenbek, J. C., Robbins, J. A., Roecker, E. B., Coyle, J. L., & Wood, J. L. (1996). A penetration-aspiration scale. *Dysphagia*, *11*(2), 93–98. DOI: 10.1007/BF00417897

Rudisch, D. M., Krasko, M. N., Burdick, R., Broadfoot, C. K., Rogus-Pulia, N., & Ciucci, M. R. (2023). Dysphagia in Parkinson Disease: Part I - Pathophysiology and diagnostic practices. *Current Physical Medicine Andand Rehabilitation Reports*, *11*(2), 176–187. DOI: 10.1007/s40141-023-00392-9

Schindler, A., Pizzorni, N., Cereda, E., Cosentino, G., Avenali, M., Montomoli, C., Abbruzzese, G., Antonini, A., Barbiera, F., Benazzo, M., Benarroch, E., Bertino, G., Clavè, P., Cortelli, P., Eleopra, R., Ferrari, C., Hamdy, S., Huckabee, M. L., Lopiano, L., & Alfonsi, E. (2021). Consensus on the treatment of dysphagia in Parkinson's disease. *Journal of the Neurological Sciences*, *430*, 120008. DOI: 10.1016/j.jns.2021.120008

Sidransky, E., & Lopez, G. (2012). The link between the GBA gene and parkinsonism. *Lancet Neurology*, *11*(11), 986–998. DOI: 10.1016/S1474-4422(12)70190-4

Simon, D. K., Tanner, C. M., & Brundin, P. (2020). Parkinson disease epidemiology, pathology, genetics, and pathophysiology. *Clinics in Geriatric Medicine*, *36*(1), 1–12. DOI: 10.1016/j.cger.2019.08.002

Simons, J. A. (2017). Swallowing dysfunctions in Parkinson's Disease. *International Review of Neurobiology*, *134*, 1207–1238. DOI: 10.1016/bs.irn.2017.05.026

Simons, J. A., Fietzek, U. M., Waldmann, A., Warnecke, T., Schuster, T., & Ceballos-Baumann, A. O. (2014). Development and validation of a new screening questionnaire for dysphagia in early stages of Parkinson's disease. *Parkinsonism & Related Disorders*, *20*(9), 992–998. DOI: 10.1016/j.parkreldis.2014.06.008

Sun, Y. M., Wang, Z. Y., Liang, Y. Y., Hao, C. W., & Shi, C. H. (2024). Digital biomarkers for precision diagnosis and monitoring in Parkinson's disease. *NPJ Digital Medicine*, *7*(1), 218. DOI: 10.1038/s41746-024-01217-2

Sung, H. Y., Kim, J. S., Lee, K. S., Kim, Y. I., Song, I. U., Chung, S. W., Yang, D. W., Cho, Y. K., Park, J. M., Lee, I. S., Kim, S. W., Chung, I. S., & Choi, M. G. (2010). The prevalence and patterns of pharyngoesophageal dysmotility in patients with early stage early-stage Parkinson's disease. *Movement disorders: Disorders. Official Journal of the Movement Disorder Society*, *25*(14), 2361–2368. DOI: 10.1002/mds.23290

Suttrup, I., & Warnecke, T. (2016). Dysphagia in Parkinson's Disease. *Dysphagia*, *31*(1), 24–32. DOI: 10.1007/s00455-015-9671-9

Takizawa, C., Gemmell, E., Kenworthy, J., & Speyer, R. (2016). A systematic review of the prevalence of oropharyngeal dysphagia in stroke, Parkinson's disease, Alzheimer's disease, head injury, and pneumonia. *Dysphagia*, *31*(3), 434–441. DOI: 10.1007/s00455-016-9695-9

Threats, T. T. (2007). Use of the ICF in dysphagia management. [). © Thieme Medical Publishers]. *Seminars in Speech and Language*, *28*(04), 323–333.

Troche, M. S., Brandimore, A. E., Okun, M. S., Davenport, P. W., & Hegland, K. W. (2014a). Decreased cough sensitivity and aspiration in Parkinson disease. *Chest*, *146*(5), 1294–1299. DOI: 10.1378/chest.14-0066

Troche, M. S., Okun, M. S., Rosenbek, J. C., Musson, N., Fernandez, H. H., Rodriguez, R., Romrell, J., Pitts, T., Wheeler-Hegland, K. M., & Sapienza, C. M. (2010). Aspiration and swallowing in Parkinson disease and rehabilitation with EMST: A randomized trial. *Neurology*, *75*(21), 1912–1919. DOI: 10.1212/WNL.0b013e3181fef115

Troche, M. S., Rosenbek, J. C., Okun, M. S., & Sapienza, C. M. (2014b). Detraining outcomes with expiratory muscle strength training in Parkinson disease. *Journal of Rehabilitation Research and Development*, *51*(2), 305–310. DOI: 10.1682/JRRD.2013.05.0101

Umay, E., Ozturk, E., Gurcay, E., Delibas, O., & Celikel, F. (2019). Swallowing in Parkinson's disease: How is it affected? *Clinical Neurology and Neurosurgery*, *177*, 37–41. DOI: 10.1016/j.clineuro.2018.12.015

Umemoto, G., & Furuya, H. (2020). Management of dysphagia in patients with Parkinson's disease and related disorders. *Internal Medicine (Tokyo, Japan)*, *59*(1), 7–14. DOI: 10.2169/internalmedicine.2373-18

Van Den Eeden, S. K., Tanner, C. M., Bernstein, A. L., Fross, R. D., Leimpeter, A., Bloch, D. A., & Nelson, L. M. (2003). Incidence of Parkinson's disease: Variation by age, gender, and race/ethnicity. *American Journal of Epidemiology*, *157*(11), 1015–1022. DOI: 10.1093/aje/kwg068

World Health Organization. (2013). How to Use the ICF: A practical manual for using the International Classification of Functioning, Disability and Health. ICF., Retrieved November 22, 2025, from.

Ws Coriolano, M.d, R Belo, L., Carneiro, D., G Asano, A., Al Oliveira, P. J., da Silva, D. M., & G Lins, O. (2012). Swallowing in patients with Parkinson's disease: A surface electromyography study. *Dysphagia*, *27*(4), 550–555. DOI: 10.1007/s00455-012-9406-0

Zhu, J., Cui, Y., Zhang, J., Yan, R., Su, D., Zhao, D., Wang, A., & Feng, T. (2024). Temporal trends in the prevalence of Parkinson's disease from 1980 to 2023: A systematic review and meta-analysis. *The Lancet. Healthy Longevity*, *5*(7), e464–e479. DOI: 10.1016/S2666-7568(24)00094-1

Zimmerman, A. S., Shune, S., Smith, K. G., Estis, J. M., & Garand, K. L. (2022). Comparison of patient-reported and caregiver-reported swallowing-related quality of life in Parkinson's disease. *Dysphagia*, *37*(2), 436–445. DOI: 10.1007/s00455-021-10301-8

Chapter 9

Feeding and Swallowing Disorders in Cerebral Palsy: Assessment and Intervention Methods

Elif Ezgi Işik
http://orcid.org/0000-0001-7722-414X
University of Health Sciences, Turkey

ABSTRACT

Cerebral Palsy (CP) is a complex group of neurodevelopmental disorders characterized by postural and movement limitations resulting from a non-progressive lesion in the developing or immature brain, with a prevalence of 2 to 3 per 1,000 live births. Motor symptoms (spasticity, ataxia, dyskinesia) often combine with comorbid conditions such as sensory, cognitive, communication, and epilepsy, aggravating the clinical picture. Feeding and swallowing disorders in children with CP, namely oropharyngeal dysphagia (OPD), are a fairly common problem with a prevalence ranging from 22% to 99%.These feeding difficulties are directly related to Oral Motor Dysfunction (OMD) (tongue thrusting, weak sucking/swallowing), seen in over 90% of cases, and poor postural control; effective feeding depends on trunk and head stability. Dysphagia reduces the efficiency of food intake by causing impairments in the oral phase and pharyngeal phase (coughing, wet voice) of swallowing.

DOI: 10.4018/979-8-3373-6405-6.ch009

INTRODUCTION

Comprehensively understanding the nature of cerebral palsy (CP) is critical for determining effective assessment and goal-oriented intervention strategies. Selecting appropriate clinical assessment and intervention methods enables the support of developmental potential across multiple domains for individuals diagnosed with CP.

This section aims to address CP from a holistic perspective. The section content will first present the definition, prevalence, etiology, and clinical classification systems of CP. Subsequently, the identification of feeding and swallowing disorders that frequently accompany CP and the assessment and intervention approaches that can be used for these conditions will be examined in detail.

OVERVIEW OF CEREBRAL PALSY

Cerebral Palsy Definition, Prevalence, and Etiology

Cerebral palsy (CP) is defined as a group of permanent disorders of the development of movement and posture, causing activity limitation. These disorders are attributed to non-progressive disturbances that occurred in the developing fetal or infant brain (Rosenbaum et. al. 2007). The diagnosis of CP is based on the identification of motor function and postural control deficits that emerge in early developmental stages and persist throughout life. Although these disorders are not progressive in nature, they may exhibit phenotypic changes depending on the individual's age. Motor limitations, which constitute the core symptoms of CP, are often accompanied by comorbid neurodevelopmental and systemic disorders. These secondary functional impairments include sensory processing, perception, cognitive abilities, communication, behavioral regulation deficits, epilepsy, and secondary musculoskeletal anomalies that develop over time (Christine et al., 2007). The average prevalence of CP is reported to be between 2 and 3 per 1,000 live births (SCPE, 2000).

CP is a complex disorder with a multifactorial etiology spanning the prenatal, perinatal, and postnatal periods (Olszak et al., 2025). The causal factors involved in the pathogenesis of this condition are listed in Table 1 (Maclennan et al., 2015; Nelson, 2008; Olszak et al., 2025; Michael-Asalu, 2019).

Table 1. Causal Factors Involved in CP Pathogenesis

Pre-pregnancy Factors	Prenatal Factors	Perinatal Factors	Postnatal Factors
Mother's age at pregnancy Assisted reproductive technology Socioeconomic status History of previous intrauterine fetal death	Genetic abnormalities Multiple pregnancy Intrauterine infections Exposure to toxins Congenital malformations	Perinatal asphyxia Mechanical trauma Infection Prematurity Low birth weight	Central nervous system infections Surgical complications Traumatic brain injury (TBI) Perinatal complications

Symptoms

The primary clinical presentation of CP is characterized by movement and posture disorders that vary in severity and type among individuals. The motor symptoms observed in individuals with CP cover a broad spectrum. These symptoms include: lack of muscle coordination in voluntary movements (ataxia), muscle rigidity, increased muscle tone and exaggerated deep tendon reflexes (spasticity), muscle weakness in the extremities, and involuntary, random movements (dystonia/tremor). In addition, abnormal gait patterns (e.g., toe-walking), muscle tone stiffness (hypertonia) or looseness (hypotonia), delays in reaching developmental motor milestones, and difficulties with activities requiring fine motor skills (writing, buttoning) are also commonly reported (Zhou et al., 2017; Wu et al., 2004).

Infants diagnosed with CP often exhibit delays in reaching developmental milestones; this results in a slowing of the acquisition of gross motor skills such as rolling over, sitting, crawling, and walking. They may also exhibit abnormal postural patterns or show a tendency to favor one side of the body when moving (National Institute of Neurological Disorders and Stroke, 2025).

In infants younger than 6 months, looseness or stiffness may be felt when held; crossing the legs into a scissor position is noteworthy. When lifted from the supine position, the head remaining behind the body (lack of head control) is a common finding.

In infants older than 6 months, unilateral reaching patterns may be observed, such as inability to turn in either direction, poor midline activity (inability to bring hands together or to mouth), and reaching with one hand held in a fist.

In infants older than 10 months, asymmetry (pushing one limb and dragging the other) or instability (imbalance) in the crawling pattern may be seen. Additionally, failure to acquire the ability to stand with support and a significant delay in gross motor development have been reported (National Institute of Neurological Disorders and Stroke, 2025; Patel et al., 2020).

Classification

Cerebral palsy is a disorder that can affect the entire developmental process. Clinically, this condition is classified using systematic criteria based on the characteristics of motor function impairments and their topographical distribution (affected areas of the body) (Jones et al., 2007). Classification based on the characteristics of motor function impairments is described in Table 2 (National Institute of Neurological Disorders and Stroke., 2025).

Table 2. Characteristics of Motor Function Impairments in Cerebral Palsy

Spastic	**When subclassifications are examined, this is the most common form of CP, accounting for 83.6% of all recorded cases. It is characterized by increased muscle tone (hypertonia), increased deep tendon reflexes, and muscle weakness. It results from upper motor neuron damage.**
Dyskinetic	This type involves involuntary, uncontrolled, repetitive, and sometimes stereotypical movement patterns. Fluctuating problems with balance and coordination are seen. It results from damage to the basal ganglia or extrapyramidal system.
Ataxic	It results from damage to the cerebellum and manifests itself in impaired voluntary movements, balance, depth perception, and coordination. Movements are poorly organized in terms of strength, rhythm, and accuracy.
Hypotonic	A rare dominant motor type, it is characterized by markedly decreased muscle tone.

Cerebral palsy is classified into five basic clinical subtypes based on the topographical involvement of the extremities. This classification is as follows: monoplegia, where a single extremity is affected; hemiplegia, where the extremities on one side of the body are affected; diplegia, where the lower extremities are typically affected symmetrically, while the upper extremities are unaffected or minimally affected; triplegia, where three extremities are affected; and quadriplegia, the most common and severe form, where all four extremities are affected and more severe involvement is often seen in the upper extremities. This topographical distinction provides critical information about the severity and prognosis of the disorder (Alireza et al., 2014). The topographical classification of cerebral palsy is shown in Figure 1.

Figure 1. Topographic Classification in Cerebral Palsy

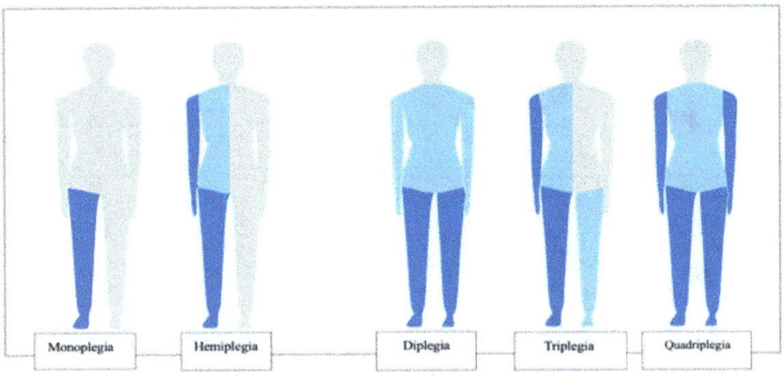

Gross Motor Function Classification System (GMFCS)

The Gross Motor Function Classification System (GMFCS) is one of the most commonly used functional classification criteria in CP. The GMFCS is a simple, five-level, sequential rating system developed to define the gross motor function level of individuals with CP (Palisano et al., 1997). This system standardizes the severity of the disorder from a functional perspective, based on the individual's mobility, use of assistive devices in daily life, and level of limitation. GMFCS was initially designed for use in the pediatric population aged 2 to 12 years. This classification tool was updated in 2008 with a revision that expanded its developmental scope to include the 6-12 and 12-18 age groups (Rosenbaum et al., 2008; Palisano et al., 2007; Paulson and Vargus-Adams, 2017). The GMFCS-E&R for children aged 6-12 with CP is shown in Figure 2.

Figure 2. GMFCS-E&R for Children Aged 6-12 With Cerebral Palsy

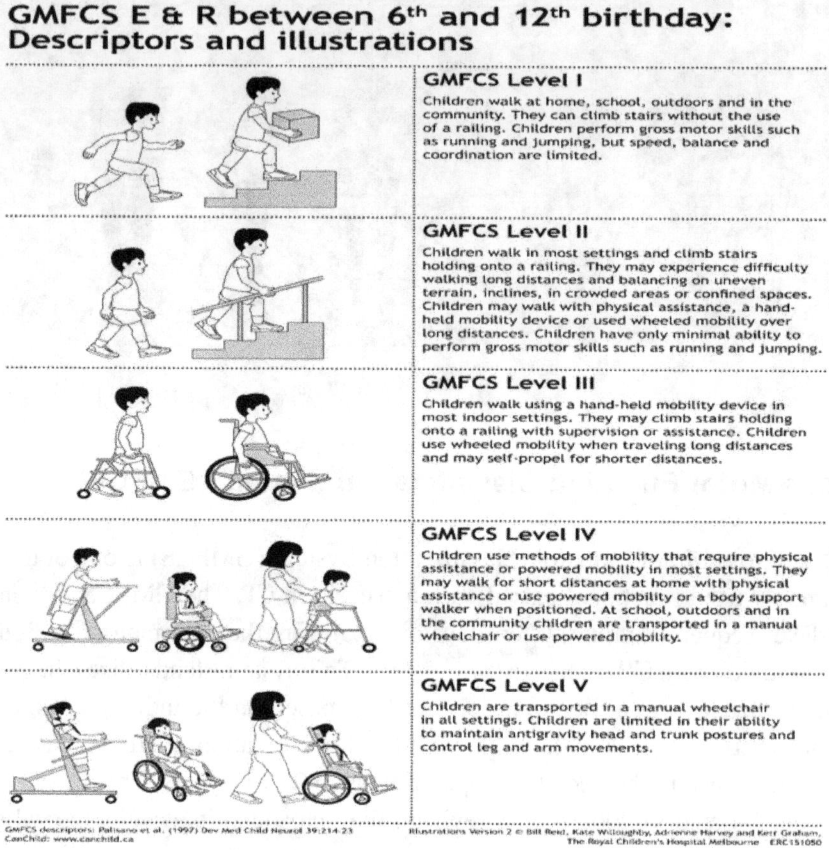
GMFCS E & R between 6th and 12th birthday: Descriptors and illustrations
GMFCS Level I
Children walk at home, school, outdoors and in the community. They can climb stairs without the use of a railing. Children perform gross motor skills such as running and jumping, but speed, balance and coordination are limited.
GMFCS Level II
Children walk in most settings and climb stairs holding onto a railing. They may experience difficulty walking long distances and balancing on uneven terrain, inclines, in crowded areas or confined spaces. Children may walk with physical assistance, a hand-held mobility device or used wheeled mobility over long distances. Children have only minimal ability to perform gross motor skills such as running and jumping.
GMFCS Level III
Children walk using a hand-held mobility device in most indoor settings. They may climb stairs holding onto a railing with supervision or assistance. Children use wheeled mobility when traveling long distances and may self-propel for shorter distances.
GMFCS Level IV
Children use methods of mobility that require physical assistance or powered mobility in most settings. They may walk for short distances at home with physical assistance or use powered mobility or a body support walker when positioned. At school, outdoors and in the community children are transported in a manual wheelchair or use powered mobility.
GMFCS Level V
Children are transported in a manual wheelchair in all settings. Children are limited in their ability to maintain antigravity head and trunk postures and control leg and arm movements.
GMFCS descriptors: Palisano et al. (1997) Dev Med Child Neurol 39:214-23
CanChild: www.canchild.ca
Illustrations Version 2 © Bill Reid, Kate Willoughby, Adrienne Harvey and Kerr Graham,
The Royal Children's Hospital Melbourne ERC151050

Manual Ability Classification System (MACS)

The Manual Ability Classification System (MACS) was developed as the upper extremity counterpart to the GMFCS. A validated measure in individuals with CP, MACS is designed to describe how children aged 4 to 18 typically use both hands and upper extremities in daily activities; It is a simple, five-level classification system similar in nature to the GMFCS (Eliasson et al., 2006; Paulson & Vargus-Adams, 2017).

Mini Manual Ability Classification System (Mini-MACS)

The Mini Manual Ability Classification System (Mini-MACS) is designed to classify the manual abilities of children aged 4 years and younger. Due to the rapidly progressive developmental nature of manual ability in the early years of life, the importance of age-related perspective and classification criteria has been reported (Eliasson et al., 2017).

Communication Function Classification System (CFCS)

The Communication Function Classification System (CFCS) is a validated measure for assessing daily communication performance in individuals with CP. The CFCS is designed to be similar to and complementary with the Gross Motor Function Classification System (GMFCS) and MACS; it is a five-level, simple, and sequential classification system (Hidecker et al., 2011).

Eating and Drinking Ability Classification System (EDACS)

The Eating and Drinking Ability Classification System (EDACS) is a validated measure for assessing eating and drinking function in individuals aged 3 years and older with a diagnosis of cerebral palsy (CP). This system is a simple, five-level, sequential classification methodology designed to be similar to and complementary with GMFCS, MACS, and CFCS. EDACS comprehensively assesses both eating and drinking efficiency, such as the amount of food lost and meal duration, as well as safety aspects like aspiration and choking risk (Sellers et al., 2014).

Feeding Disorders in Individuals with Cerebral Palsy

Feeding is a physiological activity of fundamental importance for maintaining individuals' health and ensuring their well-being. This action requires integrated cooperation between the neuromuscular coordination and motor and sensory systems (Fung et al., 2002). In typically developing children, feeding skills follow a stable and sequential pattern of development and are closely related to the acquisition of motor, language, and social development skills (Bartz and Deubler, 1990). In contrast, children with CP often have various oromotor and systemic disorders, as well as incoherent movement patterns that cause feeding difficulties (Aggarwal et al., 2015). Feeding problems are quite common in children with CP. Its prevalence varies significantly across different studies (Dahlseng et al., 2012; Fung et al., 2002; Walker et al., 2012). It has been suggested that this variation reported in the literature may primarily stem from differences in the inclusion criteria used in the studies (age range and motor skill levels) and differences in the diagnostic and technical methodologies adopted in the assessment of feeding disorders. It has been reported that feeding problems are more common in early childhood and in individuals with moderate to severe forms of CP (higher GMFCS levels) (Aggarwal et al., 2015).

FACTORS AFFECTING FEEDING DISORDERS IN INDIVIDUALS WITH CEREBRAL PALSY

Oral Motor Dysfunction (OMD)

Oromotor dysfunction is commonly seen in children with CP. It has been reported to affect more than 90% of children with CP (Reilly et al., 1996). Oral motor dysfunction reflects deficiencies in the timing, coordination, range, and strength of oral movements (Blackmore et al., 2016). Common clinical presentations of OMD include difficulties with sucking and swallowing, drooling, incomplete closure of the lips, and insensitivity/hypersensitivity around the mouth. Less common types include tongue thrusting, limited tongue movement, persistent biting reflex, jaw instability, poor respiratory coordination, weak gag reflex, lip retraction, and primitive chewing reflex (Sjakti et al., 2008).

Severity of Gross Motor Impairment

There is consensus in the literature that there is a direct and positive correlation between the severity of feeding disorders and the level of gross motor impairment (Sjakti et al., 2008; Reilly et al., 1996; Gangil et al., 2001).

Type of CP

The prevalence and severity of feeding disorders differ significantly among different types of CP. The literature reports that children with spastic quadriplegia experience dysphagia at a higher rate than children diagnosed with diplegia (Arvedson, 2013). Erkin et al. classified CP types as diplegic, hemiplegic, and quadriplegic and noted that feeding disorders and gastrointestinal problems were statistically significantly more prevalent in the quadriplegic group (Erkin et al., 2010).

Speech and Communication Disorders

The literature has linked speech intelligibility to feeding disorders. It has been observed that children with normal or mild speech intelligibility have better feeding abilities than children with severe speech disorders. One study reported that the rate of gastrostomy increased as the level of speech intelligibility decreased (Dahlseng et al., 2012).

Postural problems

An effective feeding process depends on good posture control. Neck hyperextension causes tongue retraction, downward pressure on the jawbone, swallowing disorders, and increased aspiration tendency (Larnert and Ekberg, 1995; Rose et al., 2002; Aggarwal et al., 2015). Postural abnormalities observed in children with CP have been identified as a critical factor that significantly impairs feeding abilities. Decreased posture control has been reported to increase feeding and swallowing dysfunction. In the physiological mechanism of this relationship, it has been stated that head stability is vital for jaw control and that jaw control is indirectly dependent on trunk and pelvic alignment (Redstone et al., 2004).

SWALLOWING DISORDERS IN INDIVIDUALS WITH CEREBRAL PALSY

Oropharyngeal dysphagia (OPD) is defined as a disorder of the oral-preparatory, oral (propulsive), and/or pharyngeal phases of swallowing related to eating, drinking, or saliva control (Matsuo and Pamer, 2008). OPD causes impairment in all stages of swallowing physiology: oral, pharyngeal, and esophageal. The persistence of primitive reflexes such as sucking and chewing prevents bolus formation and safe swallowing (Hirata and Santos et al., 2012). These difficulties are exacerbated by inadequate nutrition and hydration, resulting in long and stressful meal times (Çalış et al., 2008).

OPD is reported in the literature as an important factor affecting growth, nutritional status, and respiration in children diagnosed with CP (Benfer et al., 2013). OPD is commonly seen in the pediatric population with CP. OPD is reported in 22% to 99% of children with CP (Çalış et al., 2008; Parkes et al., 2010). It has been reported that 85% of children with CP aged 18 to 36 months have OPD (Benfer et al., 2013). There is broad consensus in the literature that there is a positive correlation between the prevalence and severity of OPD and the level of gross motor impairment. This indicates that as motor impairment assessed by the GMFCS increases, oral motor control and swallowing safety are also put at risk or impaired to the same extent (Fung et al., 2002; Reilly et al., 1996).

The severity of OPD in children with CP exhibits a significant and systematic correlation with the GMFCS levels. Literature provides evidence regarding this stepwise relationship; for instance, children with the most limited mobility (GMFCS V) have been found to have a 17.9-fold increased risk of OPD compared to those with higher levels of functional independence (GMFCS I-II) (Benfer et al., 2013). In cahoots with severe motor impairment, the prevalence of dysphagia reaches nearly

99%, with 76% of these cases classified as moderate-to-severe (Calis et al., 2008). Furthermore, clinical evaluations indicate that children at GMFCS levels IV and V manifest significantly higher rates of swallowing abnormalities, including a 50% incidence of aspiration, compared to only 14.3% in those with mild-to-moderate motor involvement (Kim et al., 2013). As motor function declines, the complexity and severity of dysphagia escalate, necessitating intensive and specialized nutritional monitoring.

Oral Phase Problems

The oral phase forms the basis of feeding physiology. This phase involves the individual's arousal to the bolus, the processes of bolus intake (scooping with a spoon, biting, or sucking/sipping), and the closure of the lips and nasopharynx to hold food/liquid in the mouth. It also involves manipulation of the bolus within the mouth (including chewing) to prepare it for swallowing and posterior propulsion to initiate the pharyngeal phase (Matsuo and Palmer, 2008). Oral phase disorders are the most emphasized swallowing phase in feeding literature and clinical assessments, partly because they are directly observable. The clinical significance of the oral phase primarily stems from its impact on the efficiency of nutrient intake; for example, prolongation of the oral transit time of food or liquids can lead to inadequate growth and malnutrition. Impairment of the oral phase can cause early bolus spillage into the pharynx before swallowing begins, fragmented swallowing, and residual material remaining in the mouth after swallowing; all of which can negatively affect swallowing safety (Benfer et al., 2014).

Oral phase problems are extremely common in children with CP. It has been reported that 93.8% of children with CP have directly assessed oral phase disorders. Difficulty biting, cleaning behaviors, difficulty chewing, and difficulty sipping from a cup are among the most common symptoms (Benfer et al., 2014). The severity of oral phase problems has been associated with the level of gross motor function (Benfer et al., 2013).

Pharyngeal Phase Problems

The pharyngeal phase encompasses a complex series of sensory and motor responses that occur during the passage of food or liquid through the pharynx (Matsuo and Palmer, 2008). The pharynx is a common anatomical intersection point that serves both swallowing and respiratory functions. Therefore, airway protection applied before, during, and after bolus passage through the pharynx to prevent aspiration is of vital importance for the individual's pulmonary health (Lefton-Greif and McGrath-Morrow, 2007; Benfer et al., 2015).

Pharyngeal phase problems are quite common in children with CP (Benfer et al., 2013). A study with children with CP reported that common clinical symptoms included coughing (44.7%), multiple swallows (25.2%), wheezing (20.3%), and wet breathing (18.7%) (Benfer et al., 2015). The severity of pharyngeal phase problems has been associated with the level of gross motor function (Benfer et al., 2013).

The Effects Of Swallowing Disorders On Individuals And Families

Concerns regarding dysphagia observed in children diagnosed with cerebral palsy are multifactorial and are not limited to a decrease in the volume of food and liquids consumed orally. This situation also includes problems with a limited range of food textures due to nutritional deficiencies, inadequate hydration, and slow progress in oral motor skills. These clinical outcomes create a complex risk profile that negatively affects the individual's overall growth curve and quality of life. Feeding and swallowing disorders can clinically cause inadequate growth, prolonged mealtimes, delayed acquisition of oral feeding skills, and/or recurrent respiratory tract illnesses. These symptoms can create a multidimensional clinical picture indicating an increased risk of malnutrition and pulmonary morbidity (Arvedson, 2013).

Feeding and swallowing disorders observed in children diagnosed with cerebral palsy are more than just a physiological problem; they cause significant psychological, nutritional, and social difficulties that deeply affect families. Research shows that a significant percentage of children with CP experience swallowing difficulties, which have serious negative effects on their quality of life (Calderone et al., 2025). This situation leads caregivers to experience high levels of mood disorders and chronic stress directly related to managing complex feeding difficulties (Umay et al., 2019). These disorders not only increase the risk of malnutrition and dehydration, but also negatively affect family dynamics, social interactions, and overall quality of life (Andrew et al., 2012). The psychological burden reported by caregivers is quite heavy, and they have reported significant anxiety and disruptions in their daily activities (Lefton-Greif et al., 2014). To alleviate these multidimensional challenges and support affected families, adopting comprehensive and interdisciplinary intervention approaches is critical.

ASSESSMENT OF FEEDING AND SWALLOWING DISORDERS IN INDIVIDUALS WITH CEREBRAL PALSY

Clinical Assessment Of Feeding And Swallowing Disorders In Individuals With Cerebral Palsy

The assessment of feeding and swallowing disorders in individuals diagnosed with cerebral palsy is critically important due to the high prevalence of these disorders and their significant clinical effects on health. The literature indicates that more than 90% of children with CP have clinically significant oromotor dysfunction and that 36.2% are severely disabled individuals at risk of chronic malnutrition (Reilly et al., 1996). It is emphasized that these disorders negatively affect growth, overall health, social interaction, and developmental outcomes (Andrew et al., 2012).

Table 3 lists clinically critical basic questions that should be directed to parents/caregivers to identify the risk of feeding and swallowing disorders in children with cerebral palsy and to determine the need for a comprehensive assessment (Arvedson, 2013).

Table 3. Questions to Ask Parents/Caregivers to Determine the Need for a Comprehensive Assessment of Feeding and Swallowing Disorders in Children with Cerebral Palsy

Questions	Red flags
How long does it take to feed your child?	More than 30 min, on any regular basis
Are meal times stressful to child or parent?	Yes, if one or other, or both
Is your child gaining weight adequately?	Lack of weight gain over 2–3 months in young child, not just weight loss
Are there signs of respiratory problems?	Increased congestion at meal times, 'gurgly' voice, respiratory illnesses

A comprehensive assessment is best conducted using a multidisciplinary approach involving pediatricians, neurologists, speech and language pathologists, and other specialists (Santoro et al., 2012;). Common assessment indicators include a systematic analysis of basic skills, particularly sucking, swallowing, postural control, and oral motor function (Yılmaz et al., 2004). Early diagnosis and appropriate intervention play a key role in achieving meaningful improvement in both the child's health and nutritional status (Aggarwal et al., 2015). The clinical assessment of feeding and swallowing disorders in children with CP is presented in Table 4.

Table 4. Clinical Assessment of Feeding and Swallowing Disorders in Children with Cerebral Palsy

Assessment Area	Observation Points	Purpose
Medical History		
Developmental & Medical History	Prenatal/birth history, previous surgical procedures, current medication use	Identification of etiological factors and comorbidities
Early Feeding History	Breastfeeding/bottle-feeding process, timing and type of transition to solid foods, onset of feeding difficulties.	Determining the origin of pathological feeding patterns and developmental delays
Current Dietary Patterns	Type of food and liquids taken orally, details of oral nutritional supplements or tube feeding (enteral nutrition), typical meal volume and frequency.	Quantitative determination of nutritional adequacy and hydration status
Clinical Observation and Functional Assessment		
Posture and Physiological Stability	Postural control during rest and feeding, body and pelvic alignment, observation of physiological stability (breathing pattern)	Examination of the effect of proximal stability on jaw and oral motor control
Oromotor and Sensory Assessment	Observation of facial and oral cavity structures during rest/movement, presence/persistence of oral reflexes (primitive/protective reflexes), level of oral sensitivity	Identification of mechanical and neurological components of oral phase dysfunction
Functional Skill Analysis	Examination of sucking, chewing, and swallowing skills; evaluation of the performance of structures during non-feeding tasks.	Determination of impaired stages of swallowing physiology and bolus manipulation capacity
Intervention and Interaction Observation		
Experimental Feeding Applications	Testing foods and liquids of varying consistencies/ quantities, testing different positioning and feeding equipment (spoon, cup).	Clinically testing the safest and most efficient feeding strategies.
Social and Behavioral Interaction	Observation of child behavior during meal times and meals, assessment of parent-child interaction and parent stress levels.	Determining the psychosocial and behavioral dimensions of feeding disorders and their impact on quality of life.

Children diagnosed with cerebral palsy exhibit complex and multidimensional dysfunctions in motor, sensory, and behavioral areas. In this context, it is imperative to implement protective and preventive methods before secondary complications (malnutrition, aspiration pneumonia, etc.) arise. Therefore, early and comprehensive clinical assessments are of vital importance (Akbaş, 2016). Some of the tools that can be used during the nutrition and swallowing assessment of children with cerebral palsy are listed in Table 5.

Table 5. Tools That Can Be Used During the Feeding and Swallowing Assessment of Children with Cerebral Palsy

Pediatric Eating Assessment Tool (Pedi-EAT-10) (Serel Arslan et al., 2018a)	**A quick screening tool consisting of 10 items that assesses the severity and frequency of feeding difficulties in children.**
Karaduman Chewing Performance Scale (KCPS) (Serel Arslan et al., 2018b)	A detailed tool based on observing the quality, efficiency, and motor patterns of chewing function during feeding.
Drooling Severity and Frequency Scale (DSFS) (Thomas-Stonell and Greenberg, 1988)	It assesses both the frequency and severity of drooling to determine the need for clinical intervention.
Behavioral Pediatric Feeding Assessment Scale (BPFAS) (Crist, W., & Napier-Phillips, 2001)	Focuses on assessing the behavioral and interactive aspects of feeding difficulties, namely parent-child interaction and the child's responses.
Tongue Thrust Rating Scale (Serel Arslan et al., 2017)	Used to rate the severity of abnormal tongue thrust patterns observed in children.

INSTRUMENTAL ASSESSMENT OF FEEDING AND SWALLOWING DISORDERS IN INDIVIDUALS WITH CEREBRAL PALSY

Instrumental assessment of feeding and swallowing disorders in children diagnosed with cerebral palsy is critical for comprehensively examining swallowing function and preventing potential health complications (Samy et al., 2024). These assessment methods play a vital role, considering that children with CP experience oromotor dysfunction at a high rate, which carries serious risks such as aspiration, malnutrition, and long-term feeding difficulties (Santoro et al., 2012). The main instrumental assessment techniques are as follows:

Video Fluoroscopic Swallowing Study (VFSS): This is the gold standard method that provides dynamic visualization of the oral, pharyngeal, and upper esophageal phases of swallowing. It is used for the definitive diagnosis of aspiration and to identify the mechanism of physiological dysfunction (Samy et al., 2024).

Flexible Endoscopic Swallowing Evaluation (FEES):_This allows direct examination of pharyngeal and laryngeal structures without radiation exposure. This method evaluates pre- and post-swallow residue and penetration/aspiration status (Reynolds, 2020).

Ultrasonography: A technique with the potential to quantitatively assess oral and laryngeal swallowing phases. It allows for the numerical measurement of movement ranges and timing (Samy et al., 2024).

INTERVENTION FOR FEEDING AND SWALLOWING DISORDERS IN INDIVIDUALS WITH CEREBRAL PALSY

Enteral Nutrition (EN)

Enteral nutrition (EN) serves as a critical intervention for providing essential macro- and micronutrients to individuals who are unable to meet their nutritional requirements through oral intake. In the context CP, EN is utilized as a vital supportive strategy for both short-term and long-term management. The selection of the delivery site—either gastric or post-pyloric—and the specific type of feeding tube is dictated by the anticipated duration of therapy and the patient's physiological needs. In children with CP, the requirement for EN is strongly correlated with the severity of motor impairment. As the GMFCS levels increase, the prevalence of gastrostomy tube (GT) feeding significantly rises. Specifically, research has reported GT feeding rates of 12% for GMFCS level III, 24% for level IV, and 72% for level V (Marpole et al., 2020). Within this clinical spectrum, children at GMFCS level V who utilize feeding tubes represent a particularly vulnerable cohort, facing the most significant health challenges (Trivić & Hojsak, 2019a). Furthermore, suggests that children supported by GT feeding typically exhibit lower energy expenditure and higher body fat percentages compared to their orally fed peers (Sullivan et al., 2000; Liptak et al., 2001). Given these associations, a multidisciplinary approach is essential, emphasizing early nutritional assessment and the potential for gastrostomy placement in children presenting with dysphagia and inadequate oral intake.

Ideally, nutritional assessment should be conducted by a multidisciplinary team comprising a pediatric gastroenterologist, dietitian, nurse, speech and language pathologist (SLP), physiotherapist, occupational therapist, and psychologist (Trivić & Hojsak, 2019b). A comprehensive nutritional evaluation, including body composition analysis, anthropometric measurements, and laboratory assessments, serves as a prerequisite for clinical intervention (Romano et al., 2017). Consistent with protocols for typically developing children, nutritional support should initially focus on dietary recommendations and oral intake modifications, provided they are safe and acceptable. However, in cases of unsafe swallowing or insufficient oral intake for long-term maintenance, enteral nutrition should be initiated, and early gastrostomy placement should be evaluated in consultation with parents or caregivers. Furthermore, gastrointestinal comorbidities—such as oropharyngeal dysfunction, gastroesophageal reflux disease, and constipation—are prevalent in children with CP. As these conditions can exacerbate nutritional status and feeding efficacy, they must be proactively identified and effectively managed (Romano et al., 2017; Trivić & Hojsak, 2019b).

In the field of rehabilitation, various intervention strategies have been developed to improve feeding efficiency and safety by developing oral-motor skills. These interventions can be broadly categorized into two main approaches: disorder-based and adaptive approaches:

Disorder-Based Approaches

Sensorimotor Techniques

Sensory-motor techniques aimed at increasing oral-motor control seek to decrease or increase muscle tone and inhibit abnormal reflexes that interfere with safe feeding. Additionally, training and strengthening oral muscles provides more opportunities to learn and practice feeding skills (Ganz, 1988; Snider et al., 2011). Sensory-motor approaches are used to facilitate lip closure, tongue lateralization, and rotational chewing, inhibit the tongue thrust reflex, reduce tactile hypersensitivity, and promote swallowing (Ganz, 1988; Ongkasuwan and Chiou, 2018; Snider et al., 2011).

Therapeutic applications in premature infants

- Oral stimulation
- Non-nutritive sucking
- Orocutaneous stimulation
- Oral support

Modified Beckman Oral Motor Intervention (BOMI) [Premature Infant Oral Motor Intervention (PIOMI)]

Sensory-motor methods that facilitate feeding performance in children with CP

- Lip control
- Tongue lateralization
- Strengthening chewing
- Jaw support

Apply pressure to the face and mouth muscles by hand, using a tool such as a NUK oral massage brush or an electric toothbrush

- Castillo-Morales
- Beckman Oral Motor Intervention (BOMI)
- Functional Chewing Training
- Innsbruck Sensorimotor Activator and Regulator (ISMAR)

Positioning Techniques

Poor postural alignment and decreased postural control often exacerbate feeding and swallowing disorders. Positioning techniques include applications such as stabilization of the neck and trunk, forward neck flexion, or supported lying positions to promote more effective eating behaviors (Redstone and West, 2004; Snider et al., 2011).

Adaptive Approaches

Adaptive interventions increase safety and efficiency by modifying the feeding environment or method rather than changing the child's skills. Adaptive equipment recommendations include modified pacifiers/nipples, cut cups, weighted forks and spoons, angled forks and spoons, and non-spill bowls (ASHA, 2025).

Oral Appliances

Oral appliances are used to improve orofacial sensorimotor functions such as sucking, coordination, chewing, and swallowing. Initially used for jaw stabilization, they are followed by applications aimed at activating and mobilizing oral and pharyngeal structures (Snider et al., 2011).

Modifying Food Consistency

Modifying food consistency is another important intervention strategy that affects chewing and swallowing abilities in children with CP (Snider et al., 2011). In the management of pediatric dysphagia among children with CP, modifying food and liquid consistency is fundamental to ensuring safe and efficient oral intake. To establish standardized terminology and clinical practice, the International Dysphagia Diet Standardisation Initiative (IDDSI) framework is utilized. The IDDSI pediatric framework provides an 8-level (0–7) continuum, ranging from Level 0 (Thin) to Level 4 (Extremely Thick) for liquids, and Level 3 (Liquidised) to Level 7 (Regular) for foods. Implementation of these internationally recognized standards facilitates precise communication between healthcare providers and caregivers, ultimately mitigating the risk of aspiration and enhancing nutritional outcomes (IDDSI, 2019).

Electronic Feeding Devices

Electronic feeding devices can promote self-feeding independence but also require the child's active participation. Such adaptive devices help overcome functional limitations (Snider et al., 2011).

CONCLUSION

Feeding and swallowing disorders observed in individuals with Cerebral Palsy are not merely isolated physiological problems stemming from motor deficits; they also bring about multidimensional secondary consequences such as growth retardation, malnutrition, and recurrent respiratory tract diseases. Effectively managing this complex risk profile exceeds the competence of a single specialty. Therefore, the success of early diagnosis, comprehensive clinical/instrumental assessment, and targeted intervention strategies in CP depends on adopting a multidisciplinary approach. The synergistic knowledge provided by different specialties allows for the simultaneous addressing of the child's motor, sensory-motor, psychosocial, and neurological needs. This integrated approach is essential for maximizing the quality of life and developmental potential of individuals with CP by enabling the individualization and continuous monitoring of both disorder-based and adaptive interventions.

REFERENCES

Aggarwal, S., Chadha, R. K., & Pathak, R. (2015). Feeding difficulties among children with cerebral palsy: A review. *International Journal of Health Sciences and Research, 5*(10), 297–308.

Akbas, A. N. (2016). *Assessments and outcome measures of cerebral palsy*. InTech., DOI: 10.5772/64254

Alireza, S., Amirsalari, S., Hollisaz, M. T., Rahimnia, A., & Khatibi-Aghda, A. (2014). Management of spasticity in children with cerebral palsy. *Iranian Journal of Pediatrics, 24*(4), 345–351. PMID: 25755853

American Speech-Language-Hearing Association. (2025). *Pediatric feeding and swallowing*. (Practice Portal). https://www.asha.org/practice-portal/clinical-topics/pediatric-dysphagia/

Andrew, M. J., Parr, J. R., & Sullivan, P. B. (2012). Feeding difficulties in children with cerebral palsy. *Archives of Disease in Childhood - Education and Practice, 97*(6), 222–229. DOI: 10.1136/archdischild-2011-300914 PMID: 22293504

Arvedson, J. C. (2013). Feeding children with cerebral palsy and swallowing difficulties. *European Journal of Clinical Nutrition, 67*(Suppl 2), S9–S12. DOI: 10.1038/ejcn.2013.224 PMID: 24301008

Bartz, A. H., & Deubler, D. C. (1990). Identification of feeding and nutrition problems in young children with neuromotor involvement: A self-assessment. *Journal of Pediatric & Perinatal Nutrition, 2*(2), 1–15. DOI: 10.1300/j290v02n02_01 PMID: 1703568

Benfer, K. A., Weir, K. A., Bell, K. L., Ware, R. S., Davies, P. S., & Boyd, R. N. (2013). Oropharyngeal dysphagia and gross motor skills in children with cerebral palsy. *Pediatrics, 131*(5), e1553–e1562. DOI: 10.1542/peds.2012-3093 PMID: 23589816

Benfer, K. A., Weir, K. A., Bell, K. L., Ware, R. S., Davies, P. S., & Boyd, R. N. (2014). Oropharyngeal dysphagia in preschool children with cerebral palsy: Oral phase impairments. *Research in Developmental Disabilities, 35*(12), 3469–3481. DOI: 10.1016/j.ridd.2014.08.029 PMID: 25213472

Benfer, K. A., Weir, K. A., Bell, K. L., Ware, R. S., Davies, P. S., & Boyd, R. N. (2015). Clinical signs suggestive of pharyngeal dysphagia in preschool children with cerebral palsy. *Research in Developmental Disabilities, 38*, 192–201. DOI: 10.1016/j.ridd.2014.12.021 PMID: 25562439

Blackmore, A. M., Bear, N., Blair, E., Gibson, N., Jalla, C., Langdon, K., Moshovis, L., Steer, K., & Wilson, A. C. (2016). Factors associated with respiratory ıllness in children and young adults with cerebral palsy. *The Journal of Pediatrics*, *168*, 151–157.e1. DOI: 10.1016/j.jpeds.2015.09.064 PMID: 26520916

Calderone, A., Militi, D., Cardile, D., Corallo, F., Calabrò, R. S., & Militi, A. (2025). Swallowing disorders in cerebral palsy: A systematic review of oropharyngeal dysphagia, nutritional impact, and health risks. *Italian Journal of Pediatrics*, *51*(1), 57. DOI: 10.1186/s13052-025-01903-1 PMID: 39985076

Calis, E. A., Veugelers, R., Sheppard, J. J., Tibboel, D., Evenhuis, H. M., & Penning, C. (2008). Dysphagia in children with severe generalized cerebral palsy and intellectual disability. *Developmental Medicine and Child Neurology*, *50*(8), 625–630. DOI: 10.1111/j.1469-8749.2008.03047.x PMID: 18754902

Christine, C., Dolk, H., Platt, M. J., Colver, A., Prasauskiene, A., & Krägeloh-Mann, I.SCPE Collaborative Group. (2007). Recommendations from the SCPE collaborative group for defining and classifying cerebral palsy. *Developmental Medicine and Child Neurology. Supplement*, *109*, 35–38. DOI: 10.1111/j.1469-8749.2007.tb12626.x PMID: 17370480

Crist, W., & Napier-Phillips, A. (2001). Mealtime behaviors of young children: A comparison of normative and clinical data. *Journal of Developmental and Behavioral Pediatrics: JDBP*, *22*(5), 279–286. DOI: 10.1097/00004703-200110000-00001 PMID: 11718230

Dahlseng, M. O., Finbråten, A. K., Júlíusson, P. B., Skranes, J., Andersen, G., & Vik, T. (2012). Feeding problems, growth and nutritional status in children with cerebral palsy. *Acta Paediatrica (Oslo, Norway)*, *101*(1), 92–98. DOI: 10.1111/j.1651-2227.2011.02412.x PMID: 21767308

Eliasson, A. C., Krumlinde-Sundholm, L., Rösblad, B., Beckung, E., Arner, M., Ohrvall, A. M., & Rosenbaum, P. (2006). The Manual Ability Classification System (MACS) for children with cerebral palsy: Scale development and evidence of validity and reliability. *Developmental Medicine and Child Neurology*, *48*(7), 549–554. DOI: 10.1017/S0012162206001162 PMID: 16780622

Eliasson, A. C., Ullenhag, A., Wahlström, U., & Krumlinde-Sundholm, L. (2017). Mini-MACS: Development of the Manual Ability Classification System for children younger than 4 years of age with signs of cerebral palsy. *Developmental Medicine and Child Neurology*, *59*(1), 72–78. DOI: 10.1111/dmcn.13162 PMID: 27273427

Erkin, G., Culha, C., Ozel, S., & Kirbiyik, E. G. (2010). Feeding and gastrointestinal problems in children with cerebral palsy. *International Journal of Rehabilitation Research. Internationale Zeitschrift fur Rehabilitationsforschung. Revue Internationale de Recherches de Readaptation*, *33*(3), 218–224. DOI: 10.1097/MRR.0b013e3283375e10 PMID: 20216224

Fung, E. B., Samson-Fang, L., Stallings, V. A., Conaway, M., Liptak, G., Henderson, R. C., Worley, G., O'Donnell, M., Calvert, R., Rosenbaum, P., Chumlea, W., & Stevenson, R. D. (2002). Feeding dysfunction is associated with poor growth and health status in children with cerebral palsy. *Journal of the American Dietetic Association*, *102*(3), 361–373. DOI: 10.1016/s0002-8223(02)90084-2 PMID: 11902369

Gangil, A., Patwari, A. K., Aneja, S., Ahuja, B., & Anand, V. K. (2001). Feeding problems in children with cerebral palsy. *Indian Pediatrics*, *38*(8), 839–846. PMID: 11520994

Ganz, S. F. (1988). Decreasing tongue thrusting and tonic bite reflex through nueromotor and sensory facilitation techniques. *Physical & Occupational Therapy in Pediatrics*, *7*(4), 57–76.

Hidecker, M. J., Paneth, N., Rosenbaum, P. L., Kent, R. D., Lillie, J., Eulenberg, J. B., Chester, K.Jr, Johnson, B., Michalsen, L., Evatt, M., & Taylor, K. (2011). Developing and validating the Communication Function Classification System for individuals with cerebral palsy. *Developmental Medicine and Child Neurology*, *53*(8), 704–710. DOI: 10.1111/j.1469-8749.2011.03996.x PMID: 21707596

Hirata, G. C., & Santos, R. S. (2012). Rehabilitation of oropharyngeal dysphagia in children with cerebral palsy: A systematic review of the speech therapy approach. *International Archives of Otorhinolaryngology*, *16*(3), 396–399. DOI: 10.7162/S1809-97772012000300016 PMID: 25991964

International Dysphagia Diet Standardisation Initiative. (2019). Complete IDDSI framework: Detailed definitions. https://iddsi.org/framework/

Jones, M. W., Morgan, E., Shelton, J. E., & Thorogood, C. (2007). Cerebral palsy: Introduction and diagnosis (Part I). *Journal of Pediatric Health Care*, *21*(3), 146–152. DOI: 10.1016/j.pedhc.2006.06.007 PMID: 17478303

Kim, J. S., Han, Z. A., Song, D. H., Oh, H. M., & Chung, M. E. (2013). Characteristics of dysphagia in children with cerebral palsy, related to GMFCS level. *American Journal of Physical Medicine & Rehabilitation*, *92*(10), 912–919. DOI: 10.1097/PHM.0b013e31829b4ad0 PMID: 23739271

Larnert, G., & Ekberg, O. (1995). Positioning improves the oral and pharyngeal swallowing function in children with cerebral palsy. *Acta Paediatrica (Oslo, Norway)*, *84*(6), 689–692. DOI: 10.1111/j.1651-2227.1995.tb13730.x PMID: 7670257

Lefton-Greif, M. A., & McGrath-Morrow, S. A. (2007). Deglutition and respiration: Development, coordination, and practical implications. *Seminars in Speech and Language*, *28*(3), 166–179. DOI: 10.1055/s-2007-984723 PMID: 17647129

Lefton-Greif, M. A., Okelo, S. O., Wright, J. M., Collaco, J. M., McGrath-Morrow, S. A., & Eakin, M. N. (2014). Impact of children's feeding/swallowing problems: Validation of a new caregiver instrument. *Dysphagia*, *29*(6), 671–677. DOI: 10.1007/s00455-014-9560-7 PMID: 25159316

Liptak, G. S., O'Donnell, M., Conaway, M., Chumlea, W. C., Wolrey, G., Henderson, R. C., & Stevenson, R. D. (2001). Health status of children with moderate to severe cerebral palsy. *Developmental Medicine and Child Neurology*, *43*(6), 364–370. PMID: 11409824

MacLennan, A. H., Thompson, S. C., & Gecz, J. (2015). Cerebral palsy: Causes, pathways, and the role of genetic variants. *American Journal of Obstetrics and Gynecology*, *213*(6), 779–788. DOI: 10.1016/j.ajog.2015.05.034 PMID: 26003063

Marpole, R. M., Blackmore, A. M., Gibson, N., Cooper, M. S., Langdon, K., & Wilson, A. C. (2020). Evaluation and management of respiratory illness in children with cerebral palsy. *Frontiers in Pediatrics*, *8*, 333. PMID: 32671000

Matsuo, K., & Palmer, J. B. (2008). Anatomy and physiology of feeding and swallowing: Normal and abnormal. *Physical Medicine and Rehabilitation Clinics of North America*, *19*(4), 691–707. PMID: 18940636

Michael-Asalu, A., Taylor, G., Campbell, H., Lelea, L. L., & Kirby, R. S. (2019). Cerebral Palsy: Diagnosis, Epidemiology, Genetics, and Clinical Update. *Advances in Pediatrics*, *66*, 189–208. DOI: 10.1016/j.yapd.2019.04.002 PMID: 31230694

National Institute of Neurological Disorders and Stroke. (2025). *Cerebral palsy: Hope through research.* https://www.ninds.nih.gov/Disorders/Patient-Caregiver-Education/Hope-Through-Research/Cerebral-Palsy-Hope-Through-Research

Nelson, K. B. (2008). Causative Factors in Cerebral Palsy. *Clinical Obstetrics and Gynecology*, *51*(4), 749–762. PMID: 18981800

Olszak, J., Zalewa, K., Budzyński, R., Kamieniak, A., Klepacz, N., Czuba, A., Poleszczuk, M., Poleszczuk, K., Milewska, A., & Kaus, M. (2025). Cerebral Palsy - A Comprehensive Analysis of the Causes. *Journal of Education, Health and Sport*.

Ongkasuwan, J., & Chiou, E. H. (Eds.). (2018). *Pediatric dysphagia: Challenges and controversies*. Springer.

Palisano, R., Rosenbaum, P., Bartlett, D., Livingston, M., Walter, S., & Russell, D. G. E. R. (2007). *CanChild centre for childhood disability research*. McMaster University.

Palisano, R., Rosenbaum, P., Walter, S., Russell, D., Wood, E., & Galuppi, B. (1997). Development and reliability of a system to classify gross motor function in children with cerebral palsy. *Developmental Medicine and Child Neurology*, *39*(4), 214–223. PMID: 9183258

Parkes, J., Hill, N., Platt, M. J., & Donnelly, C. (2010). Oromotor dysfunction and communication impairments in children with cerebral palsy: A register study. *Developmental Medicine and Child Neurology*, *52*(12), 1113–1119. DOI: 10.1111/j.1469-8749.2010.03765.x PMID: 20813020

Patel, D. R., Neelakantan, M., Pandher, K., & Merrick, J. (2020). Cerebral palsy in children: A clinical overview. *Translational Pediatrics*, *9*(Suppl 1), S125–S135. DOI: 10.21037/tp.2020.01.01 PMID: 32206590

Paulson, A., & Vargus-Adams, J. (2017). Overview of four functional classification systems commonly used in cerebral palsy. *Children (Basel, Switzerland)*, *4*(4), 30. DOI: 10.3390/children4040030 PMID: 28441773

Redstone, F., & West, J. F. (2004). The importance of postural control for feeding. *Pediatric Nursing*, *30*(2), 97–100. PMID: 15185730

Reilly, S., Skuse, D., & Poblete, X. (1996). Prevalence of feeding problems and oral motor dysfunction in children with cerebral palsy: A community survey. *The Journal of Pediatrics*, *129*(6), 877–882. DOI: 10.1016/s0022-3476(96)70032-x PMID: 8969730

Reynolds, J. (2020). When a child needs an instrumental swallowing assessment: How do clinicians know when it's time to move to an instrumental assessment and then choose the most appropriate one? *ASHA Leader*, *25*(1), 40–42.

Romano, C., Van Wynckel, M., Hulst, J., Broekaert, I., Bronsky, J., Dall'Oglio, L., & Gottrand, F. (2017). European Society for Paediatric Gastroenterology, Hepatology and Nutrition guidelines for the evaluation and treatment of gastrointestinal and nutritional complications in children with neurological impairment. *Journal of Pediatric Gastroenterology and Nutrition*, *65*(2), 242–264. PMID: 28737572

Rose, J., Wolff, D. R., Jones, V. K., Bloch, D. A., Oehlert, J. W., & Gamble, J. G. (2002). Postural balance in children with cerebral palsy. *Developmental Medicine and Child Neurology*, *44*(1), 58–63. DOI: 10.1017/s0012162201001669 PMID: 11811652

Rosenbaum, P., Paneth, N., Leviton, A., Goldstein, M., Bax, M., Damiano, D., & Jacobsson, B. (2007). A report: The definition and classification of cerebral palsy April 2006. *Developmental Medicine and Child Neurology. Supplement*, *109*(suppl 109), 8–14. PMID: 17370477

Rosenbaum, P. L., Palisano, R. J., Bartlett, D. J., Galuppi, B. E., & Russell, D. J. (2008). Development of the gross motor function classification system for cerebral palsy. *Developmental Medicine and Child Neurology*, *50*(4), 249–253. PMID: 18318732

Samy, H., Alawy, A. A., Ibrahim, A. F., Elsayed, S. M., Serag, A., Deen, E., & Abd-Elmonem, A. M. (2024). Objective Methods for Feeding Assessment in Children with Cerebral Palsy: Narrative Review. *The Egyptian Journal of Hospital Medicine*.

Santoro, A., Lang, M. B., Moretti, E., Sellari-Franceschini, S., Orazini, L., Cipriani, P., Cioni, G., & Battini, R. (2012). A proposed multidisciplinary approach for ıdentifying feeding abnormalities in children with cerebral palsy. *Journal of Child Neurology*, *27*(6), 708–712. PMID: 22019841

Sellers, D., Mandy, A., Pennington, L., Hankins, M., & Morris, C. (2014). Development and reliability of a system to classify the eating and drinking ability of people with cerebral palsy.

Serel Arslan, S., Aydın, G., Alemdaroğlu, I., Tunca Yılmaz, Ö., & Karaduman, A. A. (2018b). Reliability and validity of the Karaduman Chewing Performance Scale in paediatric neuromuscular diseases: A system for classification of chewing disorders. *Journal of Oral Rehabilitation*, *45*(7), 526–531. DOI: 10.1111/joor.12642 PMID: 29727486

Serel Arslan, S., Demir, N., & Karaduman, A. A. (2017). Reliability and validity of a tool to measure the severity of tongue thrust in children: The Tongue Thrust Rating Scale. *Journal of Oral Rehabilitation*, *44*(2), 119–124. DOI: 10.1111/joor.12471 PMID: 27973693

Serel Arslan, S., Demir, N., Karaduman, A. A., & Belafsky, P. C. (2018a). The Pediatric Version of the Eating Assessment Tool: A caregiver administered dyphagia-specific outcome instrument for children. *Disability and Rehabilitation*, *40*(17), 2088–2092. DOI: 10.1080/09638288.2017.1323235 PMID: 28475381

Sjakti, H. A., Syarif, D. R., & Wahyuni, L. K., & Chair, Imral. (2008). Feeding difficulties in children with cerebral palsy. *Paediatrica Indonesiana, 48*(4), 224–229. DOI: 10.14238/pi48.4.2008.224-9

Snider, L., Majnemer, A., & Darsaklis, V. (2011). Feeding interventions for children with cerebral palsy: A review of the evidence. *Physical & Occupational Therapy in Pediatrics, 31*(1), 58–77. DOI: 10.3109/01942638.2010.523397 PMID: 20950250

Sullivan, P. B., Lambert, B., Rose, M., Ford-Adams, M., Johnson, A., & Casson, D. H. (2000). Prevalence and severity of feeding and nutritional problems in children with neurological impairment: Oxford Feeding Study. *Developmental Medicine and Child Neurology, 42*(10), 674–680. PMID: 11085295

Surveillance of Cerebral Palsy in Europe (SCPE). (2000). Surveillance of cerebral palsy in Europe: A collaboration of cerebral palsy surveys and registers. *Developmental Medicine and Child Neurology, 42*(12), 816–824. DOI: 10.1017/s0012162200001511 PMID: 11132255

Thomas-Stonell, N., & Greenberg, J. (1988). Three treatment approaches and clinical factors in the reduction of drooling. *Dysphagia, 3*(2), 73–78. PMID: 3271655

Trivić, I., & Hojsak, I. (2019a). Initial evaluation of nursing and feeding difficulties in children with cerebral palsy. *Paediatrics Today (Tuzla), 15*(2).

Trivić, I., & Hojsak, I. (2019b). Evaluation and treatment of malnutrition and associated gastrointestinal complications in children with cerebral palsy. *Pediatric Gastroenterology, Hepatology & Nutrition, 22*(2), 122–131. PMID: 30899688

Umay, E., Gündoğdu, İ., & Öztürk, E. A. (2019). Reliability and validity of the pediatric feeding and swallowing disorders family impact scale for Turkish children with cerebral palsy by endoscopic evaluation. *The Turkish Journal of Pediatrics, 61*(5), 741–748. DOI: 10.24953/turkjped.2019.05.013 PMID: 32105006

Walker, J. L., Bell, K. L., Stevenson, R. D., Weir, K. A., Boyd, R. N., & Davies, P. S. (2012). Relationships between dietary intake and body composition according to gross motor functional ability in preschool-aged children with cerebral palsy. *Annals of Nutrition & Metabolism, 61*(4), 349–357. DOI: 10.1159/000342557 PMID: 23208164

Wu, Y. W., Day, S. M., Strauss, D. J., & Shavelle, R. M. (2004). Prognosis for ambulation in cerebral palsy: A population-based study. *Pediatrics, 114*(5), 1264–1271. DOI: 10.1542/peds.2004-0114 PMID: 15520106

Yilmaz, S., Basar, P., & Gisel, E. G. (2004). Assessment of feeding performance in patients with cerebral palsy. *International Journal of Rehabilitation Research. Internationale Zeitschrift fur Rehabilitationsforschung. Revue Internationale de Recherches de Readaptation, 27*(4), 325–329. DOI: 10.1097/00004356-200412000-00013 PMID: 15572999

Zhou, J., Butler, E. E., & Rose, J. (2017). Neurologic Correlates of Gait Abnormalities in Cerebral Palsy: Implications for Treatment. *Frontiers in Human Neuroscience, 11*, 103. DOI: 10.3389/fnhum.2017.00103 PMID: 28367118

Chapter 10
Simulation-Based Learning in Dysphagia Training

Namık Yücel Birol
http://orcid.org/0000-0001-7155-3591
Cappadocia University, Turkey

ABSTRACT

The practice of simulation-based learning now appears in dysphagia training because it enables healthcare professionals to practice their skills through controlled sessions which help them build their abilities while maintaining patient safety. Simulation provides essential value to competency-based training because traditional placement sites do not guarantee consistent availability of complex swallowing cases. Research findings show that participants who take part in simulated learning activities develop their diagnostic reasoning abilities and their assessment skills and their confidence levels and their communication abilities. The advantages of this technology have been documented in studies which used it for pediatric feeding, adult dysphagia assessment and treatments. The simulation environment enables students to receive directed feedback which enables them to develop their skills through multiple attempts before they interact with actual patients. Through simulation students can develop their clinical judgment while connecting theoretical knowledge to practical applications.

INTRODUCTION

The swallowing disorder known as dysphagia creates swallowing challenges which impact people from birth until old age (Shelat & Pandya, 2015). The condition

DOI: 10.4018/979-8-3373-6405-6.ch010

develops from various causes which include neurological diseases that affect stroke patients and patients with Parkinson's disease and amyotrophic lateral sclerosis and structural problems that result from head and neck cancer and normal aging processes of swallowing functions (Cichero & Murdoch, 2006; Logemann, 1998). Research indicates that dysphagia affects a large number of people because 20-30% of adults aged 50 and above and 50% of stroke survivors develop swallowing problems (Baijens et al., 2016; Martino et al., 2005).

The medical effects of dysphagia create severe problems which include starvation and body fluid depletion and lung infections from food entering the lungs and decreased life satisfaction (Clave & Shaker, 2015). The process of dysphagia management demands immediate critical choices because any wrong decision will result in dangerous medical emergencies (Reverberi et al., 2025). The complex nature of this condition requires speech–language pathologists (SLPs) and other clinicians to develop their diagnostic and therapeutic abilities (Gunasekaran et al., 2024; Hazelwood et al., 2022).

Speech–language pathology education follows a traditional approach which places students in block or weekly clinical settings under individual supervisory guidance for didactic learning and spontaneous clinical experience (Sheepway et al., 2011). The unpredictable nature of clinical exposure leads to inconsistent graduate competency levels (Hill et al., 2013). The educational model of competency-based education (CBE) was developed to address these restrictions because it focuses on teaching students the exact skills and knowledge needed to practice safely and effectively (Iobst, 2015).

The educational framework of competency-based education requires students to receive purposeful practice experience together with feedback and assessment methods which match the actual requirements of clinical practice (Frank et al., 2010). The assessment of swallowing function requires SLPs to perform accurate evaluations while they need to understand how to read results from instrumental tests including videofluoroscopic swallow study (VFSS) and fiberoptic endoscopic evaluation of swallowing (FEES) and they must use proven treatment methods (Brady et al., 2018; Edwards et al., 2024). The current educational system faces difficulties when students need to develop these competencies because it operates under standard educational boundaries (Hazelwood et al., 2022).

Simulation-based learning (SBL) has become a leading educational method in healthcare because it provides students with controlled environments to practice clinical skills without facing actual risks (Issenberg et al., 2005). Interest in SBL has been driven, in part, by rising demands and structural pressures on clinical education programs, including limited access to clinical placements, an expanding scope of practice, and disruptions to traditional training models during global health emergencies (e.g., the COVID-19 pandemic) (Dudding & Ginsberg, 2023). The SBL system enables dysphagia training through its ability to present complex scenarios which students can experience multiple times while receiving instant feedback during their practice of both medical and non-medical abilities (Ward et al., 2015).

Simulation-based education offers students a controlled environment to learn assessment techniques while they experience difficult dysphagia situations which typical clinical training sites cannot provide (Broadfoot & Estis, 2020). SBL provides support for interprofessional education which helps students from speech–language pathology and nursing and other healthcare fields to work together better for dysphagia management according to Noureddine et al. (2016). The implementation of SBL in dysphagia education follows worldwide educational developments which focus on protecting patients and developing healthcare professional competencies and maintaining their professional development (Diaz-Navarro et al., 2024; Miles et al., 2016).

The chapter presents a complete analysis of dysphagia training through simulation-based learning which combines existing research with conceptual models and operational methods and new development trends. The document presents information in a systematic order which starts with basic principles before moving to execution methods and then presents research findings and concludes with SBL in dysphagia training.

DEFINITION AND CORE PRINCIPLES OF SIMULATION-BASED LEARNING

Simulation-based learning (SBL) represents an evidence-based educational approach which uses simulated clinical environments and scenarios and technological tools to create authentic healthcare situations for training and assessment and research purposes (Gaba, 2004). SBL functions as a teaching system which uses experiential and constructivist learning theories to create a pedagogical framework that requires students to actively participate while they reflect on their work and receive feedback. The system enables students to develop their clinical abilities by working with real-world tasks which they can practice repeatedly in a protected educational space (Issenberg et al., 2005; Motola et al., 2013). The core principles of SBL include:

- **Fidelity:** The simulation achieves real-world condition replication through its complete representation of actual situations which includes physical elements and psychological aspects and conceptual elements (Tun et al., 2015).

- **Deliberate Practice:** Involves purposeful repeated practice of specific skills which receives personalized feedback to help people reach advanced levels of expertise (Ericsson, 2004).
- **Safe Learning Environment:** The simulation environment provides students with a protected learning space which allows them to practice without risking patient safety while they develop their skills through trial and error (Agha & Fowler, 2015).
- **Feedback and Debriefing:** The process of feedback and debriefing serves as a fundamental element for performance reflection which helps learners to solidify their acquired knowledge while they modify their actions (Fanning & Gaba, 2007).

Simulation-based learning provides training for both technical abilities and communication and teamwork and clinical reasoning skills which match the diverse requirements of dysphagia management (Adams et al., 2024; Miles et al., 2016). Through simulation learners can connect their theoretical education to real-world practice by using the skills they learned to develop evidence-based competent actions.

HISTORICAL DEVELOPMENT OF SIMULATION IN HEALTHCARE

Healthcare education has progressed from basic anatomical models to advanced simulation systems which create authentic clinical environments for students to learn from (Andrei et al., 2024). The first anatomical representations and task trainers emerged during the eighteenth and nineteenth centuries when Grégoire of Paris created obstetric manikins. Laerdal created Resusci Anne in 1960 as a low-fidelity simulator for teaching cardiopulmonary resuscitation (CPR) which continues to serve as a popular training tool in medical education (Bienstock & Heuer, 2022; Buck, 1991; Cooper & Taqueti, 2004).

The aviation industry began using simulation for pilot training and operational safety in the 1930s which later motivated healthcare educators to develop comparable educational approaches (Rosen, 2008). Gaba and colleagues recognized that human mistakes together with equipment breakdowns led to negative results so they applied Crisis Resource Management (CRM) from aviation to anesthesiology through team-based scenario training which focused on communication and leadership and situational awareness (Gaba et al., 2001).

The 1980s and 1990s brought about computer-based and high-fidelity simulators including Sim One and Harvey which provided authentic physiological feedback and interactive training experiences that turned traditional training models into active learning spaces (Bradley, 2006). Simulation technology started to spread quickly throughout all healthcare specialties. Simulation technology established itself as a fundamental component of competency-based medical education (CBME) during the 2000s while supporting worldwide patient safety goals (Issenberg et al., 2005; Ziv et al., 2003). Ziv et al. (2003) established simulation as an ethical requirement which enables students to practice their skills through safe patient-free errors. The Society for Simulation in Healthcare (SSH) and the International Nursing Association for Clinical Simulation and Learning (INACSL) established official standards and best practices for simulation activities.

Simulation now serves as a tool which goes past technical skill education to develop healthcare professionals who can communicate with each other and think clinically and work within healthcare systems (Lateef, 2010; Motola et al., 2013). The method serves as a teaching instrument which also functions as a transformative approach to enhance patient safety and develop lifelong learning skills and ensure competency achievement (Diaz-Navarro et al., 2024; Gaba, 2004).

The development of simulation technology for healthcare education has created new training methods which affect how healthcare providers learn to manage dysphagia (Adams & Coutts, 2025). The development of simulation technology from procedural manikins to high-fidelity interprofessional scenarios led speech-language pathology educators to implement these new technologies for teaching students to perform advanced swallowing assessments and treatment methods (Adams & Coutts, 2025; Benadom & Potter, 2011; Ward et al., 2015). The field of speech–language pathology adopted simulation as a practice method during the 2010s because clinical placement opportunities decreased while ASHA started accepting simulation hours for clinical competency (American Speech-Language-Hearing Association (ASHA), n.d.). In 2016, the Council for Clinical Certification in Audiology and Speech-Language Pathology (CFCC) updated its certification guidance to allow up to 20% of the required 375 direct clinical hours to be completed through simulation (Council for Clinical Certification in Audiology and Speech-Language Pathology [CFCC], 2018). The field now has simulation-based curricula which teach students about swallowing and voice and augmentative and alternative communication (AAC) and neurogenic communication disorders (Adams et al., 2024; Howells et al., 2019; Moineau et al., 2018; Rumbach et al., 2024).

The high-risk condition of dysphagia required educational approaches which would protect patients from harm while enabling healthcare staff to practice their skills numerous times under close supervision. The educational method of simulation proved to be the perfect solution because students could link their knowledge of anatomy and physiology with communication skills through practical training in artificial settings (Adams & Coutts, 2025). The method has developed into a fundamental element of competency-based dysphagia education since its introduction which now guides curriculum development and supports practitioners to use evidence-based reflective practice (Adams et al., 2024; Broadfoot & Estis, 2020).

The COVID-19 pandemic created an urgent need for simulation-based education which led to the development of virtual simulations and telesimulation as essential educational resources for clinical training (Nagdee et al., 2022). The post-pandemic research shows that simulation education continues to serve as an essential part of SLP curriculum development because it helps students develop their skills and learn from other healthcare professionals (Watermeyer & Kanji, 2025).

THEORETICAL FRAMEWORKS SUPPORTING SIMULATION-BASED LEARNING

The design and implementation of effective simulation-based learning experiences (SBLEs) must move beyond the allure of technology and be grounded in established educational theories. A scholarly approach to simulation ensures that curricula are goal-oriented and effective in developing professional competency (Dudding & Ginsberg, 2023). The theoretical underpinnings of SBLEs generally fall into three broad categories: behaviorist, constructivist, and cognitive science theories.

Behaviorism and Deliberate Practice

Behaviorist theories posit that learning occurs through interactions with environmental stimuli and conditioning based on observable behaviors (Skinner, 1974). In the context of communication sciences and disorders (CSD), behaviorism is particularly relevant for the development of technical and psychomotor skills, such as passing a scope or administering an oral mechanism examination. This theoretical framework supports the concept of deliberate practice (DP). DP provides learners with opportunities for repetitive performance of specific skills coupled with rigorous assessment and specific, immediate feedback (Ericsson, 2004). This repetition allows key skills to become automated, freeing up cognitive resources for more complex tasks (McGaghie et al., 2010).

Constructivism and Experiential Learning

Constructivist theory suggests that learners actively construct new knowledge by integrating new experiences with prior understanding (Dudding & Ginsberg, 2023). A central framework within this domain is Experiential Learning Theory (ELT). According to Kolb (1984), learning is the process of "grasping and transforming experience" the ELT framework consists of four stages: concrete experience, reflective observation, abstract conceptualization, and active experimentation (Dudding & Ginsberg, 2023).

In an SBLE, this cycle is operationalized through the three phases of simulation:

1. **Pre-brief and Simulation:** The learner engages in the *concrete experience.*
2. **Debriefing:** Facilitated by an educator, the learner engages in *reflective observation*, analyzing events and emotions.
3. **Schema Formation:** The learner develops cognitive schemas (*abstract conceptualization*) to bridge theory and practice.
4. **Transfer:** The learner applies these new schemas in future clinical practice (*active experimentation*).

Closely related to ELT is the concept of reflective thinking, described by Schön (1992) as "reflection-in-action" (thinking on one's feet during the simulation) and "reflection-on-action" (analyzing events after they occur, typically during the debrief).

Situated Learning Theory

Situated learning theory posits that knowledge must be presented in authentic contexts embedded within the culture of the practice (Lave, 1988). Simulation supports situated learning by providing a realistic "whole task" environment, such as a room designed to look like a clinic or hospital, where learners must integrate professional behaviors, ethics, and clinical decision-making rather than performing isolated skills in a vacuum (Dudding & Ginsberg, 2023).

Cognitive Load Theory

Derived from cognitive science, Cognitive Load Theory addresses the limitations of working memory (Dudding & Ginsberg, 2023). It distinguishes between three types of load:

- **Intrinsic load:** The inherent difficulty of the task combined with the learner's expertise.
- **Extraneous load:** The load imposed by the instructional design (which should be minimized to avoid distraction).
- **Germane load:** The mental effort required to construct long-term schemas (van Merriënboer et al. 2006).

Effective SBLE design manages these loads by matching the task complexity to the learner's level of expertise. For novice learners, introducing complex environmental distractions (extraneous load) may hinder learning, whereas for advanced learners, such complexity may generate essential germane load required for the development of expertise (Dudding & Ginsberg, 2023).

Competency-Based Education

Finally, simulation is supported by Competency-Based Education (CBE) frameworks. Unlike traditional models that focus on inputs (time spent in class), CBE focuses on outputs, the demonstrated ability to integrate knowledge, skills, and attributes (KSAs) in professional practice (McAllister et al., 2011). Simulation provides a unique platform for CBE by allowing educators to assess a learner's ability to execute professional tasks (process schemas) and recognize clinical presentations (pattern schemas) in a controlled, standardized environment (Dudding & Ginsberg, 2023).

TYPES OF SIMULATION (LOW–MEDIUM–HIGH FIDELITY)

The level of simulation fidelity exists between different points which describe how well the training environment and equipment duplicate actual clinical situations. The three categories of Fidelity include low and medium and high which deliver distinct learning experiences that produce various educational results (Kim et al., 2016).

- **Low-Fidelity Simulation (LFS):** These models consist of static models and task trainers which use rubber body parts to create simple anatomical replicas for learners to practice specific psychomotor skills (e.g., oral mechanism tasks, suctioning techniques).
- **Medium-Fidelity Simulation (MFS):** This level uses computerized manikins which run embedded software to generate some physiological responses (e.g., breathing sounds, pulse) while instructors operate them through external control.
- **High-Fidelity Simulation (HFS):** High-fidelity systems include life-sized computer-controlled manikins that duplicate human body structure and respond like people do in medical scenarios.

Hybrid simulations represent models which unite elements from multiple simulation fidelity levels to create a combined educational approach (Lateef & Too, 2019). Standardized patients (SPs) receive training to act as particular clinical situations which healthcare professionals use for educational and evaluation and practice activities (Robinson-Smith et al., 2009). SP offers specific types of fidelity through its ability to replicate human body movements and speech patterns which cannot be replicated by manikins or mechanical simulators (Kim et al., 2016).

Simulation-based learning in dysphagia training includes multiple modalities spanning written cases, standardized patients, task trainers, manikins, and technology-enabled formats. Table 1 provides an overview of these modalities and offers dysphagia-specific examples illustrating their use in training.

Table 1. Simulation Modalities and Dysphagia-Specific Examples of Use in Training

Simulation Modality	General Description	Example Applications in Dysphagia Training
Paper-based cases	Written clinical scenarios or patient records used to support clinical reasoning and decision-making	Analysis of dysphagia case histories, interpretation of VFSS/FEES reports, diet recommendation and risk stratification exercises
Task trainers	Partial anatomical or functional models designed to practice specific skills	FEES skills training using upper-airway/ endoscopy task trainers (e.g., scope handling, navigation through nasal passages, orientation and safety checks).
Manikin-based simulation	Life-sized manikins allowing procedural practice and scenario-based learning	High-fidelity scenarios to practice recognition and management of aspiration indicators (e.g., desaturation, coughing, wet voice, changes in respiratory pattern) with real-time manikin responses.
Standardized patients (SP)	Trained individuals portraying patients or caregivers in controlled scenarios	Conducting bedside swallowing assessments, patient counseling, caregiver education, informed consent discussions
Technology-enabled simulation (VR and computer-based)	Digital platforms that present interactive clinical content via computer or immersive environments (VR), allowing learners to engage with simulated cases, decision pathways, and multimedia materials.	Case-based interactive simulations to practice dysphagia assessment planning, clinical decision-making, and management recommendations across varied patient profiles. Multimedia-supported scenarios incorporating VFSS/FEES clips, case history, and structured prompts to guide interpretation and documentation.

IMPLEMENTATION PROCESS

The process of implementing simulation-based learning needs instructors to create specific educational plans while they lead students through the experience and help them analyze their learning process (Jeffers & Poling, 2019). Simulation-based learning effectiveness depends on both the degree of technological realism and the facilitator's ability to create a secure learning space which enables students to develop clinical skills (Keskitalo, 2022). The simulation process includes four connected stages which start with pre-briefing followed by simulation execution and then debriefing and finally assessment and evaluation.

Pre-briefing

The simulation-based learning process begins with pre-briefing which provides students with essential information about the simulation environment and case scenario and defines their roles and ensures academic integrity through the fiction contract. The process enables students to determine their expected results and create an execution strategy which follows the principles of experiential learning theory (Chmil, 2016).

Running the Simulation

The simulation process includes facilitators who create clinical scenarios which duplicate actual hospital environments while they adjust the level of difficulty to create an optimal learning environment for critical thinking and engagement (MacDonald et al., 2018). The facilitator maintains essential responsibility to guide the scenario progression through proper timing of cues and individualized guidance which depends on learner requirements and their achievement level to keep all participants engaged in the learning experience (Solli et al., 2022). The process of effective facilitation involves more than technical equipment management because it needs to maintain three essential elements which include fidelity and scenario pacing and interpersonal communication to support learner immersion and team collaboration and create an authentic clinical decision-making environment (Holtschneider, 2014).

Debriefing

The process of debriefing involves an educator-led structured evaluation which takes place after simulation activities to help participants evaluate their actions and link their choices to theoretical concepts and their future nursing work. The process of guided reflection together with feedback during debriefing enables students to understand experiences at a deeper level which results in knowledge acquisition and enhanced clinical performance (Burns, 2015). Simulation debriefing serves as a crucial component for improving learning results from simulation exercises because it provides students with directed thinking opportunities to enhance their performance in all healthcare training environments (Nyoni et al., 2023).

ASSESSMENT AND EVALUATION

The assessment methods in simulation-based learning systems evaluate student achievement while simultaneously evaluating the educational methods used in the process (Jeffries, 2012). The assessment method of simulation-based evaluations serves two purposes because it offers both formative and summative assessment capabilities (Buléon et al., 2022). Assessment in simulation-based training should be embedded within instructional design rather than treated as a post-hoc activity (Kibble, 2017). Simulation separates the clinical task from the patient to create a safe learning environment; however, it must also include explicit outcome indicators and evaluation checkpoints that allow learners to track progress and determine when competency (or mastery of a targeted skill) has been achieved (Dudding et al., 2019).

Defining Dysphagia-specific Learner Outcomes

Effective evaluation begins with clearly written participant objectives that guide both learners and facilitators and serve as the anchor for determining whether intended outcomes were achieved (Lioce et al., 2013). Simulation objectives should deliberately span the cognitive, psychomotor, and affective domains and specify performance levels using action verbs aligned with Bloom's taxonomy (Lioce et al., 2013).

Examples of dysphagia-focused objectives include:

- **Cognitive/clinical reasoning:** Interpret bedside and instrumental findings, identify aspiration risk and contributing factors, and justify management recommendations (e.g., diet modifications, compensatory strategies, referrals).
- **Psychomotor:** Perform structured bedside swallowing components (e.g., secretion management, bolus presentation decisions) and, where applicable, demonstrate safe procedural steps for FEES-related skills or simulator-based endoscopy handling (Benadom & Potter, 2011).
- **Affective/professional practice:** Communicate risk and recommendations to patients/families, demonstrate patient-centered counseling, and collaborate effectively within interprofessional teams (e.g., tracheostomy/airway considerations).

Objectives should be calibrated to learners' baseline knowledge and clinical exposure, remain challenging yet attainable, and be feasible within the simulation timeframe (Lioce et al., 2013).

Evaluating Learner Performance: Formative and Summative Approaches

Evaluation data may be collected during the learning process and/or at the conclusion of the activity to monitor progress toward competencies (Kulasegaram & Rangachari, 2018). Simulation assessments typically combine formative and summative approaches (Kibble, 2017; Dudding et al., 2019). Formative assessment provides feedback during skill acquisition to help learners improve, whereas summative assessment determines whether learners have met competency expectations and whether remediation is required (Sadler, 1998; Dudding et al., 2019). Learning and assessment are therefore tightly linked, and responsibility is shared: facilitators design and implement the learning environment, while learners actively engage and use feedback to improve performance (Kulasegaram & Rangachari, 2018; Reddy & Andrade, 2010).

In dysphagia simulations, formative assessment may include structured "pause-and-coach" moments and targeted debriefing prompts that focus on clinical reasoning (e.g., why a bolus choice was made), safety thresholds (e.g., when to stop oral trials), and documentation quality. Summative assessment may include proficiency check-offs or OSCE-style evaluations for a clinical swallow examination scenario, including interprofessional coordination and decision-making for complex cases.

Rubrics and Structured Scoring for Dysphagia Competencies

Rubrics can improve transparency and scoring consistency by defining expectations and performance levels. A typical rubric includes (1) evaluation criteria, (2) quality definitions/rating scale, and (3) a scoring strategy (Reddy & Andrade, 2010). In dysphagia training, rubric criteria can be organized around key competency clusters, for example:

- **Assessment process quality:** completeness and sequencing of bedside procedures; selection and rationale for tasks.
- **Clinical reasoning:** hypothesis generation, differential considerations, and evidence-based interpretation of findings.
- **Safety behaviors:** aspiration-risk recognition, stop rules, infection control, and airway/tracheostomy considerations.
- **Communication:** patient counseling, interprofessional handoff, and documentation clarity.

Rubrics can also support learner self-assessment and individualized remediation planning, particularly when each criterion is linked to observable behaviors and actionable improvement steps (Dudding et al., 2019; Reddy & Andrade, 2010).

Evaluating the Simulation Experience: Continuous Quality Improvement

In addition to assessing learners, programs should evaluate the simulation experience itself to guide continuous quality improvement. Learner feedback (Likert-type surveys and/or open-ended questions) can help identify strengths and improvement areas in scenario design, realism, facilitation, and debriefing (Dudding et al., 2019). Where appropriate, standardized measures can be used to capture perceived effectiveness, confidence, and debriefing value (e.g., the SET-M; Leighton et al., 2015) and broader perceptions of simulation design and satisfaction (e.g., instruments described by Jeffries & Rizzolo, 2006). Qualitative approaches (brief interviews or focus groups) can provide deeper insight into how simulations influence psychomotor, cognitive, and affective outcomes. Finally, facilitator evaluation is essential. Structured post-session reflection (or team debrief notes) documenting what worked, what did not, and what will be revised helps strengthen fidelity, pacing, and educational impact across iterations (Dudding & Ginsberg, 2023).

EVIDENCE BASE: EFFECTIVENESS OF SIMULATION-BASED LEARNING IN DYSPHAGIA TRAINING

Research evidence now supports the educational value of simulation for dysphagia training because it helps students develop better clinical skills and improve their diagnostic abilities and patient safety competencies and professional self-assurance (Adams & Coutts, 2025). Research conducted in speech-language pathology shows that simulated learning methods help students develop better readiness for clinical work and improve their ability to handle dysphagia cases (Adams et al., 2024) and hospital readiness for swallowing management (Miles et al., 2015). The method of simulation enables healthcare providers to practice swallowing procedures through deliberate practice while they encounter challenging swallowing situations in controlled safe environments which enhances their ability to make accurate diagnoses and clinical choices (Broadfoot & Estis, 2020). The current evidence base is presented in this section through experimental trials and observational studies and mixed-methods research and student perception studies which demonstrate simulation's wide-ranging effects on dysphagia training. The research evaluates each study based on its research methods and main results and educational findings and its connection to competency-based dysphagia teaching methods.

Research findings indicate that simulation technology enables speech-language pathology graduate students to develop essential endoscopic abilities which they can use when treating actual patients. Benadom and Potter (2011) evaluated student learning of transnasal endoscopy for FEES through two different training methods which included human patient simulation and a low-cost non-lifelike simulator for graduate students. Students achieved success in performing procedures on healthy volunteers through multiple simulation practices without any substantial variations between simulator types regarding total procedural time and intranasal time. The students achieved better speed and confidence levels during their second volunteer task which proved that practicing multiple times helps students learn psychomotor skills and build their self-efficacy. The research indicates simulation serves as a protected learning pathway which enables students to practice endoscopy through simulated experiences while maintaining patient safety and decreasing the need for instructor supervision in dysphagia training.

Potter and Allen (2013) studied an interprofessional simulation which combined speech-language pathology students with nursing students to perform a clinical bedside swallow examination on a tracheostomized patient manikin. Students learned to perform airway suctioning and conducted dysphagia evaluations while they practiced dividing their clinical work between each other. The simulation process allowed participants to observe and discuss their findings which demonstrated that the simulation improved team communication and established clear professional responsibilities and enhanced team collaboration for dysphagia treatment. The experience revealed specific skill deficiencies which became apparent only through practical assessment but not through classroom teaching or paper-based testing. The research shows that interprofessional simulation training helps students become better prepared to handle complicated dysphagia cases while they learn to work together as a team before treating actual patients.

Ward et al. (2015) studied the educational benefits of human patient simulation for teaching paediatric dysphagia management. Students who finished their lectures then participated in immersive scenarios which led to their development of better skills and increased confidence and enhanced clinical reasoning abilities. The students showed no reduction in their anxiety about pediatric dysphagia treatment until they participated in simulation activities. The post-clinic reflections demonstrated that students gained more practical readiness through simulation activities than they would have from traditional lectures yet actual clinical experience provided the most effective way to develop their capabilities. The research shows that simulation training helps students become better prepared to handle difficult paediatric dysphagia cases while building their self-assurance before working with actual patients.

Miles et al. (2015) studied how one-day simulation-based training affected hospital readiness and dysphagia management abilities of 19 new speech-language pathology students. The training program used a combination of teaching methods which included part-task skill learning stations and immersive simulated scenarios that used manikins and standardized patients to teach both pediatric and adult patient care. The research employed a mixed-methods approach to discover that students demonstrated substantial improvements in their self-assessed confidence levels and their understanding of the material and their sense of readiness right after participating in the intervention. The qualitative analysis showed that students found the simulated environment to be an ideal space for practicing and making mistakes because focus group results showed that these advantages lasted through the first three months after training when students remembered particular simulation scenarios during their hospital clinical work.

Freeland et al. (2016) studied the potential of medical mannequins to teach nurses about stroke swallowing screening administration and result interpretation. The simulation group nurses achieved better immediate accuracy than didactic-only students while needing less practice to achieve complete mastery. The study maintained high accuracy levels throughout six weeks before researchers successfully applied the learned skills to a standardized patient evaluation. The research indicates that simulation technology enables healthcare providers to practice safely multiple times which enhances their ability to perform procedures correctly while teaching them to conduct dysphagia screenings during acute stroke emergencies.

Miles et al. (2016) conducted a study to assess the effectiveness of interprofessional simulation-based dysphagia training which they delivered to speech-language pathology and dietetics students at a hospital facility. The students underwent part-task skill training and ward orientation before they experienced three immersive dysphagia scenarios which they followed with clinical vignette assessments at three different points. The study revealed substantial enhancements in healthcare providers' self-assurance and their readiness to deliver hospital-based dysphagia care and their understanding of this care. The simulation program led to substantial improvements in clinical decision-making abilities according to vignette scores which showed the most significant progress in team-based work and patient-specific planning. The research shows that simulation with structured methods enables students to learn skills safely while building their teamwork abilities and preparing them for real clinical duties with patients who have complex dysphagia.

Sia et al. (2016) studied virtual patient simulation as an educational tool which helps students learn interviewing techniques and clinical decision-making abilities during their graduate dysphagia training. Students worked with virtual dysphagia cases multiple times and they also developed their own virtual patients under specific circumstances. The research results demonstrated that simulation technology enhanced medical professionals' ability to make accurate diagnoses while they became more skilled at obtaining essential patient data and detecting patient-related issues. Students who developed virtual patients showed better reasoning abilities and provided more solid reasons for their diagnoses and displayed greater empathy than students who performed only interviews. The research findings demonstrate that virtual patient simulation provides an effective method for dysphagia assessment practice which can be used at scale during times when actual clinical experience is restricted.

The study by Broadfoot and Estis (2020) assessed how simulation-based education helps new practitioners learn to evaluate preterm infant feeding needs. The training video followed by simulated feeding scenarios helped graduate students from speech-language pathology and nursing and non-healthcare backgrounds to achieve better results in their ability to detect behavioral and physiological distress and their skills in oral feeding assessment and referral for swallowing evaluation. The research findings show that short simulation training periods enhance both assessment precision and medical choice processes which confirms simulation as an effective method for teaching newborns with fragile health to perform early dysphagia screening.

Miles et al. (2021) studied graduate speech pathology students who conducted case-history interviews with virtual patients who had dysphagia through ICF categorization to assess their questioning and communication methods. The students showed excellent understanding of the virtual patient's health literacy level because they asked numerous clinical and daily living questions about his symptoms and dietary needs and his ability to participate in meals and his environmental situation. Students demonstrated better confidence and communication and reasoning abilities through their safe participation in complex dysphagia scenarios. The research indicates that virtual patient interviewing enables complete clinical reasoning and allows students to perform detailed patient evaluations through a system which enables them to practice delicate patient interactions at any time.

The research by Clinard (2022) evaluated how high-fidelity human patient simulation (HPS) compares to traditional written case studies for teaching speech-language pathology graduate students to evaluate and treat oral feeding readiness in infants with medical complications. The research employed a sequential mixed-methods approach with two participant groups to show that both teaching approaches led to equal substantial learning of theoretical content yet the HPS intervention group showed better self-assessed confidence development than the control group. The simulation participants showed increased self-efficacy for performing hands-on clinical tasks including infant positioning and physiologic stability assessment during handling according to their reports which qualitative assessment verified through direct connection to the simulation experience. The research indicates that students can learn information through didactic teaching but simulation training provides better results for developing their ability to work with dangerous children.

The study by Adams et al. (2024) examined how students of speech-language pathology perceived their clinical abilities in dysphagia treatment through their experience with an adult manikin that simulated neurological dysphagia in a simulation laboratory. The research used a mixed-methods pilot study which involved sixteen third-year students who completed questionnaires before and after the simulation and participated in focus group interviews. The total scores together with six out of eight clinical skill and self-confidence assessment items showed substantial growth. The qualitative results showed that students developed greater self-assurance while they appreciated the chance to learn from errors in a protected educational space which helped them become better at performing dysphagia assessments in hospital environments. The authors stated that simulation training helps students develop clinical skills and build their self-efficacy but it should function as an additional educational resource instead of replacing actual patient contact.

Bauer Malandraki et al. (2025) evaluated a new hybrid computer-based simulation training system which taught 27 speech-language pathology graduate students to enhance their clinical decision-making abilities and professional confidence. The research employed a repeated measures design which included two interactive scenarios that used real-life actors who played adult patients with dysphagia through a cloud-based video assessment platform. The results showed that students demonstrated significant self-efficacy growth through their self-assessments during the three evaluation periods which spanned from the beginning to the end of the second simulation. The students maintained their ability to agree with the gold-standard rater about videofluoroscopic analysis but their performance improved substantially in clinical decision-making for cranial nerve assessments and treatment planning between the first and second simulation sessions. The results indicate that computer-based simulation proves effective for teaching adult dysphagia education.

Marshall et al. (2025) performed a pragmatic randomized controlled trial which evaluated in person simulation against telesimulation for infant feeding training with practicing speech-language pathologists. The simulation package received participation from thirty nine clinicians who had either novice or experienced status in infant feeding delivery. The simulation package included prelearning followed by didactic teaching and part task activities and an infant feeding scenario and debriefing which clinicians accessed through either on-site delivery or telepractice remote delivery. The written vignette clinical reasoning scores of both groups showed improvement throughout the study period while participants reported growing confidence and their anxiety levels decreased without any significant variation between telesimulation and in person delivery methods. The satisfaction ratings from both modalities turned out to be high while novice clinicians achieved greater confidence growth and anxiety reduction than experienced clinicians did. The authors established that telesimulation produces learning results which match traditional simulation methods while providing an effective method to deliver practical pediatric feeding and dysphagia training to healthcare providers who lack physical attendance capabilities.

CONCLUSION

The process of simulation-based learning provides students with a controlled environment to build their dysphagia skills before they start working under direct clinical supervision. The evidence from various research approaches demonstrates that simulation training leads to better diagnostic skills and enhanced communication abilities and increased clinical competence and better readiness for patient treatment. The benefits of this approach have been proven to work in different situations of dysphagia treatment which include newborn feeding and medical instrument analysis and team collaboration between healthcare professionals and virtual simulation training. Simulation enables students to develop important skills but it functions best as an additional educational tool which should not replace actual patient interactions. The implementation of simulation training within competency-based educational programs helps create standardized learning experiences which enable students to develop their skills step by step while preparing them for clinical practice despite inconsistent patient access. The research community needs to continue their work on developing better fidelity models and creating new validated assessment tools and studying how simulation affects dysphagia patient outcomes in the long run.

REFERENCES

Adams, S. N., & Coutts, K. (2025). The use of simulation in the assessment and management of dysphagia: A scoping review. *Clinical Simulation in Nursing*, *98*, 101661. DOI: 10.1016/j.ecns.2024.101661

Adams, S. N., Kater, K. A., & Seedat, J. (2024). Student perspectives of simulated learning to improve their dysphagia management. *The South African Journal of Communication Disorders = Die Suid-Afrikaanse Tydskrif vir Kommunikasieafwykings*, *71*(1), e1–e11. DOI: 10.4102/sajcd.v71i1.1060 PMID: 39354797

Agha, R. A., & Fowler, A. J. (2015). The Role and Validity of Surgical Simulation. *International Surgery*, *100*(2), 350–357. DOI: 10.9738/intsurg-d-14-00004.1 PMID: 25692441

American Speech-Language-Hearing Association (ASHA). (n.d.). *Certification Standards for Speech-Language Pathology Frequently Asked Questions: Clinical Simulation*. https://www.asha.org/certification/certification-standards-for-slp-clinical-simulation/?srsltid=AfmBOoocM-7PsYOQq13HFBu8PioqxCigga4p67BRrvry3i2Lqk7DHD-L

Andrei, R., Saratila, I., Ababii, I., Rojnoveanu, G., Dandara, O., & Spinei, L. (2024). Bridging theory and practice: enhancing medical education through simulation-based training methods. *2*(11), 68-73. https://doi.org/DOI: 10.52645/MJHS.2024.2.09

Baijens, L. W., Clave, P., Cras, P., Ekberg, O., Forster, A., Kolb, G. F., Leners, J. C., Masiero, S., Mateos-Nozal, J., Ortega, O., Smithard, D. G., Speyer, R., & Walshe, M. (2016). European Society for Swallowing Disorders - European Union Geriatric Medicine Society white paper: Oropharyngeal dysphagia as a geriatric syndrome. *Clinical Interventions in Aging*, *11*, 1403–1428. DOI: 10.2147/CIA.S107750 PMID: 27785002

Bauer Malandraki, J., Bryan, J., Wetzel, D., Schaser, A., Craig, B. A., & Malandraki, G. A. (2025). Impact of a Novel Hybrid Computer-Based Simulation Adult Dysphagia Training on the Confidence and Clinical Knowledge of Speech-Language Pathology Graduate Students. *Teaching and Learning in Communication Sciences & Disorders*, *9*(3). Advance online publication. DOI: 10.61403/2689-6443.1376

Benadom, E. M., & Potter, N. L. (2011). The use of simulation in training graduate students to perform transnasal endoscopy. *Dysphagia*, *26*(4), 352–360. DOI: 10.1007/s00455-010-9316-y PMID: 21127910

Bienstock, J., & Heuer, A. (2022). A review on the evolution of simulation-based training to help build a safer future. *Medicine*, *101*(25), e29503. DOI: 10.1097/md.0000000000029503 PMID: 35758389

Bradley, P. (2006). The history of simulation in medical education and possible future directions. *Medical Education*, *40*(3), 254–262. DOI: 10.1111/j.1365-2929.2006.02394.x PMID: 16483328

Brady, S. L., Rao, N., Gibbons, P. J., Williams, L., Hakel, M., & Pape, T. (2018). Face-to-face versus online training for the interpretation of findings in the fiberoptic endoscopic exam of the swallow procedure. *Advances in Medical Education and Practice*, *9*, 433–441. DOI: 10.2147/AMEP.S142947 PMID: 29928150

Broadfoot, C. K., & Estis, J. M. (2020). Simulation-Based Training Improves Student Assessment of Oral Feeding Skills in Preterm Infants. *Teaching and Learning in Communication Sciences & Disorders*, *4*(3). Advance online publication. DOI: 10.30707/TLCSD4.3/FVMX2142

Buck, G. H. (1991). Development of simulators in medical education. *Gesnerus*, *48*(1), 7–28. DOI: 10.1163/22977953-04801002 PMID: 1855669

Buléon, C., Mattatia, L., Minehart, R. D., Rudolph, J. W., Lois, F. J., Guillouet, E., Philippon, A.-L., Brissaud, O., Lefevre-Scelles, A., Benhamou, D., & Lecomte, F., group, t. S. A. w. s., Bellot, A., Crublé, I., Philippot, G., Vanderlinden, T., Batrancourt, S., Boithias-Guerot, C., Bréaud, J., . . . Chabot, J.-M. (2022). Simulation-based summative assessment in healthcare: An overview of key principles for practice. *Advances in Simulation (London, England)*, *7*(1), 42. DOI: 10.1186/s41077-022-00238-9 PMID: 36578052

Burns, C. L. (2015). Using debriefing and feedback in simulation to improve participant performance: An educator's perspective. *International Journal of Medical Education*, *6*, 118–120. DOI: 10.5116/ijme.55fb.3d3a PMID: 26407453

Chmil, J. V. (2016). Prebriefing in Simulation-Based Learning Experiences. *Nurse Educator*, *41*(2), 64–65. DOI: 10.1097/nne.0000000000000217 PMID: 26418838

Cichero, J. A., & Murdoch, B. E. (2006). *Dysphagia: foundation, theory and practice*. John Wiley & Sons.

Clave, P., & Shaker, R. (2015). Dysphagia: Current reality and scope of the problem. *Nature Reviews. Gastroenterology & Hepatology*, *12*(5), 259–270. DOI: 10.1038/nrgastro.2015.49 PMID: 25850008

Clinard, E. S. (2022). Increasing Student Confidence With Medically Complex Infants Through Simulation: A Mixed Methods Investigation. *American Journal of Speech-Language Pathology, 31*(2), 942–958. DOI: 10.1044/2021_AJSLP-21-00234 PMID: 35226538

Cooper, J. B., & Taqueti, V. R. (2004). A brief history of the development of mannequin simulators for clinical education and training. *Qual Saf Health Care, 13 Suppl 1*(Suppl 1), i11-18. https://doi.org/DOI: 10.1136/qhc.13.suppl_1.i11

Council for Clinical Certification in Audiology and Speech-Language Pathology. (2018). *2020 standards for the certificate of clinical competence in audiology*. American Speech-Language-Hearing Association. https://www.asha.org/certification/2020-Audiology-Certification-Standards/

Diaz-Navarro, C., Armstrong, R., Charnetski, M., Freeman, K. J., Koh, S., Reedy, G., Smitten, J., Ingrassia, P. L., Matos, F. M., & Issenberg, B. (2024). Global consensus statement on simulation-based practice in healthcare. *Advances in Simulation (London, England), 9*(1), 19. DOI: 10.1186/s41077-024-00288-1 PMID: 38769577

Dudding, C. C., Brown, D. K., Estis, J. M., Szymanski, C., Zraick, R., & Mormer, E. (2019). Best practices in healthcare simulations: Communication sciences and disorders. *Indian Hills: Council of Academic Programs in Communication Sciences and Disorders.*

Dudding, C. C., & Ginsberg, S. M. (Eds.). (2023). *Simulation-based learning in communication sciences and disorders: Moving from theory to practice*. Routledge.

Edwards, A., Holm, A., Carding, P., Steele, M., Froude, E., Burns, C., & Cardell, E. (2024). Developing novice analysts' videofluoroscopic swallowing study skills in speech-language pathology: A randomised control trial comparing blended and online training approaches. *International Journal of Speech-Language Pathology, 26*(2), 212–224. DOI: 10.1080/17549507.2023.2212142 PMID: 37294183

Ericsson, K. A. (2004). Deliberate practice and the acquisition and maintenance of expert performance in medicine and related domains. *Academic Medicine, 79*(10, Suppl), S70–S81. DOI: 10.1097/00001888-200410001-00022 PMID: 15383395

Fanning, R. M., & Gaba, D. M. (2007). The role of debriefing in simulation-based learning. *Simulation in Healthcare, 2*(2), 115–125. DOI: 10.1097/SIH.0b013e3180315539 PMID: 19088616

Frank, J. R., Snell, L. S., Cate, O. T., Holmboe, E. S., Carraccio, C., Swing, S. R., Harris, P., Glasgow, N. J., Campbell, C., Dath, D., Harden, R. M., Iobst, W., Long, D. M., Mungroo, R., Richardson, D. L., Sherbino, J., Silver, I., Taber, S., Talbot, M., & Harris, K. A. (2010). Competency-based medical education: Theory to practice. *Medical Teacher*, *32*(8), 638–645. DOI: 10.3109/0142159X.2010.501190 PMID: 20662574

Freeland, T. R., Pathak, S., Garrett, R. R., Anderson, J. A., & Daniels, S. K. (2016). Using Medical Mannequins to Train Nurses in Stroke Swallowing Screening. *Dysphagia*, *31*(1), 104–110. DOI: 10.1007/s00455-015-9666-6 PMID: 26519043

Gaba, D. M. (2004). The future vision of simulation in health care. *Qual Saf Health Care, 13 Suppl 1*(Suppl 1), i2-10. https://doi.org/DOI: 10.1136/qhc.13.suppl_1.i2

Gaba, D. M., Howard, S. K., Fish, K. J., Smith, B. E., & Sowb, Y. A. (2001). Simulation-Based Training in Anesthesia Crisis Resource Management (ACRM): A Decade of Experience. *Simulation & Gaming*, *32*(2), 175–193. DOI: 10.1177/104687810103200206

Gunasekaran, S., Murray, J., & Doeltgen, S. (2024). Clinical reasoning during dysphagia assessment and management in acute care: A longitudinal qualitative study. *International Journal of Language & Communication Disorders*, *59*(4), 1463–1477. DOI: 10.1111/1460-6984.13005 PMID: 38251794

Hazelwood, R., Bouldin, E. D., Burford, I. R., & Steffen, E. A. (2022). Speech-language pathology graduate student clinicians' self-perceived competency in dysphagia management. *Teaching and Learning in Communication Sciences & Disorders*, *6*(3), 1–15. DOI: 10.30707/TLCSD6.3.1664996985.113836

Hill, A. E., Davidson, B. J., & Theodoros, D. G. (2013). Speech-language pathology students' perceptions of a standardised patient clinic. *Journal of Allied Health*, *42*(2), 84–91. https://www.ncbi.nlm.nih.gov/pubmed/23752235 PMID: 23752235

Holtschneider, M. E. (2014). Simulation Is All About You: It Is Not About the Technology. *Journal for Nurses in Professional Development*, *30*(4), 213–214. DOI: 10.1097/nnd.0000000000000092 PMID: 25036086

Howells, S., Cardell, E. A., Waite, M. C., Bialocerkowski, A., & Tuttle, N. (2019). A simulation-based learning experience in augmentative and alternative communication using telepractice: Speech pathology students' confidence and perceptions. *Advances in Simulation (London, England)*, *4*(1), 23. DOI: 10.1186/s41077-019-0113-x PMID: 31890318

Iobst, W. F. (2015). Building the plane as we fly it. *Journal of Graduate Medical Education, 7*(2), 259–261. DOI: 10.4300/jgme-d-15-00095.1 PMID: 26221447

Issenberg, S. B., McGaghie, W. C., Petrusa, E. R., Lee Gordon, D., & Scalese, R. J. (2005). Features and uses of high-fidelity medical simulations that lead to effective learning: A BEME systematic review. *Medical Teacher, 27*(1), 10–28. DOI: 10.1080/01421590500046924 PMID: 16147767

Jeffers, J. M., & Poling, S. (2019). The development and implementation of a 12-month simulation-based learning curriculum for pediatric emergency medicine fellows utilizing debriefing with good judgment and rapid cycle deliberate practice. *BMC Medical Education, 19*(1), 22. DOI: 10.1186/s12909-018-1417-6 PMID: 30646903

Jeffries, P. R. (2012). *Simulation in Nursing Education: From Conceptualization to Evaluation* (2nd ed.). National League for Nursing.

Jeffries, P. R., & Rizzolo, M. A. (2006). *Designing and Implementing Models for the Innovative Use of Simulation to Teach Nursing Care of Ill Adults and Children: A National, Multi-Site, Multi-Method Study*. National League for Nursing and Laerdal Medical.

Keskitalo, T. (2022). Pedagogical Practices for Organizing Simulation-Based Healthcare Education. *International Journal of Learning. Teaching and Educational Research, 21*(2). Advance online publication. DOI: 10.26803/ijlter.21.4.1

Kibble, J. D. (2017). Best practices in summative assessment. *Advances in Physiology Education, 41*(1), 110–119. DOI: 10.1152/advan.00116.2016 PMID: 28188198

Kim, J., Park, J.-H., & Shin, S. (2016). Effectiveness of simulation-based nursing education depending on fidelity: A meta-analysis. *BMC Medical Education, 16*(1), 152. DOI: 10.1186/s12909-016-0672-7 PMID: 27215280

Kolb, D. A. (1984). *Experiential learning: Experience as the source of learning and development*. Prentice-Hall.

Kulasegaram, K., & Rangachari, P. K. (2018). Beyond "formative": Assessments to enrich student learning. *Advances in Physiology Education, 42*(1), 5–14. DOI: 10.1152/advan.00122.2017 PMID: 29341810

Lateef, F. (2010). Simulation-based learning: Just like the real thing. *Journal of Emergencies, Trauma and Shock, 3*(4), 348–352. DOI: 10.4103/0974-2700.70743 PMID: 21063557

Lateef, F., & Too, X. Y. (2019). The 2019 WACEM Expert Document on Hybrid Simulation for Transforming Health-care Simulation Through "Mixing and Matching". *Journal of Emergencies, Trauma and Shock, 12*(4), 243–247. DOI: 10.4103/jets.Jets_112_19 PMID: 31798236

Lave, J. (1988). *Cognition in practice: Mind, mathematics and culture in everyday life*. Cambridge University Press.

Leighton, K., Ravert, P., Mudra, V., & Macintosh, C. (2015). Updating the Simulation Effectiveness Tool: Item Modifications and Reevaluation of Psychometric Properties. *Nursing Education Perspectives, 36*(5), 317–323. DOI: 10.5480/15-1671 PMID: 26521501

Lioce, L., Reed, C. C., Lemon, D., King, M. A., Martinez, P. A., Franklin, A. E., Boese, T., Decker, S., Sando, C. R., Gloe, D., Meakim, C., & Borum, J. C. (2013). Standards of Best practice: Simulation Standard III: Participant objectives. *Clinical Simulation in Nursing*, *9*(6), S15–S18. DOI: 10.1016/j.ecns.2013.04.005

Logemann, J. A. (1998). *Evaluation and treatment of swallowing disorders* (2nd ed.). Pro-Ed Inc.

MacDonald, S., Manuel, A., Dubrowski, A., Bandrauk, N., Law, R., Curran, V., & Lee, Y. W. (2018). Emergency Management of Anaphylaxis: A High Fidelity Interprofessional Simulation Scenario to Foster Teamwork Among Senior Nursing, Medicine, and Pharmacy Undergraduate Students. *Cureus, 10*(7), e2915. DOI: 10.7759/cureus.2915 PMID: 30186720

Marshall, J., Shiu, C., Raatz, M., Penman, A., Beak, K., Clarke, S., & Ward, E. C. (2025). Telesimulation for Training in Infant Feeding: A Randomized Controlled Trial. *Dysphagia*, *40*(2), 443–453. DOI: 10.1007/s00455-024-10746-7 PMID: 39133239

Martino, R., Foley, N., Bhogal, S., Diamant, N., Speechley, M., & Teasell, R. (2005). Dysphagia after stroke: Incidence, diagnosis, and pulmonary complications. *Stroke*, *36*(12), 2756–2763. DOI: 10.1161/01.STR.0000190056.76543.eb PMID: 16269630

McAllister, S., Lincoln, M., Ferguson, A., & McAllister, L. (2011). A systematic program of research regarding the assessment of speech-language pathology competencies. *International Journal of Speech-Language Pathology, 13*(6), 469–479. DOI: 10.3109/17549507.2011.580782 PMID: 21846166

McGaghie, W. C., Issenberg, S. B., Petrusa, E. R., & Scalese, R. J. (2010). A critical review of simulation-based medical education research: 2003-2009. *Medical Education*, *44*(1), 50–63. DOI: 10.1111/j.1365-2923.2009.03547.x PMID: 20078756

Miles, A., Donaldson, S., & Friary, P. (2015). Training Hospital Readiness in Speech-Language Pathology Students through Simulation. *The Internet Journal of Allied Health Sciences and Practice*, *13*(4).

Miles, A., Friary, P., Jackson, B., Sekula, J., & Braakhuis, A. (2016). Simulation-Based Dysphagia Training: Teaching Interprofessional Clinical Reasoning in a Hospital Environment. *Dysphagia*, *31*(3), 407–415. DOI: 10.1007/s00455-016-9691-0 PMID: 26803776

Miles, A., Hayden, S., Carnell, S., Halan, S., & Lok, B. (2021). What do speech pathology students gain from virtual patient interviewing? A WHO International Classification of Functioning Disability and Health (ICF) analysis. *BMJ Simulation & Technology Enhanced Learning*, *7*(4), 239–245. DOI: 10.1136/bmjstel-2020-000616 PMID: 35516818

Moineau, S., Bennett, D., & Scheer-Cohen, A. (2018). Aphasia simulation: A perspective from the student and standardized patient. *Teaching and Learning in Communication Sciences & Disorders*, *2*(1). Advance online publication. DOI: 10.30707/TLCSD2.1Moineau

Motola, I., Devine, L. A., Chung, H. S., Sullivan, J. E., & Issenberg, S. B. (2013). Simulation in healthcare education: A best evidence practical guide. AMEE Guide No. 82. *Medical Teacher*, *35*(10), e1511–e1530. DOI: 10.3109/0142159X.2013.818632 PMID: 23941678

Nagdee, N., Sebothoma, B., Madahana, M., Khoza-Shangase, K., & Moroe, N. (2022). Simulations as a mode of clinical training in healthcare professions: A scoping review to guide planning in speech-language pathology and audiology during the COVID-19 pandemic and beyond. *The South African Journal of Communication Disorders = Die Suid-Afrikaanse Tydskrif vir Kommunikasieafwykings*, *69*(2), e1–e13. DOI: 10.4102/sajcd.v69i2.905 PMID: 36073069

Noureddine, N., Hagge, D. K., & Brady, D. (2016). Developing Simulation-based Interprofessional Education: Nursing and SLP Students. *International Journal of Nursing & Clinical Practices*, *3*(177). Advance online publication. DOI: 10.15344/2394-4978/2016/177

Nyoni, C. N., van der Merwe, A., Botha, B. S., Fourie, C., Botma, Y., Labuschagne, M. J., & van Wyk, R. (2023). Health sciences educator's simulation debriefing practice needs: A mixed methods study. *Journal of Education and Health Promotion*, *12*(1), 55. DOI: 10.4103/jehp.jehp_1011_22 PMID: 37113413

Potter, N. L., & Allen, M. (2013). Clinical Swallow Exam for Dysphagia: A Speech Pathology and Nursing Simulation Experience. *Clinical Simulation in Nursing*, *9*(10), e461–e464. DOI: 10.1016/j.ecns.2012.08.001

Reddy, Y. M., & Andrade, H. (2010). A review of rubric use in higher education. *Assessment & Evaluation in Higher Education*, *35*(4), 435–448. DOI: 10.1080/02602930902862859

Reverberi, C., Beschin, N., Barbieri, M., & Cocchini, G. (2025). The Visual Analogue Test for Anosognosia for Dysphagia: VATA-Dysphagia. *International Journal of Language & Communication Disorders*, *60*(4), e70057. DOI: 10.1111/1460-6984.70057 PMID: 40498544

Robinson-Smith, G., Bradley, P. K., & Meakim, C. (2009). Evaluating the Use of Standardized Patients in Undergraduate Psychiatric Nursing Experiences. *Clinical Simulation in Nursing*, *5*(6), e203–e211. DOI: 10.1016/j.ecns.2009.07.001

Rosen, K. R. (2008). The history of medical simulation. *Journal of Critical Care*, *23*(2), 157–166. DOI: 10.1016/j.jcrc.2007.12.004 PMID: 18538206

Rumbach, A. F., Aldridge, D., & Hill, A. E. (2024). Student Perceptions of Simulation to Enhance Clinical Readiness for Assessment and Management of Adults With Voice Disorders. *Journal of Voice*, *38*(3), 641–653. DOI: 10.1016/j.jvoice.2021.10.014 PMID: 34848106

Sadler, D. R. (1998). Formative Assessment: Revisiting the territory. *Assessment in Education: Principles, Policy & Practice*, *5*(1), 77–84. DOI: 10.1080/0969595980050104

Schön, D. A. (1992). *The reflective practitioner: How professionals think in action* (1st ed.). Routledge., DOI: 10.4324/9781315237473

Sheepway, L., Lincoln, M., & Togher, L. (2011). An international study of clinical education practices in speech-language pathology. *International Journal of Speech-Language Pathology*, *13*(2), 174–185. DOI: 10.3109/17549507.2011.491129 PMID: 20626316

Shelat, V. G., & Pandya, G. (2015). Nutritional support in dysphagia. In Speyer, R., & Bogaardt, H. (Eds.), *Seminars in Dysphagia*. IntechOpen., DOI: 10.5772/61243

Sia, I., Halan, S., Lok, B., & Crary, M. A. (2016). Virtual Patient Simulation Training in Graduate Dysphagia Management Education—A Research-Led Enhancement Targeting Development of Clinical Interviewing and Clinical Reasoning Skills. *Perspectives of the ASHA Special Interest Groups*, *1*(13), 130–139. DOI: 10.1044/persp1.SIG13.130

Skinner, B. F. (1974). *About behaviorism.* Random House.

Solli, H., Haukedal, T. A., Husebø, S. I. E., & Reierson, I. Å. (2022). Alternating between active and passive facilitator roles in simulated scenarios: A qualitative study of nursing students' perceptions. *Advances in Simulation (London, England), 7*(1), 37. DOI: 10.1186/s41077-022-00233-0 PMID: 36309736

Tun, J. K., Alinier, G., Tang, J., & Kneebone, R. L. (2015). Redefining Simulation Fidelity for Healthcare Education. *Simulation & Gaming, 46*(2), 159–174. DOI: 10.1177/1046878115576103

Van Merriënboer, J. J. G., Kester, L., & Paas, F. (2006). Teaching complex rather than simple tasks: Balancing intrinsic and germane load to enhance transfer of learning. *Applied Cognitive Psychology, 20*(3), 343–352. DOI: 10.1002/acp.1250

Ward, E. C., Hill, A. E., Nund, R. L., Rumbach, A. F., Walker-Smith, K., Wright, S. E., Kelly, K., & Dodrill, P. (2015). Developing clinical skills in paediatric dysphagia management using human patient simulation (HPS). *International Journal of Speech-Language Pathology, 17*(3), 230–240. DOI: 10.3109/17549507.2015.1025846 PMID: 25833074

Watermeyer, J., & Kanji, A. (2025). Lessons From an Exploratory Qualitative Survey on Simulation Opportunities for Clinical Education in Speech-Language Pathology and Audiology in South Africa. *Teaching and Learning in Medicine, 37*(3), 430–440. DOI: 10.1080/10401334.2024.2362878 PMID: 38850212

Ziv, A., Wolpe, P. R., Small, S. D., & Glick, S. (2003). Simulation-based medical education: An ethical imperative. *Academic Medicine, 78*(8), 783–788. DOI: 10.1097/00001888-200308000-00006 PMID: 12915366

ADDITIONAL READING

Adams, S. N., & Coutts, K. (2025). The use of simulation in the assessment and management of dysphagia: A scoping review. *Clinical Simulation in Nursing, 98*, 101661. DOI: 10.1016/j.ecns.2024.101661

Dudding, C. C., & Ginsberg, S. M. (Eds.). (2023). *Simulation-based learning in communication sciences and disorders: Moving from theory to practice.* Routledge.

KEY TERMS AND DEFINITIONS

Clinical Reasoning: Clinical Reasoning represents the mental and reflective method which healthcare providers use to detect medical issues while they analyze symptoms and evaluate potential dangers and choose suitable treatment plans according to existing research and specific circumstances.

Debriefing: The process of debriefing involves a guided discussion which takes place after simulation activities to help students evaluate their performance while linking their experiences to their knowledge base and developing strategies for applying learned skills in actual patient treatment.

Deliberate Practice: A structured learning process which requires clinical task repetition for clinical task performance while receiving goal-oriented feedback to achieve continuous improvement without endangering patient safety.

Fidelity: The simulation system demonstrates real clinical conditions through its combination of equipment realism and patient interaction authenticity and case concept accuracy.

Part-Task Trainer: The Part-Task Trainer functions as a training device which enables healthcare professionals to learn particular clinical abilities through oral suctioning and dysphagia screening and laryngeal palpation exercises while working in controlled environments that do not need complete clinical situations.

Simulation-Based Learning (SBL): Simulation-Based Learning (SBL) uses educational methods which create clinical environments through manikins and standardized patients and digital platforms to let students practice decision-making while receiving feedback in protected environments before treating actual patients.

Standardized Patient (SP): A person who receives training to create fixed clinical situations through their spoken words and their body language and their emotional reactions which help teachers and assessors evaluate clinical abilities and social interaction skills.

Telesimulation: Telesimulation allows participants to join structured learning activities and case management and debriefing sessions through telecommunication systems which enable their remote participation even when they are not physically in a simulation laboratory.

Chapter 11 Flexible Endoscopic Evaluation in Neurogenic Dysphagia for Detection and Clinical Decision-Making

İbrahim Erensoy
http://orcid.org/0000-0003-0788-3873
Ondokuz Mayıs University, Turkey

ABSTRACT

This chapter examines the diagnostic utility of Flexible Endoscopic Evaluation of Swallowing (FEES) in neurogenic dysphagia, focusing on pharyngeal phase impairments caused by neurological disorders such as stroke, traumatic brain injury (TBI), cerebral palsy (CP), multiple sclerosis (MS), Parkinson's disease (PD), and amyotrophic lateral sclerosis (ALS). FEES enables direct visualization of swallowing physiology, including secretion management, residue, penetration, and aspiration. Its portability, repeatability, and radiation-free nature make it ideal for acute and chronic settings. The chapter outlines standardized protocols using IDDSI-consistent bolus trials and validated tools like the Penetration–Aspiration Scale, Yale Pharyngeal Residue Severity Rating Scale, and the Murray Secretion Scale to support accurate diagnosis and individualized management.

DOI: 10.4018/979-8-3373-6405-6.ch011

INTRODUCTION

Swallowing is a complex neuromuscular process that begins in the embryonic period and continues throughout the lifespan, requiring precise coordination between the structures extending from the oral cavity to the stomach and the nervous system (Logemann, 1998, 2007). An average individual performs approximately 500 to 1000 swallowing events per day, with the frequency increasing during eating and fluid intake and decreasing markedly during sleep (Dodds et al., 1990). Swallowing consists of both voluntary and involuntary (reflexive) components and involves the coordinated activation of more than 30 muscles working together with central pattern generators located in the brainstem. This process necessitates the finely regulated management of physiologically critical mechanisms, such as the brief inhibition of respiration during the pharyngeal phase. Therefore, swallowing represents an anatomically, physiologically, and neurologically intricate function, and disruption at any stage of this process may result in significant clinical consequences (Miller, 2008; Shaw & Martino, 2013).

Dysphagia may occur due to motor or sensory impairments affecting the oral, pharyngeal, or esophageal phases of swallowing. When dysphagia arises from neurological disorders, it is referred to as "neurogenic dysphagia," and it most commonly affects the pharyngeal phase, leading to complications such as aspiration, penetration, residue accumulation, secretions, and silent aspiration (Panebianco et al., 2020). Central nervous system disorders—including stroke, Parkinson's disease, multiple sclerosis (MS), amyotrophic lateral sclerosis (ALS), traumatic brain injury, and cerebral palsy—are among the primary causes of neurogenic dysphagia. Neurogenic dysphagia is associated with serious outcomes such as pneumonia, malnutrition, dehydration, prolonged hospitalization, and increased mortality risk. Therefore, early, accurate, and comprehensive assessment of swallowing function in individuals with neurogenic dysphagia is of critical importance (Warnecke, Labeit, et al., 2021).

Various diagnostic tools are used in clinical practice to obtain objective information about swallowing safety and efficiency. Among these tools, Flexible Endoscopic Evaluation of Swallowing (FEES) stands out as a particularly valuable method in individuals with neurological conditions due to its ability to provide direct, real-time visualization (Burdick et al., 2024). FEES allows clinicians to observe critical components of swallowing physiology—including secretions, pharyngeal residue, penetration, and aspiration—directly. Its portability, absence of radiation exposure, repeatability, and applicability in different patient positions make it an especially suitable option for bedridden individuals and those with limited mobility (Warnecke, Dziewas, et al., 2021b).

This chapter will elaborate on the anatomical and neurophysiological foundations of swallowing and detail how FEES can be used for diagnostic purposes in individuals with neurogenic dysphagia. It will also discuss how endoscopic findings guide clinical decision-making, along with the scales and protocols used in the evaluation process. The aim is to provide clinicians with an evidence-based framework for the safe and effective assessment of neurogenic dysphagia using FEES, thereby offering a comprehensive foundation for its systematic application.

OVERVIEW OF NEUROGENIC DYSPHAGIA

Although swallowing is often perceived as a stereotyped neurological response, its variability even with identical bolus types and volumes suggests that it is not governed solely by brainstem mechanisms (Costa, 2018b). Rather, swallowing is a complex sensorimotor process involving both voluntary and reflexive components, orchestrated by the integrated activity of cortical, subcortical, brainstem, and peripheral nervous system structures (Li-Jessen & Ridgway, 2020). During the oral preparatory and oral transit phases, regions such as the primary and secondary sensorimotor cortices, premotor cortex, frontal operculum, and anterior cingulate cortex are actively engaged. These regions contribute to bolus manipulation, containment, and anterior-to-posterior propulsion within the oral cavity. In the pharyngeal phase, additional areas—such as the insular cortex, basal ganglia, amygdala, hypothalamus, and substantia nigra—play crucial roles in modulating the initiation and timing of the swallow reflex, as well as in integrating sensory feedback and emotional context. (Groher & Crary, 2015).

The involvement of these widespread cortical and subcortical regions demonstrates that swallowing is not simply a reflex but a behavior that can be influenced by attention, volition, cognitive load, and emotional state (Ertekin & Aydogdu, 2003). Disruptions in any of these neural domains—due to neurodegenerative, demyelinating, or vascular pathology—may contribute to dysphagia symptoms that manifest in diverse and sometimes unpredictable ways. Within the brainstem, the central pattern generator (CPG) serves as the neural command center responsible for regulating the reflexive phases of swallowing (Tolmachev, 2021). Located bilaterally in the medulla oblongata, the CPG integrates afferent sensory inputs and generates patterned, sequential motor output required for the safe and effective passage of the bolus. It comprises several critical motor nuclei of cranial nerves—including the trigeminal (V), facial (VII), hypoglossal (XII), glossopharyngeal (IX), and vagus (X)—which innervate the muscles of the tongue, oropharynx, larynx, and upper esophageal sphincter (Libreros-Jiménez et al., 2023). These nuclei are synchronized to ensure timely airway protection, effective pharyngeal contraction, and esophageal opening, enabling the bolus to transit safely without entering the respiratory tract (Groher & Crary, 2015; Leonard & Kendall, 2023; Shaw & Martino, 2013).

Sensory feedback also plays a vital role in the modulation and safety of the swallow. The nucleus tractus solitarius (NTS) acts as the primary relay center for afferent signals arising from the oral cavity, pharynx, and larynx, transmitted via cranial nerves VII, IX, and X. These sensory signals are processed and relayed to the dorsal swallowing group (DSG), which subsequently activates the ventral swallowing group (VSG) (Lowell et al., 2008). The VSG coordinates motor output that is distributed to the cranial nerve nuclei involved in execution. This sensorimotor integration allows the swallowing mechanism to adapt to the consistency, volume, and temperature of the bolus and to respond to threats such as penetration or aspiration (Mayerl et al., 2023). The precision of this coordination underscores how even subtle impairments in neural communication can disrupt swallowing physiology and lead to clinically significant dysphagia (Costa, 2018a; Shaw & Martino, 2013).

Neurogenic dysphagia refers to impaired swallowing function that results from structural or functional damage within the nervous system (Chandran & Doucet, 2024). It is most commonly observed in central nervous system disorders such as stroke, Parkinson's disease, multiple sclerosis (MS), amyotrophic lateral sclerosis (ALS), cerebral palsy, and traumatic brain injury. Each of these conditions may affect different components of the swallowing pathway, including voluntary motor control, reflex initiation, sensory perception, and muscular coordination (Panebianco et al., 2020). Among the various phases of swallowing, the pharyngeal phase is most frequently affected in neurogenic cases. This is particularly critical, as pharyngeal impairment can lead to penetration (entry of material into the laryngeal vestibule), aspiration (entry into the trachea), silent aspiration (without cough reflex), pharyngeal residue, and poor secretion management—all of which significantly compromise both safety and efficiency of swallowing (Warnecke, Labeit, et al., 2021)

The clinical consequences of neurogenic dysphagia are profound. Individuals may experience dehydration, malnutrition, weight loss, recurrent aspiration pneumonia, prolonged hospitalization, and reduced overall functional status. Moreover, in many cases, dysphagia contributes to loss of autonomy and reduced quality of life (Raciti et al., 2022). These risks highlight the need for early detection, comprehensive evaluation, and ongoing monitoring of swallowing function in neurologically affected populations. Neurogenic dysphagia is not simply an isolated symptom; rather, it represents a complex and dynamic clinical condition that intersects with multiple aspects of neurological function, nutrition, respiratory health, and patient-centered care (Panebianco et al., 2020; Warnecke, Labeit, et al., 2021). Understanding the neuroanatomical and neurophysiological underpinnings of swallowing is therefore essential for effective diagnosis and intervention. The clinical presentation of neurogenic dysphagia is highly variable and depends on the specific neurological disorder, the extent and location of neural damage, the phase(s) of swallowing involved, and the presence or absence of compensatory mechanisms. For example, patients with

PD often exhibit bradykinesia and reduced swallowing frequency, while those with MS may experience incoordination due to demyelination. ALS patients typically present with rapid and progressive deterioration in both voluntary and reflexive swallowing abilities, and post-stroke patients may show a wide range of impairments based on lesion location and severity (Panebianco et al., 2020)

Given this variability, assessment methods must be sensitive, individualized, and capable of capturing both overt and subtle impairments. Instrumental tools such as FEES have emerged as critical components of dysphagia evaluation, particularly in cases of neurogenic origin. FEES allows for direct visualization of pharyngeal structures before, during, and after the swallow, enabling clinicians to assess key parameters such as secretion management, pharyngeal residue, airway protection, and the effectiveness of compensatory strategies. It is particularly advantageous in patients who cannot tolerate radiation-based procedures or who require repeated bedside assessments (Dziewas et al., 2024)

In summary, the pathophysiology of neurogenic dysphagia reflects the complexity of the neural networks involved in swallowing control. It necessitates a nuanced, multidisciplinary approach to diagnosis and management. Clinicians must be well-versed in both the neuroanatomical correlates of swallowing and the clinical implications of dysfunction to deliver effective, patient-centered care.

THE ROLE OF FEES IN THE EVALUATION OF NEUROGENIC DYSPHAGIA

Dysphagia is a significant health concern that may arise from a wide range of etiological factors, including neurological disorders, head and neck cancers, traumatic brain injury, and esophageal dysfunction. It can lead to serious complications such as dehydration, malnutrition, and aspiration pneumonia. Therefore, a comprehensive and multidisciplinary assessment of swallowing disorders is essential. Swallowing evaluation typically consists of two major components: clinical (non-instrumental) assessment and instrumental assessment methods (Leonard & Kendall, 2023).

Clinical evaluation is a multifaceted process that includes detailed patient history, physical examination, oral motor assessment, clinical swallowing trials, and self-report questionnaires. According to Logemann, the primary purposes of clinical swallowing evaluation are to determine the likely cause based on medical history, generate hypotheses regarding the nature of the disorder, establish an initial treatment plan, identify questions requiring further investigation, and determine the patient's readiness for instrumental assessment (Logemann et al., 1999). Self-report tools such as the Eating Assessment Tool-10 (EAT-10) (Belafsky et al., 2008), the Swallow Quality of Life Questionnaire (SWAL-QOL) (Chen et al., 2001), and the Sydney Swallow Questionnaire (SSQ) contribute to this process by capturing swallowing-related symptoms from the patient's perspective (Shapira-Galitz et al., 2024). However, clinical methods do not allow real-time visualization of anatomical structures during swallowing. For this reason, particularly in the diagnosis and management of neurogenic dysphagia, instrumental evaluation is indispensable (Groher & Crary, 2015; Leonard & Kendall, 2023).

The Videofluoroscopic Swallow Study (VFSS) has long been considered the gold standard for dysphagia assessment because it enables radiological visualization of the oral, pharyngeal, and esophageal phases of swallowing (Scharitzer et al., 2025). By administering contrast-enhanced liquids and solids of varying consistencies, clinicians can observe bolus transit from the mouth to the esophagus, detect aspiration and penetration, evaluate residue, analyze the timing of the swallowing reflex, and assess the effects of compensatory strategies. However, VFSS has limitations: it exposes the patient to radiation, is not portable, cannot visualize secretions, and may not be easily performed in patients who are bedridden or cannot be adequately positioned (Levine & Rubesin, 2017; Scheeren et al., 2014).

In contrast, Flexible Endoscopic Evaluation of Swallowing (FEES) has emerged as an alternative or complementary method to VFSS. First described by Langmore and colleagues in 1988, FEES allows direct visualization of the nasopharynx, oropharynx, hypopharynx, and laryngeal structures via a flexible endoscope inserted transnasally (Langmore, 2017). FEES provides high sensitivity and specificity in assessing secretion management, pharyngeal residue, penetration, and aspiration. It is particularly advantageous in neurologically based dysphagia, where silent aspiration and delayed swallow initiation are common. Additional benefits include portability, lack of radiation exposure, and the ability to repeat the examination multiple times within the same day if needed (Pan & Sadoughi, 2022).

Another strength of FEES is its capacity to visualize structures before, during, and after the swallow (Warnecke, Dziewas, et al., 2021a). Clinicians can directly identify nasopharyngeal regurgitation, reduced laryngeal closure, pharyngeal muscle dysfunction, secretion pooling, and delayed swallow trigger. FEES also allows assessment of different bolus consistencies and volumes, as well as the immediate evaluation of positional adjustments or compensatory strategies. Importantly, the use of boluses standardized according to the International Dysphagia Diet Standardisation Initiative (IDDSI) enhances the reliability and reproducibility of findings (Rule et al., 2020). With these features, FEES provides valuable information for both diagnosis and management planning. In patients with neurogenic dysphagia, FEES is a powerful tool for assessing aspiration risk, laryngeal function, secretion management, and the effectiveness of compensatory strategies. It is often the preferred method in individuals with reduced consciousness, limited mobility, or when minimizing radiation exposure is essential. (Groher & Crary, 2015; Leonard & Kendall, 2023; Logemann, 1998).

FEES PROTOCOL AND IMPLEMENTATION STAGES

Fiberoptic Endoscopic Evaluation of Swallowing (FEES) is a widely recognized instrumental method that plays a pivotal role in the assessment and clinical decision-making process for dysphagia, particularly of neurogenic origin. The effective application of FEES requires a systematic protocol that ensures both technical precision and diagnostic reliability. This section outlines the essential steps of the FEES procedure, including pre-assessment considerations, bolus administration, anatomical visualization, and standardized scoring systems (Langmore & Murray, 2012; Nankivell & Pothier, 2008).

1. Pre-Assessment Preparation

Before the examination, patients must be thoroughly informed about the procedure, including its goals, potential risks, and clinical advantages. Informed consent should be obtained. Factors such as the patient's cognitive and medical status, as well as nasal anatomy, should be considered when planning the evaluation. Although topical anesthetics or vasoconstrictors may be applied to the nasal mucosa to facilitate endoscope insertion, their use is generally discouraged in swallowing evaluations due to potential suppression of reflex sensitivity and alteration of secretion visibility. Patients are seated upright in a comfortable and stable position, with appropriate head and trunk support if needed. The flexible endoscope is introduced transnasally, typically through the more patent nasal passage, and is manipulated with the dominant hand while the clinician observes the monitor for real-time visualization (Rudnick & Sie, 2008).

2. Endoscope Positioning and Visualization

The endoscope is advanced beyond the nasopharynx to provide a clear view of the soft palate, base of tongue, valleculae, piriform sinuses, epiglottis, aryepiglottic folds, and vocal folds. During the pre-swallow phase, the tip of the endoscope is positioned between the soft palate and the tip of the epiglottis, enabling optimal visualization of pharyngeal structures (Figure 1). During the swallow, transient pharyngeal constriction obscures the endoscopic image, producing a brief moment of visual whiteout. This "white-out" phenomenon, lasting approximately 0.5 seconds in healthy individuals, corresponds to pharyngeal closure and laryngeal elevation. The presence, duration, and quality of this event may provide indirect information about pharyngeal function and timing (Betito et al., 2024; Langmore & Murray, 2012).

Figure 1. A pre-swallowing image in FEES.

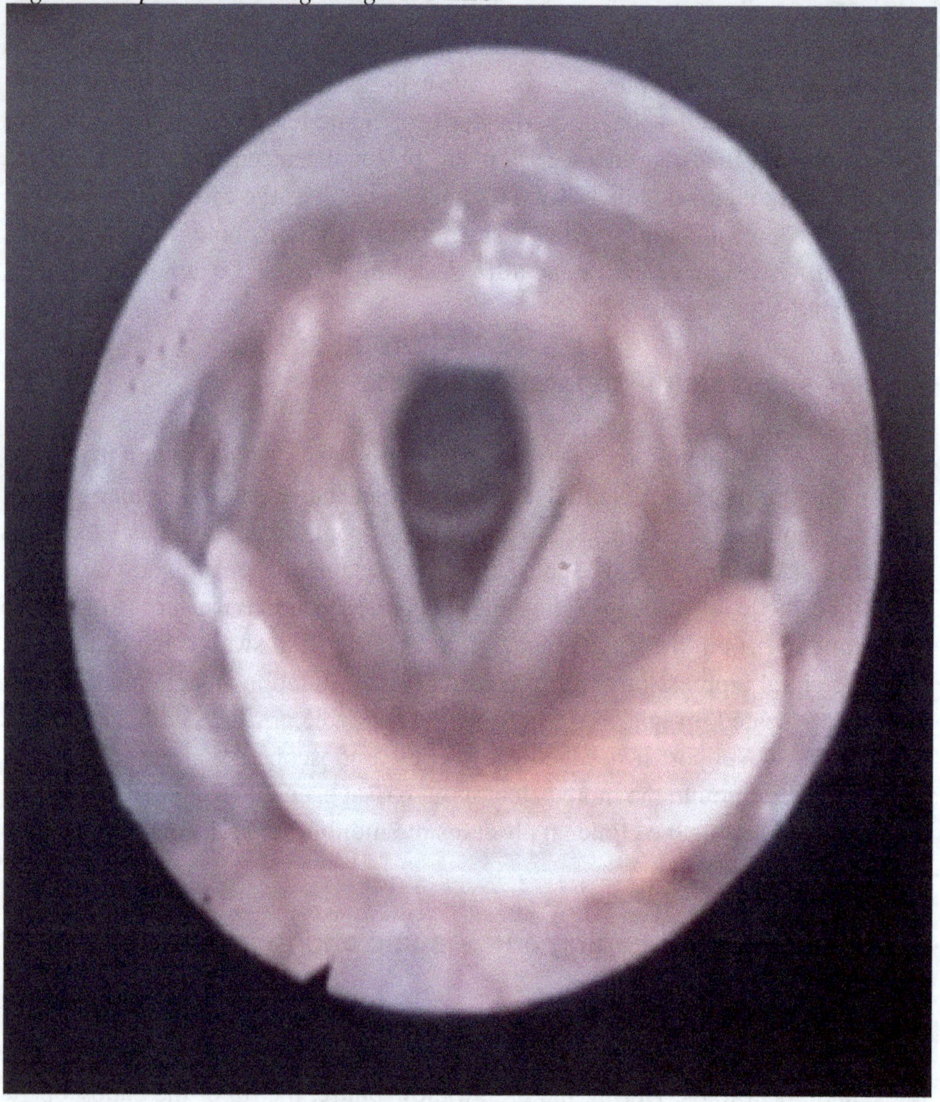

3. Secretion Assessment and Spontaneous Swallowing

Prior to bolus administration, the clinician observes for the presence, quantity, and distribution of pharyngeal and laryngeal secretions. Accumulation in the valleculae, piriform sinuses, or laryngeal vestibule may indicate reduced sensation or impaired clearance. The Murray Secretion Scale is commonly employed to rate secretion severity (0–3), factoring in both location and the patient's ability to clear them spontaneously (Kuo et al., 2017).

4. Bolus Consistencies and Volumes

Boluses are prepared in line with the IDDSI framework. Liquid consistencies are defined on a scale from 0 (thin) to 4 (extremely thick/pudding), and solid consistencies from 5 (minced) to 7 (regular) (Cichero et al., 2017). Each consistency is typically tested in increasing volumes—5 ml, 10 ml, and optionally 20 ml—to assess the influence of bolus size on swallowing physiology and safety. To enhance visualization, boluses are often dyed with blue or green food coloring to distinguish them from surrounding mucosa. Patients are instructed to hold the bolus in the oral cavity and swallow only upon cue, ensuring consistency and timing across trials (Curtis et al., 2019; Leder et al., 2005).

5. Swallowing Procedure and Clinical Observations

The clinician monitors for premature spillage, delayed swallow initiation, laryngeal closure effectiveness, penetration (Figure 2) or aspiration (Figure 3) events, and residue post-swallow (Figure 4) and (Figure 5). Observations also include compensatory strategies (e.g., chin tuck, head rotation) and their impact on bolus flow and airway protection. After each swallow, the endoscope may be advanced to the laryngeal vestibule or subglottic region to detect any silent aspiration or residual material (Langmore, 2017).

Figure 2. Penetration

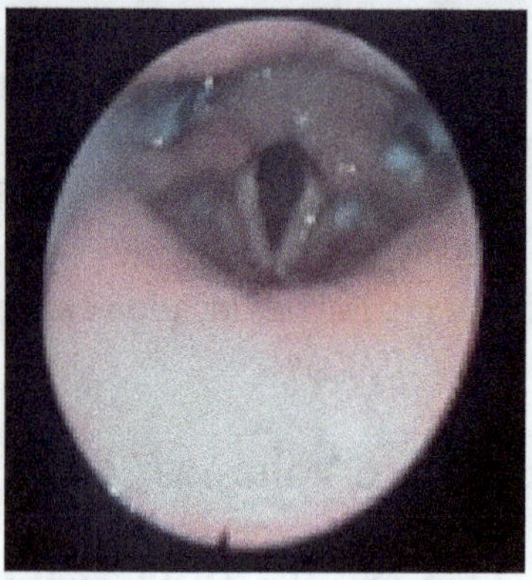

Figure 3. Aspiration

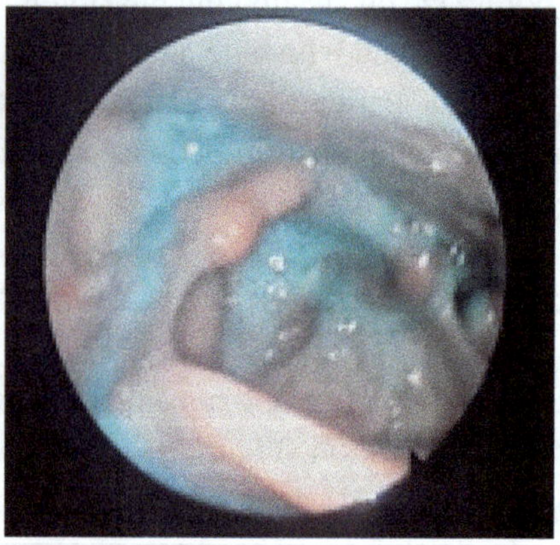

Figure 4. Valleculae residue

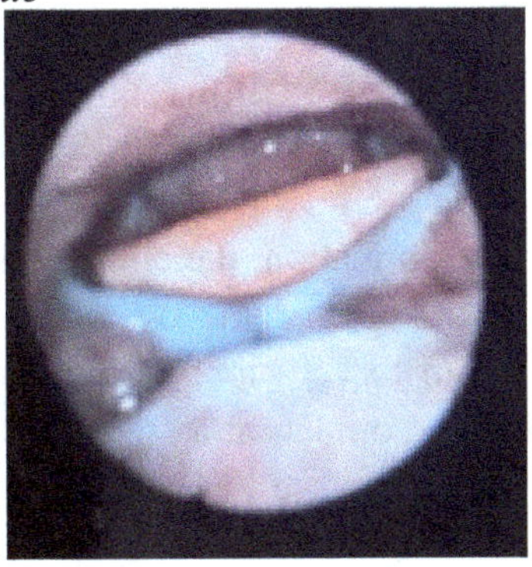

Figure 5. piriform sinus residue

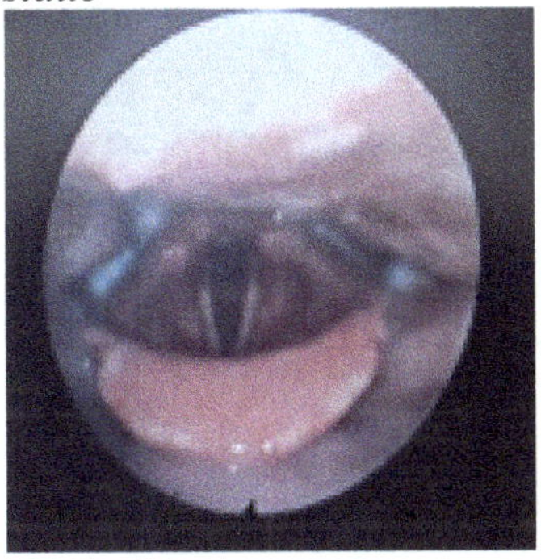

6. Standardized Scoring Systems

FEES findings are interpreted using validated clinical rating scales to enhance objectivity and inter-rater reliability:

Penetration-Aspiration Scale (PAS): Developed by Rosenbek et al., this 8-point scale quantifies the depth of airway invasion and the patient's response, ranging from no airway entry (score = 1) to silent aspiration with no response (score = 8) (Rosenbek et al., 1996). Yale Pharyngeal Residue Severity Rating Scale (YPRSRS): This 5-point visual scale is applied separately to the valleculae and piriform sinuses, assessing the amount of post-swallow residue in each location (Neubauer et al., 2015b). Murray Secretion Scale: This 4-point scale evaluates laryngeal secretion presence and the patient's ability to clear them, offering prognostic value regarding aspiration risk (Murray et al., 1996). These rating systems provide semi-quantitative data to guide treatment planning and track clinical changes over time.

7. Clinical Decision-Making and Termination of Procedure

At the conclusion of the examination, the clinician integrates structural, functional, and sensory findings with the patient's overall cognitive and physical status. The information obtained from FEES supports individualized recommendations regarding dietary modifications, compensatory techniques, rehabilitative exercises, or referral to other disciplines. Because FEES is portable, radiation-free, repeatable, and highly sensitive to pharyngeal pathophysiology, it serves as an essential tool in the comprehensive assessment of neurogenic dysphagia. When performed systematically with standardized protocols and validated outcome measures, FEES yields rich diagnostic data that inform safe and effective clinical decision-making (Cosentino et al., 2022).

INTERPRETATION OF FEES FINDINGS

FEES provides high-resolution, real-time visualization of pharyngeal swallowing physiology and has become a cornerstone assessment tool in the evaluation of dysphagia, especially in neurogenic populations. The ability to directly observe anatomical structures, secretion management, bolus flow patterns, and airway protection mechanisms offers clinicians a uniquely detailed profile of swallowing safety and efficiency. Accurate and systematic interpretation of FEES findings is essential to extract clinically relevant data and guide subsequent intervention planning(Cosentino et al., 2022; Warnecke, Dziewas, et al., 2021a). A comprehensive interpretation framework involves evaluating observations made before, during, and after swallowing, with attention to secretion pooling, swallow initiation timing, residue clearance, penetration/aspiration events, and the effectiveness of compensatory strategies. Several standardized rating scales are integrated into this process to quantify specific findings and reduce observer subjectivity (Warnecke, Dziewas, et al., 2021b).

1. Secretion Observation and the Murray Secretion Scale

Pre-swallow secretion pooling is a critical parameter that provides indirect insight into both sensory integrity and motor control of the pharynx. Accumulation of secretions in the valleculae, pyriform sinuses, or laryngeal vestibule prior to bolus delivery is often associated with impaired spontaneous swallowing frequency, poor sensation, or ineffective clearing mechanisms. FEES enables direct visualization of these secretions and their location, thickness, and movement. The Murray Secretion Scale offers a structured method to score the presence and severity of secretions, ranging from no visible secretions to copious secretions invading the laryngeal vestibule and trachea. This scale assists clinicians in stratifying aspiration risk even before test swallows are initiated (Hunting et al., 2023). In patients with neurodegenerative diseases, secretion pooling may reflect declining bulbar control and is predictive of both nutritional compromise and respiratory complications.

2. Swallow Initiation Timing and Delayed Swallow

One unique limitation of FEES is the inability to capture the exact moment of swallow onset due to the white-out phenomenon — a brief period of visual obscuration caused by pharyngeal constriction and tissue contact with the endoscope. Despite this, clinicians can indirectly assess swallow initiation timing by analyzing bolus location at the onset of white-out and whether the swallow appears to be triggered appropriately. Delayed initiation of swallowing, particularly when the bolus enters the pyriform sinuses or laryngeal vestibule without a coordinated swallow, is a hallmark of disrupted central pattern generator (CPG) functioning (Pisegna, 2022). This is especially prevalent in patients with cortical or brainstem stroke, traumatic brain injury, or Parkinsonian syndromes. Identifying such delays allows clinicians to predict silent aspiration risk and consider strategies such as sensory enhancement or bolus modification.

3. Pharyngeal Residue and YPRSRS Assessment

Post-swallow residue is a common finding in neurogenic dysphagia and can occur due to pharyngeal muscle weakness, poor base of tongue retraction, impaired hyolaryngeal excursion, or incomplete UES relaxation. The Yale Pharyngeal Residue Severity Rating Scale (YPRSRS) allows standardized scoring of residue in the valleculae and pyriform sinuses on a 5-point scale. It facilitates inter-rater agreement and supports clinical decision-making regarding bolus texture, volume, and compensatory postural strategies (Rocca et al., 2025). The presence of significant residue not only indicates impaired bolus propulsion but also increases the likelihood of secondary aspiration, particularly if the patient has impaired sensation or fails to initiate a clearing swallow. In repeated FEES evaluations, changes in YPRSRS scores can also help clinicians monitor therapeutic progress or disease progression (Neubauer et al., 2015a).

4. Penetration and Aspiration – Scored by PAS

Perhaps the most widely recognized application of FEES is the direct detection of penetration and aspiration. Penetration occurs when the bolus enters the laryngeal vestibule but remains above the vocal folds, while aspiration refers to entry of the bolus below the vocal folds into the trachea. The Penetration-Aspiration Scale (PAS) by Rosenbek et al. (1996) classifies these events on an 8-point ordinal scale based on depth of invasion and patient response (Rosenbek et al., 1996). FEES provides unparalleled sensitivity in detecting silent aspiration, defined as aspiration without a reflexive cough or throat clear — a common occurrence in patients with sensory deficits or reduced arousal. This highlights a distinct advantage over VFSS, which may fail to detect trace aspiration if occurring outside the radiographic window. PAS scoring not only quantifies risk severity but can also inform decisions about NPO status, compensatory maneuvers, or feeding route modifications (Borders & Brates, 2020).

5. Compensatory Behaviors and Protective Reflexes

During FEES, clinicians can assess the effectiveness of airway protection mechanisms, including cough, throat clearing, breath-hold, and laryngeal adduction during phonation (Langmore et al., 2022). These responses are particularly important when aspiration or penetration occurs. The presence of immediate, strong coughs may suggest sufficient protective reflexes, whereas their absence may indicate silent aspiration risk (Warnecke, Dziewas, et al., 2021b). Additionally, clinicians can introduce compensatory strategies such as effortful swallow, chin tuck, or supraglottic swallow during the examination and directly visualize their impact on bolus flow and residue clearance. This real-time feedback is critical for selecting individualized therapy techniques that are both effective and tolerable for the patient.

6. Anatomical and Functional Assessment

FEES also permits detailed evaluation of anatomical structures relevant to swallowing. Abnormalities such as reduced tongue base retraction, incomplete velopharyngeal closure, epiglottic immobility, or vocal fold paresis can all be identified. These findings contribute to the identification of the physiological source of the dysphagia and may indicate the need for further neurological workup or targeted therapy (Sasegbon & Hamdy, 2017). Functional deficits such as asymmetric pharyngeal contraction, unilateral residue, or poor glottic closure are especially relevant in stroke patients or those with focal neurological lesions. The ability to detect such patterns enhances differential diagnosis and informs prognosis.

7. Bolus-Specific Variability

Bolus consistency and volume greatly influence swallowing performance. FEES protocols increasingly utilize the IDDSI framework to standardize the testing of fluids and solids across seven consistency levels, ensuring repeatability and clinical relevance. By comparing PAS and YPRSRS scores across different IDDSI levels, clinicians can determine which textures are safest and most efficient for a given patient (Pisegna et al., 2020). For example, a patient may aspirate thin liquids (IDDSI 0) but safely tolerate mildly thick fluids (IDDSI 2) or soft solids (IDDSI 7). Alternatively, pharyngeal residue may increase disproportionately with puree (IDDSI 4), suggesting poor pharyngeal propulsion. Such findings support personalized diet recommendations that balance safety with nutritional adequacy and patient preference. Figure 6 presents the results of the liquid flow test conducted using ayran for IDDSI Level 1 (Figure 6), while Figure 7 illustrates the liquid flow test results obtained using kefir for IDDSI Level 2 (Figure 7).

Figure 6. IDDSI 1.

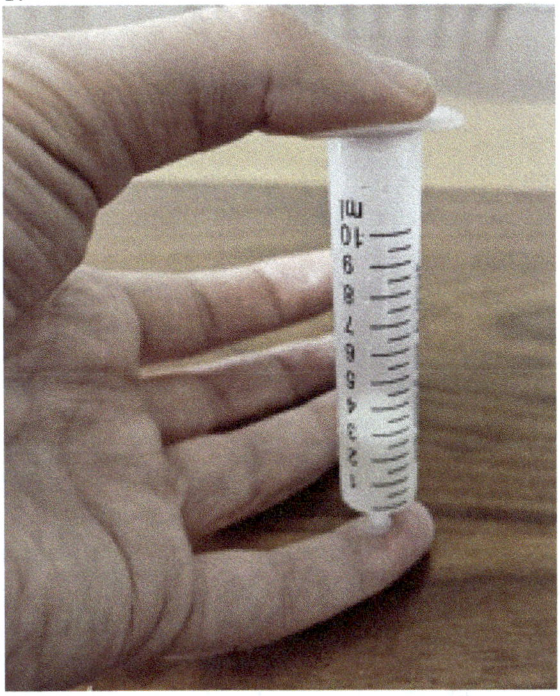

Figure 7. IDDSI 2.

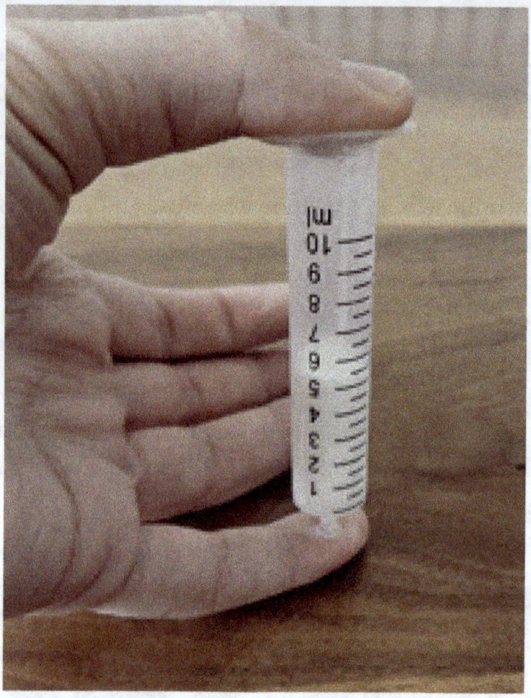

The interpretation of FEES findings is a dynamic and multifaceted process that requires both technical skill and clinical insight. Through direct visualization and structured rating scales, clinicians can assess key swallowing components including secretion management, swallow initiation, residue clearance, airway protection, and compensatory behaviors (Brady et al., 2018). Each of these parameters contributes to a comprehensive profile of dysphagia severity and helps identify the physiological impairments underlying functional deficits. When interpreted systematically, FEES findings not only inform diagnostic accuracy but also support evidence-based clinical decision-making, guide individualized therapy planning, and serve as outcome measures for rehabilitation progress. In neurogenic populations, where dysphagia is often multifactorial and progressive, the detailed data obtained through FEES is invaluable. The integration of PAS, YPRSRS, and the Murray scale—alongside observations of anatomy and function—enhances the objectivity and reliability of assessments (Neubauer et al., 2015a; Rosenbek et al., 1996). As a bedside, radiation-free, repeatable, and highly sensitive tool, FEES continues to play a pivotal role in the modern multidisciplinary approach to dysphagia management. It bridges the gap between diagnosis and intervention, offering a real-time window into the swallowing mechanism and empowering clinicians to make timely and tailored decisions that significantly improve patient outcomes.

INTERPRETATION OF TYPICAL FEES FINDINGS IN NEUROGENIC DYSPHAGIA

In individuals with neurogenic dysphagia, findings obtained through FEES vary depending on the underlying pathophysiology and the specific neurological structures affected. One of the most common observations is secretion pooling. During the examination, before any bolus is administered, secretions may accumulate in the valleculae, pyriform sinuses, or the laryngeal vestibule. This finding is associated with inadequate secretion clearance, reduced swallowing frequency, or impaired sensory awareness. In PD, bradykinesia and decreased spontaneous swallowing contribute to secretion buildup, whereas in ALS, pharyngeal muscle weakness and impaired coordination can exacerbate this accumulation (Massey et al., 2025; Nienstedt et al., 2018) The presence of secretions during FEES is considered one of the key indicators of increased risk related to swallowing safety and airway protection (Morris et al., 2025).

Delayed swallow initiation is another frequently observed finding in neurogenic dysphagia. Under typical circumstances, the swallow reflex is triggered once the bolus reaches the valleculae; however, in some individuals, this reflex is delayed, allowing the bolus to progress into the pyriform sinuses or the laryngeal vestibule. Such delay is commonly associated with cortical or subcortical lesions, including stroke and TBI (Alhashemi, 2010). When the swallow reflex begins late, the risk of silent aspiration increases, which—if unnoticed by the patient—may lead to recurrent pneumonia (Ebihara, 2022).

Pharyngeal residue results from inadequate pharyngeal contraction, insufficient tongue base retraction, or incomplete opening of the upper esophageal sphincter (UES), leading to material remaining in the valleculae or pyriform sinuses. These residues, which can be graded using the YPRSRS, indicate reduced swallowing efficiency and increased aspiration risk. In PD, pharyngeal bradykinesia may impair bolus propulsion, while in MS, lesion location can disrupt pharyngeal coordination, contributing to residue formation. This finding is particularly important in relation to aspiration, as the retained material may later be aspirated during spontaneous or involuntary inhalation (Erensoy, Yaşar, Aydınlı, Kemal, et al., 2025; Erensoy, Yaşar, Aydınlı, Tahir, et al., 2025).

Another critical finding directly observable through FEES is penetration and aspiration. Penetration refers to bolus entry down to the level of the vocal folds, while aspiration involves passage below the vocal folds into the trachea. Using the

PAS, the severity of these events and the presence of protective responses—such as coughing or throat clearing—can be evaluated. In ALS or post-stroke patients, reduced vocal fold movement or inadequate glottic closure may contribute to significant aspiration. In PD, delayed or ineffective coughing following penetration may prevent adequate airway clearance. Silent aspiration, especially common in neurodegenerative diseases with sensory impairment, represents a major risk factor for aspiration pneumonia (Falsetti et al., 2021).

Laryngeal closure insufficiency is another critical parameter assessable during FEES. Incomplete closure of the vocal folds significantly increases aspiration risk. During the examination, tasks such as phonation, coughing, and breath-holding help evaluate laryngeal closure (Song et al., 2023). Vascular or neurodegenerative impairments—as seen in PD-related vocal fold dysfunction or bilateral vocal fold paralysis in ALS—can lead to substantial deficits. Beyond contributing to aspiration, inadequate laryngeal closure also negatively affects vocal quality and overall quality of life (Patel et al., 2020).

Reduced sensory responsiveness is another notable finding during FEES. When secretions or bolus material enter the airway without eliciting reflexive responses—such as coughing—this indicates impaired sensory awareness. This finding is frequently associated with dementia, progressive neurodegenerative diseases, or brainstem lesions. When it co-occurs with silent aspiration, it represents a particularly serious clinical risk (Kamarunas et al., 2014).

Finally, differences in swallowing performance across bolus consistencies and volumes often reflect the nature of the underlying neurological disorder. Testing with IDDSI-standardized boluses allows clinicians to identify individual swallowing profiles. For example, some patients aspirate only thin liquids, while others exhibit pharyngeal residue exclusively with solid consistencies. These individual variations demonstrate how FEES contributes to personalized treatment planning (Steele et al., 2020)

Overall, the typical findings observed during FEES provide direct and reliable insight into the effects of neurological disorders on swallowing physiology. Systematic interpretation of these findings not only guides diagnostic accuracy but also plays a central role in informing appropriate therapeutic strategies.

CLINICAL DECISION-MAKING BASED ON FEES FINDINGS

Clinical decision-making in dysphagia management requires a comprehensive integration of physiological, anatomical, functional, and contextual information (Vose et al., 2018) Flexible Endoscopic Evaluation of Swallowing (FEES) has emerged as a cornerstone assessment tool in this process, particularly in individuals with neurogenic dysphagia. By enabling direct visualization of pharyngeal anatomy, secretion management, residue patterns, airway protection, and real-time bolus flow, FEES provides clinicians with high-resolution data that are essential for diagnostic accuracy, risk stratification, and individualized intervention planning (Dziewas et al., 2024).

Importantly, FEES-based clinical decision-making extends beyond the identification of impairment. It represents an iterative, hypothesis-driven process in which observed swallowing behaviors are interpreted within the broader clinical context, including neurological diagnosis, cognitive status, fatigue, medication effects, and patient-reported experiences. This section outlines a structured framework for FEES-guided decision-making across five interrelated domains: (1) diagnostic interpretation and dysphagia phenotype identification, (2) risk assessment and safety profiling, (3) implementation and evaluation of compensatory and behavioral strategies, (4) treatment planning and goal setting, and (5) interdisciplinary communication and documentation (Dziewas et al., 2016; Dziewas et al., 2024; Panebianco et al., 2020; Warnecke, Dziewas, et al., 2021a).

1. Diagnostic Interpretation and Dysphagia Phenotype Identification

The first step in FEES-based clinical reasoning involves synthesizing endoscopic findings to identify the dominant dysphagia phenotype. FEES allows clinicians to systematically evaluate both structural integrity and functional performance during swallowing, including:

- Reduced pharyngeal constriction or tongue base retraction,
- Impaired velopharyngeal closure,
- Delayed swallow initiation,
- Absent or weak protective reflexes,
- Incomplete laryngeal vestibule closure,
- Residue patterns in valleculae and pyriform sinuses,
- Presence and severity of penetration or aspiration,
- Abnormal secretion (Warnecke, Dziewas, et al., 2021b; Warnecke, Labeit, et al., 2021).

Rather than viewing these findings in isolation, clinicians integrate them with patient history, neurological diagnosis, disease stage, and cognitive profile to classify dysphagia into functional phenotypes, such as sensory-dominant, motor-deficient, coordination-impaired, or mixed presentations. These phenotypes provide a clinically meaningful framework for intervention selection. For example, individuals with pronounced pharyngeal residue due to reduced tongue base retraction may respond favorably to strength-based or effortful swallowing maneuvers, whereas patients with sensory impairment and silent aspiration may require conservative diet modification, heightened supervision, and increased emphasis on airway monitoring.

2. Risk Assessment and Safety Profiling

A central objective of FEES is the evaluation of swallowing safety and the prevention of dysphagia-related complications, including aspiration pneumonia, malnutrition, dehydration, and reduced quality of life (Giraldo-Cadavid et al., 2022; Giraldo-Cadavid et al., 2025). Clinical decisions frequently hinge on determining whether oral intake is safe, which consistencies are appropriate, and whether alternative nutrition should be considered. FEES supports these decisions through the use of validated, standardized outcome measures:

Penetration–Aspiration Scale (PAS): Assesses depth of airway invasion and patient response. High PAS scores, especially in the absence of reflexive cough, signal elevated risk and often contraindicate thin liquids or certain consistencies (Steele & Grace-Martin, 2017)

Yale Pharyngeal Residue Severity Rating Scale (YPRSRS): Quantifies residue in the valleculae and pyriform sinuses, with higher scores indicating reduced bolus clearance and increased risk for post-swallow aspiration (Leder & Neubauer, 2016).

Murray Secretion Scale: Rates secretion severity in the pharynx and larynx. Presence of pooled secretions without spontaneous clearance or reflexive response is a marker of high aspiration risk (Hunting et al., 2023).

These tools allow clinicians to develop a comprehensive safety profile for each patient. In high-risk individuals, oral intake may be withheld temporarily or modified using IDDSI-consistent thickened liquids and food textures until further improvement is observed or alternative feeding options are established (Cichero, 2020).

3. Compensatory Strategies and Therapeutic Trials

One of the most valuable aspects of FEES is the ability to conduct real-time compensatory and behavioral trials. Clinicians can test interventions during the assessment session, immediately evaluating their effectiveness in altering swallowing mechanics or airway protection. Common strategies include:

- Postural adjustments (e.g., chin tuck, head turn) to redirect bolus flow,
- Bolus modifications (e.g., smaller volumes, alternate consistencies),
- Swallowing maneuvers (e.g., supraglottic swallow, effortful swallow),

- Sensory stimulation (e.g., sour bolus, carbonation, thermal-tactile cues) (Murry et al., 2024).

By applying these techniques during FEES and observing changes in residue, penetration, aspiration, and timing, clinicians can make data-driven decisions regarding therapeutic recommendations (Schindler et al., 2022). For instance, if a chin-tuck maneuver eliminates aspiration of thin liquids during FEES, it can be prescribed as a safe strategy for use during meals (Saconato et al., 2016). Importantly, the IDDSI framework supports standardization of bolus consistencies during these trials, ensuring that observations are reliable and replicable. In clinical practice, trials should proceed from safest to riskiest consistency (e.g., thickened to thin liquids), with ongoing monitoring for adverse events (Beck et al., 2018).

4. Treatment Planning and Goal Setting

Based on the diagnostic phenotype, risk profile, and response to compensatory strategies, clinicians use FEES data to develop individualized treatment plans. These plans often include:

- Dietary modifications: Adjustments in bolus texture, volume, and pacing based on observed tolerance.
- Swallowing therapy: Exercise regimens targeting specific deficits (e.g., Mendelsohn maneuver for UES dysfunction, Shaker exercise for pharyngeal constriction).
- Compensatory strategy training: Teaching patients and caregivers maneuvers demonstrated to be effective during FEES.
- Airway protection management: Implementing protocols for oral hygiene, head-of-bed elevation, and respiratory monitoring.
- Monitoring and re-evaluation schedule: Planning future FEES or VFSS assessments to track progress or detect changes.

FEES findings are particularly useful for setting measurable, functional goals (e.g., "patient will consume IDDSI level 4 puree with no aspiration on three consecutive trials") and tracking outcomes over time. Moreover, FEES can be used at regular intervals to evaluate the efficacy of interventions, allowing for dynamic, responsive treatment (Ekberg, 2012; Groher & Crary, 2015).

5. Interdisciplinary Communication and Documentation

Clear communication of FEES findings and clinical implications is essential for coordinated care. FEES reports should be structured, concise, and include:

- Description of anatomical observations
- Severity scores from PAS, YPRSRS, and secretion scales
- Bolus types and volumes tested (IDDSI levels)
- Swallow safety and efficiency across consistencies
- Response to compensatory strategies
- Clinical impression and recommendations

Standardized templates can aid in consistency across providers and settings. Sharing findings with referring physicians, nutritionists, occupational therapists, and nursing staff ensures continuity of care and facilitates joint decision-making. In acute care, clear FEES documentation may influence discharge planning, feeding tube recommendations, and caregiver training (Majka et al., 2014)

Clinical decision-making based on FEES is a dynamic and patient-centered process that synthesizes high-resolution visual data with standardized scoring systems and real-time therapeutic trials to guide safe and individualized dysphagia management (McCoy & Bice, 2024). While FEES provides critical insight into the pharyngeal phase of swallowing—particularly secretion control, residue patterns, airway protection, and compensatory behaviors—it must be interpreted in conjunction with other assessment modalities such as VFSS and patient-reported outcome measures to ensure a comprehensive evaluation(Dewan et al., 2021). Triangulating these data sources allows clinicians to generate accurate dysphagia profiles, tailor interventions, and optimize functional outcomes. Ethical considerations, including patient preferences, cognitive status, and quality-of-life goals, must also shape clinical decisions—especially in cases where risk-reduction strategies are favored over strict dietary restrictions. Despite its limitations, such as the inability to assess the oral and esophageal phases and the transient white-out effect, FEES remains an indispensable tool in modern dysphagia care (Helliwell et al., 2023). It enables clinicians not only to detect impairments with precision but also to evaluate the real-time efficacy of therapeutic strategies, ultimately supporting evidence-based decision-making, reducing complications, and enhancing the safety, dignity, and well-being of individuals with neurogenic dysphagia.

Case-Based Interpretation Of FEES Findings

Introduction

In individuals diagnosed with neurogenic dysphagia, detailed analysis of impaired swallowing physiology constitutes a cornerstone of the clinical decision-making process. FEES provides critical data through direct, repeatable visualization, particularly for assessing pharyngeal secretion management, bolus clearance, and airway protection reflexes. This section presents four representative case examples—PD, MS, ALS, and stroke—demonstrating how FEES findings are interpreted within different neurological conditions. Bolus trials were conducted using consistencies aligned with the IDDSI, and findings were scored using the PAS, Yale Pharyngeal Residue Severity Rating Scale YPRSRS, and the Murray Secretion Scale.

Case 1 – Parkinson's Disease (PD): A 67-year-old male was evaluated using IDDSI 0 and 1 consistencies. Moderate secretion pooling was observed in the valleculae and laryngeal vestibule prior to bolus administration (Murray: 2), with no spontaneous clearance. A 5 ml thin liquid bolus (IDDSI 0) entered the laryngeal vestibule, passed the vocal folds, and silently aspirated into the trachea (PAS: 8). Post-swallow residue was severe in both the valleculae and pyriform sinuses (YPRSRS: valleculae = 5, pyriform = 4). Trials with other consistencies were not performed due to safety concerns.

Clinical Interpretation: Pooling, silent aspiration, and severe pharyngeal residue indicated significant impairment of both swallowing safety and efficiency. Oral intake was deemed high risk, and further instrumental evaluation and compensatory strategy trials were recommended.

Case 2 – Multiple Sclerosis (MS): A 45-year-old female was evaluated using IDDSI 0–4 consistencies with 5 and 10 ml boluses. No secretion pooling was observed (Murray: 0). Mild to moderate post-swallow residue was identified in the valleculae and pyriform sinuses with IDDSI 3 and 4 (YPRSRS: valleculae = 3, pyriform = 2), but not with IDDSI 0, 1, or 2. No penetration or aspiration occurred in any trial (PAS: 1). A subsequent trial with IDDSI 7 showed similar mild residue (valleculae = 3, pyriform = 2).

Clinical Interpretation: Despite reduced pharyngeal clearance, airway protection remained intact. Supported oral intake was considered appropriate, with further assessment of bolus control and pharyngeal strength recommended.

Case 3 – Amyotrophic Lateral Sclerosis (ALS): A 62-year-old male was assessed using IDDSI 0, 1, and 4 consistencies. Prior to bolus trials, significant pooling was observed in the laryngeal vestibule (Murray: 3), and the patient was unable to clear secretions. All bolus trials used 5 ml. Silent aspiration occurred with IDDSI 0 and 1 (PAS: 8), and aspiration without cough was observed with IDDSI 4 (PAS: 6).

Post-swallow residue was severe in both the valleculae and pyriform sinuses across all trials (YPRSRS: 5 for both structures).

Clinical Interpretation: Impaired secretion management, aspiration, and significant pharyngeal residue indicated a high-risk swallowing profile. FEES findings confirmed inadequate airway protection and severe dysfunction in swallowing safety and efficiency.

Case 4 – Right Hemispheric Stroke: A 72-year-old female underwent FEES with IDDSI 0, 1, 2, and 7 consistencies. No secretion pooling was observed (Murray: 0). A 5 ml mildly thick liquid (IDDSI 1) resulted in timely swallow initiation but was associated with penetration (PAS: 3). Similarly, thin liquid (IDDSI 0) led to a PAS score of 4. IDDSI 2 and 7 were associated with safe swallows (PAS: 1). Mild to moderate post-swallow residue was noted across all consistencies (YPRSRS: 2–3).

Clinical Interpretation: Swallowing efficiency and safety were mildly impaired. Although the clinical profile was considered low risk, structured dysphagia management and close follow-up were advised.

Overall Summary

Not all individuals with neurogenic dysphagia can tolerate IDDSI Level 7 (Regular) consistency safely. FEES provides individualized data on secretion management, pharyngeal clearance, and airway protection, which guide risk-based recommendations. As demonstrated in these case examples, systematic interpretation of FEES findings allows clinicians to tailor recommendations based on observed physiological deficits, ultimately supporting safer and more effective dysphagia management.

LIMITATIONS AND CONSIDERATIONS IN CLINICAL PRACTICE

FEES is widely used as a reliable, repeatable, and dynamic tool in the diagnosis and follow-up of neurogenic dysphagia. However, despite providing high-resolution visualization of the pharyngeal phase, it must be evaluated together with its technical limitations and important clinical considerations. This section addresses the major limitations encountered during the application of FEES, including patient-related factors, observer-related variability, technical constraints, challenges in clinical integration, and specific requirements unique to the neurogenic patient population (Dziewas et al., 2017).

Technical and Methodological Limitations

One of the most significant technical limitations of FEES is the transient loss of visualization during swallowing, commonly referred to as the "white-out" phenomenon. This occurs due to velopharyngeal closure and compression of the endoscope against the posterior pharyngeal wall, resulting in complete light reflection (Giraldo-Cadavid et al., 2017). Consequently, critical events such as the exact timing of bolus passage through the laryngeal vestibule and the dynamics of glottic closure cannot be directly visualized during this brief interval. This limitation complicates the precise determination of swallow initiation timing and reflex triggering. Moreover, FEES is limited to the assessment of the pharyngeal phase and does not provide direct information about the oral or esophageal phases. Key parameters such as oral bolus preparation, anterior–posterior bolus propulsion, oral residue, and esophageal transit disorders cannot be evaluated with this method. Therefore, for comprehensive swallow assessment, FEES should ideally be used in conjunction with other instrumental methods, such as VFSS (Dziewas et al., 2024; Helliwell et al., 2023; Warnecke, Dziewas, et al., 2021a).

Interpretation Errors and Interobserver Variability

The accurate interpretation of FEES findings requires advanced clinical expertise. Without sufficient training and experience, misinterpretation of critical features may occur. Distinguishing between physiological and pathological secretions, understanding the clinical significance of prolonged white-out duration, and differentiating whether pharyngeal residue results from impaired tongue base retraction or insufficient epiglottic inversion all require refined structural and functional knowledge. Additionally, interobserver reliability in scoring penetration and aspiration severity using PAS is consistently high only among clinicians who have received standardized training. Similarly, structured scales such as YPRSRS and the Murray Secretion Scale also demand advanced perceptual and analytical skills. Differences in experience levels among clinicians may result in inconsistent clinical judgments. In neurogenic disorders in particular, subtle findings such as silent aspiration may easily be overlooked, leading to direct consequences for clinical management (Pilz et al., 2016; Simon et al., 2023).

Patient-Related Factors and Tolerance

Patient cooperation, anatomical characteristics, and physiological tolerance are critical determinants of successful FEES administration. Structural nasal abnormalities such as nasal stenosis, mucosal edema, septal deviation, choanal stenosis, or heightened nasal sensitivity may hinder safe and comfortable endoscope insertion. These issues are especially prevalent among elderly patients and those with neurological deficits. Furthermore, cognitive impairment, agitation, attention deficits, or impaired behavioral control may compromise a patient's ability to remain appropriately positioned, understand instructions, and cooperate with task demands. In conditions such as dementia, delirium, or progressive neurodegenerative diseases, tolerance and procedural safety become major limiting factors. In such cases, less invasive and better-tolerated procedures should be prioritized, or FEES should be conducted following a structured preparatory and desensitization protocol (Polit et al., 2025; Schindler et al., 2022)

Challenges in Clinical Integration

The integration of FEES into routine clinical practice is dependent on infrastructure availability, trained personnel, and interdisciplinary coordination. Not all clinical settings possess adequate visualization equipment, digital recording systems, or clinicians formally trained in endoscopic assessment (Dziewas et al., 2017). These limitations may restrict the regular application of FEES. Moreover, secure data storage and protection of recorded materials pose important ethical and legal responsibilities. Equally important is the integration of FEES findings into clinical decision-making. The interpretation of FEES results should be shared within a multidisciplinary team, including speech-language therapists, neurologists, dietitians, and pulmonologists when necessary. Such collaboration maximizes patient benefit. Institutional protocols, multidisciplinary case discussions, and continuous professional training programs are strongly recommended to support this process (Denk-Linnert et al., 2023; Dziewas et al., 2024).

Training Requirements and Clinical Simulation

Effective use of FEES in neurogenic dysphagia requires structured training programs aimed at enhancing both technical and interpretive competencies (Dziewas et al., 2017). Achieving acceptable levels of interrater reliability in PAS and YPRSRS scoring is only possible through exposure to standardized video cases and simulation-based training environments. Training programs should include neurogenic dysphagia–specific symptom patterns, disorder-specific endoscopic findings, and case-based interpretation exercises. High-fidelity simulation technologies have recently gained importance in FEES education. These simulations enable clinicians to practice secretion management, recognize silent aspiration, administer boluses properly, and interpret findings in a structured manner in a controlled learning environment, thereby significantly enhancing clinical competence (Dziewas et al., 2016; Miles et al., 2016; Yoshida et al., 2020).

Impact of Neuropsychological Status

In neurogenic dysphagia evaluation, not only motor functions but also cognitive processes must be considered. During FEES, the patient's ability to execute instructed tasks—such as phonation, coughing, breath-holding, bolus containment, and command-driven swallowing—is closely related to attention, short-term memory, and auditory processing capacity (Dziewas et al., 2017; Dziewas et al., 2024). Conditions such as aphasia, frontal lobe dysfunction, dementia syndromes, and depression may significantly influence both patient performance and the accuracy of clinical interpretation. When FEES is performed in individuals with neuropsychological impairment, communication must be clear, simple, and supportive. When necessary, assistance from caregivers or healthcare staff should be utilized. The evaluation should be adapted to minimize fatigue, attentional decline, and emotional distress throughout the procedure (Braun et al., 2021).

Although FEES represents a cornerstone in the evaluation and management of neurogenic dysphagia, its application is associated with multidimensional limitations requiring careful consideration(Dziewas et al., 2016; Warnecke, Dziewas, et al., 2021a). Technical constraints, interpretation variability, patient-related factors, and system-level challenges all have the potential to influence diagnostic accuracy and patient safety. Nevertheless, through structured training, interdisciplinary collaboration, appropriate patient selection, and careful attention to neuropsychological factors, FEES can be implemented as a highly accurate, clinically effective, and patient-centered tool for assessment and clinical decision support in individuals with neurogenic dysphagia.

GENERAL CONCLUSION

Neurogenic dysphagia is a multifaceted condition that results from various disruptions across the central and peripheral nervous systems, frequently affecting swallowing physiology and increasing the risk for malnutrition, dehydration, and aspiration pneumonia. In this context, FEES has become a cornerstone assessment method, especially in clinical populations where direct, repeated, and bedside observation of pharyngeal phase dynamics is essential. This chapter has demonstrated that FEES provides robust insight into secretion management, residue clearance, airway protection, and timing of swallow initiation—parameters that are critical for assessing both the safety and efficiency of swallowing. The use of validated scoring systems such as PAS, YPRSRS, and the Murray scale enables standardized interpretation, allowing for greater consistency in diagnosis and longitudinal monitoring. The integration of IDDSI-aligned bolus consistencies has further refined the diagnostic power of FEES by offering reproducible testing conditions and enabling individualized assessment of swallow function across different textures. Case-based analyses involving PD, MS, ALS, and stroke illustrated the diverse pathophysiological mechanisms underlying neurogenic dysphagia, as well as how FEES findings can inform tailored clinical decision-making. Despite its advantages, FEES is not without limitations. The white-out phenomenon obscures real-time bolus transit through the pharynx, and the inability to visualize the oral and esophageal phases restricts the method's comprehensiveness. As such, integration with VFSS and clinical assessments is often necessary for a more holistic view. Moreover, the effectiveness of FEES is heavily reliant on clinician expertise. Interpretation errors, inter-rater variability, and procedural inconsistencies can significantly affect outcomes, particularly in the absence of structured training. Simulation-based education programs and standardized protocols are therefore crucial for enhancing scoring reliability and diagnostic precision. Patient-related factors, such as nasal anatomy, cooperation, tolerance, and cognitive status, may also limit the feasibility or success of the examination. Cognitive impairments—such as in dementia, aphasia, or frontal lobe dysfunction—can compromise task compliance and influence the validity of the findings. Furthermore, the integration of FEES findings into interdisciplinary care planning is essential. Clinical decisions must be grounded not only in instrumental results but also in broader considerations such as patient goals, nutritional needs, caregiver perspectives, and quality of life. When applied systematically and interpreted within the context of neurogenic profiles, FEES emerges as a highly sensitive, repeatable, and clinically actionable tool. It provides direct visual access to the physiology of dysphagia and supports evidence-based interventions aimed at minimizing risk, optimizing oral intake, and enhancing overall patient outcomes.

REFERENCES

Alhashemi, H. H. (2010). Dysphagia in severe traumatic brain injury. *Neuroscience Journal, 15*(4), 231–236.

Beck, A. M., Kjaersgaard, A., Hansen, T., & Poulsen, I. (2018). Systematic review and evidence based recommendations on texture modified foods and thickened liquids for adults (above 17 years) with oropharyngeal dysphagia–An updated clinical guideline. *Clinical Nutrition (Edinburgh, Lothian), 37*(6), 1980–1991.

Belafsky, P. C., Mouadeb, D. A., Rees, C. J., Pryor, J. C., Postma, G. N., Allen, J., & Leonard, R. J. (2008). Validity and reliability of the Eating Assessment Tool (EAT-10). *The Annals of Otology, Rhinology, and Laryngology, 117*(12), 919–924.

Betito, H. R., Tandler, N., Allon, R., Ganz, B., Lahav, Y., & Shapira-Galitz, Y. (2024). Evaluation of the Whiteout During Fiberoptic Endoscopic Evaluation of Swallowing and Examination of Its Correlation with Pharyngeal Residue and Aspiration. *Dysphagia*, •••, 1–9.

Borders, J. C., & Brates, D. (2020). Use of the penetration-aspiration scale in dysphagia research: A systematic review. *Dysphagia, 35*(4), 583–597.

Brady, S. L., Rao, N., Gibbons, P. J., Williams, L., Hakel, M., & Pape, T. (2018). Face-to-face versus online training for the interpretation of findings in the fiberoptic endoscopic exam of the swallow procedure. *Advances in Medical Education and Practice*, •••, 433–441.

Braun, T., Juenemann, M., Viard, M., Meyer, M., Reuter, I., Mausbach, S., Doerr, J. M., Schirotzek, I., Prosiegel, M., & Schramm, P. (2021). Flexible endoscopic evaluation of swallowing (FEES) to determine neurological intensive care patients' oral diet. *International Journal of Speech-Language Pathology, 23*(1), 83–91.

Burdick, R. J., Dallal-York, J., & Shapira-Galitz, Y. (2024). Flexible endoscopic evaluation of swallowing: A proposed checklist. *American Journal of Speech-Language Pathology, 33*(5), 2220–2229.

Chandran, S. K., & Doucet, M. (2024). Neurogenic dysphagia. *Otolaryngologic Clinics of North America, 57*(4), 589–597.

Chen, A. Y., Frankowski, R., Bishop-Leone, J., Hebert, T., Leyk, S., Lewin, J., & Goepfert, H. (2001). The development and validation of a dysphagia-specific quality-of-life questionnaire for patients with head and neck cancer: The MD Anderson dysphagia inventory. *Archives of Otolaryngology—Head & Neck Surgery, 127*(7), 870–876.

Cichero, J. A. (2020). Evaluating chewing function: Expanding the dysphagia field using food oral processing and the IDDSI framework. *Journal of Texture Studies, 51*(1), 56–66.

Cichero, J. A., Lam, P., Steele, C. M., Hanson, B., Chen, J., Dantas, R. O., Duivestein, J., Kayashita, J., Lecko, C., & Murray, J. (2017). Development of international terminology and definitions for texture-modified foods and thickened fluids used in dysphagia management: The IDDSI framework. *Dysphagia, 32*(2), 293–314.

Cosentino, G., Todisco, M., Giudice, C., Tassorelli, C., & Alfonsi, E. (2022). Assessment and treatment of neurogenic dysphagia in stroke and Parkinson's disease. *Current Opinion in Neurology, 35*(6), 741–752.

Costa, M. M. B. (2018a). Neural control of swallowing. *Arquivos de Gastroenterologia, 55*, 61–75.

Costa, M. M. B. (2018b). Neural control of swallowing. *Arquivos de Gastroenterologia, 55*(Suppl 1), 61–75.

Curtis, J., Perry, S., & Troche, M. S. (2019). Detection of airway invasion during flexible endoscopic evaluations of swallowing: Comparing barium, blue dye, and green dye. *American Journal of Speech-Language Pathology, 28*(2), 515–520.

Denk-Linnert, D.-M., Farneti, D., & Nawka, T., am Zehnhoff-Dinnesen, A., Moerman, M., Zorowka, P., Farahat, M., Schindler, A., & Geneid, A. (2023). Position statement of the Union of European Phoniatricians (UEP): Fees and phoniatricians' role in multidisciplinary and multiprofessional dysphagia management team. *Dysphagia, 38*(2), 711–718.

Dewan, K., Clarke, J. O., Kamal, A. N., Nandwani, M., & Starmer, H. M. (2021). Patient reported outcomes and objective swallowing assessments in a multidisciplinary dysphagia clinic. *The Laryngoscope, 131*(5), 1088–1094.

Dodds, W. J., Stewart, E. T., & Logemann, J. (1990). Physiology and radiology of the normal oral and pharyngeal phases of swallowing. *AJR. American Journal of Roentgenology, 154*(5), 953–963.

Dziewas, R., Baijens, L., Schindler, A., Verin, E., Michou, E., Clave, P., & Disorders, E. S. S. (2017). European Society for Swallowing Disorders FEES accreditation program for neurogenic and geriatric oropharyngeal dysphagia. *Dysphagia, 32*(6), 725–733.

Dziewas, R., Glahn, J., Helfer, C., Ickenstein, G., Keller, J., Ledl, C., Lindner-Pfleghar, B. G., Nabavi, D., Prosiegel, M., & Riecker, A. (2016). Flexible endoscopic evaluation of swallowing (FEES) for neurogenic dysphagia: Training curriculum of the German Society of Neurology and the German stroke society. *BMC Medical Education*, *16*(1), 70.

Dziewas, R., Warnecke, T., Labeit, B., Claus, I., Muhle, P., Oelenberg, S., Ahring, S., Wüller, C., Jung, A., & von Itter, J. (2024). Systematic approach to contextualize findings of flexible endoscopic evaluation of swallowing in neurogenic dysphagia–towards an integrated FEES report. *Neurological Research and Practice*, *6*(1), 26.

Ebihara, T. (2022). Comprehensive approaches to aspiration pneumonia and dysphagia in the elderly on the disease time-axis. *Journal of Clinical Medicine*, *11*(18), 5323.

Ekberg, O. (2012). *Dysphagia: diagnosis and treatment*. Springer Science & Business Media.

Erensoy, İ., Yaşar, Ö., Aydınlı, F. E., Kemal, Ö., & Terzi, M. (2025). The discriminant ability of the Eating Assessment tool-10 to detect swallowing efficiency in neurogenic dysphagia. *Logopedics, Phoniatrics, Vocology*, *50*(2), 95–103.

Erensoy, İ., Yaşar, Ö., Aydınlı, F. E., Tahir, E., & Terzi, M. (2025). The Ability of DYMUS and EAT-10 to Detect Pharyngeal Residue, Penetration, and Aspiration in Individuals with Multiple Sclerosis. *Multiple Sclerosis and Related Disorders*, •••, 106597.

Ertekin, C., & Aydogdu, I. (2003). Neurophysiology of swallowing. *Clinical Neurophysiology*, *114*(12), 2226–2244.

Falsetti, L., Viticchi, G., Zaccone, V., Tarquinio, N., Nobili, L., Nitti, C., Salvi, A., Moroncini, G., & Silvestrini, M. (2021). Chronic respiratory diseases and neurodegenerative disorders: A primer for the practicing clinician. *Medical Principles and Practice : International Journal of the Kuwait University, Health Science Centre*, *30*(6), 501–507.

Giraldo-Cadavid, L. F., Bastidas, A. R., Maldonado-Lancheros, J., Gasca-Zuluaga, D. A., Aguilar-Farias, M. J., & Bohorquez-Tibavisco, L. (2022). Pneumonia, mortality, and other outcomes associated with unsafe swallowing detected via fiberoptic endoscopic evaluation of swallowing (FEES) in patients with functional oropharyngeal dysphagia: A systematic review and meta-analysis. *Dysphagia*, *37*(6), 1662–1672.

Giraldo-Cadavid, L. F., Insignares, D., Velasco, V., Londoño, N., Galvis, A. M., Rengifo, M. L., & Bastidas-Goyes, A. R. (2025). Fiberoptic endoscopy evaluation of swallowing (FEES) findings associated with high pneumonia risk in a cohort of patients at risk of dysphagia. *Dysphagia*, *40*(1), 282–291.

Giraldo-Cadavid, L. F., Leal-Leaño, L. R., Leon-Basantes, G. A., Bastidas, A. R., Garcia, R., Ovalle, S., & Abondano-Garavito, J. E. (2017). Accuracy of endoscopic and videofluoroscopic evaluations of swallowing for oropharyngeal dysphagia. *The Laryngoscope*, *127*(9), 2002–2010.

Groher, M. E., & Crary, M. A. (2015). *Dysphagia: clinical management in adults and children*. Elsevier Health Sciences.

Helliwell, K., Hughes, V., Bennion, C., & Manning-Stanley, A. (2023). The use of videofluoroscopy (VFS) and fibreoptic endoscopic evaluation of swallowing (FEES) in the investigation of oropharyngeal dysphagia in stroke patients: A narrative review. *Radiography*, *29*(2), 284–290.

Hunting, A., Steffanoni, B., Jacques, A., & Miles, A. (2023). Accumulated secretions and Associated Aerodigestive function in patients with Dysphagia. *American Journal of Speech-Language Pathology*, *32*(6), 2691–2702.

Kamarunas, E. E., McCullough, G. H., Guidry, T. J., Mennemeier, M., & Schluterman, K. (2014). Effects of topical nasal anesthetic on fiberoptic endoscopic examination of swallowing with sensory testing (FEESST). *Dysphagia*, *29*(1), 33–43.

Kuo, C.-W., Allen, C. T., Huang, C.-C., & Lee, C.-J. (2017). Murray secretion scale and fiberoptic endoscopic evaluation of swallowing in predicting aspiration in dysphagic patients. *European Archives of Oto-Rhino-Laryngology*, *274*(6), 2513–2519.

Langmore, S. E. (2017). History of fiberoptic endoscopic evaluation of swallowing for evaluation and management of pharyngeal dysphagia: Changes over the years. *Dysphagia*, *32*(1), 27–38.

Langmore, S. E., & Murray, J. (2012). Fiberoptic endoscopic evaluation of swallowing (FEES). In *Manual of diagnostic and therapeutic techniques for disorders of deglutition* (pp. 85-101). Springer.

Langmore, S. E., Scarborough, D. R., Kelchner, L. N., Swigert, N. B., Murray, J., Reece, S., Cavanagh, T., Harrigan, L. C., Scheel, R., & Gosa, M. M. (2022). Tutorial on clinical practice for use of the fiberoptic endoscopic evaluation of swallowing procedure with adult populations: Part 1. *American Journal of Speech-Language Pathology*, *31*(1), 163–187.

Leder, S. B., Acton, L. M., Lisitano, H. L., & Murray, J. T. (2005). Fiberoptic endoscopic evaluation of swallowing (FEES) with and without blue-dyed food. *Dysphagia*, *20*(2), 157–162.

Leder, S. B., & Neubauer, P. D. (2016). *The Yale pharyngeal residue severity rating scale*. Springer.

Leonard, R., & Kendall, K. (2023). *Dysphagia assessment and treatment planning: a team approach*. Plural publishing.

Levine, M. S., & Rubesin, S. E. (2017). History and evolution of the barium swallow for evaluation of the pharynx and esophagus. *Dysphagia*, *32*, 55–72.

Li-Jessen, N. Y., & Ridgway, C. (2020). Neuroanatomy of voice and swallowing. *Neurologic and neurodegenerative diseases of the larynx*, 21-40.

Libreros-Jiménez, H. M., Manzo, J., Rojas-Durán, F., Aranda-Abreu, G. E., García-Hernández, L. I., Coria-Ávila, G. A., Herrera-Covarrubias, D., Pérez-Estudillo, C. A., Toledo-Cárdenas, M. R., & Hernández-Aguilar, M. E. (2023). On the cranial nerves. *NeuroSci*, *5*(1), 8–38.

Logemann, J. A. (1998). The evaluation and treatment of swallowing disorders. *Current Opinion in Otolaryngology & Head & Neck Surgery*, *6*(6), 395–400.

Logemann, J. A. (2007). Swallowing disorders. *Best Practice & Research. Clinical Gastroenterology*, *21*(4), 563–573.

Logemann, J. A., Veis, S., & Colangelo, L. (1999). A screening procedure for oropharyngeal dysphagia. *Dysphagia*, *14*, 44–51.

Lowell, S. Y., Poletto, C. J., Knorr-Chung, B. R., Reynolds, R. C., Simonyan, K., & Ludlow, C. L. (2008). Sensory stimulation activates both motor and sensory components of the swallowing system. *NeuroImage*, *42*(1), 285–295.

Majka, A. J., Wang, Z., Schmitz, K. R., Niesen, C. R., Larsen, R. A., Kinsey, G. C., Murad, A. L., Prokop, L. J., & Murad, M. H. (2014). Care coordination to enhance management of long-term enteral tube feeding: A systematic review and meta-analysis. *JPEN. Journal of Parenteral and Enteral Nutrition*, *38*(1), 40–52.

Massey, C., Griffiths, A. W., McDermott, C., & Hobson, E. (2025). How healthcare professionals support cough and secretion management in amyotrophic lateral sclerosis (ALS): A UK national survey. *Amyotrophic Lateral Sclerosis & Frontotemporal Degeneration*, •••, 1–12.

Mayerl, C., Gould, F., Adjerid, K., Edmonds, C., & German, R. (2023). The pathway from anatomy and physiology to diagnosis: A developmental perspective on swallowing and dysphagia. *Dysphagia*, *38*(1), 33–41.

McCoy, Y. M., & Bice, E. M. (2024). *Adult Dysphagia Clinical Reasoning and Decision-making Guide* (Vol. 1). Plural Publishing.

Miles, A., Friary, P., Jackson, B., Sekula, J., & Braakhuis, A. (2016). Simulation-based dysphagia training: Teaching interprofessional clinical reasoning in a hospital environment. *Dysphagia*, *31*(3), 407–415.

Miller, A. J. (2008). The neurobiology of swallowing and dysphagia. *Developmental Disabilities Research Reviews*, *14*(2), 77–86.

Morris, K., Taylor, N. F., & Freeman-Sanderson, A. (2025). Safety-related outcomes for patients with a tracheostomy and the use of flexible endoscopic evaluation of swallowing (FEES) for assessment and management of swallowing: A systematic review. *International Journal of Speech-Language Pathology*, *27*(1), 70–80.

Murray, J., Langmore, S. E., Ginsberg, S., & Dostie, A. (1996). The significance of accumulated oropharyngeal secretions and swallowing frequency in predicting aspiration. *Dysphagia*, *11*(2), 99–103.

Murry, T., Chan, K., & Walsh, E. H. (2024). *Clinical management of swallowing disorders*. Plural Publishing.

Nankivell, P., & Pothier, D. (2008). Nasal and instrument preparation prior to rigid and flexible nasendoscopy: A systematic review. *The Journal of Laryngology and Otology*, *122*(10), 1024–1028.

Neubauer, P. D., Rademaker, A. W., & Leder, S. B. (2015a). The yale pharyngeal residue severity rating scale: An anatomically defined and image-based tool. *Dysphagia*, *30*(5), 521–528.

Neubauer, P. D., Rademaker, A. W., & Leder, S. B. (2015b). The yale pharyngeal residue severity rating scale: An anatomically defined and image-based tool. *Dysphagia*, *30*, 521–528.

Nienstedt, J., Buhmann, C., Bihler, M., Niessen, A., Plaetke, R., Gerloff, C., & Pflug, C. (2018). Drooling is no early sign of dysphagia in Parkinson′ s disease. *Neurogastroenterology and Motility*, *30*(4), e13259.

Pan, S., & Sadoughi, B. (2022). Effectiveness of injection laryngoplasty for aspiration in acute iatrogenic vocal fold paralysis: A systematic review. *The Laryngoscope*, *132*(4), 813–821.

Panebianco, M., Marchese-Ragona, R., Masiero, S., & Restivo, D. (2020). Dysphagia in neurological diseases: A literature review. *Neurological Sciences*, *41*(11), 3067–3073.

Patel, B., Legacy, J., Hegland, K. W., Okun, M. S., & Herndon, N. E. (2020). A comprehensive review of the diagnosis and treatment of Parkinson's disease dysphagia and aspiration. *Expert Review of Gastroenterology & Hepatology*, *14*(6), 411–424.

Pilz, W., Vanbelle, S., Kremer, B., van Hooren, M. R., van Becelaere, T., Roodenburg, N., & Baijens, L. W. (2016). Observers' agreement on measurements in fiberoptic endoscopic evaluation of swallowing. *Dysphagia*, *31*(2), 180–187.

Pisegna, J. M. (2022). What's the evidence? A commentary on FEES research. *Perspectives of the ASHA Special Interest Groups*, *7*(6), 1941–1959.

Pisegna, J. M., Kaneoka, A., Coster, W. J., Leonard, R., & Langmore, S. E. (2020). Residue ratings on FEES: Trends for clinical application of residue measurement. *Dysphagia*, *35*(5), 834–842.

Polit, M., Chmielewska-Walczak, J., Sobol, M., Domitrz, I., & Niemczyk, K. (2025). Safety of FEES Performed by Speech-Language Pathologists and Physicians–Evidence Supporting Task Sharing from a Retrospective Observational Study of 964 Consecutive Examinations. *Nutrients*, *17*(20), 3193.

Raciti, L., Raciti, G., Pulejo, G., Conti-Nibali, V., & Calabrò, R. S. (2022). Neurogenic dysphagia and nutrition in disorder of consciousness: An overview with practical advices on an "old" but still actual clinical problem. *Medicines (Basel, Switzerland)*, *9*(2), 16.

Rocca, S., Negri, L., Valenza, N., Schindler, A., & Pizzorni, N. (2025). Pharyngeal residues scoring through the Yale pharyngeal residue severity rating scale (YPRSRS): Efficacy of training. *Dysphagia*, *40*(1), 271–281.

Rosenbek, J. C., Robbins, J. A., Roecker, E. B., Coyle, J. L., & Wood, J. L. (1996). A penetration-aspiration scale. *Dysphagia*, *11*, 93–98.

Rudnick, E. F., & Sie, K. C. (2008). Velopharyngeal insufficiency: Current concepts in diagnosis and management. *Current Opinion in Otolaryngology & Head & Neck Surgery*, *16*(6), 530–535.

Rule, D. W., Kelchner, L., Mulkern, A., Couch, S., Silbert, N., & Welden, K. (2020). Implementation strategies for the International Dysphagia Diet Standardisation Initiative (IDDSI), part I: Quantitative analysis of IDDSI performance among varied participants. *American Journal of Speech-Language Pathology*, *29*(3), 1514–1528.

Saconato, M., Chiari, B. M., Lederman, H. M., & Gonçalves, M. I. R. (2016). Effectiveness of chin-tuck maneuver to facilitate swallowing in neurologic dysphagia. *International archives of otorhinolaryngology, 20*(01), 013-017.

Sasegbon, A., & Hamdy, S. (2017). The anatomy and physiology of normal and abnormal swallowing in oropharyngeal dysphagia. *Neurogastroenterology and Motility*, *29*(11), e13100.

Scharitzer, M., Schima, W., Walshe, M., Verin, E., Doratiotto, S., Ekberg, O., Farneti, D., Pokieser, P., Quaia, E., & Woisard, V. (2025). ESSD–ESGAR best practice position statements on the technical performance of videofluoroscopic swallowing studies in adult patients with swallowing disorders. *European Radiology*, *35*(6), 3169–3180.

Scheeren, B., Maciel, A. C., & Barros, S. G. S. d. (2014). Videofluoroscopic swallowing study: Esophageal alterations in patients with dysphagia. *Arquivos de Gastroenterologia*, *51*, 221–225.

Schindler, A., Baijens, L. W., Geneid, A., & Pizzorni, N. (2022). Phoniatricians and otorhinolaryngologists approaching oropharyngeal dysphagia: An update on FEES. *European Archives of Oto-Rhino-Laryngology*, *279*(6), 2727–2742.

Shapira-Galitz, Y., Anderson, A., Balou, M., & Collaborative, F. (2024). Patient-reported outcome measures for swallowing: A proposed checklist. *American Journal of Speech-Language Pathology*, *33*(5), 2167–2176.

Shaw, S. M., & Martino, R. (2013). The normal swallow: Muscular and neurophysiological control. *Otolaryngologic Clinics of North America*, *46*(6), 937–956.

Simon, S. R., Wieland, M. W., Hendriks, C., Pilz, W., Schindler, A., Winkens, B., & Baijens, L. W. (2023). Intra and interobserver agreement of the Dynamic Imaging Grade of Swallowing Toxicity Scale (DIGEST) in fiberoptic endoscopic evaluation of swallowing (FEES): The importance of observer-tailored training. *European Archives of Oto-Rhino-Laryngology*, *280*(6), 2865–2876.

Song, J., Wan, Q., Wang, Y., & Zhou, H. (2023). Establishment of a multi-parameter evaluation model for risk of aspiration in dysphagia: A pilot study. *Dysphagia*, *38*(1), 406–414.

Steele, C. M., & Grace-Martin, K. (2017). Reflections on clinical and statistical use of the penetration-aspiration scale. *Dysphagia*, *32*(5), 601–616.

Steele, C. M., Peladeau-Pigeon, M., Barrett, E., & Wolkin, T. S. (2020). The risk of penetration–aspiration related to residue in the pharynx. *American Journal of Speech-Language Pathology*, *29*(3), 1608–1617.

Tolmachev, P. (2021). *Modelling The Interaction Between The Respiratory And Swallowing Central Pattern Generators*. University of Melbourne.

Vose, A. K., Kesneck, S., Sunday, K., Plowman, E., & Humbert, I. (2018). A survey of clinician decision making when identifying swallowing impairments and determining treatment. *Journal of Speech, Language, and Hearing Research: JSLHR, 61*(11), 2735–2756.

Warnecke, T., Dziewas, R., & Langmore, S. (2021a). FEES and other instrumental methods for swallowing evaluation. In *Neurogenic Dysphagia* (pp. 55–107). Springer.

Warnecke, T., Dziewas, R., & Langmore, S. (2021b). Using FEES in the treatment and management of neurogenic dysphagia: General principles and methodologies. In *Neurogenic Dysphagia* (pp. 223–240). Springer.

Warnecke, T., Labeit, B., Schroeder, J., Reckels, A., Ahring, S., Lapa, S., Claus, I., Muhle, P., Suntrup-Krueger, S., & Dziewas, R. (2021). Neurogenic dysphagia: Systematic review and proposal of a classification system. *Neurology, 96*(6), e876–e889.

Yoshida, M., Kagaya, H., Kamakura, Y., Miura, Y., Saitoh, E., Okawa, Y., & Sanada, H. (2020). Safety and the effectiveness of a new education program for nurses to assess swallowing function using fiberoptic endoscopic evaluation of swallowing (FEES). *Japan Journal of Nursing Science, 17*(2), e12313.

Chapter 12
The Cognitive Dimension of Swallowing Disorders:
Assessment and Clinical Implications

Samet Tosun
http://orcid.org/0000-0002-9604-7430
Biruni University, Turkey

ABSTRACT

This chapter per the authors conceptualizes swallowing as a cognitively mediated sensorimotor process rather than a purely brainstem reflex or peripheral biomechanical act. It synthesizes evidence from neuroimaging, electrophysiology, and dual-task paradigms to describe cortical, subcortical, and cerebellar networks supporting attentional control, executive regulation, and memory processes in swallowing. The chapter demonstrates how cognitive load, aging, and neurodegenerative conditions disrupt these networks, resulting in reduced swallowing safety, efficiency, and therapeutic adherence. An integrative assessment framework is presented, combining instrumental swallowing evaluations (VFSS, FEES, BRACS-Tr) with cognitive-linguistic measures (MoCA, TDQ-30/60 Tr, BECLA-Tr, DVAQ-30 Tr, DTLA-Tr), with emphasis on Turkish-adapted tools and cross-cultural normative data. Clinical implications focus on cognition-informed intervention planning, individualized cueing strategies, and multidisciplinary management, concluding with future directions for technology-assisted dysphagia care.

DOI: 10.4018/979-8-3373-6405-6.ch012

1. BACKGROUND

1.1. The Connection Between Brain Function and Swallowing

Swallowing is not just a simple reflex controlled by the brainstem. Instead, it is a complex cognitive-motor action that involves several distributed neural networks, including both cortical and subcortical regions. Traditional models of swallowing emphasized its peripheral sensory-motor components; however, contemporary research using neuroimaging and behavioral paradigms has clearly demonstrated the crucial contribution of cognitive processes such as attention, executive functioning, and working memory (Humbert & Robbins, 2008; Daniels & Huckabee, 2014). Evidence from dual-task paradigms further supports the notion that swallowing performance is significantly influenced by cognitive load and the allocation of attentional resources.

Suntrup-Krueger and colleagues demonstrated through functional magnetic resonance imaging (fMRI) investigations that concurrent cognitive task performance alters activation patterns within cortical swallowing networks, particularly in healthy older adults, highlighting the role of attentional control in maintaining swallowing safety (Suntrup-Krueger et al., 2025). Similarly, Muhle et al. (2020) reported that simultaneous cognitive or motor task engagement during swallowing significantly compromises swallowing efficiency and safety, resulting in increased pharyngeal residue and penetration-aspiration events. These findings supported the view that swallowing is not merely an automatic reflex but a cognitively modulated sensorimotor process dependent on central resource management.

Functional neuroimaging studies have further reinforced this notion. Cheng, Hamdy, and Mistry (2022) identified a distributed cortical-subcortical network comprising the insula, anterior cingulate cortex, prefrontal cortex, and basal ganglia as central to voluntary swallowing control. These regions, known for their roles in attentional regulation, decision-making, and interoception, underscore the cognitive governance of swallowing. In particular, the insula has been repeatedly identified as a critical integration hub linking sensory input with motor execution and affective-cognitive modulation of swallowing behavior (Lowell et al., 2008).

When cognitive load increases either through multitasking or environmental distraction swallowing safety demonstrably declines. This phenomenon was especially pronounced in older adults and individuals with cognitive impairment (Suntrup-Krueger et al., 2025). Thus, swallowing vulnerability becomes evident in clinical populations such as stroke survivors, individuals with Parkinson's disease (PD), mild cognitive impairment (MCI), and Alzheimer's disease (AD), where dysphagia frequently co-occurs with declines in executive function and disrupted cortical connectivity (Alagiakrishnan et al., 2013; Smithard et al., 2007; Easterling & Robbins, 2008; Tosun et al., 2024).

Accordingly, swallowing should no longer be conceptualized solely as a peripheral biomechanical process but as a cognitively mediated activity requiring sustained attention, conscious control, and dynamic coordination across distributed neural systems. Efficient and safe swallowing thus depends on intact executive attention, working memory, and cognitive flexibility, positioning dysphagia firmly within the domain of cognitive-neurophysiological dysfunction.

Taken together, converging evidence from neuroimaging and dual-task paradigms indicates that swallowing is governed by a distributed cortical–subcortical network in which attentional regulation, executive monitoring, and sensorimotor integration are functionally indispensable. Across studies, increased cognitive load reliably alters cortical recruitment and degrades swallowing safety and efficiency, particularly in older adults and clinical populations, underscoring that dysphagia cannot be fully explained by peripheral biomechanics alone.

1.2. Literature Gaps

Despite growing evidence of how cognition affects swallowing, there are still significant gaps in our understanding. First, the cognitive aspects of swallowing performance was not studied in detail. Existing dual-task studies often use small, homogenous cohorts of young adults (Muhle et al., 2020). This limits the generalisability of findings to older adults or those with neurological conditions. Moreover, there is a lack of longitudinal research examining how cognitive decline and swallowing dysfunction evolve together across disease stages. Martínez-Peña et al. (2025) reported a high prevalence of swallowing impairment among older adults attending a memory clinic, highlighting the early vulnerability of swallowing function in cognitive decline. Systematic review and meta-analytic evidence further supports this association, demonstrating a robust relationship between cognitive impairment and swallowing disorders across clinical populations (Dehaghani et al., 2021).

Thirdly, assessment methods that integrate cognitive and swallowing evaluation are still under development. Current clinical tools such as videofluoroscopic swallowing study (VFSS), fibre-optic endoscopic evaluation of swallowing (FEES), and residue/clearance scales primarily target biomechanical aspects of swallowing. They do not systematically assess patients' cognitive capacities. Consequently, critical dimensions such as attentional control, executive monitoring, and cognitive flexibility remain largely overlooked in routine dysphagia evaluation protocols. Research linking cognitive screening instruments (MoCA, MMSE) (Nasreddine et al., 2005; Folstein et al., 1975) with swallowing outcomes is limited. Studies utilising cognitive-linguistic tools validated for cultural/linguistic differences (TDQ, DVAQ, BECLA, DTLA) are even rarer (Karalı et al., 2025; Eskioglu et al., 2025; Tosun et al., 2024).

Additionally, there is a paucity of cross-cultural research exploring the interplay among language, cognition and swallowing. Turkish adaptations of BECLA (Karalı et al., 2025), TDQ-60/TDQ-30 (Eskioglu et al., 2025; Karalı et al., 2025) and DVAQ-30 (Tosun et al., 2025) provide vital insights into cognitive-linguistic profiles influencing swallowing safety and therapy adherence. Yet, their integration in international dysphagia research remains minimal.

Finally, evidence-based guidelines on tailoring dysphagia therapy to patients' cognitive profiles are lacking. A systematic review by Serra-Prat et al. (2020) found that intervention protocols for people living with dementia (PLWD) remain heterogeneous and under-validated, underscoring the need for therapy models sensitive to cognitive functioning. Hence, the discipline urgently requires a comprehensive framework linking cognitive mechanisms, assessment instruments and therapeutic strategies for dysphagia management.

1.3. Objectives and Contributions of This Chapter

This chapter aims to address these gaps by introducing a cognitive-neurophysiological paradigm. This framework will be used to analyse, assess, and treat swallowing difficulties. The primary objective is to conceptualise swallowing not merely as a peripheral mechanical action but as a process modulated and governed by higher-order cognitive mechanisms. This conceptualisation is grounded in evidence derived from neuroimaging studies, dual-task paradigm research, and investigations exploring cross-linguistic variability in swallowing-related cognitive processing. Importantly, this framework advances existing models by explicitly operationalizing cognitive control as a clinically actionable dimension by linking measurable cognitive–linguistic profiles to instrumental swallowing findings and to tailored rehabilitation parameters such as cueing, pacing, and strategy complexity rather than treating cognition as a background correlate.

The chapter will first describe the neural substrates involved in swallowing, with a particular emphasis on cortical and subcortical networks responsible for cognitive control, resource allocation, and sensory integration. Subsequently, specific cognitive domainsincluding attention, working memory, and executive functioningwill be examined in relation to swallowing safety, efficiency, and rehabilitation outcomes. A third focus will be the proposal of an integrative assessment framework combining cognitive-linguistic instruments (BECLA-Tr, TDQ-30/60 Tr, DVAQ-30, DTLA-Tr) with instrumental swallowing evaluations (VFSS, FEES, BRACS-Tr). This perspective aligns with emerging Turkish research demonstrating the clinical utility of cognitive-language assessments in differentiating MCI from AD and in predicting therapeutic adherence and rehabilitation responsiveness (Tosun et al., 2024; Eskioglu et al., 2025).

Furthermore, the chapter integrates theoretical and clinical insights from the authors' empirical work, including hierarchical cluster analysis revealing associations between swallowing efficiency and cognitive performance (Tosun et al., 2024) and the psychometric validation of the BRACS-Tr scale highlighting its clinical reliability in assessing residue and clearance patterns (Tosun, Topbaş, & Aksoy, 2025). Collectively, these findings underscored the pivotal role of cognitive mechanismsparticularly attentional regulation and executive controlin both the onset and recovery processes of dysphagia.

The chapter concludes by discussing the clinical and future implications of cognition-informed dysphagia management. Emphasis is placed on rehabilitation approaches responsive to cognitive changes, the necessity of interdisciplinary collaboration, and the integration of culturally sensitive assessment tools. These strategies are essential for optimising therapeutic outcomes in neurodegenerative disorders and post-stroke populations. By synthesising perspectives from neuroscience, speech-language pathology, and neuropsychology, the chapter aims to advance a holistic understanding of swallowing disorders beyond biomechanical explanations, situating them within the broader framework of human cognitive functioning.

2. THE NEUROCOGNITIVE BASES OF SWALLOWING

2.1. Cortical and Subcortical Systems in Swallowing Control

Swallowing involves a complex network of neurons, extending beyond the brainstem's primary control centres. It is represented bilaterally in the cortex, though with partial hemispheric asymmetry. The primary motor cortex (M1), primary somatosensory cortex (S1), supplementary motor area (SMA), insula, anterior cingulate cortex (ACC), and prefrontal cortices all contribute to swallowing control (Cheng et al., 2022; Lowell et al., 2008). These cortical regions interact with subcortical structures such as the basal ganglia, thalamus, and cerebellum, which are essential for temporal coordination, motor sequencing, and error correction during swallowing (Humbert & Robbins, 2008; Jean, 2001).

The insula plays a particularly central role. Functional connectivity studies demonstrate that the anterior insula integrates visceral sensory input with motor planning and affective-cognitive processing, making it a key node in swallowing regulation (Hamdy et al., 2000; Cheng et al., 2022). Clinical neuroimaging studies have consistently linked insular damage to aspiration, delayed swallow initiation, and impaired bolus propulsion (Daniels & Huckabee, 2014). The anterior cingulate cortex contributes to attentional monitoring and motivational aspects of feeding, while the prefrontal cortex supports goal-directed initiation and voluntary modulation of swallowing.

Subcortically, the basal ganglia regulate initiation and termination of motor patterns by integrating sensory, motivational, and reward-related information, which is crucial for adaptive swallowing control. In Parkinson's disease, disruption of these pathways results in delayed swallow initiation, repetitive swallows, and impaired coordination (Kalf et al., 2009; Miller et al., 2006). Although historically associated with coordination, the cerebellum is now recognised as essential in predictive timing and adaptive motor learning during swallowing. Neurophysiological evidence demonstrates that cerebellar activity modulates responsiveness to altered bolus consistency and supports compensatory swallowing strategies (Malandraki et al., 2011).

Recent comprehensive reviews further emphasize that swallowing is governed by distributed cortical–subcortical networks integrating sensorimotor control with higher-order cognitive processes, reinforcing the conceptualization of swallowing as a cognitively modulated behavior (Cheng et al., 2022).

Collectively, these findings indicated that swallowing is a distributed, network-based function embedded within broader neural systems for sensory integration, motor coordination, and cognitive control. Safe and efficient bolus transfer therefore depends on dynamic interactions between attentional systems, working memory processes, and somatosensory feedback.

2.2 Cognitive Load and Dual-Task Modulation

The use of dual-task paradigms has become a key method for investigating how cognitive load affects swallowing ability. The underlying premise is grounded in the concept of limited cognitive capacity, whereby simultaneous performance of a cognitive and motor task requires shared attentional resources.

The resource-competition paradigm is strongly supported by empirical evidence. In healthy adults, concurrent cognitive tasks such as mental arithmetic or auditory reaction tasks seemed to to significantly prolong swallow duration and increase pharyngeal residue volume (Muhle et al., 2020).

Similarly, Suntrup-Krueger et al. demonstrated that increased cognitive demands during swallowing result in altered cortical activation patterns, particularly within SMA and insular cortex, reflecting reduced neural efficiency under attentional strain (Suntrup-Krueger et al., 2025). These effects are more pronounced in older adults and individuals with cognitive impairment, who exhibit diminished adaptive capacity and reduced compensatory potential.

Therefore, the relationship between attention and swallowing represents a critical regulatory mechanism. Event-related potential (ERP) studies indicate that preparatory attentional shifts precede swallow initiation, and impaired attentional disengagement is associated with delayed or unsafe swallowing responses (Hamdy et al., 2000; Cheng et al., 2022). Consequently, cognitive fatigue or environmental distraction common during mealtimes and rehabilitation sessions may significantly elevate aspiration risk.

Executive functions, including task-switching and inhibitory control, play an equally important role. In individuals with Parkinson's disease, deficits in executive control contribute to premature swallow initiation and reduced adaptability to changing bolus properties (Miller et al., 2006; Kalf et al., 2009). In populations with MCI and AD, declines in processing speed and working memory are associated with delayed swallow initiation, poor strategy implementation, and reduced adherence to compensatory techniques (Easterling & Robbins, 2008; Tosun et al., 2024). This reciprocal relationship suggests that cognitive dysfunction both exacerbates dysphagia and may itself be aggravated by the nutritional deficits resulting from swallowing impairment.

Neuroimaging studies have substantially expanded understanding of cognitive-motor integration in swallowing. fMRI consistently demonstrates bilateral activation of the precentral and postcentral gyri, insula, ACC, supplementary motor area, and cerebellum during volitional swallowing (Hamdy et al., 1999; Lowell et al., 2008). Positron emission tomography (PET) findings further support these observations, indicating coordinated metabolic activity between prefrontal and motor regions during complex swallowing tasks (Hamdy et al., 1998).

Beyond activation patterns, functional connectivity analyses reveal dynamic interactions between cognitive networks and swallowing motor circuits. Altered connectivity involving the insula and medial prefrontal cortex has been linked to impaired swallow planning and reduced anticipatory control, suggesting a role for emotional and cognitive preparedness in swallowing performance (Cheng et al., 2022). Moreover, neuromodulation studies using transcranial magnetic stimulation (TMS) and transcranial direct current stimulation (tDCS) demonstrate that stimulation of the dorsolateral prefrontal cortex (DLPFC) and SMA enhances swallowing coordination and recovery, particularly when combined with behavioural therapy.

Electrophysiological data provide complementary support for these neuroimaging findings. Electroencephalography (EEG) studies have shown increased beta-band synchronisation between frontal and central regions during voluntary swallowing preparation, reflecting heightened attentional engagement (Hamdy et al., 2000). Conversely, reduced frontal-central coherence has been associated with aspiration risk in individuals with neurodegenerative disorders, reinforcing the notion that safe swallowing relies on intact executive-attentional networks (Tosun et al., 2024).

Collectively, these data converge on the conclusion that swallowing safety is predicated on the integrity of distributed cognitive networks responsible for attentional allocation, executive monitoring, and sensory-motor coordination. Disruption of these systems compromises the efficiency and safety of the swallowing process.

2.3. Integrative Perspective: Connecting Cognitive-Linguistic and Swallowing Networks

Neuroimaging, behavioral studies, and linguistic analyses together support a unified paradigm. This model suggests that swallowing and language share similar neurological bases, particularly in the insula, inferior frontal gyrus, and anterior temporal lobe. These brain areas are involved in both planning speaking movements and coordinating the oropharynx for swallowing, as shown by Humbert and Robbins (2008). Therefore, language activities that require retrieving action-related verbs, as those measured by the DVAQ-30, engage networks near those involved in swallowing (Tosun et al., 2025).

The overlap in anatomy and function has important clinical implications. Cognitive-linguistic evaluations, such as the TDQ-30/60, BECLA-Tr, and DTLA-Tr, are capable of detecting nuanced executive and semantic impairments. These deficits could potentially jeopardize swallowing safety indirectly, stemming from difficulties in strategy acquisition or adherence to tasks (Karalı et al., 2025; Eskioglu et al., 2025). Patients with difficulties retrieving words and those with working-memory problems often struggle to remember compensatory strategies like "double swallow" or "chin tuck." Recognizing this shared brain structure allows clinicians to create combined assessment methods that include both cognitive-linguistic and swallowing evaluations.

Recent investigations in Turkey support this combined viewpoint. Tosun and colleagues' (2024) hierarchical cluster analysis revealed a connection between cognitive assessments (MoCA, EAT-10, EdFED) and swallowing function, indicating that patient groupings were determined by integrated cognitive-motor profiles, as opposed to solely physiological factors. This research provides a basis for a cognitive-motor classification of dysphagia. It suggests that the intensity, complexity, and cueing methods used in therapy should be adjusted based on a person's cognitive abilities.

In summary, the neurocognitive processes that control swallowing involve a network that is both physically scattered and functionally interconnected. The initiation, sequencing, and safety of swallowing are controlled by the dynamic interactions of cortical, subcortical, and cerebellar nodes with attentional and executive systems. Swallowing difficulties can arise from cognitive overload, disease-related decline, or diminished connections within this network. Understanding these connections is important, as it creates the basis for personalized, cognition-focused assessment and therapeutic approaches, which will be described later.

From a clinical standpoint, this integrative perspective suggests that impairments observed in cognitive–linguistic tasks may signal vulnerability within shared neural networks that also support swallowing. Such insights allow clinicians to interpret language-based cognitive findings as functionally relevant indicators when planning dysphagia assessment and intervention. Taken together, these neurocognitive and cognitive–linguistic mechanisms provide the conceptual foundation for systematic assessment. Building on this framework, the following section focuses on how cognitive factors can be operationalized within dysphagia assessment and clinical decision-making.

Key Points:

1. Swallowing is supported by distributed cortical–subcortical networks that overlap with attentional and executive systems.
2. Cognitive load and impaired executive control reliably compromise swallowing safety and efficiency.
3. Disruption of these networks provides a neurocognitive explanation for dysphagia in neurodegenerative and cerebrovascular conditions.

Together, these mechanistic insights provide a rationale for integrating cognitive–linguistic measures into dysphagia assessment, enabling clinicians to align evaluation strategies with underlying neurocognitive constraints.

3. COGNITIVE PROCESSES AFFECT THE ACT OF SWALLOWING

3.1. Attention and Resource Allocation

Swallowing is a complex operation that requires attention, which is a basic cognitive function. This function regulates the timing, coordination, and safety of swallowing. Swallowing needs constant monitoring of internal sensory information and external stimuli, which necessitates flexible use of attentional resources. Studies employing dual-task methods show that when attention is divided between swallowing and another task, the efficiency and safety of swallowing are reduced. For instance, doing an auditory reaction-time task while swallowing leads to more pharyngeal residue and aspiration episodes. This shows that safe swallowing depends on maintaining attention throughout the process. Neuroimaging studies consistently show that ACC, DLPFC, and parietal association regions are active during voluntary swallowing. These areas together form a fronto-parietal network, which is crucial for directing, maintaining, and changing attention. In both healthy aging and MCI, the decreasing efficiency of this network explains the increased difficulty with swallowing when cognitive demands are high. In clinical practice, changes in attention are seen as inconsistent use of swallowing methods or feeding routines. Patients with attention problems, including those recuperating from a stroke or in the early stages of dementia, might not be able to use compensatory strategies or respond to caregivers' instructions. Therapeutic settings that reduce distractions and use short, repeated prompts can help stabilize attention and improve safety.

For example, an individual with mild cognitive impairment may demonstrate safe swallowing during structured VFSS evaluation but fail to consistently initiate compensatory strategies during everyday meals due to reduced executive monitoring. In such cases, dysphagia risk emerges not from biomechanical impairment but from diminished cognitive control in unstructured contexts. From a clinical perspective, these findings underscored the importance of evaluating attentional capacity when planning dysphagia assessment conditions and structuring therapy sessions, particularly in environments with high cognitive load.

3.2. Executive Functions and Cognitive Control

As described earlier in the chapter, increased cognitive load places additional demands on attentional and executive systems, which may compromise swallowing safety. Executive functions (EF) cover a set of higher-level cognitive abilities needed for goal-directed behavior, including planning, inhibition, task switching, and cognitive flexibility. These skills are essential for controlling swallowing voluntarily, particularly when people need to start, stop, or change their swallowing actions on purpose. Problems with executive functions can impede the capacity to control the time and order of swallowing. In situations like Parkinson's disease or after a stroke in the frontal lobe, problems in the frontostriatal circuits lead to swallowing that is either repeated or delayed, along with a reduced ability to respond to stimuli. Neurophysiological studies show that DLPFC and SMA send top-down control signals.

These signals then affect the excitability of the cortex in the swallowing motor cortex. Improved swallowing performance after stimulating these areas supports the idea that executive-control networks directly influence how we carry out sensorimotor tasks. In contrast, reduced activity in the prefrontal cortex is linked to swallowing difficulties, including delayed or hazardous swallowing, in people with neurodegenerative illnesses.

Executive function deficiencies also influence the cognitive and behavioral aspects of managing dysphagia. People who have trouble with planning may struggle to manage their meal schedules or implement plans that include changing food textures. People with weak cognitive flexibility could resist moving from compensatory strategies to rehabilitative tasks. Including EF screening in dysphagia assessments, using basic trail-making or verbal-fluency tasks, helps clinicians predict potential problems with patient compliance. This allows them to adjust the structure and pace of therapy to better fit each patient's abilities. Accordingly, identifying executive monitoring mechanisms limitations supports more informed decisions regarding strategy complexity, cueing frequency, and the pacing of swallowing rehabilitation. For example, a patient with executive dysfunction may demonstrate adequate swallowing safety during structured therapy tasks but show inconsistent adherence to compensatory strategies such as chin tuck or double swallow across sessions. This difficulty often reflects impaired planning, monitoring, or task initiation rather than a lack of understanding, underscoring the need for simplified strategies and increased external cueing.

3.3. Memory Processes and Learning in Swallowing Rehabilitation

Swallowing rehabilitation depends on learning and memory, which are based on both procedural and declarative processes. Procedural memory facilitates the incremental automation of secure motor sequences via repetition and feedback mechanisms. Conversely, declarative and working memory are essential for comprehending, retaining, and sequencing therapeutic directives, exemplified by instructions like "hold, swallow, cough, re-swallow." Limitations in working memory capacity hinder the transient storage of these sequential steps, thereby contributing to erratic performance. Long-term memory is essential for consolidating methods over time. However, in conditions like mild MCI and AD, problems with declarative memory hinder retention, even while short-term improvements are still present. This difference explains why some individuals do well during therapy but later struggle to sustain safe behaviors. Improving memory function in clinical settings is linked to better rehabilitation results. Retention is improved by using techniques like spaced repetition, external cues, and multimodal reinforcement, which includes visual, verbal, and tactile methods. External memory aids, such as illustrated instruction cards, caregiver checklists, and digital reminders, are used to help people with cognitive loss. Moreover, combining cognitive-linguistic training with swallowing therapy could involve overlapping brain networks, which would promote the simultaneous activation of memory and motor systems. Studies in Turkey, using action-verb naming tests like the TDQ-60 and DVAQ-30, have shown that the ability to retrieve verbs, a linguistic skill related to motor function, declines early in neurodegenerative diseases. Because the brain regions that process action verbs are similar to those that govern the mouth and throat, early language difficulties might be linked to problems with swallowing. Recognizing these similarities allows doctors to include cognitive-linguistic assessments in dysphagia evaluations. This, in turn, helps them create therapeutic programs that use the learning methods that are still functioning.

Key Points:

1. Cognitive load and executive dysfunction directly shape swallowing safety in everyday contexts.
2. Cognitive profiles influence assessment sequencing, cueing strategies, and therapy adherence.
3. Integrating cognitive screening with instrumental swallowing assessment improves clinical decision-making.

4. ASSESSMENT AND CLINICAL TOOLS

4.1. Reasons for Using Integrative Assessment

Swallowing is a complex behavior that involves the integration of thinking, language, and movement systems. Traditional assessment methods have mostly concentrated on physiological indicators, including aspiration, residue, and bolus transit, sometimes overlooking the patient's cognitive ability to comprehend and execute compensatory techniques. However, the efficacy of therapy and its long-term safety depend as much on cognitive processes and learning as they do on the biomechanics of the oropharynx. Therefore, a thorough assessment of dysphagia requires combining tests that measure swallowing function with standardized examinations of thinking and language skills. This approach helps create a complete picture of a person's abilities in daily life.

The integration principle is based on two main ideas:

1. Cognitive deficiencies, such as those affecting attention, executive function, or memory, directly influence how safe swallowing is and how well people follow treatment plans.
2. Understanding a patient's cognitive and language skills helps doctors customize cueing, pacing, and feedback throughout therapy. Therefore, assessment should be done across three interconnected areas: physical health, mental control, and the ability to communicate effectively.

4.2. Instrumental and Observational Assessment of Swallowing

The best way to understand the biomechanics of dysphagia is through instrumental assessment. VFSS and FEES are the two most common methods used to objectively visualize how food moves through the throat, how much remains after swallowing, and how the airway is protected. VFSS allow for a detailed, frame-by-frame investigation of how the mouth and throat move during swallowing. The Modified Barium Swallow Impairment Profile (MBSImP) and the Penetration–Aspiration Scale are examples of quantitative rating systems that are extensively used in clinical practice around the world. In contrast, FEES offers a portable and repeatable method for bedside assessment. This is especially valuable for patients who are medically fragile or have cognitive impairments, making them unable to undertake traditional imaging tests. In Turkish clinical settings, the Boston Residue and Clearance Scale (BRACS-Tr) has proven to be a dependable and validated instrument for assessing both residue and clearance efficiency (Tosun et al., 2024). The BRACS-Tr's psychometric evaluation showed a high level of agreement amongst different raters (an ICC above 0.9) and its capacity to detect minor changes in the pharynx. Importantly, the scale can be used alongside a brief cognitive screening, allowing for a simultaneous evaluation of cognitive and biomechanical components during the analysis. In addition, observational and screening technologies provide further support for instrumental methods. The Eating Assessment Tool (EAT-10) (Belafsky et al., 2008) and the Edinburgh Feeding Evaluation in Dementia Scale (EdFED) (Watson,1994) are both used to assess symptoms and eating behaviors, based on information from the person or their caregiver. Combining these subjective assessments with objective data creates a multi-faceted diagnostic view, reflecting both actual performance and personal perceptions.

4.3. Cognitive Screening and Neuropsychological Assessment

A thorough assessment of cognitive function is crucial for accurately identifying swallowing difficulties in people with neurological conditions. Standardized cognitive screening techniques, such as the Montreal Cognitive Assessment (MoCA) and the Mini-Mental State Examination (MMSE), are still useful as first assessments. However, their ability to identify executive dysfunction related to language is limited. More sophisticated assessment tools, particularly those that evaluate word meaning and thinking skills, are critical for distinguishing mild cognitive impairment from normal aging and for predicting how well someone would follow a treatment plan.

In this context, various Turkish-adapted assessments produced in recent years have addressed a significant methodological need.

The TDQ-30 and TDQ-60 tests, which assess color picture-naming, are used to evaluate noun retrieval, semantic memory, and lexical access in both adults and older people (Eskioglu et al., 2025; Karalı et al., 2025). These tests are sensitive to early signs of cognitive impairment and have shown convergent validity with global cognitive assessments, such the MoCA.

The DVAQ-30 Tr is a video-based task that assesses verb-naming abilities, focusing on action semantics and motor cognition. Because the brain areas involved in processing verbs overlap with those that control swallowing, success on the DVAQ might indirectly indicate the condition of networks associated with action.

BECLA-Tr: A comprehensive battery testing executive and linguistic components of cognition. Subtests addressing working memory, sentence comprehension, and verbal fluency allow physicians to measure attentional and planning capacities essential to swallowing rehabilitation.

DTLA-Tr: A fast bedside screening tool which is ideal for older persons or medically complex patients.

Together, these measures enable doctors to create a cognitive–linguistic baseline before commencing dysphagia therapy. Identifying impairments in attention, inhibition, or memory directs the clinician's choice of educational strategies (repetition versus explanation) and anticipates future carry-over difficulties. For instance, a patient with intact motor swallowing but reduced working memory may perform well during structured assessment yet demonstrate inconsistent strategy use during meals, prompting clinicians to prioritize simplified instructions and external cueing.

4.4. Interpreting Cognitive Profiles in the Context of Swallowing

Combining cognitive exams with swallowing evaluations provides important diagnostic information. A patient with normal motor skills but weak working memory could show inconsistent use of techniques across several sessions. In contrast, a patient with executive dysfunction might show safe swallowing during a test, but they could struggle to start swallowing when they should, due to problems with their ability to control their actions. By comparing scores from the TDQ, DVAQ, or BECLA assessments with the results of instrumental tests like VFSS or BRACS-Tr, doctors can identify whether a swallowing problem is mostly caused by cognitive or physical issues. This kind of interpretation across different modes can also help with predicting outcomes. Tosun et al. (2024) used cluster analysis, and their results showed a substantial relationship between swallowing efficiency and the MoCA, EAT-10, and EdFED scores. This led to the identification of cognitive-motor groups that might predict how well patients will respond to rehabilitation. These findings support the idea of a cognitive-motor continuum, rather than a rigorous separation between "neurological" and "mechanical" causes of swallowing difficulties.

Clinically, this integrative interpretation allows clinicians to anticipate therapy adherence difficulties—for instance, adjusting cueing frequency or simplifying strategy sets in patients with reduced working memory or attentional endurance. From a clinical decision-making perspective, such cognitive–motor profiling supports more targeted choices regarding assessment sequencing, cueing strategies, and the anticipated intensity of rehabilitation. For example, reduced performance on executive or verb-naming tasks may prompt clinicians to anticipate difficulties with strategy initiation or adherence, guiding the selection of simplified compensatory techniques and increased external cueing during rehabilitation.

4.5. Practical Guidelines for Clinicians

These criteria represent the best practices for conducting a comprehensive dysphagia assessment:

1. Cognitive examination should be the first step. Administer the MoCA or DTLA-Tr to measure initial attention, memory, and executive functioning capabilities.
2. Selecting the right instrumental evaluation is crucial. When a thorough physiological assessment is needed, VFSS is the go-to. For situations where bedside convenience or the ability to take repeated measurements is more important, FEES or BRACS-Tr are the better choices.
3. Integrate quantitative and qualitative metrics. Combine scores from objective residue analyses with behavioral observations and caregiver reports.
4. Organize data in a hierarchical manner. Determine if the observed deficiencies originate from biomechanical factors, cognitive control processes, or a combination of the two.
5. Keep a record of interactions. When you see fatigue, attention, or confusion occurring alongside risky swallowing, it's important to take note. These observations can reveal how cognitive factors impact swallowing ability.
6. Using these combined methods improves diagnosis accuracy and guarantees that therapy recommendations are realistic from a cognitive perspective.

Together, these steps provide a structured pathway for translating neurocognitive assessment findings into individualized rehabilitation planning.

4.6. Standardization and Cross-Cultural Adaptation

To ensure fairness in clinical research, it's vital to adjust cognitive and swallowing assessments for different cultures. The creation of Turkish versions of BECLA, TDQ, DVAQ, and BRACS exemplify this procedure, ensuring they are both linguistically and culturally relevant. The translation process followed international norms, including forward and backward translation, assessment by experts, pilot testing, and statistical evaluation to confirm reliability and construct validity. These adaptations do more than just localize instruments; they also generate comparative data, which strengthens the global evidence base. For example, the normative data for the TDQ-60 Tr show how education and age affect how quickly words are retrieved. These same factors also determine how well someone swallows. By including these demographic factors, researchers can create culturally relevant standard values and analyze how cognition and swallowing interact in different groups. By grounding assessment and intervention decisions in culturally validated cognitive–linguistic tools, clinicians can apply the proposed framework more consistently across diverse clinical populations.

4.7. Future Directions in Assessment Research

New technologies provide the potential to improve how we analyze the connections between cognition and swallowing. In addition, recent systematic reviews and meta-analyses highlight the growing role of brain neuromodulation techniques, such as rTMS and tDCS, in dysphagia rehabilitation, underscoring the relevance of cognition-informed and network-based therapeutic approaches (Speyer et al., 2022). Artificial intelligence can automatically analyze VFSS and FEES recordings to measure timing and movement. At the same time, digital cognitive-screening tools offer a way to test attention and memory from a distance. Using these tools could soon allow for real-time connections between cognitive load and how well someone swallows. Another important area to consider is ecological validity. Most lab studies of swallowing are done in controlled circumstances. However, eating in real life happens with talking and other distractions in the environment. Using virtual reality or dual-task setups that mimic real-world situations will provide more accurate information about the cognitive demands of eating. Ultimately, large-scale, multi-center research using standardized tools could create international reference frameworks. These frameworks would connect cognitive performance profiles with swallowing outcomes in various neurodegenerative diseases.

An additional consideration concerns the ecological validity of dysphagia assessment and intervention. While most swallowing evaluations are conducted under controlled clinical conditions, real-world eating frequently involves social interaction, background noise, multitasking, and environmental distractions. These contextual factors impose additional cognitive demands that may exacerbate swallowing risk, particularly in individuals with attentional or executive dysfunction. Incorporating ecologically valid paradigms such as dual-task mealtime simulations or socially embedded assessment contexts may therefore improve the clinical applicability of cognition-informed dysphagia models.

To facilitate clinical application, the assessment approaches discussed above can be conceptually summarized along three complementary dimensions: (1) biomechanical integrity, (2) cognitive control and learning capacity, and (3) functional communication abilities. This integrative view supports clinicians in selecting assessment tools and intervention strategies appropriate to the patient's overall profile.

5. THERAPEUTIC AND MULTIDISCIPLINARY IMPLICATIONS

5.1. Therapeutic Frameworks that Consider Cognition

Building on the neurocognitive mechanisms and assessment principles outlined earlier, this section focuses on how cognition-informed trends directly shape therapeutic decision-making in dysphagia management. Effective dysphagia management entails recognizing that swallowing is more than just a physical action; it's a process that involves thinking. The success of therapy depends on a person's ability to pay attention, plan, recall, and adapt, all of which are controlled by executive and attentional systems. Therefore, modern rehabilitation approaches emphasize cognitive-aware therapy, where treatment is tailored to the patient's cognitive abilities instead of following a standard plan. For a patient with good attention but low memory, using massed practice inside sessions, along with visual aids, could be helpful. In contrast, someone with concentration problems might benefit from short, frequent sessions in environments with few distractions. Therefore, cognitive-aware treatment uses assessment results to create personalized intervention plans, taking into account both neurocognitive strengths and weaknesses. Moreover, the complexity of a task should be matched to the cognitive burden it creates. In this way, cognitive profiling directly informs intervention selection, determining whether therapy should emphasize repetition, environmental modification, or compensatory strategy training. Using dual-task difficulties, such swallowing while answering simple questions, can be a helpful way to improve attentional resilience. On the other hand, for people with decreased working memory or executive function, multitasking too much could pose a safety risk. Therefore, therapists must adjust the difficulty of therapy in real-time, guided by constant observation and cognitive evaluation. In practical terms, identifying specific neurocognitive constraints—such as reduced attentional endurance or executive monitoring—guides clinicians in adapting task complexity, session structure, and feedback frequency to maximize therapeutic effectiveness.

5.2. Integrating Cognitive-Linguistic Training

Because the brain areas involved in swallowing and language overlap, therapies that improve language skills or executive function could also indirectly help with swallowing. Cognitive-linguistic dual training is based on this premise. It combines activities like retrieving action verbs or categorizing words semantically with exercises that involve swallowing. For example, patients using the effortful swallow technique might also do verb-generation tasks at the same time. This could help stimulate the fronto-insular circuits, which are involved in both actions. Initial findings from Turkish studies on the DVAQ-30 and TDQ-60 reveal that activities involving action verbs activate brain areas involved in controlling the oropharynx. This combined approach encourages the brain's ability to change and helps apply learned motor skills to real-world swallowing situations. Cognitive-linguistic training also enhances how well patients follow strategies. This is because they better grasp the reasons behind therapeutic instructions when cognitive understanding is developed with motor skills.

5.3. Improving Adherence and Knowledge Acquisition

Cognitive impairments commonly hamper commitment to therapy, especially in older persons with MCI or dementia. Therefore, interventions should include errorless learning, spaced retrieval, and external cueing strategies, they improve the retention of procedural memories. Using visual symbols, video demonstrations, and simpler directions reduces cognitive strain, which in turn promotes autonomous application. The involvement of family members and caregivers remains a vital factor. When caregivers understand cognitive limitations, they can give consistent cues and feedback outside of formal clinical settings. Using different types of cues helps people remember strategies better and ensures that therapy suggestions are used in daily life. Therapists also need to assess cognitive exhaustion. Fatigue can reduce both the ability to control attention and the efficiency of swallowing. Breaking sessions into bite-sized, purpose-driven chunks can keep people interested and avoid overwhelming them mentally. From an outcome prediction perspective, preserved attentional control and procedural learning capacity are associated with greater carry-over of swallowing strategies, whereas executive and memory impairments signal the need for increased external support and caregiver involvement.

5.4. Multidisciplinary Collaboration

Managing dysphagia requires a team approach, which means that speech-language pathologists, neurologists, physiatrists, dietitians, neuropsychologists, and occupational therapists must work together. The combined experience of several professionals helps to address the complex biological, psychological, and social aspects of swallowing difficulties. The neuropsychologist is crucial in defining cognitive profiles, recognizing executive or memory problems that could affect the safety of eating or the opportunity for rehabilitation. Speech and language therapists (SLTs) use these data to guide their therapy plans, choosing communication methods and how quickly they speak based on the patient's cognitive abilities. Physiatrists and neurologists work together to improve the medical treatment of the underlying illness. At the same time, dietitians adjust nutritional plans to promote healthy eating habits, avoiding too much mental strain. This collaborative approach shows the necessary combination of biological, psychological, and social factors, which is essential for lasting change. Interdisciplinary case conferences, along with shared digital documentation and cross-training sessions, help maintain consistency across different environments. This approach ensures that cognitive and swallowing goals stay on the same page. Such interdisciplinary coordination ensures that emerging cognition-informed trends are operationalized into coherent, functionally meaningful rehabilitation plans.

6. FUTURE DIRECTIONS AND CONCLUSION

The study of swallowing, viewed through a cognitive lens, has significantly changed dysphagia research. However, there are still many conceptual and methodological issues that need to be addressed. Current evidence suggests that swallowing efficiency and safety depend on the integrity of attention, executive function, and memory. However, the association between cognitive decline and swallowing difficulties is still incompletely defined. Most studies have focused on either biomechanics or cognition, but they haven't looked at how these two areas interact in real time. Therefore, future research should use combined approaches that measure cognitive load, brain activity, and the physical processes of swallowing at the same time. To advance this goal, multimodal neuroimaging and dual-task behavioural paradigms will be crucial. fMRI, electroencephalography (EEG), and TMS stimulation are techniques that can be used to study how brain activity changes with different cognitive tasks. They can help us understand how attention affects the motor control of swallowing. Longitudinal studies are particularly critical for determining whether cognitive problems appear before swallowing difficulties, or if they develop later due to starvation, dehydration, or diminished sensory feedback. Understanding this specific trend will help us create early intervention strategies and cognitive therapies to avoid swallowing problems in groups at risk.

Future research should focus on collaboration that crosses both disciplines and cultures. Combining datasets from speech-language pathology, neurology, and neuropsychology will allow researchers to find cognitive markers that can predict swallowing outcomes. Using standardized tools like the TDQ-60 Tr, DVAQ-30 Tr, BECLA-Tr, and BRACS-Tr in large, multi-center studies can help create standard guidelines. These guidelines would connect cognitive profiles with different types of swallowing difficulties. Therefore, using artificial intelligence for analysis could reveal hidden connections between cognitive and motor networks, which would then support rehabilitation programs tailored to individual needs. It's essential to keep cultural and linguistic variety as a key focus. The Turkish versions of important cognitive and swallowing assessments show how important it is to consider context. Expanding this research to include other languages and populations will increase the global applicability of neurocognitive models related to swallowing. Comparative studies of different languages can help us understand how the structures of language and cultural eating habits affect both thinking and the physical actions involved in swallowing.

To successfully apply study findings in practical settings, cognitive assessment should be systematically included in the management of dysphagia. Including short cognitive exams in regular examinations helps identify attention, memory, and executive function problems before starting treatment. This allows physicians to customize feedback, adjust the speed of sessions, and change the environment to fit each person's cognitive abilities. Therefore, speech-language therapy training programs should include neurocognitive content. This will help clinicians understand behavioral differences, such as distractibility or non-compliance, as signs of cognitive load, rather than just viewing them as resistance or lack of motivation. To improve the consistency of care, it's important to create multidisciplinary dysphagia teams within organizations. These teams should comprise neuropsychologists, neurologists, and nutritionists. Shared digital records, interprofessional discussions, and combined reporting systems can help synchronize cognitive and swallowing goals across different healthcare settings, including acute care, sub-acute care, and community-based services. This integration ensures that treatment plans remain consistent as patients go through different levels of care.

Technological advancements will continue to change the sector. Using wearable sensors, smartphone apps, and AI-assisted VFSS/FEES analysis for real-time monitoring allows us to connect cognitive states, such weariness or inattention, with physiological swallowing parameters. Virtual reality and brain-computer interface technologies will offer immersive training settings. These environments will use feedback to help rehabilitate both cognitive and motor functions at the same time. These advancements suggest a shift in therapeutic practice, moving from occasional, clinic-based therapies to ongoing, ecologically valid rehabilitation integrated into daily life.

Integrating neurocognitive findings into dysphagia management allows clinicians to move beyond descriptive diagnosis toward predictive and adaptive care. Cognitive profiles inform not only risk stratification but also the selection, timing, and expected durability of therapeutic strategies, thereby linking assessment results directly to rehabilitation planning and functional outcomes.

Therefore, swallowing should be understood as more than just a reflex or mechanical action. It is a complicated cognitive-motor process that involves the combined effects of attention, memory, and executive resources involved in task regulation. Recognizing and evaluating this integration will change how doctors assess and treat dysphagia in patients with neurological and developmental disorders. By incorporating cognitive science into dysphagia research and clinical practice, future approaches will likely shift toward a swallowing rehabilitation model that considers cognition. This model aims to not only make eating safe again but also to support independence, respect, and involvement throughout a person's life.

Although the present chapter primarily focuses on adult and aging populations, similar cognition–swallowing interactions are likely relevant in pediatric and neurodevelopmental conditions, where attentional regulation, executive control, and learning mechanisms are still maturing. High-level integration of developmental perspectives may offer valuable insights into early risk identification and the longitudinal evolution of swallowing–cognition interactions across the lifespan.

Finally, the increasing use of advanced technologies, including AI-assisted VFSS/FEES analysis and digital cognitive screening tools, raises important ethical and practical considerations. Issues related to data privacy, algorithmic transparency, clinical interpretability, and equitable access must be carefully addressed to ensure responsible implementation. Integrating ethical awareness into future dysphagia research frameworks will be essential as technology-driven assessment and intervention models continue to evolve. By maintaining a balance between theoretical rigor and applied guidance, the chapter is intended to support both experienced clinicians and readers at earlier stages of professional training.

Key Clinical Implications

1. Swallowing safety and efficiency are closely linked to attentional capacity, executive control, and memory processes.
2. Cognitive profiling supports more accurate risk stratification and informs individualized assessment planning.

3. Cognition-informed rehabilitation facilitates realistic strategy selection, improved adherence, and more predictable outcomes.
4. Integrating cognitive screening into routine dysphagia management enhances clinical decision-making across care settings.

REFERENCES

Alagiakrishnan, K., Bhanji, R. A., & Kurian, M. (2013). Evaluation and management of oropharyngeal dysphagia in different types of dementia: A systematic review. *Archives of Gerontology and Geriatrics*, *56*(1), 1–9. DOI: 10.1016/j.archger.2012.04.011 PMID: 22608838

Belafsky, P. C., Mouadeb, D. A., Rees, C. J., Pryor, J. C., Postma, G. N., Allen, J., & Leonard, R. J. (2008). Validity and reliability of the Eating Assessment Tool (EAT-10). *The Annals of Otology, Rhinology, and Laryngology*, *117*(12), 919–924. DOI: 10.1177/000348940811701210 PMID: 19140539

Cheng, I., Takahashi, K., Miller, A., & Hamdy, S. (2022). Cerebral control of swallowing: An update on neurobehavioral evidence. *Journal of the Neurological Sciences*, *442*, 120434. DOI: 10.1016/j.jns.2022.120434 PMID: 36170765

Daniels, S. K., & Huckabee, M.-L. (2014). *Dysphagia following stroke* (2nd ed.). Plural Publishing.

Dehaghani, S. E., Khosropoor, Z., Yousefzadeh, H., & Hamedanchi, A. (2021). Association between swallowing disorders and cognitive impairment: A systematic review and meta-analysis. *Dysphagia*, *36*(6), 1085–1096. DOI: 10.1007/s00455-021-10265-9

Easterling, C., & Robbins, E. (2008). Dementia and dysphagia. *Geriatric Nursing*, *29*(4), 275–285. DOI: 10.1016/j.gerinurse.2007.10.015 PMID: 18694703

Eskioglu, E. İ., Karali, F. S., Tosun, S., Cinar, N., & Macoir, J. (2025). Normative Data for the Adult Turkish Population and Validation Study in Mild Cognitive Impairment and Alzheimer's Disease of the TDQ-30 Tr, a Color Picture-naming Test for Adults and the Elderly. *Brain and Behavior*, *15*(8), e70718. DOI: 10.1002/brb3.70718 PMID: 40792495

Folstein, M. F., Folstein, S. E., & McHugh, P. R. (1975). "Mini-mental state". A practical method for grading the cognitive state of patients for the clinician. *Journal of Psychiatric Research*, *12*(3), 189–198. DOI: 10.1016/0022-3956(75)90026-6 PMID: 1202204

Hamdy, S., Aziz, Q., Rothwell, J. C., Power, M., Singh, K. D., Nicholson, D. A., Tallis, R. C., & Thompson, D. G. (1998). Recovery of swallowing after dysphagic stroke relates to functional reorganization in the intact motor cortex. *Gastroenterology*, *115*(5), 1104–1112. DOI: 10.1016/s0016-5085(98)70081-2 PMID: 9797365

Hamdy, S., Mikulis, D. J., Crawley, A., Xue, S., Lau, H., Henry, S., & Diamant, N. E. (1999). Cortical activation during human volitional swallowing: An event-related fMRI study. *The American Journal of Physiology*, *277*(1), G219–G225. DOI: 10.1152/ajpgi.1999.277.1.G219 PMID: 10409170

Hamdy, S., Rothwell, J. C., Aziz, Q., & Thompson, D. G. (2000). Organization and reorganization of human swallowing motor cortex: implications for recovery after stroke. Clinical science (London, England: 1979), 99(2), 151–157.

Humbert, I. A., & Robbins, J. (2008). Dysphagia in the elderly. *Physical Medicine and Rehabilitation Clinics of North America*, *19*(4), 853–866. DOI: 10.1016/j.pmr.2008.06.002 PMID: 18940645

Jean, A. (2001). Brain stem control of swallowing: Neuronal network and cellular mechanisms. *Physiological Reviews*, *81*(2), 929–969. PMID: 11274347

Kalf, J. G., de Swart, B. J. M., Borm, G. F., Bloem, B. R., & Munneke, M. (2009). Prevalence and definition of drooling in Parkinson's disease: A systematic review. *Journal of Neurology*, *256*(9), 1391–1396. DOI: 10.1007/s00415-009-5098-2 PMID: 19288042

Karalı, F. S., Eskioğlu, E. İ., Tosun, S., Çınar, N., & Macoir, J. (2025). Turkish adaptation, reliability, and validity of the detection test for language impairments in adults and the aged. *Applied Neuropsychology. Adult*, *32*(6), 1662–1669. DOI: 10.1080/23279095.2023.2301393 PMID: 38241752

Karalı, F. S., Tosun, S., Eskioğlu, E. İ., Çınar, N., & Macoir, J. (2025). The TDQ-60 Tr-a Picture-Naming Test to Assess Anomia in Turkish Adults and the Elderly: Normative Data and Validation Study in Alzheimer's Disease and Mild Cognitive Impairment. Archives of clinical neuropsychology: the official journal of the National Academy of Neuropsychologists, 40(3), 529–540. DOI: 10.1093/arclin/acaf005

Lowell, S. Y., Poletto, C. J., Knorr-Chung, B. R., Reynolds, R. C., Simonyan, K., & Ludlow, C. L. (2008). Sensory stimulation activates both motor and sensory components of the swallowing system. *NeuroImage*, *42*(1), 285–295. DOI: 10.1016/j.neuroimage.2008.04.234 PMID: 18515150

Malandraki, G. A., Johnson, S., & Robbins, J. (2011). Functional MRI of swallowing: from neurophysiology to neuroplasticity. Head & neck, 33 Suppl 1(0 1), S14–S20. DOI: 10.1002/hed.21903

Martínez-Peña, G., Mimenza-Alvarado, A. J., & Aguilar-Navarro, S. G. (2025). Dysphagia in older adults with mild cognitive impairment and dementia through fluoroscopic study with barium swallow in a memory clinic. *Frontiers in Neurology*, *15*, 1461239. DOI: 10.3389/fneur.2024.1461239 PMID: 39882370

Miller, N., Noble, E., Jones, D., & Burn, D. (2006). Hard to swallow: Dysphagia in Parkinson's disease. *Age and Ageing*, *35*(6), 614–618. DOI: 10.1093/ageing/afl105 PMID: 17047007

Muhle, P., Claus, I., Labeit, B., Ogawa, M., Dziewas, R., Suntrup-Krueger, S., & Warnecke, T. (2020). Effects of cognitive and motor dual-tasks on oropharyngeal swallowing assessed with FEES in healthy individuals. *Scientific Reports*, *10*(1), 20403. Advance online publication. DOI: 10.1038/s41598-020-77421-3 PMID: 33230259

Nasreddine, Z. S., Phillips, N. A., Bédirian, V., Charbonneau, S., Whitehead, V., Collin, I., Cummings, J. L., & Chertkow, H. (2005). The Montreal Cognitive Assessment, MoCA: A brief screening tool for mild cognitive impairment. *Journal of the American Geriatrics Society*, *53*(4), 695–699. DOI: 10.1111/j.1532-5415.2005.53221.x PMID: 15817019

Serra-Prat, M., Palomera, E., Gómez, C., & Clavé, P. (2020). Dysphagia treatment in dementia: A systematic review. *Clinical Nutrition (Edinburgh, Lothian)*, *39*(11), 3297–3305. DOI: 10.1016/j.clnu.2020.03.022

Smithard, D. G., Smeeton, N. C., & Wolfe, C. D. A. (2007). Long-term outcome after stroke: Does dysphagia matter? *Age and Ageing*, *36*(1), 90–94. DOI: 10.1093/ageing/afl149 PMID: 17172601

Speyer, R., Sutt, A.-L., Bergström, L., Hamdy, S., Pommée, T., Balaguer, M., & Cordier, R. (2022). Neurostimulation in people with oropharyngeal dysphagia: A systematic review and meta-analysis of randomised controlled trials—Part II: Brain neurostimulation. *Journal of Clinical Medicine*, *11*(4), 993. DOI: 10.3390/jcm11040993 PMID: 35207265

Suntrup-Krueger, S., Muhle, P., & Slavik, J.. (2025). Cognitive decline limits compensatory resource allocation within the aged swallowing network. *GeroScience*, *47*, 5481–5491. DOI: 10.1007/s11357-025-01649-y PMID: 40202551

Tosun, S., Karalı, F. S., Eskioğlu, E. İ., Çınar, N., & Macoir, J. (2025). Turkish Version of the Video-Naming Test for Assessing Verb Anomia (DVAQ-30): Normative Data for the Adult Turkish Population and Validation Study in Mild Cognitive Impairment and Alzheimer's Disease. *International Journal of Language & Communication Disorders*, *60*(4), e70068. DOI: 10.1111/1460-6984.70068 PMID: 40570084

Tosun, S., Karali, F. S., Kacar Kutukcu, D., Cinar, N., Kendirli, S., Sen Aksut, M., Albayrak, I., & Celik, Y. (2024). Assessment of swallowing performance in patients with neurodegenerative disease: A hierarchical cluster analysis. *Brain and Behavior*, *14*(9), e70005. DOI: 10.1002/brb3.70005 PMID: 39197023

Tosun, S., Topbaş, S. S., & Aksoy, E. (2025). A Tool for the Assessment of Swallowing Safety and Efficiency in Adults: Turkish Adaptation of Boston Residue and Clearance Scale. *Dysphagia*, *40*(1), 88–97. DOI: 10.1007/s00455-024-10706-1 PMID: 38703232

Watson, R. (1994). Measuring feeding difficulty in patients with dementia: Developing a scale. *Journal of Advanced Nursing*, *19*(2), 257–263. DOI: 10.1111/j.1365-2648.1994.tb01079.x PMID: 8188956

Chapter 13
Developmental Processes, Comorbidities, and Quality of Life of Autism Spectrum Disorders:
Clinical and Neuropsychological Perspectives

Maria Theodoratou
http://orcid.org/0000-0003-4200-4643
Hellenic Open University, Greece

Dimitra Katsarou
http://orcid.org/0000-0001-8690-0314
University of the Aegean, Greece

Evangelos Mantsos
http://orcid.org/0009-0002-8490-2660
University of Western Macedonia, Greece

Kalliopi D. Megari
http://orcid.org/0000-0002-5861-7199
York University, Greece

Elpida Denazi
Hellenic Open University, Greece

Soultana Papadopoulou
http://orcid.org/0000-0002-0950-1456
University of Ioannina, Greece

Efthymia Efthymiou
http://orcid.org/0000-0003-0411-1720
Zayed University, UAE

ABSTRACT

Autism Spectrum Disorders (ASD) are complex neurodevelopmental conditions marked by social communication difficulties, restricted interests, and repetitive

DOI: 10.4018/979-8-3373-6405-6.ch013

behaviors. This chapter examines developmental trajectories, emphasizing genetic, neurobiological, and environmental influences on symptom emergence and progression. Comorbidities—including intellectual disabilities, ADHD, anxiety, epilepsy, gastrointestinal disorders, and dysphagia—are discussed regarding their prevalence, functional impact, and implications for diagnosis and intervention. The chapter also explores quality of life in ASD, highlighting the importance of adaptive skills, social support, educational inclusion, and access to individualized interventions. By integrating research and clinical insights, it provides a comprehensive overview of how developmental processes and comorbidities shape experiences of individuals with ASD and offers guidance for improving outcomes across the lifespan.

INTRODUCTION TO AUTISM SPECTRUM DISORDER

Autism Spectrum Disorder (ASD) represents a complex neurodevelopmental condition characterized by a multidimensional involvement that manifests through decreased social interaction, deficiencies in both verbal and nonverbal communication, and behavioral inflexibility often presenting as repetitive behaviors and restricted interests (*Alcal & Madrigal, 2023*). This pervasive developmental condition affects how individuals perceive and relate to the world and other people, making it a lifelong challenge (Ostrowski et al., 2024; Sala et al., 2020). The term "spectrum" aptly highlights the vast heterogeneity in the clinical presentation, severity, and associated features among individuals diagnosed with ASD (Ostrowski et al., 2024). Symptoms can vary significantly from patient to patient, with differing levels of severity in communication and cognitive functioning (Ostrowski et al., 2024). Historically, research and clinical attention have predominantly focused on the behavioral and cognitive manifestations of ASD, which, while crucial, have sometimes overshadowed the recognition of its common association with a wide array of physical and mental health conditions (Sala et al., 2020). These co-occurring conditions can exacerbate the core symptoms, further impairing social communication and behavior, leading to a diminished quality of life, increased morbidity, and even premature mortality (Sala et al., 2020).

The global prevalence of ASD underscores its significance as a growing public health concern, with estimates from the World Health Organization suggesting that approximately 1 in 100 children have ASD, although these figures can vary depending on the diagnostic methodology employed (Ostrowski et al., 2024). Other reports indicate a prevalence of around 1 in 160 children globally (*Alcal & Madrigal, 2023*) and even up to 2% of the population in the US (Ma et al., 2022). Despite this considerable prevalence, ASD is often underdiagnosed or identified late, frequently only upon the emergence of significant comorbidities like anxiety or depression

(*Alcal & Madrigal, 2023*). Early detection and the initiation of appropriate, comprehensive therapy are deemed essential for enhancing the continued functioning of patients and supporting their families (Ostrowski et al., 2024). This chapter aims to provide a comprehensive overview of ASD, integrating clinical and neuropsychological perspectives to explore its developmental processes, the extensive range of comorbidities, and their cumulative impact on the quality of life, emphasizing the critical need for integrated, multidisciplinary care across the lifespan.

ATYPICAL DEVELOPMENTAL PROCESSES IN ASD

The developmental trajectory in Autism Spectrum Disorder is marked by profound deviations from typical development, emerging from dynamic interactions among neural activity networks, behavioral systems, and experience-dependent processes (Bradshaw et al., 2022). These atypical developmental processes begin very early in life and critically shape an individual's abilities and challenges over time. Understanding these unique pathways is fundamental for early identification, accurate diagnosis, and the implementation of effective, targeted interventions. The complexity and heterogeneity of ASD, with its biological and behavioral features cutting across multiple developmental domains—including motor, cognitive, sensory, and bioregulatory—make a developmental cascades framework ideal for illustrating how interconnected systems have far-reaching effects in atypical development (Bradshaw et al., 2022).

Neurobiological Foundations of Atypical Development

From a neurobiological standpoint, ASD is increasingly understood as a connectopathy, a syndrome of neurobiological origin characterized by alterations in neural connectivity that impact cortical network organization and the excitation-to-inhibition ratio (Beopoulos et al., 2022*; Grañana, 2022*). This concept of abnormal brain connectivity is supported by a growing body of evidence from functional imaging, diffusion tensor imaging, and high-definition fiber tracking studies, which suggest that altered microstructure in axonal tracts connecting cortical areas may underpin many of the cognitive manifestations of ASD (McFadden & Minshew, 2013). These studies indicate that regions that should work together smoothly and efficiently to perform information-processing tasks are affected, leading to a "disconnection syndrome" (Williams & Minshew, 2010). Initial evidence for this comes from fMRI studies showing reduced coordination between brain areas involved in sentence-reading comprehension (Williams & Minshew, 2010).

Large-scale genomic studies further implicate numerous gene candidates known or suspected to mediate neuritic outgrowth and guidance during fetal and perinatal life (McFadden & Minshew, 2013). Neuropathological observations from postmortem ASD samples also support this model, revealing subtle disturbances in lamination and subcortical morphology (McFadden & Minshew, 2013). A relatively common finding is poor differentiation of the gray-white junction, associated with an excess of superficial white matter "interstitial" neurons (INs), which are thought to be remnants of the subplate—a transient structure playing a key role in the morphogenesis of thalamocortical and cortico-cortical connections and the organization of columnar architecture (McFadden & Minshew, 2013). These findings suggest that abnormal development of the brain's neuronal architecture, including synaptogenesis and dendritic arborization, occurs *in utero* (Williams & Minshew, 2010). Some theories postulate that sudden changes in environmental conditions, specifically linked to serotonin/kynurenine supply to the developing fetus during critical gestational weeks, are likely to promote ASD pathogenesis during fetal brain development (Beopoulos et al., 2022). This appears to be driven by discrete alterations in differentiation and patterning mechanisms arising from *in utero* RNA editing, favoring vulnerability outcomes over plasticity outcomes (Beopoulos et al., 2022). Recent advancements in single-cell brain organoid screening have identified developmental defects in autism, showing that perturbing high-risk ASD genes related to transcriptional regulation uncovers their effects on cell fate determination, with dorsal intermediate progenitors, ventral progenitors, and upper-layer excitatory neurons being among the most vulnerable cell types (Li et al., 2022).

Cognitive and Sensory Manifestations

Neuropsychological assessments provide an in-depth analysis of cognitive functioning in individuals with ASD, revealing a unique profile of intact and impaired abilities (Williams & Minshew, 2010; Zwick, 2017). Simpler skills, often relying on lower-order brain circuitry, such as basic attention, elementary motor skills, sensory perception, simple memory, formal language elements (phonological and grammatical), rule-learning, and visuospatial processing, may be intact or even enhanced in ASD (Williams & Minshew, 2010). In stark contrast, higher-order cognitive functions that necessitate integrative processing are disproportionately affected across various domains, including complex sensory integration and concept formation (Williams & Minshew, 2010). This "disconnection syndrome" means individuals with ASD often rely on their intact lower-order functions, leading to different ways of thinking and learning compared to neurotypical individuals (Williams & Minshew, 2010).

For example, they may struggle with prototype formation, such as automatically categorizing faces or emotional expressions, instead developing idiosyncratic strategies for discrimination tasks (Williams & Minshew, 2010).

A significant aspect of atypical cognition in ASD is inflexible thinking, also referred to as cognitive inflexibility, rigidity, insistence on sameness, intolerance of uncertainty, set-shifting deficits, brooding rumination, or black-and-white thinking (Hollander & Ferretti, 2023). This is a transdiagnostic endophenotype, or vulnerability factor, present in ASD and other disorders, profoundly affecting an individual's ability to adapt to a constantly changing world and contributing to difficulties in relationships and the workplace (Hollander & Ferretti, 2023). Inflexible thinking is a core component of the restricted and repetitive behavior (RRB) domain, a symptom required for an ASD diagnosis, where insistence on sameness and intolerance of uncertainty can lead to extreme discomfort, protests, tantrums, self-injury, or aggression in response to unexpected environmental changes (Hollander & Ferretti, 2023). Neurocognitive studies suggest individuals with ASD can recognize and learn rules, patterns, and routines but tend to maintain them over longer periods rather than flexibly switching (Hollander & Ferretti, 2023). This preference for rules underlies a strong need for environmental predictability, and the severity of RRBs is linked to impairments in adaptive skills, social communication, and interpersonal challenges (Hollander & Ferretti, 2023).

Sensory anomalies are also a hallmark of ASD, with individuals often experiencing hyper- or hypo-sensitivity to various sensory inputs (Esposito et al., 2023; Hollander & Ferretti, 2023). This can manifest as visual fascination with lights or movement, or aversions to certain smells, textures, or sounds (Hollander & Ferretti, 2023). These sensory processing differences can significantly impact daily functioning, contributing to challenging behaviors and influencing attention patterns, as a child might be drawn to bright colors or specific auditory input (Williams & Minshew, 2010).

Motor and Language Development

Atypical motor development is frequently observed in individuals with ASD, including delays in achieving gross motor milestones and unusual movement patterns (Wiley & Moeller, 2007). These motor challenges can impact a child's ability to explore their environment and engage in play, and may include low muscle tone, affecting their ability to maintain an upright posture and attend to communication-related tasks (Wiley & Moeller, 2007). Such motor difficulties necessitate specialized support, including physical therapy, to promote functional independence (Wiley & Moeller, 2007).

Language development in ASD is highly variable. While some individuals may develop language skills within typical ranges, many experience significant delays or deficits (Venker & Stronach, 2017). Research has identified various contributing factors, including difficulties with auditory processing and motor speech planning (Chenausky et al., 2021; Williams & Minshew, 2010). For instance, a notable proportion of minimally verbal children with ASD may have a comorbid motor speech disorder, such as childhood apraxia of speech, which affects their ability to produce speech sounds consistently and variably within and between tokens (Chenausky et al., 2021). Some children may also present with both motor speech and auditory processing disorders, leading to highly centralized, schwa-like speech (Chenausky et al., 2021). These challenges are further compounded by difficulties in processing the rapid stream of connected speech, discriminating words, and relating objects to actions in the environment (Williams & Minshew, 2010). Individuals with ASD may also struggle with interpreting meaning based on contextual cues, often failing to respond to their names or lacking a preference for their mother's voice in infancy (Williams & Minshew, 2010). The propensity to process linguistic information in the right hemisphere, rather than the left, may also contribute to these difficulties (Williams & Minshew, 2010). The variability in language outcomes underscores the heterogeneity of ASD and the need for individualized assessment and intervention approaches that target specific underlying deficits, such as using visual aids or explicitly teaching concepts that neurotypical individuals acquire automatically (Williams & Minshew, 2010).

MEDICAL COMORBIDITIES: A FOCUS ON FEEDING AND GASTROINTESTINAL ISSUES

The clinical landscape of Autism Spectrum Disorder is frequently complicated by a high prevalence of co-occurring medical conditions, many of which can significantly impact an individual's physical health, behavior, and overall quality of life (Ferrara et al., 2025; Sala et al., 2020). Among these, feeding problems and gastrointestinal (GI) disorders are particularly common and relevant to the broader context of dysphagia, necessitating a focused, multidisciplinary approach to assessment and management (Beaudry-Bellefeuille et al., 2021; Leader, OReilly, et al., 2020). These conditions are not merely secondary concerns but can actively worsen the clinical course of autism and contribute to resistance to pharmacological treatments (Ferrara et al., 2025).

Prevalence and Types of Gastrointestinal Issues

Gastrointestinal symptoms are highly prevalent in children and adolescents with ASD, with studies reporting rates ranging from 30% to 70% (James et al., 2021; Penzol et al., 2019). A retrospective study of patients admitted to a comprehensive medical program for ASD found that at least one functional GI disorder (fGID) was present in 30.5% of patients, with constipation being the most prevalent (47.4% of fGID patients) (Penzol et al., 2019). Other commonly reported GI issues include dyspepsia, reflux, pica, abdominal pain, and diarrhea (Prabhakaran et al., 2025). These GI symptoms are not only common but can also be severe, negatively impacting quality of life for both individuals with ASD and their caregivers (James et al., 2021). Specific feeding problems are also frequently endorsed by caregivers, including food refusal, limited variety of food, single food intake, or liquid diets (Esposito et al., 2023; Leader, OReilly, et al., 2020). These dysfunctional behaviors at mealtime are often multifactorial, stemming from medical, sensory, or behavioral origins (Esposito et al., 2023). In particular, oral motor issues or dysphagia can make it physically difficult for individuals with ASD to manage certain food consistencies, further contributing to feeding difficulties (Freeland, 2012).

Interplay with Core Symptoms and Exacerbation of Behavioral Problems

The presence of GI issues is not isolated but is intricately linked to the core symptoms and challenging behaviors often seen in ASD (Neuhaus et al., 2018). Studies have revealed that GI problems are significantly associated with intellectual disability, sleep disorders, and the prescription of psychopharmacological treatments, indicating their connection to behavioral problems (Penzol et al., 2019). For individuals with ASD, especially those who are minimally verbal or nonverbal, physical distress from GI discomfort or food allergies may manifest as increased irritability, aggression, or self-injurious behaviors, rather than verbally expressed pain (McDougle, 2018; Neuhaus et al., 2018). This highlights the critical importance of a thorough medical evaluation to rule out identifiable medical causes for aberrant behaviors before proceeding with treatments solely focused on behavior modification (McDougle, 2018).

The link between GI symptoms and psychiatric outcomes in children with ASD is further supported by research, where higher levels of GI symptoms are associated with increased internalizing, externalizing, and self-injurious behaviors, even after accounting for ASD symptoms and psychosocial factors (Neuhaus et al., 2018). For instance, constipation can increase by 20% for unit increases in speech-language communication scores, and pica can increase by 23.2% for unit increases in sensory patterns scores (Prabhakaran et al., 2025). These findings suggest that GI distress may exacerbate defining behavioral symptoms such as irritability, social withdrawal, stereotypy, and hyperactivity (James et al., 2021). Consequently, recognizing and treating these medical conditions can lead to an improvement in behavioral symptoms and overall quality of life for individuals with autism and their caregivers (Ferrara et al., 2025).

Underlying Mechanisms and the Gut-Brain Axis

Emerging research highlights a significant role for alterations in the gut in the pathoetiology and/or pathophysiology of ASD (Seo & Anderson, 2020). The relationship between GI disorders and ASD is thought to be bidirectional, involving shared mechanisms related to gut-brain axis abnormalities and immune dysregulation (McDougle, 2018; Seo & Anderson, 2020). The gut microbiome, for example, has been shown to have a significant impact on amygdala development in infancy, suggesting that alterations in the gut microbiome may modulate not only amygdala development but also how the amygdala influences the development of the frontal cortex and other brain regions (Seo & Anderson, 2020). Genetic, epigenetic, and environmental factors interact in early development to regulate these gut-mediated changes, potentially involving microRNA (miR)-451, 14-3-3 proteins, cytochrome P450 (CYP)1B1, and melatonergic pathways (Seo & Anderson, 2020). These factors can contribute to hyperserotonemia, which is often evident in ASD, affecting mitochondrial functioning and exosome content (Seo & Anderson, 2020).

Dysphagia Connection

In the context of dysphagia, feeding and GI issues in ASD are directly relevant. Difficulties with chewing and swallowing, the presence of drooling, impaired automatic lip closure and lingual mobility, and oral asymmetries are all indicators of potential praxis issues that can interfere with feeding (Wiley & Moeller, 2007). A study noted that almost 30% of screened patients with developmental disabilities had problems with swallowing difficulties (Freeland, 2012). These challenges, combined with sensory sensitivities to food textures, tastes, and smells, can make mealtimes a significant source of stress and can lead to inadequate nutrition (Esposito et al., 2023; Trambacz-Oleszak, 2019). The high prevalence of GI distress, manifesting as constipation, abdominal pain, and reflux, further complicates feeding by causing discomfort that can lead to food refusal or aversion (Bresciani et al., 2023; Prabhakaran et al., 2025). Therefore, a comprehensive assessment of dysphagia in individuals with ASD must consider the intricate interplay of sensory, motor, behavioral, nutritional, and gastrointestinal factors (Beaudry-Bellefeuille et al., 2021).

PSYCHIATRIC COMORBIDITIES

Psychiatric comorbidities are a critical aspect of Autism Spectrum Disorder, significantly affecting the quality of life, prognosis, and functional outcomes for individuals across the lifespan (Ferrara et al., 2025; Mutluer et al., 2022). Most studies report a high prevalence of these co-occurring disorders, with nearly half of individuals with ASD receiving at least one psychiatric diagnosis (Hollander & Ferretti, 2023). Recognizing and addressing these conditions is paramount because they can worsen the clinical course of autism and contribute to treatment resistance (Ferrara et al., 2025).

Prevalence and Types of Psychiatric Conditions

A wide range of psychiatric disorders are frequently observed in individuals with ASD. A meta-analysis examining population-based studies found significant prevalence rates: 22.9% for intellectual disability, 26.2% for attention-deficit hyperactivity disorder (ADHD), 11.1% for anxiety disorders, 19.7% for sleep-wake disorders, 7% for disruptive mood dysregulation disorder, 2% for bipolar disorder, 2.7% for depression, 1.8% for obsessive-compulsive disorder (OCD), and 0.6% for psychosis (Mutluer et al., 2022). These population-based estimates are often lower than those found in clinical or treatment referral samples, which may overestimate frequency and severity (Mutluer et al., 2022). Another study on children and adolescents with high-functioning ASD in an Italian sample found that 32.2% had a comorbid psychiatric condition, with ADHD being most frequent among preschoolers (20.4%) and ADHD and anxiety/OCD being common in school-age children (21% and 10.6% respectively) (*Fucà et al., 2023*). Adolescents showed a higher prevalence of anxiety/OCD (21.8%) (*Fucà et al., 2023*).

The co-occurrence of ASD and ADHD is well-established, with ASD diagnosis being associated with elevated ADHD traits and symptoms (Dupuis et al., 2022). Children with co-occurring ASD and ADHD also have a higher prevalence of most other mental, behavioral, and developmental disorders (MBDDs), including anxiety, depression, and behavior or conduct problems, compared to children with ASD without ADHD or children with ADHD without ASD (Casseus et al., 2023). This highlights the complex needs of this population, often requiring a multidisciplinary approach (Casseus et al., 2023).

Impact on Functioning and Quality of Life

Psychiatric comorbidities contribute substantially to additional functional impairment, increased treatment costs, and a greater burden on caregivers (Chandrasekhar & Sikich, 2015). For example, greater autism symptoms are associated with more parent- and teacher-reported peer problems, emotional problems, and conduct problems in children with ADHD (Green et al., 2016). Every standard deviation increase in autism symptom scores is linked to increased internalizing and externalizing disorders, a decrease in quality of life, and an increase in moderate/severe sleep problems (Green et al., 2016). Individuals with ASD and intellectual disability, particularly those with comorbid challenging behavior, experience higher psychological distress and lower quality of family life (Staunton et al., 2020).

High alexithymic traits, characterized by difficulty describing emotions, are frequently observed among adults with ASD and are linked to increased depression and social phobia (Albantakis et al., 2020). These traits, along with autistic traits, are predictive risk factors for depressive and phobic symptoms, highlighting the importance of assessing these in individuals with ASD (Albantakis et al., 2020). The presence of psychiatric comorbidities can lead to poorer psychosocial functioning and quality of life, often creating a vicious cycle of negative experiences, stigma, maladjustment, and exclusion (Eapen et al., 2016).

Diagnostic Challenges

Diagnosing comorbid neuropsychiatric illnesses in individuals with ASD can be particularly challenging due to communication deficits inherent in ASD, the atypical presentation of psychiatric symptoms, and a lack of standardized diagnostic tools tailored for this population (Chandrasekhar & Sikich, 2015). Clinicians may struggle to differentiate between core ASD symptoms and those of a co-occurring psychiatric disorder, leading to diagnostic overshadowing where symptoms are inappropriately attributed to ASD rather than being treated as separate conditions (Freeland, 2012). For instance, depression in individuals with developmental disabilities may not present with typical sadness or loss of appetite but rather through acting out or aggression (Freeland, 2012). This necessitates careful and comprehensive assessment, often involving a multidisciplinary team, to identify these conditions accurately (*Fucà et al., 2023;* Hollander & Ferretti, 2023). Better targeted tools are needed to detect psychiatric comorbidities in youth with ASD for future studies, which are essential for providing new insights into their nature and underlying mechanisms (Mutluer et al., 2022).

OTHER SIGNIFICANT MEDICAL COMORBIDITIES

Beyond feeding and gastrointestinal issues, individuals with Autism Spectrum Disorder frequently experience a broad spectrum of other medical comorbidities that significantly impact their health, daily functioning, and overall quality of life. These conditions often contribute to the complexity of ASD presentation, further emphasizing the need for a holistic and integrated approach to care.

Sleep Disturbances

Sleep problems are recognized as a common and significant comorbid condition in ASD, affecting a substantial majority of individuals across the lifespan (Ballester et al., 2018; Mazzone et al., 2018). Studies indicate that between 50% and 80% of children with ASD experience sleep problems, which are also prevalent in adults with ASD, both with and without intellectual disability (Ballester et al., 2018; Mazzone et al., 2018). These disturbances include longer sleep latency, frequent night awakenings, and circadian rhythm sleep-wake disorders (Ballester et al., 2018). The impact of sleep problems extends beyond the individual, increasing parental stress and adversely affecting family quality of life (Mazzone et al., 2018). Parents of children with ASD and poor sleep report higher levels of parenting stress, anxiety, and depression, along with a lower quality of life in physical health, psychological well-being, and environmental domains (Mannion & Leader, 2023).

The underlying causes of sleep disorders in ASD are complex and likely multifactorial. Neurobiological alterations and genetic mutations are considered possible etiological explanations (Mazzone et al., 2018). For example, deficiency of the autism-related *Scn2a* gene in mice, which encodes the voltage-gated sodium channel NaV1.2, disrupts sleep patterns and circadian rhythms, leading to increased wakefulness and reduced non-rapid-eye-movement (NREM) sleep (Ma et al., 2022). This suggests a possible mechanism for sleep disturbances related to this genetic deficiency (Ma et al., 2022). Sleep problems can also be exacerbated by other comorbidities, such as gastrointestinal issues, which contribute to increased irritability and can aggravate core autism symptoms (Bresciani et al., 2023; McKenna et al., 2024).

Effective management of sleep disturbances is crucial, as they can significantly worsen behavioral problems (Mazzone et al., 2018). Pharmacological options, such as prolonged-release melatonin (PedPRM), have shown efficacy and safety in improving sleep parameters in children and adolescents with ASD, leading to longer sleep duration, faster sleep onset, fewer awakenings, and better overall sleep quality (Maras et al., 2018). Improvements in sleep also translate to statistically significant and clinically relevant improvements in caregiver satisfaction and overall quality of life (Maras et al., 2018). Exercise programs have also been shown to substantially decrease sleep disturbances in children and adolescents with ASD (Toscano et al., 2022).

Otolaryngological Manifestations

Individuals with ASD commonly experience otolaryngological comorbidities, particularly auditory disorders, which can negatively impact their ability to communicate effectively and further impair their functioning (McKenna et al., 2024). These include hearing loss, auditory processing disorders such as central auditory processing disorder (CAPD), and both chronic and recurrent otitis media (McKenna et al., 2024). Such challenges can interfere with language acquisition and social communication, making it even more difficult for individuals with ASD to engage with their environment (McKenna et al., 2024). The higher rate of sinusitis also contributes to a worsening of the autism phenotype (McKenna et al., 2024). The high prevalence of these comorbidities necessitates better collaboration between various healthcare providers, including otolaryngologists, to improve the quality of life for affected individuals and their families/caregivers (McKenna et al., 2024).

Neurological Comorbidities

Epilepsy and seizure disorders are frequently observed in individuals with ASD, representing another significant neurological comorbidity (Hollander & Ferretti, 2023). Some studies cite that 41% of individuals with developmental disabilities, including ASD, have a seizure diagnosis (Freeland, 2012). Developmental regression followed by epilepsy and aggression is a hypothesized syndrome, with patients experiencing developmental regression showing a non-significantly higher rate of epilepsy and aggression when evaluated separately, but a statistically significant combined rate of aggression and epilepsy (Gaitanis et al., 2023). These comorbidities can profoundly inhibit habilitation in language and social function and severely impact quality of life, effectively causing a second regression in individuals who experienced an earlier developmental regression as toddlers (Gaitanis et al., 2023). Autonomic dysfunction, characterized by alterations in neural connectivity, is also noted, with previous reports indicating enhanced sympathoexcitation in ASD (Owens et al., 2021). There is a strong association between ASD and joint hypermobile Ehlers-Danlos syndrome (hEDS), which may be overrepresented in ASD and is linked to orthostatic-related dysfunction (Owens et al., 2021). Intermittent autonomic dysfunction affecting blood pressure is overrepresented in ASD and can further impair quality of life, especially for those unable to adequately express their symptoms (Owens et al., 2021).

IMMUNE AND METABOLIC ISSUES

Immune dysregulation and inflammation are increasingly recognized as significant underlying mechanisms in the pathogenesis of both allergic diseases and neurodevelopmental disorders, including Autism Spectrum Disorder . This suggests a converging pathophysiology, where shared biological pathways contribute to the co-occurrence of these conditions. Epidemiological studies have provided compelling evidence for a direct link between various allergic conditions and ASD . For example, Regina Sala, Lorene Amet, Natasa Blagojevic-Stokic, Paul Shattock, and Paul Whiteley highlight key comorbidities affecting the immune system in ASD populations, noting that many conditions appear with greater frequency in individuals with ASD compared to non-ASD populations (Sala et al., 2020).

Further substantiating this connection, research by Xu and colleagues, as detailed by C. McDougle, has provided new data supporting an immune-mediated subtype of ASD (McDougle, 2018). Their analysis of the National Health Interview Survey data, encompassing a large sample of children, revealed that children with ASD were significantly more likely to have food allergies (11.25% vs 4.25%), respiratory allergies (18.73% vs 12.08%), and skin allergies (16.81% vs 9.84%) compared to those without ASD (McDougle, 2018). The likelihood of a child having an ASD diagnosis more than doubled among children with food allergy, while respiratory and skin allergies also showed a significant, though lesser, association (McDougle, 2018). Interestingly, sex differences were observed, with boys with ASD being significantly more likely than girls with ASD to have respiratory and skin allergies, though no sex difference was found for food allergy (McDougle, 2018). These findings align with recent reports suggesting differences in vulnerability to early-life immune insult between male and female mice in animal models of ASD (McDougle, 2018).

The presence of these immune-mediated conditions has profound clinical implications, particularly for individuals with ASD who are minimally verbal or nonverbal. Such individuals may be unable to articulate the pain and discomfort stemming from food allergies and subsequent gastrointestinal inflammation (McDougle, 2018). Instead, their physical distress may manifest as increased irritability, aggression, or self-injurious behaviors, which can be easily misinterpreted as purely behavioral problems (McDougle, 2018). Therefore, it is crucial for healthcare professionals to conduct a thorough medical history and physical examination to identify and rule out these underlying medical causes of aberrant behavior before initiating treatments solely aimed at behavior modification (McDougle, 2018). The interconnectedness of these conditions is further highlighted by the observation that gastrointestinal dysfunction, seizures, and sleep disorders—all common comorbidities in ASD—have also been associated with inflammatory processes, potentially characterizing an immune-mediated subtype of ASD (McDougle, 2018). The exploration and understanding of these shared mechanisms are critical for elucidating the complex comorbidity in ASD .

In addition to immune dysregulation, metabolic issues represent another significant cluster of comorbidities in individuals with ASD, contributing to a complex health profile (Hollander & Ferretti, 2023). Studies indicate a high prevalence of unhealthy body weight, including overweight and obesity, within the ASD population (Trambacz-Oleszak, 2019). This trend is influenced by a multitude of factors that are often interconnected with the core features of ASD and its other comorbidities. For instance, treatment modalities, encompassing behavioral and medical interventions, dietary practices, and the use of psychotropic medications, can all play a role in weight management challenges (Trambacz-Oleszak, 2019). Many psychotropic medications, while beneficial for managing behavioral symptoms, can predispose individuals to weight gain, increases in lipids, blood sugar, hepatic enzymes, and prolactin levels, necessitating careful monitoring by providers (Freeland, 2012).

Psychological comorbidities such as depression and anxiety, which are highly prevalent in ASD, can also influence eating habits and activity levels, thereby contributing to weight issues (Trambacz-Oleszak, 2019). Furthermore, various somatic comorbidities exacerbate the risk for unhealthy weight. These include feeding problems, which can lead to selective eating or limited food variety, sensory processing disorders that make certain food textures or tastes aversive, and gastrointestinal problems that cause discomfort and affect nutrient absorption (Trambacz-Oleszak, 2019). Sleep issues and physical inactivity are also significant contributors, as disturbed sleep can disrupt metabolic regulation, and sedentary lifestyles, often observed in individuals with ASD due to social isolation or restricted interests, reduce energy expenditure (Trambacz-Oleszak, 2019). Emma Staunton, Claire Kehoe, and Louise Sharkey's research, for instance, highlights how conditions like intellectual disability and ASD, particularly with comorbid challenging behavior, can decrease family quality of life, which may indirectly affect lifestyle factors related to weight (Staunton et al., 2020).

The long-term consequences of unaddressed metabolic issues are severe, potentially leading to chronic complications and increased mortality. Conditions such as hypertension, hyperlipidemia, and obesity are major public health concerns in the general population, and their elevated prevalence in individuals with ASD underscores the urgent need for targeted interventions (Freeland, 2012). Healthcare professionals, therefore, have a crucial duty to recognize these needs and actively promote routine medical assessments that encompass not only screening for ASD-related behaviors but also for these widespread medical disorders (Muskens et al., 2017; Sala et al., 2020). A comprehensive approach to care must integrate nutritional guidance, promotion of physical activity, and careful management of medications to mitigate these risks and improve overall well-being. This integrated strategy is vital for bridging the gap between physical health and ASD, ultimately delivering equality of experiences and reducing the likelihood of early mortality (Sala et al., 2020).

IMPACT ON QUALITY OF LIFE AND THE NEED FOR INTEGRATED CARE

The complex interplay between the core symptoms of Autism Spectrum Disorder, atypical developmental processes, and the extensive range of medical and psychiatric comorbidities profoundly impacts the quality of life (QoL) for individuals with ASD and their families across the lifespan. QoL is a multifaceted construct encompassing physical health, psychological well-being, social relationships, personal independence, and environmental factors, all of which can be significantly affected by the unique challenges associated with ASD (Ozonoff et al., 2005; Perkins & Berkman, 2012).

Multidimensional Impact on Individuals with ASD

The persistent deficits in social communication and interaction, a defining feature of ASD, often lead to social isolation, difficulties in forming and maintaining friendships, and challenges in navigating social nuances (*Alcal & Madrigal, 2023;* Eapen et al., 2016). These social difficulties, combined with restricted and repetitive behaviors and interests, can limit participation in community activities, educational settings, and vocational opportunities, thereby constraining personal growth and independence (Francis et al., 2021; Hollander & Ferretti, 2023). For instance, despite intellectual giftedness, individuals with ASD may struggle in school due to slowness, stress, and difficulty with homework assignments, as exemplified by a case study where an individual dropped out of private school in 10th grade (Hollander & Ferretti, 2023). Inflexible thinking, a core component of restricted and repetitive behaviors, further exacerbates these challenges by contributing to workplace and relationship difficulties (Hollander & Ferretti, 2023).

The high rates of co-occurring psychiatric conditions, such as anxiety, depression, ADHD, and obsessive-compulsive disorder, add a significant emotional and functional burden (Chandrasekhar & Sikich, 2015; Mutluer et al., 2022). Clinically anxious children with ASD, for example, often experience similar numbers and types of anxiety disorders as clinically anxious children without ASD, but may have higher total anxiety, social anxiety disorder, and panic disorder scores, further impacting their QoL (*Steensel et al., 2012*). Rumination, a dysfunctional coping strategy often seen in ASD, can lead to poorer emotion regulation and higher burnout, contributing to increased internalizing (anxiety) and externalizing (explosive episodes) symptoms (Hollander & Ferretti, 2023). These challenges can lead to poorer psychosocial functioning, stigma, maladjustment, and exclusion, creating a vicious cycle of negative experiences (Eapen et al., 2016). Adam Helles, I. Carina Gillberg, Christopher Gillberg, and Eva Billstedt's study on adults with Asperger syndrome found great variability in objective quality of life, noting that while diagnostic stability was associated with some outcomes, comorbidity had a significant impact on QoL (Helles et al., 2016).

Medical comorbidities, particularly feeding and gastrointestinal problems, exert a direct and substantial impact on QoL. The discomfort and pain associated with GI issues can manifest as increased irritability, challenging behaviors, and sleep disturbances, which in turn negatively affect the individual's daily life (Bresciani et al., 2023*;* Neuhaus et al., 2018). A research highlighted that high rates of feeding problems, gastrointestinal symptoms, challenging behavior, and sensory issues were endorsed by caregivers, and these comorbid conditions significantly impact quality of life and adaptive behavior (Leader, OReilly, et al., 2020). Feeding problems not only pose risks for nutritional deficiencies and poor growth but also transform mealtimes into significant sources of stress and conflict for both the child and their caregivers (Esposito et al., 2023*; Leader, O"Reilly, et al., 2020*). Sleep problems, prevalent in 50-80% of children with ASD, increase parental stress and negatively affect family quality of life (Mazzone et al., 2018). Furthermore, otolaryngological issues like auditory disorders can impair communication and overall functioning (McKenna et al., 2024). The cumulative effect of these interconnected challenges can be profound, leading to a significantly lower overall QoL for individuals with ASD (Leader, OReilly, et al., 2020*;* Sala et al., 2020).

Impact on Families and Caregivers

The burden of care for individuals with ASD and their numerous comorbidities significantly affects the mental health and well-being of their families and caregivers. Parents of children with intellectual disability and ASD, especially when challenging behaviors are present, experience increased psychological distress and a lower quality of family life (Staunton et al., 2020). Keith Pecor, Georgia Barbayannis, Max Yang, Jacklyn Johnson, Sarah Materasso, Mauricio Borda, D. Madariaga Garcia, Varsha Garla, and Xue Ming's study revealed that caregivers of children with ASD and/or ADHD reported lower quality of life, particularly during challenging times like the COVID-19 pandemic, experiencing greater decreases in QoL compared to caregivers of neurotypical children (Pecor et al., 2021). Sleep problems in children with ASD are particularly impactful, leading to higher levels of parenting stress, anxiety, and depression in parents, and a lower perceived quality of life across multiple domains (Mannion & Leader, 2023). This highlights that the impact of ASD extends far beyond the individual, affecting the entire family unit's well-being.

Improving knowledge about sleep patterns, for instance, might help in designing targeted interventions that reduce family stress and improve overall quality of life (Ballester et al., 2018).

The Need for Integrated, Multidisciplinary Care

Given the complex, heterogeneous, and multifaceted nature of ASD, an integrated, multidisciplinary approach to care is absolutely essential for optimizing outcomes and significantly improving QoL across the lifespan (Ferrara et al., 2025; Francis et al., 2021). This approach must be person-centered and family-focused, taking into account the individual's unique strengths, needs, and preferences, as well as their developmental stage (Francis et al., 2021; Ozonoff et al., 2005). Effective management requires seamless collaboration among a wide range of professionals, including pediatricians, gastroenterologists, neurologists, psychologists, psychiatrists, speech-language pathologists, occupational therapists, nutritionists, and educators (Beaudry-Bellefeuille et al., 2021; Prabhakaran et al., 2025; Stanciu et al., 2021). This collaborative model ensures that all aspects of the individual's health—core ASD symptoms, developmental delays, medical comorbidities (including dysphagia, GI issues, sleep problems), and psychiatric conditions—are comprehensively addressed (*Fucà et al., 2023;* Muskens et al., 2017).

Interventions should be evidence-based, individually tailored, and adapted to the specific needs and developmental stage of the person with ASD (*Grañana, 2022;* Hollander & Ferretti, 2023). This may involve a combination of behavioral therapies, educational supports, medical treatments, and family support services (Francis et al., 2021; Lordan et al., 2021). For example, behavior-oriented treatments include programs that aim to re-condition target behaviors and develop vocational, social, cognitive, and living skills (Lordan et al., 2021). While no single or combination of treatments has been able to reverse ASD completely, therapeutic and pharmacological options can improve the quality of life for individuals with ASD (*Alcal & Madrigal, 2023*). Pharmacological interventions, such as risperidone and aripiprazole, are FDA-approved for managing irritability in pediatric patients with ASD, and other medications can address attention, mood, and anxiety difficulties (Hollander & Ferretti, 2023). Prolonged-release melatonin (PedPRM) has also shown to be a safe and efficacious option for long-term insomnia in children and adolescents with ASD, subsequently improving their quality of life (Maras et al., 2018).

Beyond conventional treatments, exercise programs have demonstrated substantial benefits for children and adolescents with ASD, decreasing social interaction problems, attention deficits, emotional reactivity, stereotypical verbal and motor behavior, and sleep disturbances (Toscano et al., 2022). Nutritional interventions, such as gluten- and casein-free diets, show promise for some subgroups, complementing the evolving view of "plural autisms" and suggesting a possible diet-related phenotype (Whiteley, 2014). The success of early diagnosis and comprehensive intervention is evident in outcomes where, with professional help, more than 25% of individuals can achieve an independent life, and 50% can complete primary school with fewer disruptive behaviors in adulthood, allowing them to continue living with their families (*Grañana, 2022*).

The ultimate goal of such integrated interventions is to promote the individual's overall well-being, enhance their functional independence, and empower them to lead fulfilling and meaningful lives (Grañana, 2022), (Francis et al., 2021). By adopting a holistic and integrated approach to care, healthcare systems can better support individuals with ASD and their families in navigating the multifaceted challenges of the condition, thereby achieving the best possible quality of life outcomes (Sala et al., 2020). This requires ongoing research to identify effective prevention strategies from preconception through adulthood, as well as to develop better targeted diagnostic tools and treatment algorithms for this vulnerable group (Francis et al., 2021; Muskens et al., 2017).

DISCUSSION

The preceding sections delineate Autism Spectrum Disorder as a profoundly complex and heterogeneous neurodevelopmental condition, characterized not only by its core diagnostic features but also by a pervasive influence on developmental trajectories and an extensive array of co-occurring medical and psychiatric conditions (Alcal & Madrigal, 2023; Sala et al., 2020;Ostrowski et al., 2024). This discussion aims to synthesize these interconnected elements, providing a holistic perspective on the challenges faced by individuals with ASD and their families, with particular attention to the implications for dysphagia. Understanding ASD requires acknowledging its nature as a lifelong condition, where symptoms and challenges evolve and interact across developmental stages, from early childhood through adulthood (Ostrowski et al., 2024; Hollander & Ferretti, 2023). The initial focus on behavioral and cognitive manifestations, while important, has increasingly broadened to encompass the critical role of physical and mental health comorbidities in shaping the overall clinical picture and long-term outcomes (Sala et al., 2020).

The neurobiological underpinnings of ASD highlight fundamental alterations in brain connectivity and organization that begin in prenatal development (Grañana, 2022; Beopoulos et al., 2022). These structural and functional differences, evidenced by studies on axonal tracts and brain organoids, directly contribute to the atypical cognitive processing observed in individuals with ASD (McFadden & Minshew, 2013; Li et al., 2022; Williams & Minshew, 2010). The "disconnection syndrome" theory posits that the brain regions responsible for complex, integrative processing are less coordinated, leading individuals to rely more heavily on intact lower-order functions (Williams & Minshew, 2010). This manifests as a unique profile of strengths and weaknesses, where basic attention or rule-learning may be preserved or even enhanced, while higher-order functions like concept formation or flexible thinking are significantly impaired (Williams & Minshew, 2010). Inflexible thinking, a core aspect of restricted and repetitive behaviors, is a pervasive vulnerability factor that affects adaptation, relationships, and vocational success throughout life (Hollander & Ferretti, 2023). The insistence on sameness and intolerance of uncertainty can lead to significant distress and challenging behaviors.

The pervasive and multifaceted nature of Autism Spectrum Disorder, characterized by its inherent heterogeneity and lifelong impact, necessitates a comprehensive understanding that extends beyond its core behavioral and communication deficits (Sala et al., 2020 ; Alcal & Madrigal, 2023). As this chapter has meticulously detailed, the atypical developmental processes—ranging from foundational neurobiological alterations in brain connectivity and cellular development (McFadden & Minshew, 2013), (Li et al., 2022) to distinct cognitive profiles marked by inflexible thinking and sensory processing differences (Hollander & Ferretti, 2023) —are inextricably linked with a vast spectrum of medical and psychiatric comorbidities (Bradshaw et al., 2022). Conditions such as prevalent gastrointestinal issues, feeding difficulties including dysphagia, chronic sleep disturbances, neurological complications like epilepsy, and a high incidence of anxiety, depression, and ADHD, collectively contribute to a significantly diminished quality of life for individuals with ASD and their families (Neuhaus et al., 2018; Mazzone et al., 2018; Mutluer et al., 2022). The cumulative burden of these interconnected challenges—from the physical discomfort of GI problems and the functional limitations imposed by motor and sensory anomalies to the emotional distress of psychiatric disorders and social isolation—underscores the profound impact on daily functioning, well-being, and overall independence across the lifespan (Ozonoff et al., 2005; Pecor et al., 2021).

Therefore, an integrated, person-centered, and multidisciplinary approach to care is not merely beneficial but absolutely essential, fostering collaborative efforts among pediatricians, gastroenterologists, neurologists, psychologists, speech-language pathologists, and other specialists to provide tailored, evidence-based interventions that address the entire spectrum of an individual's needs (Beaudry-Bellefeuille et al., 2021; Stanciu et al., 2021). This holistic strategy, encompassing early detection, accurate diagnosis, and continuous support, aims not only to alleviate specific symptoms but ultimately to enhance functional independence, promote overall well-being, and empower individuals with ASD to lead fulfilling lives, while also supporting their caregivers in navigating this complex journey (Grañana, 2022 ; Ferrara et al., 2025).

CONCLUSION

Autism Spectrum Disorder stands as a profoundly complex and heterogeneous neurodevelopmental condition, characterized by enduring deficits in social communication and interaction, coupled with restricted, repetitive patterns of behavior, interests, or activities that impact individuals throughout their entire lifespan.

As demonstrated throughout this chapter, optimizing outcomes for individuals with ASD hinges on adopting an integrated, multidisciplinary approach. This person-centered and family-focused model requires seamless collaboration across a diverse team of healthcare professionals (Francis et al., 2021; Grañana, 2022). By coordinating efforts, the team can holistically address the complex and varied challenges—including core symptoms, developmental delays, and common comorbidities such as dysphagia and psychiatric conditions (Beaudry-Bellefeuille et al., 2021; Stanciu et al., 2021). The strategic use of evidence-based, individualized interventions based on this integrated understanding is the key to unlocking potential. Therefore, continued commitment to comprehensive, coordinated support is paramount to achieving the ultimate goal: empowering individuals with ASD toward greater functional independence and enhanced quality of life.

REFERENCES

Albantakis, L., Brandi, M.-L., Zillekens, I. C., Henco, L., Weindel, L., Thaler, H., Schliephake, L., Timmermans, B., & Schilbach, L. (2020). Alexithymic and autistic traits: Relevance for comorbid depression and social phobia in adults with and without autism spectrum disorder. *Autism*, *24*(8), 2046–2056. DOI: 10.1177/1362361320936024 PMID: 32662285

Ballester, P., Martínez, M. J., Javaloyes, A., Inda, M., Fernández, N., Gázquez, P., Aguilar, V., Pérez, A., Hernández, L., Richdale, A. L., & Peiró, A. M. (2018). Sleep problems in adults with autism spectrum disorder and intellectual disability. *Autism Research*, *12*(1), 66–79. DOI: 10.1002/aur.2000 PMID: 30273974

Beaudry-Bellefeuille, I., Pomoni, M., Welch, A., Moriyón-Iglesias, T., Suárez-González, M., & Ramos-Polo, E. (2021). Multidisciplinary approach to assessment and intervention of feeding problems in children with autism spectrum disorders: A clinical perspective. *Irish Journal of Occupational Therapy*, *49*(2), 77–83. DOI: 10.1108/ijot-12-2020-0019

Beopoulos, A., Géa, M., Fasano, A., & Iris, F. (2022). Autism spectrum disorders pathogenesis: Toward a comprehensive model based on neuroanatomic and neurodevelopment considerations. *Frontiers in Neuroscience*, *16*. Advance online publication. DOI: 10.3389/fnins.2022.988735 PMID: 36408388

Bradshaw, J., Schwichtenberg, A. J., & Iverson, J. M. (2022). Capturing the complexity of autism: Applying a developmental cascades framework. *Child Development Perspectives*, *16*(1), 18–26. DOI: 10.1111/cdep.12439 PMID: 36407945

Bresciani, G., Da Lozzo, P., Lega, S., Bramuzzo, M., Di Leo, G., Dissegna, A., Colonna, V., Barbi, E., Carrozzi, M., & Devescovi, R. (2023). Gastrointestinal disorders and food selectivity: Relationship with sleep and challenging behavior in children with autism spectrum disorder. *Children (Basel, Switzerland)*, *10*(2), 253. DOI: 10.3390/children10020253 PMID: 36832380

Casseus, M., Kim, W. J., & Horton, D. B. (2023). Prevalence and treatment of mental, behavioral, and developmental disorders in children with co-occurring autism spectrum disorder and attention-deficit/hyperactivity disorder: A population-based study. *Autism Research*, *16*(4), 855–867. DOI: 10.1002/aur.2894 PMID: 36644987

Chandrasekhar, T., & Sikich, L. (2015). Challenges in the diagnosis and treatment of depression in autism spectrum disorders across the lifespan. *Dialogues in Clinical Neuroscience*, *17*(2), 219–227. DOI: 10.31887/dcns.2015.17.2/tchandrasekhar PMID: 26246795

Chenausky, K. V., Brignell, A., Morgan, A. T., Norton, A. C., Tager-Flusberg, H. B., Schlaug, G., & Guenther, F. H. (2021). A modeling-guided case study of disordered speech in minimally verbal children with autism spectrum disorder. *American Journal of Speech-Language Pathology, 30*(3S), 1542–1557. DOI: 10.1044/2021_ajslp-20-00121 PMID: 33852328

Dupuis, A., Mudiyanselage, P., Burton, C. L., Arnold, P. D., Crosbie, J., & Schachar, R. J. (2022). Hyperfocus or flow? Attentional strengths in autism spectrum disorder. *Frontiers in Psychiatry, 13*. Advance online publication. DOI: 10.3389/fpsyt.2022.886692 PMID: 36276327

Eapen, V., Cavanna, A. E., & Robertson, M. M. (2016). Comorbidities, social impact, and quality of life in tourette syndrome. *Frontiers in Psychiatry, 7*. Advance online publication. DOI: 10.3389/fpsyt.2016.00097 PMID: 27375503

Esposito, M., Mirizzi, P., Fadda, R., Pirollo, C., Ricciardi, O., Mazza, M., & Valenti, M. (2023). Food selectivity in children with autism: Guidelines for assessment and clinical interventions. *International Journal of Environmental Research and Public Health, 20*(6), 5092. DOI: 10.3390/ijerph20065092 PMID: 36982001

Ferrara, F., Vaira, F., D'Agostino, L., Fiorilli, L., Ottaviano, M., & Marini, S. (2025). MEDICAL COMORBIDITIES IN AUTISM SPECTRUM DISORDER: A NARRATIVE REVIEW. *Global Journal for Research Analysis, 67–71*. Advance online publication. DOI: 10.36106/gjra/4007041

Francis, K., Karantanos, G., Al-Ozairi, A., & AlKhadhari, S. (2021). Prevention in autism spectrum disorder: A lifelong focused approach. *Brain Sciences, 11*(2), 151. DOI: 10.3390/brainsci11020151 PMID: 33498888

Freeland, K. (2012). Medical and psychiatric conditions in patients with developmental disabilities. *The Mental Health Clinician, 2*(3), 56–59. DOI: 10.9740/mhc.n115483

Fucà, E., Guerrera, S., Valeri, G., Casula, L., Novello, R. L., Menghini, D., & Vicari, S. (2023). Psychiatric comorbidities in children and adolescents with high-functioning autism spectrum disorder: A study on prevalence, distribution and clinical features in an italian sample. *Journal of Clinical Medicine, 12*(2), 677. DOI: 10.3390/jcm12020677 PMID: 36675606

Gaitanis, J., Nie, D., Hou, T., & Frye, R. (2023). Developmental regression followed by epilepsy and aggression: A new syndrome in autism spectrum disorder? *Journal of Personalized Medicine, 13*(7), 1049. DOI: 10.3390/jpm13071049 PMID: 37511662

Grañana, N. (2022). Espectro autista: Una propuesta de intervención a la medida, basada en la evidencia. *Revista Médica Clínica Las Condes, 33*(4), 414–423. DOI: 10.1016/j.rmclc.2022.06.006

Green, J. L., Sciberras, E., Anderson, V., Efron, D., & Rinehart, N. (2016). Association between autism symptoms and functioning in children with ADHD. *Archives of Disease in Childhood, 101*(10), 922–928. DOI: 10.1136/archdischild-2015-310257 PMID: 27117836

Helles, A., Gillberg, I. C., Gillberg, C., & Billstedt, E. (2016). Asperger syndrome in males over two decades: Quality of life in relation to diagnostic stability and psychiatric comorbidity. *Autism, 21*(4), 458–469. DOI: 10.1177/1362361316650090 PMID: 27233289

Hollander, E., & Ferretti, C. J. (2023). Special report: Autism spectrum disorder and inflexible thinking—affecting patients across the lifespan. *Psychiatric News, 58*(04). Advance online publication. DOI: 10.1176/appi.pn.2023.04.4.34

James, D. M., Davidson, E. A., Yanes, J., Moshiree, B., & Dallman, J. E. (2021). The gut-brain-microbiome axis and its link to autism: Emerging insights and the potential of zebrafish models. *Frontiers in Cell and Developmental Biology, 9*. Advance online publication. DOI: 10.3389/fcell.2021.662916 PMID: 33937265

Leader, G., O'Reilly, M., Gilroy, S. P., Chen, J. L., Ferrari, C., & Mannion, A. (2020). Comorbid feeding and gastrointestinal symptoms, challenging behavior, sensory issues, adaptive functioning and quality of life in children and adolescents with autism spectrum disorder. *Developmental Neurorehabilitation, 24*(1), 35–44. DOI: 10.1080/17518423.2020.1770354 PMID: 32496834

Li, C., Fleck, J. S., Martins-Costa, C., Burkard, T. R., Stuempflen, M., Vertesy, Á., Peer, A. M., Esk, C., Elling, U., Kasprian, G., Corsini, N. S., Treutlein, B., & Knoblich, J. A. (2022). *Single-cell brain organoid screening identifies developmental defects in autism.* Cold Spring Harbor Laboratory. https://doi.org/DOI: 10.1101/2022.09.15.508118

Lordan, R., Storni, C., & De Benedictis, C. A. (2021). Autism spectrum disorders: Diagnosis and treatment. In *Autism Spectrum Disorders* (pp. 17–32). Exon Publications., DOI: 10.36255/exonpublications.autismspectrumdisorders.2021.diagnosis

Ma, Z., Eaton, M., Liu, Y., Zhang, J., Chen, X., Tu, X., Shi, Y., Que, Z., Wettschurack, K., Zhang, Z., Shi, R., Chen, Y., Kimbrough, A., Lanman, N. A., Schust, L., Huang, Z., & Yang, Y. (2022). Deficiency of autism-related Scn2a gene in mice disrupts sleep patterns and circadian rhythms. *Neurobiology of Disease, 168*, 105690. DOI: 10.1016/j.nbd.2022.105690 PMID: 35301122

Mannion, A., & Leader, G. (2023). Relationship between child sleep problems in autism spectrum disorder and parent mental health and well-being. *Sleep Medicine*, *109*, 4–10. DOI: 10.1016/j.sleep.2023.05.009 PMID: 37379630

Maras, A., Schroder, C. M., Malow, B. A., Findling, R. L., Breddy, J., Nir, T., Shahmoon, S., Zisapel, N., & Gringras, P. (2018). Long-Term efficacy and safety of pediatric prolonged-release melatonin for insomnia in children with autism spectrum disorder. *Journal of Child and Adolescent Psychopharmacology*, *28*(10), 699–710. DOI: 10.1089/cap.2018.0020 PMID: 30132686

Mazzone, L., Postorino, V., Siracusano, M., Riccioni, A., & Curatolo, P. (2018). The relationship between sleep problems, neurobiological alterations, core symptoms of autism spectrum disorder, and psychiatric comorbidities. *Journal of Clinical Medicine*, *7*(5), 102. DOI: 10.3390/jcm7050102 PMID: 29751511

McDougle, C. J. (2018). Another step toward defining an immune-mediated subtype of autism spectrum disorder. *JAMA Network Open*, *1*(2), e180280. DOI: 10.1001/jamanetworkopen.2018.0280 PMID: 30646065

McFadden, K., & Minshew, N. J. (2013). Evidence for dysregulation of axonal growth and guidance in the etiology of ASD. *Frontiers in Human Neuroscience*, *7*. Advance online publication. DOI: 10.3389/fnhum.2013.00671 PMID: 24155705

McKenna, K., Prasad, S., Cooper, J., King, A. M., Shahzeidi, S., Mittal, J., Zalta, M., Mittal, R., & Eshraghi, A. A. (2024). Incidence of otolaryngological manifestations in individuals with autism spectrum disorder: A special focus on auditory disorders. *Audiology Research*, *14*(1), 35–61. DOI: 10.3390/audiolres14010005 PMID: 38247561

Muskens, J. B., Velders, F. P., & Staal, W. G. (2017). Medical comorbidities in children and adolescents with autism spectrum disorders and attention deficit hyperactivity disorders: A systematic review. *European Child & Adolescent Psychiatry*, *26*(9), 1093–1103. DOI: 10.1007/s00787-017-1020-0 PMID: 28674760

Mutluer, T., Aslan Genç, H., Özcan Morey, A., Yapici Eser, H., Ertinmaz, B., Can, M., & Munir, K. (2022). Population-Based psychiatric comorbidity in children and adolescents with autism spectrum disorder: A meta-analysis. *Frontiers in Psychiatry*, *13*. Advance online publication. DOI: 10.3389/fpsyt.2022.856208 PMID: 35693977

Neuhaus, E., Bernier, R. A., Tham, S. W., & Webb, S. J. (2018). Gastrointestinal and psychiatric symptoms among children and adolescents with autism spectrum disorder. *Frontiers in Psychiatry*, *9*. Advance online publication. DOI: 10.3389/fpsyt.2018.00515 PMID: 30405456

Ostrowski, J., Religioni, U., Gellert, B., Sytnik-Czetwertyński, J., & Pinkas, J. (2024). Autism spectrum disorders: Etiology, epidemiology, and challenges for public health. *Medical Science Monitor, 30*. Advance online publication. DOI: 10.12659/msm.944161 PMID: 38833427

Owens, A. P., Mathias, C. J., & Iodice, V. (2021). Autonomic dysfunction in autism spectrum disorder. *Frontiers in Integrative Neuroscience, 15*. Advance online publication. DOI: 10.3389/fnint.2021.787037 PMID: 35035353

Ozonoff, S., Goodlin-Jones, B. L., & Solomon, M. (2005). Evidence-Based assessment of autism spectrum disorders in children and adolescents. *Journal of Clinical Child and Adolescent Psychology, 34*(3), 523–540. DOI: 10.1207/s15374424jccp3403_8 PMID: 16083393

Pecor, K., Barbayannis, G., Yang, M., Johnson, J., Materasso, S., Borda, M., Garcia, D., Garla, V., & Ming, X. (2021). Quality of Life Changes during the COVID-19 Pandemic for Caregivers of Children with ADHD and/or ASD. *International Journal of Environmental Research and Public Health, 18*(7), 3667. DOI: 10.3390/ijerph18073667 PMID: 33915884

Penzol, M. J., Salazar de Pablo, G., Llorente, C., Moreno, C., Hernández, P., Dorado, M. L., & Parellada, M. (2019). Functional gastrointestinal disease in autism spectrum disorder: A retrospective descriptive study in a clinical sample. *Frontiers in Psychiatry, 10*. Advance online publication. DOI: 10.3389/fpsyt.2019.00179 PMID: 31024351

Perkins, E. A., & Berkman, K. A. (2012). Into the unknown: Aging with autism spectrum disorders. *American Journal on Intellectual and Developmental Disabilities, 117*(6), 478–496. DOI: 10.1352/1944-7558-117.6.478 PMID: 23167487

Prabhakaran, N., Jestine, S., Chandran, S., Shiva, L., & Moncy, A. M. (2025). Gastrointestinal manifestations and associated comorbidities in children with autism spectrum disorder: A cross-sectional analysis from south india. *Indian Journal of Psychological Medicine*. Advance online publication. DOI: 10.1177/02537176251331152 PMID: 40255413

Sala, R., Amet, L., Blagojevic-Stokic, N., Shattock, P., & Whiteley, P. (2020). Bridging the gap between physical health and autism spectrum disorder. *Neuropsychiatric Disease and Treatment, 16*, 1605–1618. DOI: 10.2147/ndt.s251394 PMID: 32636630

Seo, M., & Anderson, G. (2020). Gut-Amygdala Interactions in Autism Spectrum Disorders: Developmental Roles via regulating Mitochondria, Exosomes, Immunity and microRNAs. *Current Pharmaceutical Design, 25*(41), 4344–4356. DOI: 10.2174/1381612825666191105102545 PMID: 31692435

Stanciu, A. C., Rad, F., Mihailescu, I., Mateescu, L., Grozavescu, R., Andrei, E., Budisteanu, B., Linca, F., Ioana, D., Iliescu, C., Papuc, S., Arghir, A., Dobrescu, I., & Budisteanu, M. (2021). Multidisciplinary approach in children with autism spectrum disorder. *European Psychiatry : the Journal of the Association of European Psychiatrists*, *64*(S1), S86–S86. DOI: 10.1192/j.eurpsy.2021.256

Staunton, E., Kehoe, C., & Sharkey, L. (2020). Families under pressure: Stress and quality of life in parents of children with an intellectual disability. *Irish Journal of Psychological Medicine*, *40*(2), 192–199. DOI: 10.1017/ipm.2020.4 PMID: 32106892

Toscano, C. V. A., Ferreira, J. P., Quinaud, R. T., Silva, K. M. N., Carvalho, H. M., & Gaspar, J. M. (2022). Exercise improves the social and behavioral skills of children and adolescent with autism spectrum disorders. *Frontiers in Psychiatry*, *13*. Advance online publication. DOI: 10.3389/fpsyt.2022.1027799 PMID: 36620673

Trambacz-Oleszak, S. (2019). Why are individuals with autism spectrum disorder at risk group for unhealthy weight? *Anthropological Review*, *82*(3), 313–326. DOI: 10.2478/anre-2019-0023

van Steensel, F. J. A., Bögels, S. M., & Dirksen, C. D. (2012). Anxiety and quality of life: Clinically anxious children with and without autism spectrum disorders compared. *Journal of Clinical Child and Adolescent Psychology*, *41*(6), 731–738. DOI: 10.1080/15374416.2012.698725 PMID: 22775580

Venker, C. E., & Stronach, S. T. (2017). When Is Simplified too…Simple? *ASHA Leader*, *22*(1), 42–47. DOI: 10.1044/leader.ftr1.22012017.42

Whiteley, P. (2014). Nutritional management of (some) autism: A case for gluten- and casein-free diets? *The Proceedings of the Nutrition Society*, *74*(3), 202–207. DOI: 10.1017/s0029665114001475 PMID: 25311313

Wiley, S., & Moeller, M. P. (2007). Red Flags for Disabilities in Children who are Deaf/ Hard of Hearing. *ASHA Leader*, *12*(1), 8–29. DOI: 10.1044/leader.ftr3.12012007.8

Williams, D. L., & Minshew, N. J. (2010). How the brain thinks in autism: Implications for language intervention. *ASHA Leader*, *15*(5), 8–11. DOI: 10.1044/leader.ftr1.15052010.8

Zwick, G. P. (2017). Neuropsychological assessment in autism spectrum disorder and related conditions. *Dialogues in Clinical Neuroscience*, *19*(4), 373–379. DOI: 10.31887/dcns.2017.19.4/gzwick PMID: 29398932

Chapter 14
Formulation Science in Dysphagia Care:
Advances in Oral Drug Delivery Systems for Swallowing Disorders

Charuwan Thanawiroon
http://orcid.org/0009-0004-9076-3219
Faculty of Pharmaceutical Sciences, Ubon Ratchathani University, Thailand

Rojjares Netthong
http://orcid.org/0000-0001-9751-7564
Faculty of Pharmaceutical Sciences, Ubon Ratchathani University, Thailand

Soultana Papadopoulou
http://orcid.org/0000-0002-0950-1456
Department of Speech and Language Therapy, University of Ioannina, Greece

Bancha Yingngam
http://orcid.org/0000-0001-7215-9123
Faculty of Pharmaceutical Sciences, Ubon Ratchathani University, Thailand

ABSTRACT

Dysphagia is common in children and elderly individuals, making conventional oral forms of medication such as tablets or capsules inappropriate for these patients. The inflexibility of these dosage forms is fraught with potential dangers; they cannot be altered without the potential for loss of their therapeutic effect. This rigidity of the systems can lead to dosing inaccuracies and potentially an insufficient therapeutic effect or aspiration. To overcome these limitations, several novel drug delivery systems have been proposed. These include rapidly dissolving films, gels with drugs, hydrogels and complex 3D-printed formulations, as well as a number of

DOI: 10.4018/979-8-3373-6405-6.ch014

nanoengineering methodologies. These improvements lead to better swallowability and lung deposition. Moreover, the bioavailability of a given pharmaceutical and patient acceptance are maintained. This chapter concentrates on these new systems for drug delivery, their clinical implications and regulation considerations, specifically in compliance with medication errors in patients with dysphagia.

INTRODUCTION

Dysphagia, a common dysmotility of swallowing observed in elderly and neurological patients, is an important barrier to the use of oral therapy with drugs. Despite the common use of tablets and capsules as standard dosage forms, they are not applicable in many patients because of their perceived unsafe consumption (Harnett et al., 2023). The incidence of dysphagia is highly variable, but it affects an estimated 30–40% of older adults living in the community and over 70% of those living in institutions (Atkin et al., 2024; Can, 2025). High prevalence rates, such as these, have serious consequences, including low compliance with drug therapy, malnutrition, aspiration pneumonia and failure of treatment (Rivelsrud et al., 2023). In the absence of suitable drug formulations, crushing or opening tablets is commonly performed by carers to aid administration. Almost half of these changes are hazardous: 13% have the potential for toxicity, and 8% have the potential for reduced drug efficiency (Blaszczyk et al., 2023). These unsafe behaviors are commonly documented within the ecosystem of geriatric and long-term care, thereby increasing the risk for medication errors. This represents a pressing requirement for bedside swallow-engineered therapies to improve treatment efficacy for this high-risk population.

In pharmaceutical technology, the development allows the development of tailored products (i.e., products adapted for an individual patient), such as orodispersible tablets and films, drug-loaded gels and jellies, multiparticulates (e.g., mini-tablets, granules) or even personalized 3D-printed medicines (Yingngam, 2024). New technologies, such as nanocarrier systems and additive manufacturing, allow the development of mouth-dispersible formulations that dissolve quickly into the oral cavity or require a minimum amount of water to take, which can be adjusted in size and/or dosage according to various patients (Maheshwari et al., 2024; Topuz & Uyar, 2025). These novel solutions not only increase swallowability but also aim to achieve sustained therapeutic performance.

Figure 1 summarizes the relationship between dysphagia and limitations of conventional dosage forms and their corresponding patient-tailored solutions, such as orodispersible tablets, gels, mini-tablets, and 3D-printed medicines (Yingngam, 2025). This figure provides an overview of integrated dysphagia care and the four interconnected scientific domains crucial for multidisciplinary consideration when developing oral formulations for patients with swallowing disorders. It starts with the mechanics of swallowing and reiterates that, for safety, any formulary must meet the patient's neural precipitants and anatomic coordination. This physiological need directly impacts how a product will behave rheologically (i.e., its viscosity, yield stress) to control bolus transit time and reduce the risk of aspiration. The rheological properties of such thickened or texture-modified fluid or solid, in turn, become the physical characteristics that influence drug delivery and activity, namely, altering drug dissolution kinetics and bioavailability. Moreover, a sensory and palatability profile, e.g., taste and mouth feel, contributes largely to patient compliance. The outer arrows illustrate an ongoing circular connection: mechanoregulation of the nervous system controls transit, which in turn influences drug release delivered in a sensory sense that facilitates conditionally essential engagement with a therapeutic strategy.

In this chapter, the latest developments in terms of formulation strategies for dysphagia are presented. This chapter first outlines the pathophysiological basis of dysphagia and the limitations of conventional dosage forms, followed by a review of novel technologies such as orodispersible tablets (ODTs), gels, multiparticulates, 3D printing, and nanotechnology. Pharmaceutical development considerations such as excipient safety, manufacturing feasibility, and regulatory requirements are also presented. Case studies and trial data are included to demonstrate clinical translation, and future directions are discussed, covering AI-based design, 4D printing, and personalized medicine for dysphagia care.

Figure 1. Conceptual framework of formulation science in dysphagia care

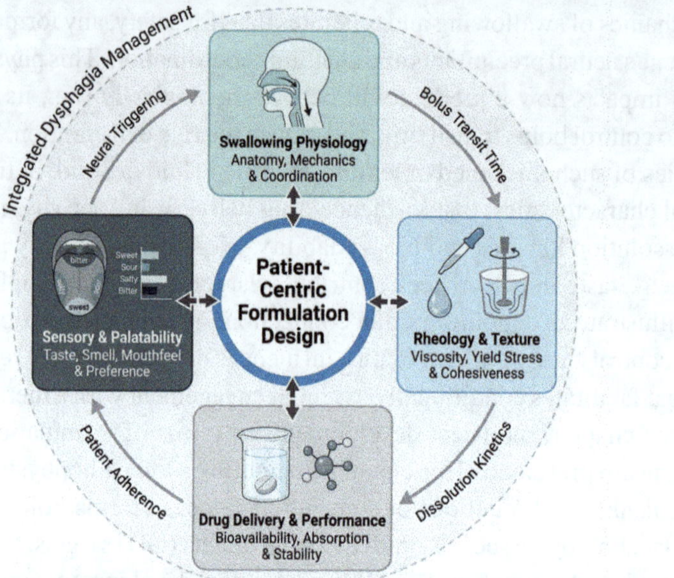

PATHOPHYSIOLOGICAL CONSIDERATIONS IN DYSPHAGIA

Dysphagia, or difficulty swallowing, can occur when any phase of the swallowing process is disrupted. Typically, swallowing progresses through oral (bolus transport), pharyngeal (involuntary propulsion with airway protection), and esophageal (peristaltic transport) phases. Dysphagia can be classified as oropharyngeal, affecting initiation and oral–pharyngeal transit, or esophageal, involving impaired passage owing to motility or structural problems.

Videofluoroscopy and endoscopic studies have shown that approximately 65% of stroke patients experience oropharyngeal dysphagia acutely, with 10–15% still affected months later (Maciejewska et al., 2024). Reduced tongue strength, delayed reflexes, and poor airway protection make solid dosage forms hazardous, as even small tablets may cause coughing or aspiration (Harnett et al., 2023). Postural adjustments or thickened liquids offer only partial safety. In esophageal dysphagia, large tablets or capsules may lodge above strictures, leading to pain, mucosal damage, or impaired absorption. Certain groups are especially vulnerable. In older adults, sarcopenia and polypharmacy increase swallowing difficulty and medication errors.

Stroke survivors and patients with Parkinson's disease often face multifactorial dysphagia, with both neurological deficits and medications (e.g., anticholinergics) contributing. Head and neck cancer survivors frequently struggle with structural changes or dry mouth from surgery and radiotherapy, further complicating oral drug administration (Bhidayasiri et al., 2024; Watanabe et al., 2025).

Figure 2 shows the important interplay between the three swallowing phases (oral, pharyngeal and esophageal) in relation to the safety of drugs administered orally. Such a diagram demonstrates where particular physiological impairments, such as poor tongue control during the oral phase or dysmotility and strictures in the esophageal stage, directly lead to difficulties with drug administration. These adverse events include immediate physical hazards (e.g., aspiration, choking) and decreases in exposure to active agents from local mucosal irritation or impaired transit of the medication owing to poor mouth cleaning. To minimize these risks, the scheme maps three main management options: modifying texture (crushing tablets), considering alternative delivery methods (liquid medications and parenteral administration) and adopting postural interventions to maximize safety during the transition of the medication bolus.

Figure 2. Pathophysiological influences on medication use in dysphagia patients

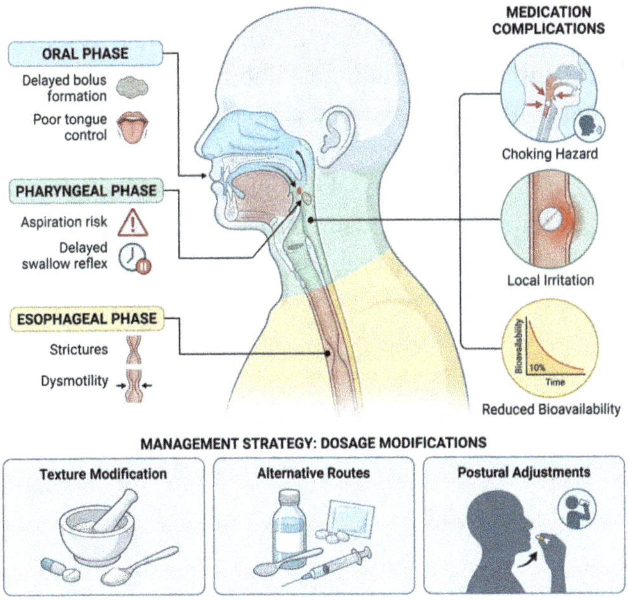

Table 1 also outlines some specific patient groups who are affected by dysphagia, including the etiology of their condition, the difficulties associated with adminis-

tering medications to them, and medication formulation considerations with regard to such patients. In children, congenital abnormalities and developmental delays frequently contribute to pill rejection or the increased risk of gagging and the need to employ suitable pediatric dosage forms (e.g., mini-tablets, flavored liquids, or orodispersible films). Delayed swallow reflexes and increased risk of aspiration are common in poststroke adults; orodispersible tablets, thickeners and medicated gels might improve safety, as well as efficacy, for these patients. For patients with Parkinson's disease, there are additional limitations based on bradykinesia as well as oropharyngeal rigidity, which affect the ability to take oral medications in a timely manner; thus, quickly dissolving formulations, mini-tablets or transdermal systems may be appropriate for these patients to ensure ongoing therapeutic coverage. These obstructions and xerostomia are common in survivors of head and neck cancer, and nonspecific treatments, such as medicated gels, mouth-dissolving films and topical sprays, are considered to be more patient friendly. Impairment is present in older people with the combined burdens of sarcopenia, cognitive decline, and polypharmacy, causing manipulation errors and poor adherence. Innovative applications, including 3D-printed polypills, multiparticulate systems and mini-tablets, seem to be promising in the management of dysphagia-related risks. As such, these swallow-sensitive formulations mitigate swallowing difficulties in addition to improving patient convenience and providing a means for imparting expeditious therapy. Beyond the near-term issues of overcoming poor swallowing function, dysphagia is associated with greater clinical problems, including aspiration pneumonia, suboptimal efficacy from expectoration or refusal to take medications and adherence challenges related to pill aversion. To meet these challenges satisfactorily, or fit-for-purpose, dosage forms that are easy to swallow, such as ODTs, mini-tablets and concentrated solutions that are formulated for swallowing without risk, need to be used. For this reason, predictable and efficient oral drug delivery is essential.

Table 1. Patients with dysphagia, its etiology, pharmaceutical problems and formulations

Population	Common causes of dysphagia	Medication-related issues	Formulation strategies	Reference
Pediatric (infants, children)	Congenital anomalies, cerebral palsy, developmental delay	Pill aversion, choking risk, need for flexible dosing	Min-tablets, orodispersible films, flavored oral liquids	Münch et al. (2023a); Münch et al. (2023b) ;Wargenau et al. (2022)
Poststroke adults	Neurological impairment of swallow reflex	Aspiration of solids, inability to swallow large tablets	Orodispersible tablets, gels/jellies, thickened liquids	Balcerak et al. (2022)
Parkinson's disease	Bradykinesia, oropharyngeal rigidity	Irregular intake of time-sensitive medications	Rapid dissolving formulations, mini-tablets, patches	Bhidayasiri et al. (2024)
Head and neck cancer	Surgery, radiotherapy-induced fibrosis/ xerostomia	Structural obstruction, dry mouth causing swallowing difficulty	Gels, mouth-dissolving films, local sprays	Watanabe et al. (2025)
Geriatric polypharmacy	Sarcopenia, cognitive decline	Pill burden, manipulation errors, poor adherence	3D-printed polypills, multiparticulates, mini-tablets	Harnett et al. (2023)

LIMITATIONS OF CONVENTIONAL DOSAGE FORMS FOR DYSPHAGIC PATIENTS

The commonly used tablets, capsules and solutions assume that patients can swallow them with water, which is also frequently not present in cases of dysphagia. These conventional dosage forms may be difficult to use and can have safety concerns. There are concerns about the size and shape of tablets, the need for fluids and an upright position during swallowing and the hazardous nature of crushing or dividing medications. Liquid formulations, however, have their own disadvantages. The use of feeding tubes also complicates the administration of medications (Drumond & Stegemann, 2021; Harnett et al., 2023). These issues create challenges in achieving consistent dosing as well as reducing the therapeutic benefit and health consequences. The clinical inadequacy of a "one-size-fits-all" approach to ODF dosages for people with dysphagia is illustrated in *Figure 3*. This discrepancy leads to numerous hazards that are directly attributed to irregular on-demand drug delivery (e.g., choking during intake, chronic pulmonary complications postaspiration) or treatment failure due to nonuniform drug uptake. Thus, new drug delivery platforms such as ODTs or buccal-film-forming systems that can capitalize on the physiological act of swallowing should be developed urgently.

Figure 3. Mismatch between conventional oral dosage forms and the needs of dysphagic patients, showing the risks of oversized tablets, water dependence, aspiration, and inconsistent absorption

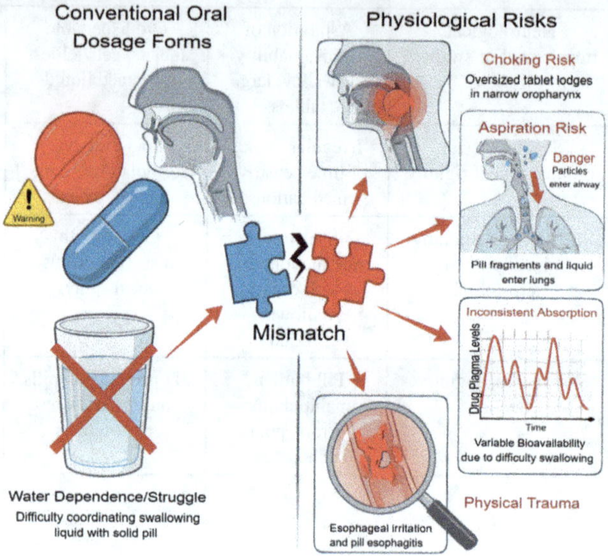

Table Size and Shape

Many commercial tablets are still too large in size or inappropriate in shape for patients with dysphagia to swallow comfortably. There is evidence that tablets approximately 6–7 mm in diameter, especially those with oval or round shapes, are better taken by elderly adults. In comparison, larger and/or nonround tablets are a potential cause of clustering and pain (Hummler et al., 2023). A controlled trial in young (19–36 years) and elderly (65–94) adults revealed that none of the oval tablets at a dose of 250 mg obtained the judgment "swallowable" from more than 80% of the participants. Inadequacies in such benefits are of concern, as seen with 500 mg oval round-shaped tablets, particularly among the elderly (Hauber et al., 2024). However, numerous dosage forms are intended for adult use, e.g., sustained release and combination tablets may be greater than these swallowable volumes. Jelly caplets also have problems: if patients suffer from dry mouth or low or no intake of fluids, these caps may adhere to the walls of the oropharynx and esophagus if swallowing is not possible with a certain amount of vigilance. It can cause a gag feeling or pressure on the chest, and it can even be harmful to the lining of the throat. Tablet-induced esophagitis is a well-established consequence of the impaction of some tablets—e.g., doxycycline or alendronone—in the esophagus and occurs particularly in dysphagic patients (Hummler et al., 2023). More generally, tablets that stick to the lining of the esophagus—especially when taken without a sufficient amount of water or just before lying down—can lead to mucosal inflammation, ulceration and severe pain (Ahmed et al., 2024).

Water Requirements and Postural Dependence

The majority of solid oral formulations are designed to administer 30–100 mL of water to patients seated in an upright position. These barriers are insurmountable for the majority of dysphagic patients. While thickened liquids are believed to be safer with respect to the risk of aspiration, they could hinder the dissolution of tablets and thus affect their pharmacokinetics. Similarly, although thin fluids are less difficult to swallow, they are also associated with a higher incidence of aspiration. The use of thickened fluids, which are often indicated to increase patient safety, can slow the break-up time of tablets and prolong drug release (Atkin et al., 2024; Cho et al., 2024). In addition, patients with limited mobility may have difficulty ingesting large amounts of liquid or staying upright, which could lead to tablets being retained in the esophagus (Matías Ambiado-Lillo, 2025). The carer's response is often to crush tablets and mix them with soft foods, e.g., apple sauce or pudding. Nevertheless, this new practice might bring forth uncertainty in dosing accuracy and drug–food interactions (Watanabe et al., 2025).

Manipulation by Crushing or Splitting

Crushing or splitting tablets and opening capsules are common in the hospital environment and nursing home setting, where the medication administration of patients who have difficulty swallowing is facilitated. In hospitals, nurses report crushing of medications on a daily basis between 28% and 67%, even soaring two-thirds in geriatric units (Blaszczyk et al., 2023). In skilled nursing facilities, 27% of the residents even receive crushed medication, whereas the prevalence in Australian aged-care homes is ~18%. This reveals, on the one hand, the variability and constancy of this behavior (Brunemann et al., 2025). Some formulations, such as controlled release opioids, beta-blockers, antiepileptics or enteric-coated agents, should not be crushed, as this may result in dose dumping with a loss of therapeutic effect. However, inappropriate crushing is common, especially when managing the sustained release of morphine, oxycodone and enteric-coated proton pump inhibitors (Harnett et al., 2023). Even if crushable preparations are possible, the risk of drug loss during preparation or suboptimal mixing with food may lead to inaccurate dosing. Studies have reported between 4–38% drug loss depending on the crushing device used and the aseptic technique used (Tosun et al., 2021).

With respect to safety and dosing, stripped protective coatings can expose patients to the unpleasant bitterness and abrasiveness of many drugs. Products including metronidazole and perindopril are recognized to be particularly unpalatable, with associated refusals or rejection of doses. Caregivers may also try to cover these unpleasant tastes with sweet substances, such as honey or jam, but this is an inexact strategy carrying the risk of food–drug interactions (e.g., decreased antibiotic absorption with dairy products). In some facilities, drugs are also occasionally "cocktailed" into a single food vehicle to facilitate administration. This can increase the likelihood of drug–drug incompatibilities and make it cumbersome for nurses to verify if all medications have been consumed if a patient only eats part of the mixture. Thus, although crushing or splitting tablets offers a temporary method for those with swallowing difficulties, it is considered a dangerous alternative for patients with dysphagia.

Liquid Formulation Limitations

While liquids (solutions and suspensions) are commonly prescribed for dysphagia, they have limitations. Sorbitol, which is used as an excipient in many of these products, may cause gastrointestinal intolerance (bloating and diarrhea) when it is consumed in large amounts. Furthermore, high osmolality preparations are frequently not well tolerated in frail or elderly patients and may lead to worsening of abdominal pain. One major problem is that many medications do not have liquid preparations, and the majority, which can be formulated in solid dosing forms and compounded in extemporaneous preparations for liquids, may have problems regarding stability and dosing accuracy (Harnett et al., 2023).

In addition, palatability is a major challenge where bitter taste or lingering aftertaste may cause patients to refuse a dose, especially patients with cognitive impairment. Certain liquid dosage forms are not bioequivalent to their solid counterparts, which can lead to safety concerns, particularly for medicines with a narrow therapeutic range (Klang, 2023). Compared with unit-dose tablets, liquids require dosing devices and are associated with a greater risk of dosing errors in clinical practice (Zhu et al., 2025). As a result, the addition of viscosity-enhancing agents to liquid medications ingested per os may retard breakdown and absorption even more for patients who need thickeners for prevention from aspiration after swallowing.

Feeding Tube Administration

Medications are often administered via enteral feeding tubes, such as nasogastric or percutaneous endoscopic gastrostomy (PEG) tubes, when oral intake is severely limited. Although this approach bypasses the problem of swallowing dysfunctions, it raises both formulation and safety issues. In most cases, solid forms of the drug must be crushed and suspended in liquid; otherwise, there is significant potential for the tube to become clogged. In fact, studies have shown that errors in drug administration by feeding lead to enteral tube occlusion, gastrointestinal intolerance, a reduced therapeutic effect of the administered drugs or active ingredients, adverse reactions and death (Zhu et al., 2025). In addition, Klang broadly characterized over 300 oral medications for potential enteral application and found 36 formulations inappropriate for feeding-tube delivery owing to disintegration, pH-induced coagulation, or incompatibility with lumen dynamics (Klang, 2023). Formulations, such as enteric-coated beads or liquid-filled soft capsules, may not fully disperse and/or stick to the sidewall of a tube, particularly narrow (small bore) tubes, which may increase the potential for clogging (Zhu et al., 2025).

The simultaneous or sequential delivery of multiple drugs via a single feeding tube is particularly problematic. Physical and chemical incompatibilities may compromise the stability of drugs and reduce their bioavailability, while some drug/nutrient combinations have been shown to precipitate within the tube, increasing the risk of blockade. Regardless of formulation-specific issues, a lack of and incomplete knowledge among healthcare workers is still a main source of error. Almost 50% of nurses in survey studies reported no formal enteral drug therapy training. However, >50% of these patients experienced tube blockage and needed replacement, typically due to insufficient flushing, dilution or inappropriate dosage forms (Ahmed Abdulmohsen et al., 2024). Clinical studies also emphasize how medication errors related to unrecognized drug-like incompatibilities or nonadherence to protocols are common in tube-fed patients (Bifari et al., 2024; Zhu et al., 2025). Although the feeding tube is essential for delivering medications and nutrition to dysphagic patients, commercially available oral formulations are often unsuitable for enteral use, requiring careful considerations before management to ensure safe and effective delivery.

EMERGING ORAL DRUG DELIVERY TECHNOLOGIES FOR DYSPHAGIES

In recent years, oral drug delivery has given new hope to people who have difficulty swallowing pills. This new method is designed to make drug administration easier for patients, eliminate the need to crush tablets or open capsules for fewer doses and ensure that consistent as-prescribed dosages are delivered in a consistent release pattern while also making them more patient friendly. Over the past few years, several potential strategies have approached the bench-to-bedside scenario. Notable advancements include orodispersible tablets and films, drug-loaded gels, multiparticulates such as mini-tablets and 3D printed and nanoenabled medicated delivery platforms. All of these approaches address particular aspects of dysphagia, and an increasing evidence base from laboratory to clinical work clearly underscores the potential of making therapy much safer—patients are more likely now than in previous decades to swallow their meds so to speak, which will markedly increase the quality of life for millions of people coping every day with this ailment one way or another.

Orodispersible Tablets and Films

Orodispersible tablets (ODTs) and orodispersible films (ODFs) are solid oral dosage forms designed to disintegrate spontaneously in the mouth without the need for water or chewing, making them particularly suitable for dysphagic patients. In accordance with the regulatory definitions of the U.S. Food and Drug Administration (FDA) and the European Medicines Agency (EMA), ODTs are defined as products that disintegrate within 30 seconds *in vitro* (EMA, 2025; U.S. FDA, 2008). In practice, however, many commercial products have an even shorter dissolution time. For example, olanzapine and risperidone ODTs disintegrate in less than 10 seconds and present a more patient-friendly option for those unable to swallow traditional tablets. Disintegration within 3–4 s has been achieved via technologies such as Zydis® (Chue et al., 2002), whereas for some ODFs formulated via hot-melt extrusion, complete melt disintegration has been established in 6–11 s *in vitro* (Jacob et al., 2023). Compared with conventional tablets, ODTs reduce the swallowing burden and aspiration risk. The results remain inconclusive with respect to long-term adherence of the patient. These formulations have several advantages, such as ease of administration, fewer potential risk methods during rehabilitation and patient compliance (Yingngam, 2024).

Figure 4 shows the mechanism and benefits of orodispersible tablets (ODTs) and orodispersible films (ODFs) with respect to fast disintegration in the oral cavity and subsequent drug release. This concept is based on the ability of orodispersible dosage forms to come into contact with saliva to allow immediate release of the active drug without chewing and water. As illustrated at the top of the figure, ODTs predominantly function by rapid disintegration. The figure shows how saliva penetrates into the porous matrix particles of an orally disintegrating tablet by wicking (capillary action), which results in swelling, leading to pressure inside the tablet and breaking it into smaller granules with an increased surface area for absorption. ODFs, on the other hand, rely on their immediate dissolution. These films are designed to stick on the surface of the tongue by mucoadhesion, and following contact with saliva, a thin polymeric matrix dissolves quickly, releasing a liquid solution that enhances drug penetration through the body.

Four key benefits that benefit patient adherence and drug effectiveness are indicated at the bottom of the illustration. First, they provide a convenient way to take medicine without the need for water so that it can be taken in multiple settings. Second, they are designed for dysphagia treatment and are especially useful in pediatric or geriatric patients with anatomical or psychological disorders related to the swallowing of typical solid dosage forms. Pharmacologically, the chart highlights rapid onset; once dissolved, drugs may be rapidly absorbed via well-vascularized oral mucosa. Finally, this pathway may enable pregastric absorption. Because the drug travels directly into systemic circulation from the mouth, it is able to bypass the acidic milieu of the stomach and liver first-pass metabolism, which can dramatically improve bioavailability when compared with traditional oral delivery. Representative marketed products include Zydis® olanzapine ODT, which dissolves in under 10 seconds, and Spritam® levetiracetam ODT, the first 3D-printed high-dose orodispersible medicine. These development features show the benefits of ODTs/ODFs in terms of improving swallowability and dosing safety for the dysphagic population and, accordingly, patient compliance with conventional oral tablets.

Figure 4. Orodispersible tablets and films: Mechanisms and advantages

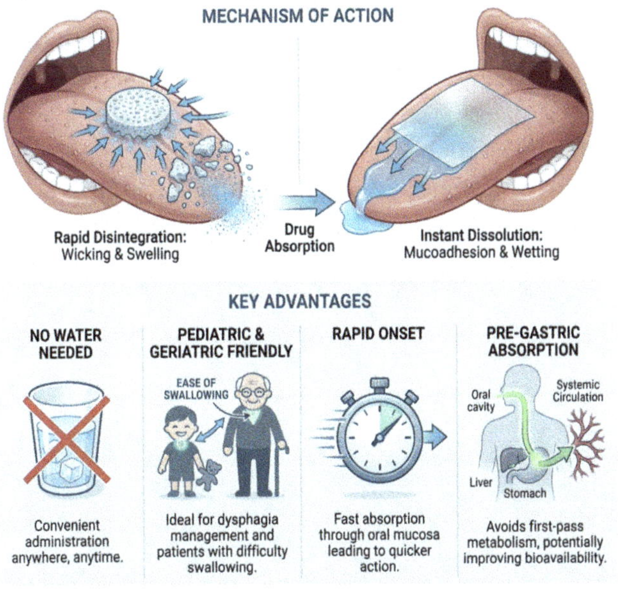

Table 2 summarizes a comparative analysis of ODTs and ODFs with those of conventional tablets. Unlike conventional tablets, which require the use of water and the risk of aspiration, ODTs and ODFs dissolve rapidly in saliva, obviating the requirement for liquids and increasing their safety profile for patients. Apart from considerations of practical administration, the conceptual design and patient comfort between these dosage forms are also chasmic at 30 seconds, as a rule, and the ODFs at 15--30 seconds depend on the kind of formula and thickness. In view of the large surface areas, efficient taste masking is needed to achieve patient acceptability. Advanced palatability-improving technologies such as ion exchange resins and polymer-enveloped and taste-masked medicaments have significantly improved the acceptability of such dosage forms, especially for bitter drugs. While conventional tablets can contain several hundred milligrams of active pharmaceutical ingredient (API), ODFs are typically limited to < 50 mg, making them more suitable for potent actives or for buccal delivery. Recent developments, such as Spritam® (levetiracetam up to 1000 mg), which is the first 3D-printed ODT, have demonstrated that high-dose ODTs can be practically applied. These developments demonstrate that ODTs and ODFs would be a well-suited remedy for many of the restrictions resulting from conventional tablets, particularly in dysphagic patients. Despite this, considerations such as the susceptibility of disintegration to moisture, physical frailty and, possibly, the need for caregiver support persist in the clinical application of appropriate dosage forms (Yingngam, 2024).

ODTs and ODFs are continually advancing with new technologies. Technologies such as electrospinning have allowed the development of nanofiber-based films that dissolve ultrafastly, whereas taste-masking approaches—such as ion-exchange resins and cyclodextrins—have increased the palatability of bitter APIs, including donepezil (Sapiee et al., 2023; Yingngam, 2024). Furthermore, 3D printing technology (Aprecia's ZipDose®) has facilitated the formation of high-dose ODTs, such as Spritam® (1000 mg levetiracetam), which disintegrate quickly despite containing large quantities of API, leading to a simple treatment regimen, especially in patients receiving several medications simultaneously (Kömür et al., 2025).

Table 2. Comparison of conventional tablets with ODTs and ODFs in dysphagia management, focusing on swallowability, disintegration, taste masking, dose capacity, and acceptability

Feature	Conventional tablets	Orally disintegrating tablets (ODTs)	Oral dissolvable films (ODFs)	Clinical significance for dysphagia
Swallowing mechanism	Must be swallowed intact with ≥150 mL water; high aspiration risk in dysphagia (Harnett et al., 2023)	Disintegrate in saliva (15–30 s), no water needed; patient swallows dissolved solution (Juan et al., 2024; Sato et al., 2025)	Dissolve on tongue/buccal mucosa (10–25 s), no water needed; ultrathin format (Jacob et al., 2023)	Critical advantage: Eliminates choking risk and water dependency (Atkin et al., 2024)
Disintegration kinetics	Not designed to disintegrate before gastric arrival (typically >15 min) (Harnett et al., 2023)	Rapid disintegration (<30 s United States Pharmacopeia (USP) limit); marketed products: 3–15 s (Juan et al., 2024; U.S. FDA, 2008)	Ultrarapid dissolution (5–20 s); thickness-dependent (50–200 μm films) (Jacob et al., 2023; Paipa-Jabre-Cantu et al., 2025)	Performance metric: Faster disintegration = reduced oral retention time (Fouad et al., 2025)
Physical manipulation	Cannot be chewed without compromising release profile (may damage release properties or taste awful unless chewable) (Drumond & Stegemann, 2021)	No chewing needed; fragile structure demands careful handling (Juan et al., 2024)	No manipulation needed; flexible film adheres and dissolves completely (Jacob et al., 2023)	Safety consideration: Eliminates inappropriate crushing practices (Blaszczyk et al., 2023)
Fluid requirements	Requires 150–250 mL per dose; problematic for fluid-restricted diets (Hummler et al., 2023)	None needed; compatible with all diet textures (Harnett et al., 2023; Juan et al., 2024)	None needed; saliva sufficient (Jacob et al., 2023; Paipa-Jabre-Cantu et al., 2025)	Compliance factor: Reduces administration barriers (Lura et al., 2025)
Taste management	Protected by coating until gastric dissolution (Harnett et al., 2023)	Requires active taste-masking (sweeteners, flavors, ion-exchange resins) (Juan et al., 2024; U.S. FDA, 2008)	Extensive taste-masking needed due to large surface area exposure (Jacob et al., 2023; Paipa-Jabre-Cantu et al., 2025)	Patient acceptance: Taste quality directly impacts adherence (Trofimiuk et al., 2024)
Dose capacity	High capacity (50-1000 mg API) (Harnett et al., 2023)	Moderate capacity (<500 mg); high-dose via 3D printing (Spritam® 1000 mg) (Denis et al., 2024; U.S. FDA, 2008)	Limited capacity (<50 mg per film); suitable for potent drugs (Jacob et al., 2023; Paipa-Jabre-Cantu et al., 2025)	Formulation constraint: Limits drug selection possibilities (Kim et al., 2024)

continued on following page

Table 2. Continued

Feature	Conventional tablets	Orally disintegrating tablets (ODTs)	Oral dissolvable films (ODFs)	Clinical significance for dysphagia
Administration in dysphagia	Often requires crushing creating dosing inaccuracy and aspiration risk (Blaszczyk et al., 2023; Brunemann et al., 2025)	Direct oral administration; reduces medication errors by 30–60% (Harnett et al., 2024)	Easy tongue placement; caregiver-friendly administration (Paipa-Jabre-Cantu et al., 2025; Yingngam, 2024)	Clinical outcome: Measurable reduction in administration errors (Harnett et al., 2024)
Stability profile	Stable in low-moisture environments (Harnett et al., 2023)	Moisture-sensitive; requires protective blister packs (Juan et al., 2024; U.S. FDA, 2008)	Highly moisture-sensitive; sealed foil pouches essential (Jacob et al., 2023; Paipa-Jabre-Cantu et al., 2025)	Storage requirement: More stringent packaging protocols (Yingngam, 2024)
Representative products	Metoprolol extended release, atorvastatin (not dysphagia-friendly)(Harnett et al., 2023)	Zydis® (olanzapine), Spritam® (levetiracetam), Aricept® (donepezil) (Huang et al., 2025; Juan et al., 2024; U.S. FDA, 2008)	Zuplenz® (ondansetron), Exservan® (riluzole) (Huang et al., 2025; Jacob et al., 2023; Paipa-Jabre-Cantu et al., 2025)	Clinical applications: Specific therapeutic areas show adoption (Huang et al., 2025)

Medicated Oral Gels and Jelly

Medicated oral gels and jellies combine some viscoelastic properties familiar to patients when they consume food with accurate pharmaceutical dosing, resulting in cohesiveness that improves swallowing safety and ease of delivery. This product conforms to the International Dysphagia Diet Standardization Initiative (IDDSI) Level 4 requirements for viscosity, which suggest that a cohesive texture may be used to help reduce the risk of aspiration. Clinical evidence bolsters this assertion. For example, >90% of mothers were satisfied with propranolol gels based on gellan gum as a matrix for uniform dosing among toddlers with epilepsy. This underlines the ease of use and safety features maintained through improved delivery methods based on semisolid pharmaceutical products, such as medicated jelly. In elderly individuals, a jelly based formulation of donepezil resulted in compliance rates close to 95%, as opposed to the 72% rate achieved by crushed-tablet preparations. This further implies their potential use to facilitate the uptake of drugs, e.g., drugs for Alzheimer's disease therapy, such as drugs that are not able to be administered through conventional tablets. These systems have been continually refined in recent years. "Instant jellies", which are produced by dissolving powders in water, offer more convenience and better stability. Combinations of hydrocolloids, such as Konjac and gellan gum, contribute to texture uniformity and reduce syneresis so that the product is palatable and does not separate over time. The development of sustained-release microparticles in jellies has also offered an appealing means for long-acting release worthy of evaluation in dysphagic patients (Kállai-Szabó et al., 2024; Li et al., 2025; Patel et al., 2020).

The anatomy and clinical application of medicated gels and jellies for the treatment of dysphagia are described in *Figure 5*. Pharmaceutical gels and jellies are carefully formulated with 3D polymer networks that provide both high viscosity and physical integrity. This complex microscopic structure acts like a net that catches the API, which would otherwise fall out of solution over time in a thinner liquid form. These gels ensure that each dose of drug is chemically uniform. Because they are spoonable semisolid formulas, the gel does not flow like a liquid; instead, its shape can be maintained as it leaves the spoon, reducing spill risk—an especially positive aspect for elderly patients or those with tremors because accurate dosing is possible. They are important for differential diagnosis of speech disorders, of which the most common or prominent is dysphagia (impaired swallowing). Unlike thin liquids, which have a high flow velocity and can prematurely pass through the airway until the epiglottis is closed for protection, this gel has a cohesive bolus and transits slowly, which makes it safe during ingestion. This controlled transit time allows the patient's reflexes enough time to properly and safely deliver the medication into the esophagus. The inherent mucoadhesive properties of the gel may also serve to extend the contact time of the drug with mucosal surfaces and enhance local therapeutic action via local administration.

Figure 5. Structural and clinical applications of medicated gels and jellies. Their cohesive texture slows bolus flow, reduces aspiration risk, and supports consistent dosing in dysphagic patients.

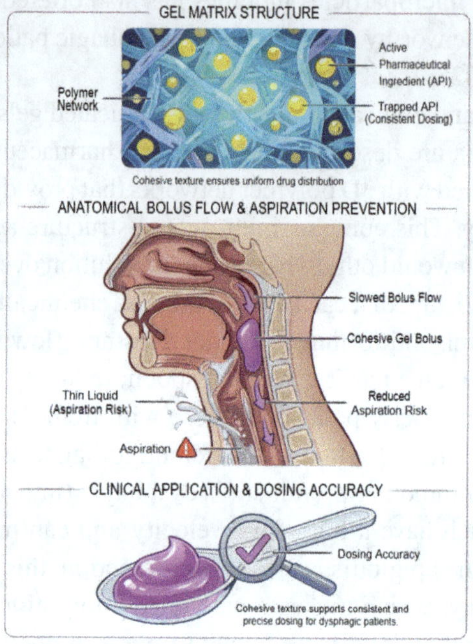

In contrast to ODTs/ODFs, which dissolve quickly, gels and jellies produce a semisolid bolus that is cohesive enough to slide easily down the pharynx and trachea with less risk of aspiration than liquids and therefore improve the swallow response. The comparison of medicated gels/jellies and conventional tablets/liquids with respect to formulations, rheological properties, swallowability and patient satisfaction is presented in *Table 3*. These systems produce a cohesive bolus that travs the pharynx safely, reduces the risk of aspiration and delivers each dose consistently. Nevertheless, some difficulties in formulation remain regarding the low shelf-life and the necessity of incorporating preservatives for microbiological stability. Gels and jellies are smoother than tablets are, and choking hazards are lower than intact swallowing reflexes. Although liquids are easier to swallow, thin fluids frequently, if not always, increase the risk of aspiration unless they have thickened (Patel et al., 2020). Medicated gels and jellies are a compromise — they are scoopable and hold together and safer for swallowing than thin liquids or solids are. Their clinical evaluation thus endorses their use as an easily perceptible reduction in safety and efficiency in people with dysphagia (Huang et al., 2025).

In addition to their desirable taste, flexible gels and jellies can be formulated as follows: one can prepare formulations with virtually any desired viscosity, flavor or level of loading with active ingredients that are mouth tolerant 15; lozenges are less cumbersome and easier to administer than an oral liquid by hand, such as a patient or care giver. In this context, a study conducted in Japan suggested that medication adherence could be enhanced in elderly patients with dementia by proper administration of traditional drugs (yokukansan) as jelly formulations and might be beneficial for those whose drugs are routinely rejected if dispensed as tablets. Another illustrative example is iluzole, which has been resolubilized in an orodispersible gel film formulation (Exservan®) for patients with amyotrophic lateral sclerosis who experience frequent dysphagia. These cases highlight the importance of semisolid dosage forms as alternative oral dosage forms in the presence of severe intolerance to standard oral medications (Huang et al., 2025). The drawbacks of medicated gels and jellies may be their susceptibility to microbial contamination, as their shelf life is generally shorter than that of solid formulations, and they often rely on the presence of preservatives to maintain stability (EMA, 2025). However, despite being structurally suboptimal for their intended purpose, they increase safety (as a choking hazard is reduced), convenience and patient acceptance, confirming that function can be compromised in these species when conventional tablets and liquids are no longer suitable.

Table 3. Comparing medicated gels/jellies with traditional tablets and liquids in terms of swallowability, texture, handling, stability and acceptability

Feature	Conventional tablets/ capsules	Conventional oral liquids (syrups/ solutions)	Oral medicated gels/jellies	Reference
Swallowing requirement	Must be swallowed intact with water; high aspiration risk in dysphagia.	Easier than tablets but thin liquids often unsafe for dysphagic patients.	Smooth, cohesive texture; glides down easily, reducing choking risk.	Patel et al. (2020)
Consistency	Solid, rigid; cannot be modified without crushing (may alter pharmacokinetics).	Thin, flowable; viscosity too low for safe swallowing in many patients.	Semisolid; viscosity can be tailored for safer swallowing.	Li et al. (2025)
Ease of administration	Requires intact swallowing reflex and water.	Requires measuring device; dosing errors or spillage possible.	Spoonable or squeezable; caregiver-friendly; no additional water needed.	Patel et al. (2020)

continued on following page

Table 3. Continued

Feature	Conventional tablets/ capsules	Conventional oral liquids (syrups/ solutions)	Oral medicated gels/jellies	Reference
Dose capacity	High; can carry several hundred mg API.	Moderate; limited by solubility and stability.	Moderate; drugs can be suspended or dissolved in the gel matrix.	Kállai-Szabó et al. (2024)
Stability	Stable under dry conditions; humidity-sensitive.	At risk of microbial growth; preservatives needed.	Moisture-sensitive; requires preservatives; generally shorter shelf-life.	EMA (2025)
Patient acceptabilility	Poor for dysphagia; large tablets often refused.	Better than tablets but thin fluids remain unsafe for many.	High acceptability; flavored jellies improve palatability and compliance.	Huang et al. (2025)
Examples	Metformin tablets; multivitamins	Paracetamol syrup; antibiotic suspensions	Tsumura yokukansan jelly (Japan); Exservan® riluzole jelly/film for ALS.	Huang et al. (2025)

Multiparticulates and Mini-Tablets

Most multiple-unit dosage forms, such as granules, beads or mini-tablets, disperse the drug over many small units, which reduces the risk of choking and allows for flexible dosing. This technique has been rigorously adopted in pediatric studies. In a randomized crossover study, 80% of infants aged 6–11 months successfully swallowed two-millimeter minitablets without chewing, whereas only 35% swallowed liquids in the oral cavity and left no residue. This further highlights the improved swallowing ability of mini-tablets (Mitsui et al., 2022). There is further clinical evidence that mini-tablets are widely accepted throughout early childhood and, therefore, offer a convenient and efficacious alternative to traditional formulations for pediatric patients (Lazic et al., 2025). These findings are also relevant for older patients. A 2025 study reported that mini-tablets were easier to swallow than conventional tablets were but still supported modified release profiles suitable for geriatric patients with dysphagia (Hida et al., 2025; Lura et al., 2025). Multiparticulates are also compatible with automated multidose dispensing, reducing medication errors in institutional care (Martín-Oliveros et al., 2024).

The use of multiparticulates depends on manufacturing and administration methods. *Figure 6* presents the manufacturing process, as well as the utilization of mini-tablets (2–3 mm in diameter) and coated pellets, in production by predosing and using standard tablet presses equipped with multitipdies. Functional film coatings allow such small forms to continue to have modified release properties, even when they are miniaturized. Multiparticulates are highly versatile for administration with or without water, as they can be swallowed directly. They can also be sprinkled onto soft food and administered along with it or be suspended and given through enteral tubes to cater to a variety of swallowing abilities. The commercial preparations Zispin SolTab® and Kappaprox® pellets offer a perspective on the clinical implications of such technologies. Multicompartment systems also minimize choking hazard, and they allow for dosage to be titrated, as the multicomponent doses can be spread across multiple small units instead of relying on a single large tablet. Importantly, they maintain pharmacokinectic reproducibility without compromising. Such product resistance to discontinuation and the safety of doing so, as well as the ease of dosage, are particularly beneficial for children and elderly patients who have trouble swallowing or need accurate dosing adjustments.

Figure 6. Multiparticulates and mini-tablets distribute medication into small units, improving swallowability and dosing flexibility for pediatric and geriatric patients

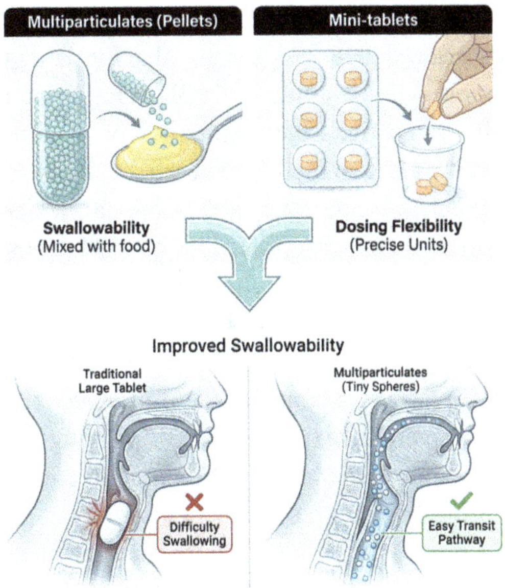

3D-Printed Personalized Dosage Forms

Three-dimensional (3D) printing is promising for the customization of oral medication products, providing accurate drug dosing as well as multiple tablet sizes, shapes, combination medicines and programmed drug release. This manufacturing technique is especially attractive for tailoring the porosity and internal structure to meet patient-specific requirements, particularly for patients with dysphagia (Abdullah et al., 2025; Denis et al., 2024; Karalia et al., 2021; Milliken et al., 2024). Polypills, which contain several drugs within layered structures and may have immediate or controlled release, are among the most appealing potential applications for improving therapy. These formulations provide a feasible solution to pill burden and foster patient compliance, particularly among the geriatric population that is taking multiple drugs (Vaz & Kumar, 2021).

The acceptability study revealed that tableau shape has an impact on swallowing. For example, toroidal (ring)-shaped tablets are claimed to have been rated higher in terms of swallowability than conventional round or spheroid shapes when the fused deposition modeling (FDM) technique is used (Goyanes et al., 2017). These results illustrate the potential of 3D-printed personalized dosages, which use the flexibility they allow for spectral design, as tools and approaches not only for the development of tailor-made radiation doses but also for patient comfort and safety. Thus, adjustable therapies can be applied via 3D printing on the basis of detailed data per patient with dysphagia. Some examples of swallowing-focused ODFs prepared via 3D printing are depicted in *Figure 7*. Of these, fast disintegrating and swallowable orodispersible porous tablets are fabricated via the binder jet process. Moreover, polymedicine polypills built by fused deposition modeling also offer the possibility of incorporating multiple drugs into one single dosage form with independent release patterns. Selective laser sintering (SLS) takes the design freedom a step further, which allows for torus-shaped tablets that are specifically designed to enhance oropharyngeal transit. The figure also illustrates the potential for point-of-care integration, where on-demand 3D printing in clinical or pharmacy settings could facilitate tailored treatment regimens and reduce the medication load and adherence burden for those with swallowing issues.

Figure 7. 3D-printed oral dosage forms such as porous ODTs, torus-shaped tablets, and polypills, showing how personalized design can improve swallowing ability and adherence

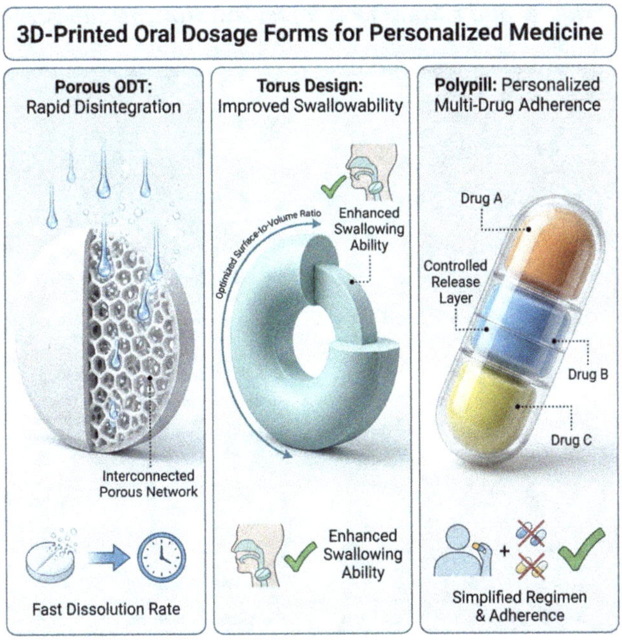

In addition to medicine in solid dosage forms (tablets), 3D printing has been studied for the production of integrated, nutritionally enriched "medifoods". *Figure 8* shows one of the pediatric-friendly formats, e.g., animal shapes, ultrathin oro-dispersible films, and texture modified purees, that may provide total medication with necessary nutrients. This technology solves swallowing difficulties and dietary needs, especially in patients with dysphagia. These developments represent an important amalgamation of pharmaceutical science and food technology, addressing both means for drug delivery and nutritional support that are appropriate for people living with complex swallowing problems.

Figure 8. Three-dimensional (3D)-printed personalized oral dosage forms and food-based carriers designed to support patients with dysphagia. These novel systems integrate precision medicine with patient-friendly delivery, allowing the customization of dose, shape, and texture to enhance swallowing safety and adherence.

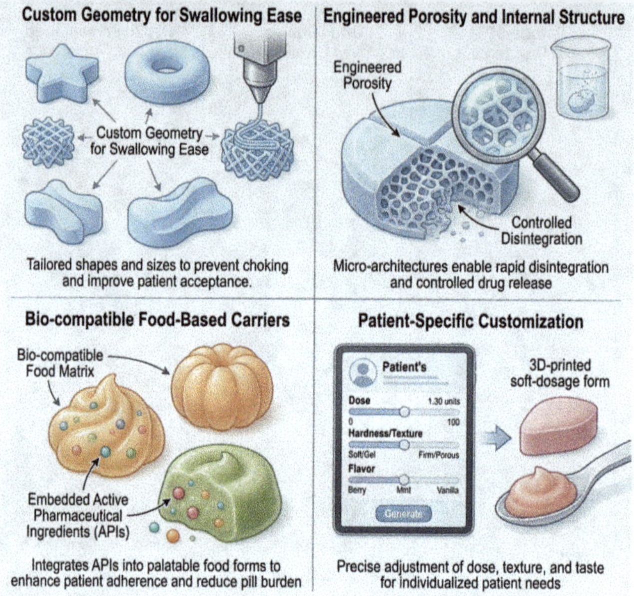

Nanotechnology and NanEnabled Formulations

Nanotechnology offers many potential benefits in the development of personalized formulations intended for patients with dysphagia, especially by minimizing the dose–volume ratio, increasing the solubility and improving palatability. One frequently used strategy in the field is nanocrystal technology, which increases the drug surface area and dissolution rates. Recent reports suggest that nanocrystals can improve absorption even in thickened fluids frequently used with dysphagia diets, one of the major challenges when conventional tablet forms are used (Macedo et al., 2024; Mobaleghol Eslam et al., 2024). Similarly, nanotechnology-based taste masking is another unique approach. The encapsulation of bitter APIs in lipid or polymeric nanoparticles has been shown to improve taste profiles and, thus, patient compliance with ODS. This research is still in its experimental stage or dedicated to pediatric pharmaceuticals; however, it establishes a solid foundation for the future development of dysphagia-friendly ODTs and ODFs (Al-kasmi et al., 2017).

Nanoemulsion delivery systems have received much attention because of their ability to increase the solubility and systemic bioavailability of lipophilic drugs, which can be administered in small volumes. Despite the lack of extensive use in patients with swallowing problems, their ability to deliver a therapeutically effective dose using reduced fluid volume is promising, especially for elderly or neurologically impaired patients limited by <100 ml of fluid per meal (Mobaleghol Eslam et al., 2024) In parallel, mucoadhesive nanocarrier systems have become a new approach to completely avoid swallowing and to facilitate buccal or sublingual drug absorption. Initial preclinical reports have shown significant enhancement of the bioavailability of small-molecule drugs delivered through these routes, although very little evidence has supported extensive clinical validation in the dysphagic population. This option could offer a clinical treatment alternative to the very few patients who have severe swallowing problems and are no longer able to safely take solid or semisolid oral dosage forms. Overall, delivery systems based on nanotechnology are adaptable and promising platforms for improving the safety, acceptability and therapeutic efficacy of oral treatment in dysphagic patients, albeit with a desperate need for extensive translational research and clinical assessment.

A schematic representation of the major nanotechnology-enabled approaches for enhanced drug delivery in patients with swallowing dysfunction is shown in *Figure 9*. Enabling core nanoparticle systems can be formulated in any dosage form, e.g., a nanoemulsion, a lipid nanoparticle encapsulate, a nanoparticle tablet or a nanoparticle suspension. The ability to utilize these novel technologies greatly improves solvent drug solubility and controlled release mechanisms and is more acceptable to patients who are looking for safer or more versatile alternatives to existing formulations. Finally, these developments help drive the aims of precision medicine and patient-centered therapeutic strategies.

Figure 9. Nanotechnology strategies for dysphagia care, including the use of nanocrystals, nanoemulsions, and mucoadhesive nanoparticles to increase the solubility, release, and patient acceptability

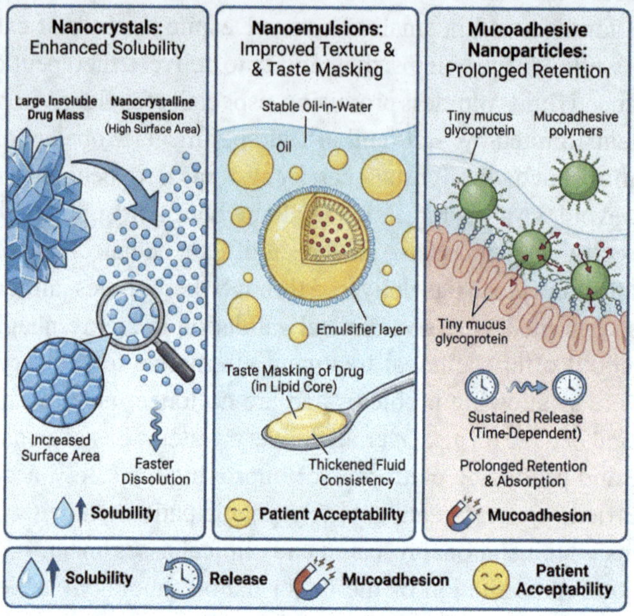

With the detailed study of individual techniques, a comprehensive multiplatform comparison can promote evidence-based selection in patients and for different situations. From a comparison of manufacturing, clinical benefits and relevant applications, *Table 4* summarizes how each dysphagia-adaptable technology, such as ODTs and ODFs, medicated gel systems, multiparticulate products, 3D printing drug delivery systems (DDSs) or nanonized DDSs, is compared. These comparisons provide insight into how different technology infrastructures address different components of the dysphagia problem. For example, ODTs stress disintegration speed, gels pay attention to rheology controllability, multiplication provides dosing flexibility, 3D printing achieves a personalized shape, and nanotechnology promotes dissolution. This systematic approach provides formulators and clinicians with a rigorous framework to identify technologies that best match patient needs and treatment goals.

Table 4. Comprehensive comparison of emerging dysphagia-friendly oral drug delivery technologies

Technology	Mechanism of action	Key performance metrics	Clinical advantages	Limitations	Representative products	Patient population	Reference
Orodispersible tablets (ODTs)	Rapid disintegration via superdisintegrants; drug dissolution in saliva (Juan et al., 2024; U.S. FDA, 2008)	Disintegration: <30 s (USP); marketed products: 3–15 s; patient acceptance: 85–95% (Juan et al., 2024; Sato et al., 2025)	Water-free administration; reduced aspiration risk; familiar tablet format; regulatory acceptance (Fouad et al., 2025)	Moisture sensitivity; limited dose capacity (<500 mg typical); higher cost; fragile handling (U.S. FDA, 2008; Yingngam, 2024)	Zydis® (olanzapine); Spritam® (levetiracetam); Aricept® (donepezil) (Chue et al., 2002; Juan et al., 2024)	Poststroke; pediatric; geriatric; psychiatric patients	Jacob et al. (2023); Yingngam (2024)
Oral dissolvable films (ODFs)	Ultrathin polymer matrix dissolves on tongue/buccal mucosa (Jacob et al., 2023; Paipa-Jabre-Cantu et al., 2025)	Dissolution: 5–20 s; thickness: 50–200 μm; dose limit: <50 mg per 4 cm²; acceptance: 90–95% (Jacob et al., 2023; Topuz & Uyar, 2025)	Fastest dissolution; no choking risk; precise dosing; portable format; buccal absorption possible (Paipa-Jabre-Cantu et al., 2025; Visser et al., 2020)	Very limited dose capacity; extensive taste-masking needed; complex manufacturing; moisture sensitive (Jacob et al., 2023; Morath et al., 2022)	Zuplenz® (ondansetron); Exservan® (riluzole); nicotine replacement films (Goyanes et al., 2017; Jacob et al., 2023)	ALS patients; severe dysphagia; pediatric; traveling patients	Yingngam (2024)
Medicated oral gels/jellies	Controlled rheology via hydrocolloid matrix; cohesive bolus formation (Huang et al., 2025; Malouh et al., 2024)	Viscosity: 50–500 Pa·s (optimal: 73–200 Pa·s); transit time: 0.8–2.1 s; acceptance: 90–95%; aspiration reduction: 40% (Aii et al., 2024; Huang et al., 2025)	Safest swallowing profile; IDDSI compliant; enhanced bioavailability (120–280%); sustained release possible (Huang et al., 2025; Patel et al., 2020)	Shorter shelf-life (6–24 months); preservatives needed; higher cost; refrigeration needed (Huang et al., 2025; Li et al., 2025)	Tsumura yokukansan jelly; experimental propranolol gels; chitosan swallowing aids (Malouh et al., 2024; Watanabe et al., 2025)	Moderate-severe dysphagia; nursing home residents; polypharmacy patients	Huang et al. (2025); Li et al. (2025)
Multiparticulates and mini-tablets	Dose distribution across 2–3 mm units; administration via direct swallowing, sprinkling on food, or suspension for tube feeding (Kállai-Szabó et al., 2024; Lura et al., 2025)	Size: 1–3 mm diameter; swallow success up to 90% in infants; flexible dose 0.5–50 mg; 60% reduction in administration errors (Harnett et al., 2024; Lura et al., 2025)	Flexible dosing; preserved modified-release; reduced choking; feeding tube compatible; scalable manufacturing (Kállai-Szabó et al., 2024; Mitra et al., 2017)	Requires soft food vehicle; potential grittiness; complex counting/ dispensing; limited palatability options (Lura et al., 2025; Meruva et al., 2024)	Losartan mini-tablets; hydrocortisone taste-masked minitabs; experimental multiparticulates (Harnett et al., 2024; Trofimiuk et al., 2024)	Pediatric (6-23 months); geriatric; enteral feeding patients; dose titration needs	Lazic et al. (2025); Lura et al. (2025)

continued on following page

Table 4. Continued

Technology	Mechanism of action	Key performance metrics	Clinical advantages	Limitations	Representative products	Patient population	Reference
3D printed systems	Additive manufacturing; personalized geometry and drug loading (Denis et al., 2024; Karalia et al., 2021)	Production time: 15–45 min/unit; geometries tested: 6+ shapes; optimal: torus (30% faster transit); dose range: 1–1000 mg (Denis et al., 2024; Kim et al., 2024)	Complete personalization; complex geometries; polypill capabilities; point-of-care production; optimized swallowability (Karalia et al., 2021; Milliken et al., 2024)	High equipment cost; regulatory complexity; limited material options; production time; quality control challenges (Denis et al., 2024; Saleh-Bey-Kinj et al., 2025)	Spritam® levetiracetam (FDA-approved); experimental polypills; hospital-based platforms (Karalia et al., 2021; Vaz & Kumar, 2021)	Complex polypharmacy; rare diseases; pediatric special needs; clinical trials	Abdullah et al. (2025)
Nanoenabled formulations	Nanoparticle encapsulation; enhanced dissolution and targeting (Alebachew, 2025; Macedo et al., 2024)	Particle size: 10–200 nm; solubility enhancement: 5–50×; encapsulation efficiency: 75–95%; bioavailability improvement: 15–300% (Alebachew, 2025; Hunt et al., 2024)	Superior dissolution in thickened fluids; enhanced bioavailability; taste masking; controlled release; targeting capabilities (Al-kasmi et al., 2017; Macedo et al., 2024)	Complex manufacturing; regulatory uncertainty; potential toxicity concerns; high development cost; limited long-term data (Alebachew, 2025; Atkin et al., 2024)	Oral nanoinsulin (clinical trials); nanocrystal formulations; experimental mucoadhesive systems (Hunt et al., 2024; Mobaleghol Eslam et al., 2024)	Diabetes; severe malabsorption; drug-resistant conditions; precision medicine applications	Al-kasmi et al. (2017); Macedo et al. (2024)

As a demonstration of clinical translation and current lines of research in dysphagia-friendly formulations, Table 5 summarizes original research recently conducted from 2024–2025 that has used each of the five technological approaches detailed above. These trials provide considerable evidence of the improvements in safety, effectiveness and patient compliance that can be achieved via innovative oral drug delivery technologies.

Table 5. Recent original research and review articles (2024–2025) on formulation science in dysphagia care: Advances in oral drug delivery systems for swallowing disorders

No.	Formulation technology	Parameter investigated	Key findings	Reference
1	Orally disintegrating tablets (ODTs)	PDC ≥80%, cardiovascular events (n=2,246 matched pairs), aspiration pneumonia incidence, 1-year follow-up	Large-scale retrospective cohort study (15,000 patients) found comparable adherence rates between ODT and non-ODT users, suggesting patient preference rather than clinical superiority drives ODT selection	Sato et al. (2025)
2	Medicated oral gels/jellies	Patient acceptance (90–95% vs 72%), viscosity (50–500 Pa·s), gel strength (200–800 g), bioavailability enhancement (1.2–2.8×)	Comprehensive review demonstrating >90% patient acceptance rates for medicated jellies vs. 72% for conventional tablets; enhanced bioavailability through controlled rheological properties	Huang et al. (2025)
3	3D printing for central nervous system disorders	Publication analysis (747 papers, 2019–2024), esophageal transit time (30% reduction), printlet geometries (torus, sphere, cylinder)	Analysis of 747 publications showing FDM as predominant 3D printing technique; novel torus-shaped printlets demonstrated 30% faster esophageal transit for dysphagia patients	Paipa-Jabre-Cantu et al. (2025)
4	Mini-tablets (2–3 mm)	Tablet diameter (1–3 mm), swallow success (90% in 6–23 months), dose flexibility (0.5–50 mg), choking incidents (0% vs 8% conventional)	Review highlighting 90% swallow success in infants; flexible dosing capabilities with reduced choking risk compared to conventional tablets	Lura et al. (2025)
5	Dual porogenic ODTs	Disintegration time (<10 s), porosity (15–4 5%), dissolution enhancement (Q30 = 85–95%), bioavailability AUC (2.5× increase)	Novel dual porogenic approach achieved <10 second disintegration time with 2.5-fold enhanced bioavailability compared to conventional tablets	Fouad et al. (2025)
6	Nanotechnology platforms	Nanoparticle size (10–200 nm), solubility enhancement (5–50×), encapsulation efficiency (75–95%), targeting index (2-8×)	Comprehensive review of nanoenabled oral delivery systems showing enhanced drug solubility and targeting for patients with swallowing difficulties	Alebachew (2025)
7	Hospital-based 3D printing	Production time (15–45 min/unit), quality parameters (weight ±5%, content 95–105%), regulatory compliance (GMP standards)	First clinical implementation of point-of-care 3D printing platform producing personalized medicines for dysphagia patients with regulatory compliance	Denis et al. (2024)

continued on following page

Table 5. Continued

No.	Formulation technology	Parameter investigated	Key findings	Reference
8	Direct compression ODTs	Disintegration time (15–20 s), hardness (30–50 N), friability (<1%), pediatric acceptance scores (8.5/10), cost reduction (40%)	Cost-effective direct compression method achieved <20 second disintegration with improved pediatric compliance; suitable for patients with dysphagia	Juan et al. (2024)
9	Multiparticulate systems assessment	Swallowing difficulty prevalence (28%), error rates (conventional: 21.1% vs mini-tablets: 8.4%), patient age (65–95 years)	Hospital survey revealed 28% prevalence of swallowing difficulties; mini-tablets showed 60% reduction in administration errors compared to crushed tablets	Harnett et al. (2024)
10	Gelatin-based jelly technology	NRRSv (0.02–0.18), NRRSp (0.01–0.15), PAS (1–3), PTT (0.8–2.1 s), jelly volume (3–5 mL), gelatin concentration (1.5–2.5%)	Clinical study of 50 patients demonstrated sliced gelatin jellies reduce aspiration risk by 40% compared to thickened liquids while maintaining drug delivery integrity	Aii et al. (2024)
11	3D-printed mini-tablets	Tablet geometries (6 shapes), release kinetics (t50: 15–120 min), swallowability scores (7–9/10), surface area/volume ratios (0.8–2.4)	Polyhedral-shaped mini-tablets demonstrated controlled release profiles; torus geometry showed optimal swallowability for dysphagic patients	Kim et al. (2024)
12	Taste-masked mini-tablets	Tablet diameter (2 mm), taste scores (bitter: 1–2/10), disintegration time (25–30 s), drug content (98–102%), palatability index (8.2/10)	Ball milling technique achieved effective taste masking in 2 mm mini-tablets with maintained rapid disintegration (<30 seconds) for pediatric dysphagia	Trofimiuk et al. (2024)
13	Medication lubricants/gels	Viscosity (73.74 ± 3.20 Pa·s), tube diameter (8–12 mm), transit time (6 s vs. 3 s reference), chitosan concentration (6.25% w/w)	Novel chitosan-based swallowing gel demonstrated 73.74 ± 3.20 Pa s viscosity with enhanced pill transit through 300 mm tube in 6 seconds	Malouh et al. (2024)
14	Thickened formulations	Thickener concentrations (0.5–3% w/v), disintegration delay (250% increase), dissolution rates (Q30: 45–85%), IDDSI levels (2–4)	Systematic review showed xanthan gum-based thickeners delayed tablet disintegration by 250% but nanocrystal formulations maintained dissolution rates	Atkin et al. (2024)
15	Nanoenabled oral insulin	Nanoparticle size (10 nm, 1/10,000th hair width), glucose responsiveness (5–25 mM), hypoglycemia reduction (70%), bioavailability (15–25%)	Revolutionary nanoscale insulin delivery system (1/10,000th width of human hair) enabling oral administration through glucose-responsive release mechanism	Hunt et al. (2024)

Abbreviations: AUC = Area Under the Curve; CNS = Central Nervous System; FDM = Fused Deposition Modeling; g = grams; GMP = Good Manufacturing Practice; IDDSI = International Dysphagia Diet Standardization Initiative; mg = milligrams; min = minutes; mL = milliliter; mm = millimeter; mM = millimolar; N = Newton; nm = nanometer; NRRSp = Normalized Residue Ratio Scale (pyriform sinus);

NRRSv = Normalized Residue Ratio Scale (vallecula); ODTs = Orally Disintegrating Tablets; Pa·s = Pascal-seconds; PAS = Penetration-Aspiration Scale; PDC = Proportion of Days Covered; PTT = Pharyngeal Transit Time; Q30 = Amount released at 30 minutes; s = seconds; t50 = Time for 50% release; w/v = weight/volume; w/w = weight/weight.

PHARMACEUTICAL ENGINEERING AND FORMULATION DESIGN CONSIDERATIONS

The successful translation of dysphagia-friendly oral formulations from conceptual design to clinical application relies on the integration of pharmaceutical engineering principles tailored to specific swallowing impairments. *Figure 10* summarizes the normal trajectory of swallow and the different perturbations that could disrupt how medication is delivered to its intended location, possibly compromising both its efficacy and safety. This mechanism can be a major pathophysiological challenge, where for example, failure to swallow solid doses makes patients more vulnerable to aspiration, and changes in drug transit and dissolution profiles further complicate this. This clinical consideration is crucial to strategy. ODTs and film-coated tablets require excipient systems that rapidly disintegrate the tablets, provide effective taste masking and maintain physical stability over time. While ensuring that powders (multiparticulates/gel preparations) of each dose are flowable, they must adhere to one another sufficiently so that a user can pick up a predetermined amount and swallow it safely. Moreover, such progress in technology permits dosing according to individual requirements and maximizes drug release as well as the design of tablet geometries. However, these advances also pose critical questions such as reproducibility, regulation, scale and how to assemble a pill. All these prospective hazards, product stability for some methods and groups, including alternative storage properties, and quality control of products still remain basic principles that patients anticipate when applying any therapy as well as with which doctors feel confident (Klang, 2023).

Figure 10. Pathophysiological Impairments in Dysphagia and Their Implications for Formulation Design

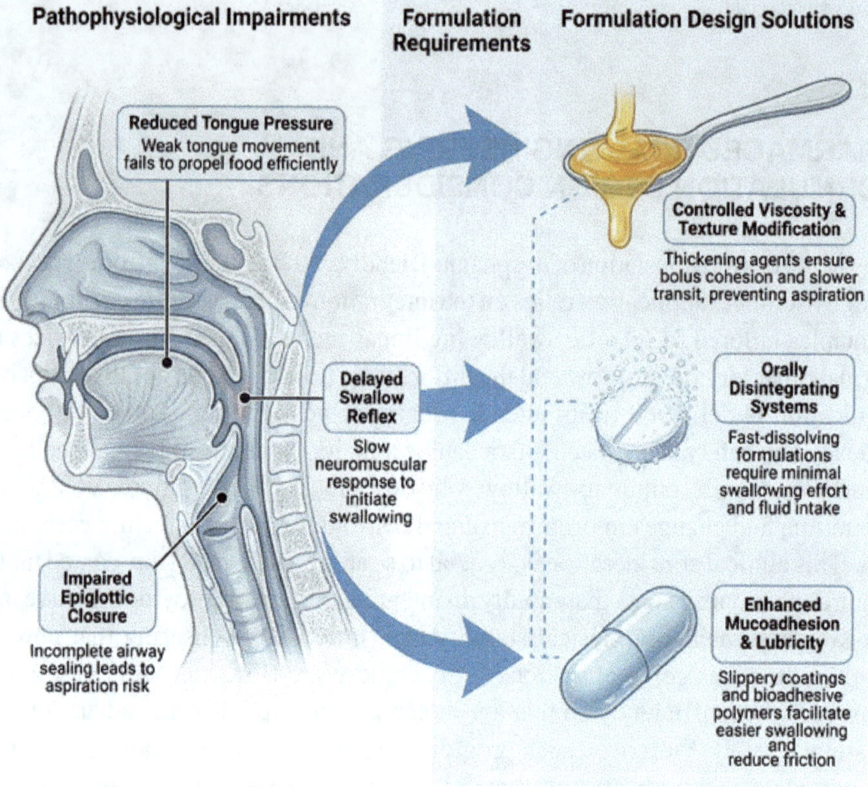

Excipients and Safety

The formulation of dysphagia-friendly dosage forms will routinely involve unusual excipient inclusion in dedicated dosage forms, such as gelatin in medicated jellies, superdisintegrants at high loading, orodispersible tablets or bespoke polymers, when 3D printing drugs. The safety and biocompatibility of these excipients are highly important in medically sensitive or vulnerable populations. Photopolymers in photopolymers in stereolithography (SLA) and selective laser sintering (SLS) 3D printing processes are becoming a focus of scientific interest; these materials often contain residual monomers, plasticizers, or other impurities that are not suitable for oral ingestion. Recent reviews have highlighted the lack of toxicity data for most 3DP resins and powders that are currently available, confirming the use of pharmaceutical-grade materials designed to be ingested (Bernatoniene et al., 2025; Racaniello et al., 2024; Saleh-Bey-Kinj et al., 2025). In line with this trend, food-grade polymers (including maltodextrin, diverse sugars, and Eudragit®) have recently been studied as materials for safe 3D-printed drug delivery systems aligned with patient preferences. Although the use of these materials has improved safety profiles, the common use of 3D printing in hospital or care settings has been less widely adopted. Bottlenecks include limited access to approved excipients and a lack of economically feasible combined processes with online, real-time quality control for product consistency, safety and regulatory compliance.

For ODTs and films, the selection of excipients is also an important issue and affects the balance between taste, mechanical strength and fast disintegration in the oral cavity. In another embodiment, the composition includes mannitol for a sweet taste and a cool feeling and superdisintegrants such as crospovidone or croscarmellose sodium to help immediate disintegration. For example, in *in vitro* studies, formulations optimized to contain approximately 5% crospovidone can disintegrate within six seconds, indicating potential utility for treating dysphagic patients (Szakonyi & Zelkó, 2013). Moreover, medicated gels commonly employ food-grade thickeners such as xanthan and carrageenans, although the latter has raised concern for gastrointestinal distress upon ingestion in relatively large amounts. Recently, an alternative to konjac-only systems was proposed (konjac–gellan gum blends) to offer better textural stability and less water syneresis (Huang et al., 2025). Nonetheless, these results require validation. It is also important to consider excipient–drug compatibility, e.g., ionic gels may react with basic drugs requiring the addition of a pH modifier or the release of enhancers. Another obstacle was the preservative (parabens) used for gel application, and it was also noted during the study that this compound can induce sensitization in some patients; single-dose preservative free gel sachets were developed to facilitate safer administration.

Manufacturing Processes

Conventional manufacturing technologies such as direct compression and granulation are not sufficient for the fabrication of more recent, dysphagia-friendly dose forms. For example, Zydis® freeze-drying technology results in ODTs that are very porous and undergo rapid dispersion but have high fragility and costly production steps, requiring special blister packaging to be stable on the shelf (Carou-Senra et al., 2024). To mitigate these challenges, scalable technology alternatives such as melting granulation and electrospinning are being investigated for film-type products. Industrial players such as DuPont are also developing continuous manufacturing platforms that can process heat-sensitive APIs without degradation. Dose uniformity is a critical quality control feature of thin films; each 2×2 cm film unit should represent its labeled dose. Print-based technologies, particularly inkjet printing, can provide accurate drug deposition and have the potential for personalized on-demand dosing. New developments include the use of handheld inkjet printers for the preparation of drug-containing buccal films from hydroxypropyl cellulose under field conditions (Carou-Senra et al., 2025).

Multiparticulates and mini-tablets also introduce challenges in both manufacturing and dosing. High-speed fill-by-weight systems and specialized mini-tablet dispensers have been developed to reduce errors by supplying unit-dose sachets, which lowers the risk of manual counting mistakes in care facilities. Advances in coating methods have further improved performance: electrostatic spray coating, for example, has been shown to enhance the uniformity of 2 mm mini-tablets while also supporting taste masking and controlled-release properties. Quality control remains essential. ODTs are generally tested according to pharmacopeial specifications such as USP <701> for disintegration in simulated saliva (Cerveto et al., 2024; Yingngam, 2024). Unlike other oral dosage forms, ODFs undergo a number of mechanical tests, including tensile strength and elongation tests, to ensure that they are able to withstand normal handling. Packaging is equally important, particularly for moisture-sensitive formulations. ODTs are typically provided in alu-alu blisters or desiccant-containing containers to protect their integrity; oral films are typically packed in pouches formed of foil to maintain stability during shelf life. Recent developments A multiunit calendar blister package, which is designed specifically for geriatric patients to improve convenience and provide protection, offers both ease of use and moisture barrier properties by combining elderly friendly design and moisture barrier technology.

Compatibility and Stability

The inclusion of new dosage forms such as complex oral solid dosage forms (such as 3D-printed polypills combining several APIs in a single dosage unit) presents important issues in terms of drug stability and compatibility between components. Robles-Martinez et al. (2019) demonstrated this in practice by successfully printing a six-drug polypill using SLA, but their phenomenal diffusion between drug layers highlighted the dangers of such multilayered systems. Structural diffusion is not the only stability issue. Hygroscopic APIs are particularly challenging in the formulation of orodispersible tablets and thin films, as they may take up water with subsequent softening, deformation or too fast disintegration of the dosage form. The potential risk associated with such drawbacks has been addressed by, for example, controlling drying induction during thermoplastic production and the use of excipients that enable the formation of moisture barrier layers. Masking of taste is also an added difficulty in convenient patient dose forms. For example, taste-masking films or coatings that are designed to mask flavors may deteriorate and release offensive tastes over periods of time, which will cause patients to be less compliant. It is therefore essential to carry out stability studies widely, such as accelerated studies, which are also relevant to ICH guidelines. Ultimately, however, the evaluation should not be limited to the physical and chemical stability of an active substance but should also consider the integrity of the coating, release kinetics and organoleptic properties to ensure uniform therapeutic efficacy throughout the shelf-life of the product.

Regulatory Aspects in Formulation Design

Regulatory bodies are increasingly prioritizing patient-centric criteria—particularly swallowability and overall acceptability—when novel oral dosage forms are being evaluated. The International Council for Harmonization (ICH) guideline Q8(R2) emphasizes the application of quality-by-design (QbD) principles throughout pharmaceutical development. These principles advocate for the systematic identification of control strategies, design space, and critical quality attributes (CQAs) to ensure that drug products meet both therapeutic performance requirements and user-related requirements (refer to *Table 6*) (ICH, 2009; Simões et al., 2024). In the United States, a recent FDA review by McGuire et al. (2024) revealed that swallowability is increasingly considered in generic drug submissions. However, evaluation methods remain inconsistent: most rely on patient-reported questionnaires, with only approximately half assessing multiple doses and few treating swallowability as a primary endpoint. These findings highlight the urgent need for standardized, validated assessment tools—such as visual analog scales and structured participant training—to clearly differentiate swallowability from related factors such as palatability. From a formulation development perspective, incorporating human factors into product design is becoming essential. The evidence suggests that oval, film-coated tablets are generally favored by patients, as both peer-reviewed studies and regulatory data confirm that specific shapes and coatings increase the ease of swallowing. In response, some manufacturers now proactively conduct small-scale swallowability studies in healthy volunteers, particularly when a product's physical characteristics differ from those of the reference formulation. Adapting QbD frameworks for dysphagic populations also necessitates the definition of new CQAs. These may include rapid disintegration in simulated saliva, gel viscosities consistent with IDDSI guidelines, and dimensional thresholds for mini-tablets on the basis of maximum swallowable size. As noted by Atkin et al. (2024), common food thickeners used in dysphagia diets can significantly delay drug dissolution, underscoring the need for formulation strategies that maintain therapeutic release profiles while ensuring safe and efficient swallowing.

Table 6. Critical quality attributes (CQAs) of dysphagia-friendly formulations and their patient-centered benefits

Dosage form	Key CQA	Patient-centered benefit	Limitation/risk
ODTs/ODFs	Disintegration ≤30 seconds in simulated saliva	Rapid swallowability, no water needed	Fragility, moisture sensitivity
Gels/Jellies	IDDSI Level 4 cohesive texture; viscosity 50–500 Pa·s	Reduced aspiration risk, improved acceptability	Microbial contamination, preservative need
Multiparticulates	Size ≤3 mm; uniform dose distribution	Flexible dosing, reduced choking	Potential grittiness, counting errors
3D-printed tablets	Shape/geometry optimization; porosity control	Personalized swallowability and dosing	High cost, regulatory uncertainty
Nanoformulations	Particle size 10–200 nm; encapsulation efficiency >75%	Dose-volume reduction, taste masking, buccal delivery	Toxicity risk, limited clinical data

REGULATION AND SAFETY CONSIDERATIONS

The safe and efficacious use of medicines in people with dysphagia requires good collaboration between both the pharmaceutical industry and regulatory authorities. Regulatory agencies (the FDA (United States), EMA (European Union), PMDA (Japan), and national authorities) now emphasize swallowing ability and acceptability in dosage form design for vulnerable populations. In recent years, submissions of novel dosage forms have increasingly included swallowability studies and patient-centric clinical data for ODTs, oral films, and mini-tablets (McGuire et al., 2024). Harmonized pathways for innovative systems (e.g., 3D-printed medicines) remain limited, highlighting the need for international alignment among industry, regulators, and academia.

Patient safety also relies on more detailed knowledge of the risks related to each formulation type. Nearly half of crushed or dispersed formulations are unsuitable for manipulation, leading to pharmacokinetic variability, dose imprecision, and aspiration risk (Blaszczyk et al., 2023). Mini-tablets and multiparticulates offer safer, more versatile alternatives. Figure 1 Nevertheless, the lack of conformity in definitions and classification of mini-tablets among regulatory regions raises potential concerns for both clinical application and regulatory acceptance (Meruva et al., 2024).

However, the introduction of dysphagia-friendly products in practice could be multidisciplinary only. Recommendations tend to focus on the pharmacist (e.g., do not crush lists) and personalize administration mandates. Both in the form of BANS and AAS, they will ultimately need to merge with clear frameworks for integration that are underpinned by rigorous evaluations, shared professional teaching, and regulation with safety and clinical practice in balanced harmony to ensure that downstream innovation outputs can indeed be turned into real patient gains. A patient-focused model of the regulatory and safety context surrounding dysphagia-tailored pharmaceutical care is illustrated in *Figure 11*. From the regulatory and safety perspective, this model offers a constricted view of dysphagia care management into layers radiating from the highest levels of governance to the individual patient. The second layer, regulatory coherence, provides the basic conditions for coherent and legally sound rules. This involves compliance with the IDDSI Standard (International Dysphagia Diet Standardization Initiative), ensuring consistent terminology on food texture and drink thickness, as evidenced by the pyramid icon, as well as meeting labeling standards and pharmacopoeia requirements. The moderate band (focused on criteria of safety and efficacy) is limited by external considerations. Here, we consider the physiological merits of a formulation: nutritional sufficiency, swallowing ability, and, importantly, the prevention of aspiration to guard against possible lung risk for patients.

For clinical application and patient convergence, the internal layers aside from transposing the operational translation of these safety guidelines to everyday healthcare. The clinical practice ring highlights the ability-to-touch tasks performed by clinicians (e.g., bedside assessments) and the exact magnitude of texture modification of food/liquid for each patient's one-of-a-kind physiological threshold. The converging arrows are saying that everything out there—money, data sharing and research templates—all point to this centered care. Patient preference is a meta-center of this center, since a formulation that will not be taken by the patient can have no effect. The model shows that effective dysphagia care requires constant alignment between one-size fits all global standards (IDDSI) and the flexible, personal needs of individuals.

Figure 11. Patient-centered model linking regulatory requirements, safety, and clinical practice in dysphagia-friendly formulations (IDDSI, the International Dysphagia Diet Standardization Initiative)

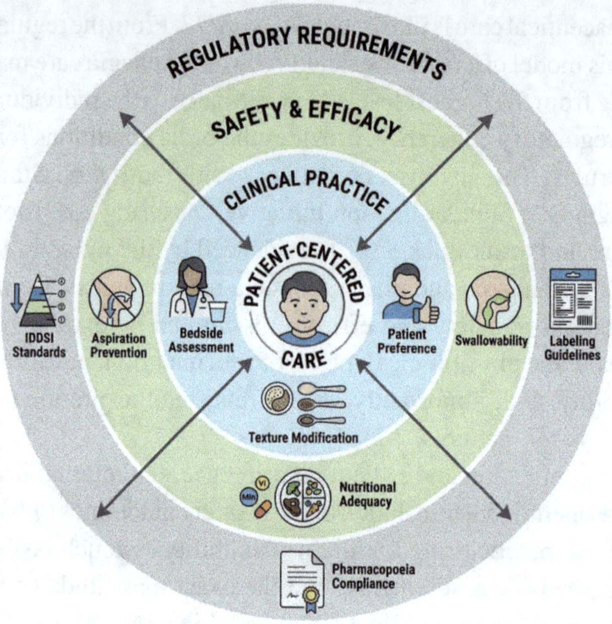

Figure 12 illustrates the transformation from a rectilinear legacy oral dose (on the left side) to patient-focused, dysphagia-based dosing. The conventional workflow is a typical drug development process, expecting stability and efficient manufacturing and not necessarily being designed to address specific patient needs. At the stages of preformulation and design, standard solid dosage forms, including compressed tablets or capsules, are generally made that are best suited for shelf-life storage and mass production. The main drawback of this model system is that studies concerning clinical trials are usually conducted on healthy adults with normal swallowing function, so handling problems in the administration rarely occurs during development. Therefore, patient acceptability is only evaluated postmarket, and standard formulations that are not appropriate or safe for vulnerable populations are approved, as they appear to be red warning symbols. In contrast, the dysphagia-oriented workflow adopts a patient-centric approach that includes end-user physiology right from inception. The preformulation stage is extended to investigate rheology and texture so that the physical characteristics of the drug allow safe bolus formation and swallowing. This methodology provides for the development of special formulations that are easy to swallow, such as gels, films or multiparticulate liquids. Importantly, this

workflow adapts clinical trials to incorporate subjects with impaired swallowing and progresses patient acceptability testing upstream in development. This proactive approach ensures that the final regulatory submission includes dosage forms validated to be safe and palatable for the targeted population, leading to improved medication adherence while reducing the risk of choking.

Figure 12. Conventional versus dysphagia-oriented workflows in oral drug development

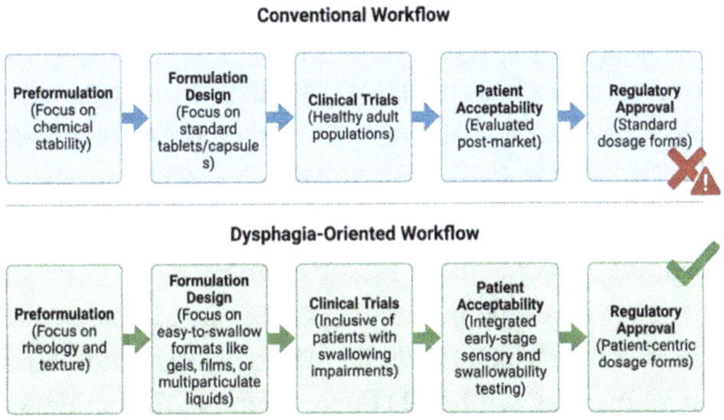

CLINICAL CASE STUDIES AND REAL-WORLD APPLICATIONS

New case histories and clinical reports are reviewed to illustrate the use of new developments in formulation science. They also reinforce the evidence that novel dosages from vehicles for those with swallowing difficulties are promoted with such technology because of their safety, adherence and therapeutic benefits. They also raised ongoing concerns — including problems with implementation, regulatory hurdles and variation in clinical adoption — that must be addressed lest they relegate these new approaches to little-used curiosities.

Poststroke Dysphagia and the Use of ODTs

A nationwide retrospective cohort study in Japan reported an association between ODT and adherence to medication therapy and between ODT and clinical outcome among elderly individuals suffering from poststroke dysphagia (Sato et al., 2025). In a large commercial claims database of approximately 15,000 patients, researchers have applied high-dimensional propensity score (hd-PS) matching to adjust for confounding characteristics between ODT users and individuals taking conventional oral formulations. At follow-up, 2246 matched pairs were analyzed over a 1-year time frame. Adherence, assessed by the PDC, was greater than 80% for both groups, and there was no statistically significant difference between the groups (0.902 among ODT users, 0.889 among non-ODT users; $p = 0.977$). Clinical outcomes, such as cardiovascular events and aspiration pneumonia, were also comparable between the groups. Subgroup analyses within therapeutic domains—hypertension, diabetes, and hyperlipidemia—further confirmed the absence of significant differences, suggesting that while ODTs may offer practical advantages in terms of administration, these advantages did not translate into measurable differences in adherence or clinical endpoints within the study population.

The implications are twofold. First, ODTs did not confer measurable superiority in terms of adherence or safety outcomes over standard formulations, suggesting that Japan's generally high adherence rates may overshadow formulation-specific benefits. Second, clinicians may base the choice between ODTs and conventional tablets on patient preference, palatability, and administration convenience rather than expectations of improved clinical outcomes. This large-scale evidence highlights earlier clinical impressions that ODTs inherently reduce aspiration risk or substantially enhance adherence. Instead, while ODTs are valuable for patient comfort and ease of administration, their real-world effectiveness is context dependent. For patients struggling with pill swallowing, ODTs remain a viable strategy, but they should be integrated into individualized care plans rather than being assumed to provide universal benefits (Sato et al., 2025).

Medications Underdosing from Tablet Crushing in Geriatric Units

A survey of the general practice of crushing tablets in geriatric wards across French hospitals was conducted in 2023 and raised concerns about the accuracy of dosing and patient safety when crushing tablets as part of a dysphagia management plan (Blaszczyk et al., 2023). With the traditional method, approximately 70% of administrations cause significant underdosage owing to the retention of residual drug in the crushing device. However, to address this problem, scientists have tested 24 tablet crushers for sale on the UK market. The degree of drug loss was between 1.9% and 13.3%, depending on the device type. Even with rinsing, losses remained at 0.5–10.4%, and in some cases, one rinse left up to 42.5% of the active product behind. These results highlight the real and clinical risks of crushing tablets in older people. While this form of drug delivery is employed commonly to aid in the management of dysphagia, incomplete dosing may result and subsequently contribute to subtherapeutic treatment effects, underscoring the dire need for new, safer forms of accurate administration among older adults.

Posthead and Neck Cancer Surgery – 3D-Printed Nutrient–Drug Hybrid Foods

Head and neck cancer survivors often face severe dysphagia, making drug and nutrient intake difficult. Advances in 3D food printing now allow the creation of hydrogel-based meals that are safe to swallow and nutritionally balanced. Although medicines are not yet integrated into such foods clinically, the concept of "med-nutrient" products—combining therapy and nutrition—has strong potential to simplify administration and improve adherence. In the future, carefully designed clinical trials and clear regulatory pathways will be essential to translate these concepts into safe, legitimate options for patients.

Balabram et al. (2025) described the fabrication of 3D-printed, hydrogel model foods that could be modeled to resemble a bolus for individuals with dysphagia. Nothing pharmacologically was contained in these formulations, but they introduced the concept of texture-optimized, nutritionally tailored systems as a starting basis for future nutrient–drug combination products. Gelatin- and starch-based hydrogels were developed by the research team and were loaded with bioactive compounds obtained from annatto seeds via natural deep eutectic solvents (NADES). Structures produced could be printed into cohesive, International Dysphagia Diet Standardization Initiative (IDDSI)-compliant gels of increased softness and spreadability characteristics crucial for safe swallowing in patients with oral or pharyngeal compromise, especially for cancer treatment.

The sequential building work of Chao et al. (2024) also demonstrated the feasibility of 3D food printing for geriatric nutrition. With the use of hydrocolloids to adjust viscoelasticity, texture-adapted meals with different macronutrient compositions have been developed to minimize the risk of malnutrition in head and neck cancer patients. Together, these developments demonstrate the potential for 3D printing to be used to create safe texture, nutrient-dense meals-on-demand and provide a path to personalized nutritional and therapeutic care for patients with complex swallowing disorders.

Clinical Outcome Evidence

However, these case reports provide some knowledge regarding the risk of adaptation of the formulation being performed by individual patients and the potential benefits. Larger-scale observational and interventional research will provide stronger evidence to clarify the balance of risk and benefit for the pharmaceutical industry in adapting pharmaceutical products for those with swallowing difficulties. A multicenter European study revealed that medication errors were far more common in dysphagic patients (21.1%) than in those without swallowing problems

(5.9%) (Kelly et al., 2011). Most errors stem from inappropriate tablet crushing, which compromises stability, dosing accuracy, and safety. These findings highlight the increased risk of drug-related harm in dysphagic populations.

Later reviews confirmed the favorable effects of pharmacist-led interventions. For example, Bourdenet et al. (2015) conducted a review of geriatric care units in France, and a reduced rate of incorrect crushing of tablets was demonstrated when the recommendations of the pharmacist, such as alternative formulations and methods of administration, were received. This led to improved dosing accuracy, bedside safety and interprofessional practice by offering nurses explicit evidence-based recommendations. Current reviews of the literature reinforce that interprofessional care—frequently involving a combined effort from pharmacists, nurses and speech-language pathologists—is essential for promoting proper medication use for patients with dysphagia. Blaszczyk et al. (2023) described how unsupervised tablet crushing was still widespread in both hospitals and long-term care, despite the resulting underdosing, with altered pharmacokinetics being potential risks. The authors suggest that such problems could be addressed through the use of specific protocols, staff education and increased availability of dysphagia-appropriate formulations (such as ODTs, minitablets and liquids). The findings of this study show that technological progress should not be the unique justification for the success of pharmaceutical innovations (including ODT, film, mini-tablet and 3D printing-based nutrient–drug hybrids, which are still in development). The true standard is clinical impact, including fewer medication errors, improved compliance and safer administration. Therefore, systems changes — such as provider education and regulatory support — that allow for safe prescribing, access to and use of preparations specifically formulated for patients with swallowing issues.

FUTURE DIRECTIONS IN DYSPHAGIA-FRIENDLY PHARMACEUTICS

Dysphagia-focused therapeutics are rapidly evolving at the intersection of pharmaceutical science, digital innovation, and biomedical engineering. Technologies such as artificial intelligence (AI)-assisted design, 4D printing, and advanced nanotechnology are driving increasingly personalized, adaptable, and effective therapies. *Figure 13* shows a variety of novel pharmaceutical approaches to the treatment of dysphagia, which impair swallowing and therefore either place patients at risk for unsafe swallowing practices or result in poor medication adherence. To diminish the choking and aspiration hazards of traditional solid tablets, methods that significantly affect the physical properties and flow behavior of the dosage forms are shown. Multiparticulate systems in the form of pellets or granules offer a great deal of versatility, as subunits can be individually dosed with less difficulty than a single large tablet and can frequently be sprinkled onto soft food to assist in the formation of an easily swallowed bolus. Similarly, medicated gels and jellies utilize semisolid networks to produce a soft homogenous consistency that not only lubricates the esophageal passageway but also effectively masks the bitter tastes of medications. This figure also adds oral liquid foams as a new tool, whereby a gas is mixed with a liquid base. The result is a stick pack with a lower density and volume, with faster disintegration and less muscular exertion to swallow than regular liquid medications do.

In addition to texture manipulation, the figure highlights the importance of advanced manufacturing and microtechnology for improving individualized dysphagia care. 3D-printed doses have had a material impact on the field of personalized medicine. Recent developments include the formulation of tablets with noncentrifuged geometries and an internal porous microstructure to increase the dissolution rate. In addition, the use of polypills, which combine several medication regimens into a single pill, makes it easier to swallow. At the microscale, the figure highlights the contribution of nanotechnology-enabled carriers (e.g., liposomes and polymeric nanoparticles) to this field. These carriers are especially important for bioavailability, whose goal is to protect medicaments from degradation and enhance their efficacy in a body that could suffer from gastrointestinal dysfunction to overcome physiological barriers. Altogether, five novel delivery systems that differ from the "one-size-fits-all" pill offer customizable patient formulations without sacrificing swallowability but provide therapeutic benefits specific to each individual. Taken together, these innovations represent a sea change toward a patient-centric care model for those with dysphagia that leverages technology. If proven effective in the clinical domain, these applications may strongly contribute to an ealier and higher adherence (and therefore therapeutic efficacy) of prescribed treatments, as well as to a better life standard for patients with swallow disorders.

Figure 13. Emerging formulation strategies for oral drug delivery in dysphagia patients

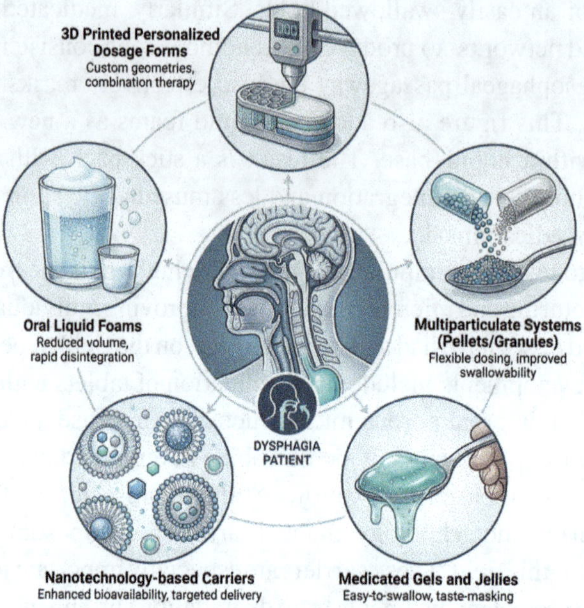

AI-Driven Formulation Design

AI plays a greater role in dysphagia-friendly products. Currently, predictive models predict disintegration, hardness and stability with stunning accuracy, significantly reducing the need for trial-and-error testing. For example, the DisCoNet model yielded a predictive accuracy of 73% for tablet disintegration and 99% for hardness based on more than 2,000 formulations (Momeni et al., 2024) and helps to make product development faster and more individualized for patients who have difficulty swallowing. AI is also being applied to 3D printing platforms within hospitals to help make individualized medicines for patients in a very fast and affordable way. While published data are scarce, preliminary pilot studies have revealed significant decreases in the time required for formulation compared with conventional practice (Malamatari et al., 2024). Additionally, market trends suggest that up to 25% of personalized geriatric drugs will be AI-derived by 2030, representing a new era in data-driven/agile drug development instead of trial- and error-based formulations (Serrano et al., 2024). This progress implies that AI has the potential to serve as a fundamental driver for scaling and patient-centering innovations in dysphagia-focused drug delivery, more specifically relating technological breakthroughs to improved efficiency and clinical application levels.

Four-Dimensional (4D) Printing

4D printing consists of 3D-printed dosage forms that are designed to change shape or function in response to an environmental stimulus over time (e.g., pH or temperature). This will create opportunities for dynamic drug delivery, such as the use of gastroretentive devices or stimuli-sensitive hydrogels that can respond to changes under physiological conditions *in vivo*. Recent studies point to its promise for dynamic delivery systems such as gastroretentive constructs that swell in gastric media and increase mucosal adhesion and transit regulation (Mahmoud & Schulz-Siegmund, 2023) or responsive hydrogels, including shape memory materials, which could perhaps be used for site-selective or extended release dosing. While specific performance parameters such as "250% volume expansion in gastric fluid" still remain experimentally or formulation dependent, these studies validate the ability of shape-altering dosage forms.

Nanotechnology and Mucoadhesive Systems

Nanotechnology is very useful in drug delivery, especially for improving drug solubility and formulation stability and increasing drug absorption in mucosal barriers. For example, nanocrystal preparations can sufficiently delay drug release in viscous media, leading to constant availability of the drug (Gadhiya et al., 2021). Additionally, mucoadhesive nanogels are advantageous for buccal delivery, thereby being an attractive option for patients experiencing difficulties in swallowing conventional oral dosage forms (Almeida et al., 2024). These novel approaches are promising developments in dysphagia treatment and integrate the effectiveness of therapy with patient-oriented experience. Although there are few bioavailability studies focusing directly on amyotrophic lateral sclerosis, similar studies in mucoadhesive delivery systems have shown a marked improvement in systemic drug uptake. This enhancement in mucosal adhesion is attributed mainly to increased residence time on the mucosal surface (Hua, 2019). From an economic standpoint, nanomedicine is experiencing exponential growth in market size (expectedly reaching 410.15 billion USD by 2030), with an overall average compound annual growth rate (CAGR) of ~11.6%. This expansion is influenced mainly by developments in drug delivery technologies that are finding parallel movements in dysphagia patients (Grand View Research, 2023). Although the detailed market figures regarding dysphagia are limited, these estimates highlight rising commercial opportunities and the potential market volume for oral nanotherapeutics. Thus, the use of dissolution-enhancing nanocrystals and patient-friendly mucoadhesive formulations is a promising approach to enhance drug efficacy for those who rely on texture-modified diets. Existing market indications also support the future viability of nanotherapeutics for the treatment of dysphagia.

Convergence of Technologies

The merging of AI technology with 4D printing and nanotechnology has given rise to what is called "medifoods", essentially food products, which store concentrated amounts of nutrients or pharmaceuticals that are easy to swallow. The results of a European Union (EU) project validated the practical feasibility of mass production of standardized meals designed according to individual nutritional requirements and swallowing capability (Smith et al., 2022). Developments such as this have the potential to help fuse treatment and nutrition into a complementary, patient-focused plan. In addition to mere demonstrations of technical feasibility, holistic system-level analyses suggest that these innovations might bring sizeable clinical and economic benefits. Marin et al. (2020) assessed the effects of replacing commercial tablets with dysphagia-friendly medicines), which included osmotically dispersed tablets, medicated jelly, and multiparticulate preparations. Their results indicated that there was a 20% lower incidence of aspiration pneumonia for patients who had difficulty swallowing standard tablets. This savings corresponds to approximately US$1,200–1,500 per patient/year, which becomes particularly relevant if we take into account the implications in an elderly population that usually presents a high prevalence of dysphagia. A reduction in the cost of healthcare could represent significant financial support, especially for a growing middle-aged population with difficulty swallowing. Collectively, these developments demonstrate how AI-driven formulation design, 4D-printed texture and release control and nanoenabled delivery systems may be disruptor technologies. When working collectively as a group, they partner to advance interdisciplinary patient-centered innovations that combine the provision of medication and nutritional care. By increasing safety, palatability, compliance and aesthetics while reducing health care utilization and hence the costs of health care, these 2nd generation dysphagia-medifoods may be considered pathfinders for personalized, cost-effective solutions.

CONCLUSION

Formulation science is reshaping the traditional landscape of dysphagia care from reactive treatments to an oral amenable system that focuses on patient experience. Emerging applications, such as ODTs and ODFs, medicated jellies, multiparticulates,

3D/4D-printed formulations, and nanoenabled systems, are highly advantageous to consumers. For example, ODTs and jellies have compliance rates of more than 90%, multiparticulates can reduce medication errors by 30–60%, and the use of 3D-printed regimens has been linked with a shorter length of hospital stay. These technical improvements have resulted in safer and more standardized products for therapy and have relieved caregivers of some workload with both direct and indirect positive clinical and financial impacts. International health agencies, such as the FDA, EMA and PMDA, are also moving quickly to increase their level of expectations, especially in the areas of swallowing safety, excipient tolerance and label clarity. The recent recognition of swallowing as a critical quality attribute requires that pharma companies consider what this means for product development as the environment changes. Further development of personalized dysphagia-focused treatments may be facilitated through AI-assisted formulation tools, 4D printing and nanotechnology. For example, approximately 2030, the order of 1 in 10 new oral entities may be associated with adapting designs or individualized patient product forms on the basis of precise bioassays. Predictions interpret a move to patient-oriented pharmacology in pharmaceuticals, and dysphagia care is a case-in-point approach. The direction of this evolution will depend on further positive developments in science and not the continuation of current technological advances. This transformation may be driven by greater funding of evidence-based medicines, global regulatory cooperation, and the creation of an environment conducive to patient access to and innovation in medical treatments. Novel formulation approaches that encompass pharmaceutical engineering, patient care and regulatory science will therefore be key to bridging the current gap between laboratory-based excellence and safe effective drug delivery for several million adults with dysphagia.

REFERENCES

Abdullah, M. R., Peng, Z., Rajendren, V. b., Ahmad, F., Shah, S. S. A., Zia, A. W., & Shehzad, K. (2025). Comprehensive review of 3D/4D printing of soft materials, methods and applications. *Applied Materials Today*, *43*, 102667. DOI: 10.1016/j.apmt.2025.102667

Ahmed, M. M., DeSantis, M., FarrowCypel, B., Hossain, T., Weaver, M., Harasym, E., & Diener, M. (2024). S3399 Pill swallowing: a case of misdirection - hydroxychloroquine induced pill esophagitis complicated by an aberrant right subclavian artery. *Official journal of the American College of Gastroenterology | ACG, 119*(10S), S3399. DOI: DOI: 10.14309/01.ajg.0001042964.68079.34

Ahmed Abdulmohsen, A., Mohammed Dawood, A., Nahlah Mubark, A., Ali Nassir Al, A., Meshal Saeed, A., Zahra Hussain Ali Bu, H., & Murtadha Essa Ali, A. (2024). An examination of nurses' understanding and experience with enteral tube drug delivery. *International Journal of Medical Toxicology and Legal Medicine*, *27*(2S), 402–405. https://ijmtlm.org/index.php/journal/article/view/494

Aii, S., Fujishima, I., Shigematsu, T., Ohno, T., Kunieda, K., & Yamawaki, M. (2024). Sliced jelly whole swallowing reduces deglutition risk: A novel feeding method for patients with dysphagia. *Dysphagia*, *39*(5), 940–947. DOI: 10.1007/s00455-024-10674-6 PMID: 38568345

Al-kasmi, B., Alsirawan, M. H. D. B., Bashimam, M., & El-zein, H. (2017). Mechanical microencapsulation: The best technique in taste masking for the manufacturing scale - effect of polymer encapsulation on drug targeting. *Journal of Controlled Release*, *260*, 134–141. DOI: 10.1016/j.jconrel.2017.06.002 PMID: 28603029

Alebachew, M. (2025). The advancements of nanobiotechnology in novel drug delivery system: Current trends and future directions. *International Journal of Biomedical Science and Engineering*, *13*(3), 57–65. DOI: 10.11648/j.ijbse.20251303.12

Almeida, S. L., Lazo, R. L., Carneiro, J., Caldonazo, A., Pires, C., Andreazza, I. F., & Murakami, F. S. (2024). Cellulose nanocrystals as an innovative superdisintegrant for oral dispersible tablets. *Journal of Drug Delivery Science and Technology*, *96*, 105694. DOI: 10.1016/j.jddst.2024.105694

Atkin, J., Devaney, C., Yoshimatsu, Y., & Smithard, D. (2024). Modified medication use in dysphagia: The effect of thickener on drug bioavailability—a systematic review. *European Geriatric Medicine*, *15*(1), 19–31. DOI: 10.1007/s41999-023-00896-6 PMID: 38280090

Balabram, S. K., Tessaro, L., Astolfo, M. E., Sponchiado, P. A., Bogusz, S.Junior, & Maniglia, B. C. (2025). Development of NADES–annatto seed extract for enhancing 3d printed food designed for dysphagia patients. *Foods, 14*(9), 1604. DOI: 10.3390/foods14091604 PMID: 40361685

Balcerak, P., Corbiere, S., Zubal, R., & Kägi, G. (2022). Poststroke dysphagia: Prognosis and treatment–a systematic review of RCT on interventional treatments for dysphagia following subacute stroke. *Frontiers in Neurology, 13*, 823189. DOI: 10.3389/fneur.2022.823189 PMID: 35547370

Bernatoniene, J., Stabrauskiene, J., Kazlauskaite, J. A., Bernatonyte, U., & Kopustinskiene, D. M. (2025). The future of medicine: How 3D printing is transforming pharmaceuticals. *Pharmaceutics, 17*(3), 390. DOI: 10.3390/pharmaceutics17030390 PMID: 40143052

Bhidayasiri, R., Chaisongkram, A., Anan, C., & Phuenpathom, W. (2024). User-centered design, validation and clinical testing of an anti-choking mug for people with Parkinson's disease. *Scientific Reports, 14*(1), 14165. DOI: 10.1038/s41598-024-65071-8 PMID: 38898235

Bifari, N., & Bifari, N., I., & Ahmed Alharbi, Y. (2024). Unraveling medication errors in enteral tube administration: A cross-sectional study in geriatric patients receiving home health care. *Saudi Pharmaceutical Journal : SPJ : the Official Publication of the Saudi Pharmaceutical Society, 32*(2), 101938. DOI: 10.1016/j.jsps.2023.101938 PMID: 38261870

Blaszczyk, A., Brandt, N., Ashley, J., Tuders, N., Doles, H., & Stefanacci, R. G. (2023). Crushed tablet administration for patients with dysphagia and enteral feeding: Challenges and considerations. *Drugs & Aging, 40*(10), 895–907. DOI: 10.1007/s40266-023-01056-y PMID: 37707775

Bourdenet, G., Giraud, S., Artur, M., Dutertre, S., Dufour, M., Lefèbvre-Caussin, M., & Doucet, J. (2015). Impact of recommendations on crushing medications in geriatrics: From prescription to administration. *Fundamental & Clinical Pharmacology, 29*(3), 316–320. DOI: 10.1111/fcp.12116 PMID: 25789404

Brunemann, A., Schifano, A., Fenwick, S., & Seibert, C. (2025). Assessing the rate of inappropriately crushed medications in skilled nursing facilities. *The Senior Care Pharmacist, 40*(2), 72–96. DOI: 10.4140/TCP.n.2025.72 PMID: 39891323

Can, B. (2025). Characteristics of patients with oropharyngeal dysphagia in a geriatric outpatient clinic. *Clinical Science of Nutrition, 7*(1), 30–36. DOI: 10.62210/ClinSciNutr.2025.102

Carou-Senra, P., Awad, A., Basit, A. W., Alvarez-Lorenzo, C., & Goyanes, A. (2025). Harnessing handheld inkjet printing technology for rapid and decentralized fabrication of drug-loaded hydroxypropyl cellulose buccal films. *Carbohydrate Polymer Technologies and Applications*, *9*, 100724. DOI: 10.1016/j.carpta.2025.100724

Carou-Senra, P., Rodríguez-Pombo, L., Awad, A., Basit, A. W., Alvarez-Lorenzo, C., & Goyanes, A. (2024). Inkjet printing of pharmaceuticals. *Advanced Materials*, *36*(11), e2309164. DOI: 10.1002/adma.202309164 PMID: 37946604

Cerveto, T., Denis, L., Stoops, M., Lechanteur, A., Jérôme, C., Leenhardt, J., & Choisnard, L. (2024). The promising role of semisolid extrusion technology in custom drug formulation for pediatric medicine. *International Journal of Bioprinting*, *10*(6), 4063. DOI: 10.36922/ijb.4063

Chao, C., Nam, H. K., Park, H. J., & Kim, H. W. (2024). Potentials of 3D printing in nutritional and textural customization of personalized food for elderly with dysphagia. *Applied Biological Chemistry*, *67*(1), 25. DOI: 10.1186/s13765-023-00854-7

Cho, W. H., Yoo, W., & Yoo, B. (2024). Effect of thickened beverage and swallowing aid jelly used for dysphagic patients on the disintegration of orally administered tablets. *Clinical Nutrition Research*, *13*(2), 89–95. DOI: 10.7762/cnr.2024.13.2.89 PMID: 38784854

Chue, P., Jones, B., Taylor, C. C., & Dickson, R. (2002). Dissolution profile, tolerability, and acceptability of the orally disintegrating olanzapine tablet in patients with schizophrenia. *Canadian Journal of Psychiatry*, *47*(8), 771–774. DOI: 10.1177/070674370204700809 PMID: 12420656

Denis, L., Jørgensen, A. K., Do, B., Vaz-Luis, I., Pistilli, B., Rieutord, A., & Annereau, M. (2024). Developing an innovative 3D printing platform for production of personalized medicines in a hospital for the OPERA clinical trial. *International Journal of Pharmaceutics*, *661*, 124306. DOI: 10.1016/j.ijpharm.2024.124306 PMID: 38871137

Drumond, N., & Stegemann, S. (2021). Better medicines for older patients: Considerations between patient characteristics and solid oral dosage form designs to improve swallowing experience. *Pharmaceutics*, *13*(1), 32. DOI: 10.3390/pharmaceutics13010032 PMID: 33379258

EMA. (2025). *ICH M13A Guideline on bioequivalence for immediaterelease solid oral dosage forms*. Retrieved 18 August from https://www.ema.europa.eu/en/documents/scientific-guideline/ich-m13a-guideline-bioequivalence-immediaterelease-solid-oral-dosage-forms-step-5_en.pdf

Fouad, S. A., Abdelaziz, N., Teaima, M. H., El-Nabarawi, M., Taha, A. A., Abdelmonem, R., & El-Refai, K. (2025). Engineering orally disintegrating tablets for buccal delivery of cilostazol with enhanced dissolution and bioavailability: A novel dual porogenic approach, *in vitro* characterization, and *in vivo* evaluation in rats. *Pharmaceutical Development and Technology, 30*(3), 280–294. DOI: 10.1080/10837450.2025.2472887 PMID: 40007241

Gadhiya, D. T., Patel, J. K., & Bagada, A. A. (2021). An impact of nanocrystals on dissolution rate of Lercanidipine: Supersaturation and crystallization by addition of solvent to antisolvent. *Future Journal of Pharmaceutical Sciences, 7*(1), 128. DOI: 10.1186/s43094-021-00271-x

Goyanes, A., Scarpa, M., Kamlow, M., Gaisford, S., Basit, A. W., & Orlu, M. (2017). Patient acceptability of 3D printed medicines. *International Journal of Pharmaceutics, 530*(1), 71–78. DOI: 10.1016/j.ijpharm.2017.07.064 PMID: 28750894

Grand View Research. (2023). *Nanomedicine market size projected to reach USD 410.15 billion by 2030; CAGR 11.57%. May 2023.* Retrieved 18 August from https://www.prnewswire.com/news-releases/nanomedicine-market-to-be-worth-410-15-billion-by-2030-grand-view-research-inc-301833021.html

Harnett, A., Byrne, S., O'Connor, J., Burke, E., South, L., Lyons, D., & Sahm, L. J. (2024). Point prevalence survey of acute hospital patients with difficulty swallowing solid oral dose forms. *Pharmaceutics, 16*(5), 584. DOI: 10.3390/pharmaceutics16050584 PMID: 38794246

Harnett, A., Byrne, S., O'Connor, J., Lyons, D., & Sahm, L. J. (2023). Adult patients with difficulty swallowing oral dosage forms: A systematic review of the quantitative literature. *Pharmacy (Basel, Switzerland), 11*(5), 167. DOI: 10.3390/pharmacy11050167 PMID: 37888511

Hauber, B., Hand, M. V., Hancock, B. C., Zarrella, J., Harding, L., Ogden-Barker, M., & Watt, S. J. (2024). Patient acceptability and preferences for solid oral dosage form drug product attributes: A scoping review. *Patient Preference and Adherence, 2024*, 1281–1297. DOI: 10.2147/PPA.S443213 PMID: 38919378

Hida, N., Serizawa, F., Sambe, T., Nakamura, A., & Harada, T. (2025). The Feasibility of the repeated administration of acetylsalicylic acid mini-tablets to children with Kawasaki disease: A pilot study. *Pharmaceutics, 17*(3), 333. DOI: 10.3390/pharmaceutics17030333 PMID: 40142997

Hua, S. (2019). Advances in nanoparticulate drug delivery approaches for sublingual and buccal administration. *Frontiers in Pharmacology, 10*, 1328. DOI: 10.3389/fphar.2019.01328 PMID: 31827435

Huang, X., Mu, Y., Shen, L., & Zhao, L. (2025). Advantages, progress, and future trends in oral medicated jellies/gels: Focus on adherence aspects. *Drug Discovery Today*, *30*(8), 104431. DOI: 10.1016/j.drudis.2025.104431 PMID: 40653263

Hummler, H., Stillhart, C., Meilicke, L., Grimm, M., Krause, E., Mannaa, M., & Page, S. (2023). Impact of tablet size and shape on the swallowability in older adults. *Pharmaceutics*, *15*(4), 1042. DOI: 10.3390/pharmaceutics15041042 PMID: 37111528

Hunt, N. J., Lockwood, G. P., Heffernan, S. J., Daymond, J., Ngu, M., Narayanan, R. K., & Cogger, V. C. (2024). Oral nanotherapeutic formulation of insulin with reduced episodes of hypoglycemia. *Nature Nanotechnology*, *19*(4), 534–544. DOI: 10.1038/s41565-023-01565-2 PMID: 38168926

ICH. (2009). *ICH harmonized tripartite guideline pharmaceutical development Q8(R2)* Retrieved 18 August from https://database.ich.org/sites/default/files/Q8_R2_Guideline.pdf?utm_source=chatgpt.com

Jacob, S., Boddu, S. H. S., Bhandare, R., Ahmad, S. S., & Nair, A. B. (2023). Orodispersible films: Current innovations and emerging trends. *Pharmaceutics*, *15*(12), 2753. DOI: 10.3390/pharmaceutics15122753 PMID: 38140094

Juan, C., Gallo, L., & Gonzalez Vidal, N. (2024). Development of losartan orally disintegrating tablets by direct compression: A cost-effective approach to improve pediatric patient's compliance. *AAPS PharmSciTech*, *25*(4), 79. DOI: 10.1208/s12249-024-02796-9 PMID: 38589718

Kállai-Szabó, N., Farkas, D., Lengyel, M., Basa, B., Fleck, C., & Antal, I. (2024). Microparticles and multiunit systems for advanced drug delivery. *European Journal of Pharmaceutical Sciences*, *194*, 106704. DOI: 10.1016/j.ejps.2024.106704 PMID: 38228279

Karalia, D., Siamidi, A., Karalis, V., & Vlachou, M. (2021). 3D-printed oral dosage forms: Mechanical properties, computational approaches and applications. *Pharmaceutics*, *13*(9), 1401. DOI: 10.3390/pharmaceutics13091401 PMID: 34575475

Kelly, J., Wright, D., & Wood, J. (2011). Medicine administration errors in patients with dysphagia in secondary care: A multicenter observational study. *Journal of Advanced Nursing*, *67*(12), 2615–2627. DOI: 10.1111/j.1365-2648.2011.05700.x PMID: 21615463

Kim, Y.-J., Choi, Y.-R., Kang, J.-H., Park, Y.-S., Kim, D.-W., & Park, C.-W. (2024). Geometry-driven fabrication of mini-tablets via 3D printing: Correlating release kinetics with polyhedral shapes. *Pharmaceutics*, *16*(6), 783. DOI: 10.3390/pharmaceutics16060783 PMID: 38931904

Klang, M. G. (2023). Developing guidance for feeding tube administration of oral medications. *JPEN. Journal of Parenteral and Enteral Nutrition*, *47*(4), 519–540. DOI: 10.1002/jpen.2490 PMID: 36847617

Kömür, M., Kıyan, H. T., & Öztürk, A. A. (2025). Development of donepezil hydrochloride-loaded PLGA-based nanoparticles for Alzheimer's disease treatment. *Scientific Reports*, *15*(1), 13184. DOI: 10.1038/s41598-025-95792-3 PMID: 40240764

Lazic, M., Djukic, M., Vukomanovic, V., Bijelic, M., Obarcanin, E., & Bajcetic, M. (2025). Acceptability and palatability of novel orodispersible minitablets of enalapril in children up to the age of 6 with heart failure. *Journal of Clinical Medicine*, *14*(3), 915. PMID: 39941586

Li, S., Han, W., Li, J., & Li, B. (2025). Improving the edible quality of deacetylated konjac glucomannan gel: Synergistic ethanol immersion and low-temperature pretreatment. *Innovative Food Science & Emerging Technologies*, *104*, 104130. DOI: 10.1016/j.ifset.2025.104130

Lura, V., Lura, A., Breitkreutz, J., & Klingmann, V. (2025). The revival of the mini-tablets: Recent advancements, classifications and expectations for the future. *European Journal of Pharmaceutics and Biopharmaceutics*, *210*, 114655. DOI: 10.1016/j.ejpb.2025.114655 PMID: 39922507

Macedo, L. D., Masiero, J. F., & Bou-Chacra, N. A. (2024). Drug nanocrystals in oral absorption: Factors that influence pharmacokinetics. *Pharmaceutics*, *16*(9), 1141. DOI: 10.3390/pharmaceutics16091141 PMID: 39339178

Maciejewska, O., Kępczyńska, K., Polit, M., & Domitrz, I. (2024). Dysphagia in ischemic stroke patients: One center retrospective study. *Nutrients*, *16*(8), 1196. DOI: 10.3390/nu16081196 PMID: 38674886

Maheshwari, S., Singh, A., Varshney, A. P., & Sharma, A. (2024). Advancing oral drug delivery: The science of fast dissolving tablets (FDTs). *Intelligent Pharmacy*, *2*(4), 580–587. DOI: 10.1016/j.ipha.2024.01.011

Mahmoud, D. B., & Schulz-Siegmund, M. (2023). Utilizing 4D printing to design smart gastroretentive, esophageal, and intravesical drug delivery systems. *Advanced Healthcare Materials*, *12*(10), 2202631. DOI: 10.1002/adhm.202202631 PMID: 36571721

Malamatari, M., Wan, K. W., & Baxevanis, F. (2024). Regulatory Aspects of 3D-Printed Medicinal Products. In D. A. Lamprou, D. Douroumis, & S. Qi (Eds.), *3D Printing of Pharmaceutical and Drug Delivery Devices: Progress from Bench to Bedside* (pp. 211-225). John Wiley & Sons. DOI: DOI: 10.1002/9781119836001.ch11

Malouh, M. A., Cichero, J. A. Y., Sun, Y., Lau, E. T. L., Nissen, L. M., & Steadman, K. J. (2024). Medication lubricants for oral delivery of drugs: Oral processing reduces thickness, changes characteristics, and improves dissolution profile. *Pharmaceutics*, *16*(3), 417. DOI: 10.3390/pharmaceutics16030417 PMID: 38543311

Marin, S., Serra-Prat, M., Ortega, O., & Clavé, P. (2020). Healthcare-related cost of oropharyngeal dysphagia and its complications pneumonia and malnutrition after stroke: A systematic review. *BMJ Open*, *10*(8), e031629. DOI: 10.1136/bmjopen-2019-031629 PMID: 32784251

Martín-Oliveros, A., Plaza Zamora, J., Monaco, A., Anitua Iriarte, J., Schlageter, J., Ducinskiene, D., & Donde, S. (2024). Multidose drug dispensing in community healthcare settings for patients with multimorbidity and polypharmacy. *Inquiry : a Journal of Medical Care Organization, Provision and Financing*, *61*, 469580241274268. DOI: 10.1177/00469580241274268 PMID: 39373170

Matías Ambiado-Lillo, M. (2025). Impact of head and neck posture on swallowing kinematics and muscle activation: A systematic review. *Dysphagia*, *40*, 1049–1054. DOI: 10.1007/s00455-025-10821-7 PMID: 40085151

McGuire, M. R., Mostofa, A., Shon, J., Frost, M., Kim, M.-J., & Li, K. (2024). Designs of clinical swallowability assessments of solid oral dosage forms in regulatory submissions. *International Journal of Pharmaceutics*, *659*, 124229. DOI: 10.1016/j.ijpharm.2024.124229 PMID: 38762166

Meruva, S., Singaraju, A. B., Vinjamuri, B. P., Ternik, R., & Stagner, W. C. (2024). Current state of minitablet product design: A review. *Journal of Pharmaceutical Sciences*, *113*(5), 1123–1154. DOI: 10.1016/j.xphs.2024.02.016 PMID: 38369020

Milliken, R. L., Quinten, T., Andersen, S. K., & Lamprou, D. A. (2024). Application of 3D printing in early phase development of pharmaceutical solid dosage forms. *International Journal of Pharmaceutics*, *653*, 123902. DOI: 10.1016/j.ijpharm.2024.123902 PMID: 38360287

Mitra, B., Chang, J., Wu, S.-J., Wolfe, C. N., Ternik, R. L., Gunter, T. Z., & Victor, M. C. (2017). Feasibility of mini-tablets as a flexible drug delivery tool. *International Journal of Pharmaceutics*, *525*(1), 149–159. DOI: 10.1016/j.ijpharm.2017.04.037 PMID: 28432019

Mitsui, N., Hida, N., Kamiya, T., Yamazaki, T., Miyazaki, K., Saito, K., & Harada, T. (2022). Swallowability of minitablets among children aged 6–23 months: An exploratory, randomized crossover study. *Pharmaceutics, 14*(1), 198. DOI: 10.3390/pharmaceutics14010198 PMID: 35057092

Mobaleghol Eslam, H., Hataminia, F., Esmaeili, F., Salami, S. A., Ghanbari, H., & Amani, A. (2024). Preparation of a nanoemulsion containing active ingredients of cannabis extract and its application for glioblastoma: *In vitro* and *in vivo* studies. *BMC Pharmacology & Toxicology, 25*(1), 73. DOI: 10.1186/s40360-024-00788-w PMID: 39375818

Momeni, M., Afkanpour, M., Rakhshani, S., Mehrabian, A., & Tabesh, H. (2024). A prediction model based on artificial intelligence techniques for disintegration time and hardness of fast disintegrating tablets in preformulation tests. *BMC Medical Informatics and Decision Making, 24*(1), 88. DOI: 10.1186/s12911-024-02485-4 PMID: 38539201

Morath, B., Sauer, S., Zaradzki, M., & Wagner, A. H. (2022). Orodispersible films – recent developments and new applications in drug delivery and therapy. *Biochemical Pharmacology, 200*, 115036. DOI: 10.1016/j.bcp.2022.115036 PMID: 35427572

Münch, J., Kloft, C., Farhan, M., Fishman, V., Leng, S., Bosse, H. M., & Klingmann, V. (2023a). Acceptability, swallowability, palatability, and safety of multiple film-coated mini-tablets in children aged ≥2-<7 years: Results of an open-label randomized study. *Pharmaceutics, 15*(2), 701. DOI: 10.3390/pharmaceutics15020701 PMID: 36840023

Münch, J., Sessler, I., Bosse, H. M., Wargenau, M., Dreesen, J. D., Loforese, G., & Klingmann, V. (2023b). Evaluating the acceptability, swallowability, and palatability of film-coated mini-tablet formulation in young children: Results from an open-label, single-dose, crossover study. *Pharmaceutics, 15*(6), 1729. DOI: 10.3390/pharmaceutics15061729 PMID: 37376177

Paipa-Jabre-Cantu, S. I., Rodriguez-Salvador, M., & Castillo-Valdez, P. F. (2025). Revealing three-dimensional printing technology advances for oral drug delivery: Application to central-nervous-system-related diseases. *Pharmaceutics, 17*(4), 445. DOI: 10.3390/pharmaceutics17040445 PMID: 40284440

Patel, S., Scott, N., Patel, K., Mohylyuk, V., McAuley, W. J., & Liu, F. (2020). Easy to swallow "instant" jelly formulations for sustained release gliclazide delivery. *Journal of Pharmaceutical Sciences, 109*(8), 2474–2484. DOI: 10.1016/j.xphs.2020.04.018 PMID: 32360661

Racaniello, G. F., Silvestri, T., Pistone, M., D'Amico, V., Arduino, I., Denora, N., & Lopedota, A. A. (2024). Innovative pharmaceutical techniques for pediatric dosage forms: A systematic review on 3D printing, prilling/vibration and microfluidic platform. *Journal of Pharmaceutical Sciences*, *113*(7), 1726–1748. DOI: 10.1016/j.xphs.2024.04.001 PMID: 38582283

Rivelsrud, M. C., Hartelius, L., Bergström, L., Løvstad, M., & Speyer, R. (2023). Prevalence of oropharyngeal dysphagia in adults in different healthcare settings: A systematic review and meta-analyses. *Dysphagia*, *38*(1), 76–121. DOI: 10.1007/s00455-022-10465-x PMID: 35639156

Robles-Martinez, P., Xu, X., Trenfield, S. J., Awad, A., Goyanes, A., Telford, R., & Gaisford, S. (2019). 3D printing of a multilayered polypill containing six drugs using a novel stereolithographic method. *Pharmaceutics*, *11*(6), 274. DOI: 10.3390/pharmaceutics11060274 PMID: 31212649

Saleh-Bey-Kinj, Z., Heller, Y., Socratous, G., & Christodoulou, P. (2025). 3D printing in oral drug delivery: Technologies, clinical applications and future perspectives in precision medicine. *Pharmaceuticals*, *18*(7), 973. DOI: 10.3390/ph18070973 PMID: 40732263

Sapiee, N. H., Mat Saufi, M. H., Abu Bakar, N. F., & Adam, F. (2023). Fabrication and characterization of electrospun κ-carrageenan based oral dispersible film with vitamin C. *Materials Today: Proceedings*. Advance online publication. DOI: 10.1016/j.matpr.2023.04.030

Sato, S., Sasabuchi, Y., Okada, A., & Yasunaga, H. (2025). Do orally disintegrating tablets facilitate medical adherence and clinical outcomes in patients with poststroke dysphagia? *Dysphagia*, *40*(2), 381–387. DOI: 10.1007/s00455-024-10737-8 PMID: 39096331

Serrano, D. R., Luciano, F. C., Anaya, B. J., Ongoren, B., Kara, A., Molina, G., & Lalatsa, A. (2024). Artificial intelligence (AI) applications in drug discovery and drug delivery: Revolutionizing personalized medicine. *Pharmaceutics*, *16*(10), 1328. DOI: 10.3390/pharmaceutics16101328 PMID: 39458657

Simões, A., Veiga, F., & Vitorino, C. (2024). Question-based review for pharmaceutical development: An enhanced quality approach. *European Journal of Pharmaceutics and Biopharmaceutics*, *195*, 114174. DOI: 10.1016/j.ejpb.2023.114174 PMID: 38160986

Smith, R., Bryant, L., & Hemsley, B. (2022). Allied health professionals' views on the use of 3D food printing to improve the mealtime quality of life for people with dysphagia: Impact, cost, practicality, and potential. *American Journal of Speech-Language Pathology*, *31*(4), 1868–1877. DOI: 10.1044/2022_AJSLP-21-00391 PMID: 35613623

Szakonyi, G., & Zelkó, R. (2013). Prediction of oral disintegration time of fast disintegrating tablets using texture analyzer and computational optimization. *International Journal of Pharmaceutics*, *448*(2), 346–353. DOI: 10.1016/j.ijpharm.2013.03.047 PMID: 23558313

Topuz, F., & Uyar, T. (2025). Recent developments in nanofiber-based fast-disintegrating drug delivery systems. *Expert Opinion on Drug Delivery*, *22*(7), 957–969. DOI: 10.1080/17425247.2025.2497831 PMID: 40285755

Tosun, B., Nursemin, Ü., Nurten, Ö., & Atalay, F. (2021). Comparison of dosage loss between medications crushed with two different methods by two nurses: An *in vitro* study. *Bezmialem Science*, *9*, 106–111. DOI: 10.14235/bas.galenos.2020.4016

Trofimiuk, M., Olechno, K., Trofimiuk, E., Czajkowska-Kośnik, A., Ciosek-Skibińska, P., Głowacz, K., & Winnicka, K. (2024). Utilization of the drug–polymer solid dispersion obtained by ball milling as a taste masking method in the development of orodispersible minitablets with hydrocortisone in pediatric doses. *Pharmaceutics*, *16*(8), 1041. DOI: 10.3390/pharmaceutics16081041 PMID: 39204386

U.S. FDA. (2008). *Guidance for Industry: Orally Disintegrating Tablets*. Retrieved 18 August 2025 from https://www.gmp-compliance.org/files/guidemgr/Orally Disintegrating_Tablets_Final_FDA_8528fnl.pdf

Vaz, V. M., & Kumar, L. (2021). 3D printing as a promising tool in personalized medicine. *AAPS PharmSciTech*, *22*(1), 49. DOI: 10.1208/s12249-020-01905-8 PMID: 33458797

Visser, J. C., Wibier, L., Mekhaeil, M., Woerdenbag, H. J., & Taxis, K. (2020). Orodispersible films as a personalized dosage form for nursing home residents, an exploratory study. *International Journal of Clinical Pharmacy*, *42*(2), 436–444. DOI: 10.1007/s11096-020-00990-w PMID: 32052239

Wargenau, M., Reidemeister, S., Klingmann, I., & Klingmann, V. (2022). A composite endpoint for acceptability evaluation of oral drug formulations in the pediatric population. *Therapeutic Innovation & Regulatory Science*, *56*(6), 903–909. DOI: 10.1007/s43441-022-00406-z PMID: 35471561

Watanabe, N., Ebisujima, M., Ichihara, T., Ando, M., & Kawahara, M. (2025). Survey of dysphagia and related medications in nursing home residents using the Eating Assessment Tool (EAT-10) applied by community pharmacists: A single-center retrospective study. *Journal of Pharmaceutical Health Care and Sciences, 11*(1), 38. DOI: 10.1186/s40780-025-00447-0 PMID: 40329345

Yingngam, B. (2024). Advances in Electrospinning Technology for Fast-Dissolving Oral Film Applications. In Javed, R., Chen, J.-T., & Khalil, A. T. (Eds.), *Nanomaterials for Biomedical and Bioengineering Applications* (pp. 133–176). Springer Nature Singapore., DOI: 10.1007/978-981-97-0221-3_6

Yingngam, B. (2025). Carbon-based nanocomposites for 3D printing. In Khanna, V. (Ed.), *Carbon-based nanocomposites for sustainable applications* (Vol. 1, pp. 201–227). Springer., DOI: 10.1007/978-3-031-95306-4_9

Zhu, Y., Zhu, B., & Jin, P. (2025). Medication administration through feeding tubes in a tertiary hospital: A retrospective observational study. *Risk Management and Healthcare Policy, 2025*, 319–328. DOI: 10.2147/RMHP.S500557 PMID: 39911206

APPENDIX

Abbreviations

3D - Three-dimensional
4D - Four-dimensional
AI - Artificial intelligence
API - Active pharmaceutical ingredient
AUC - Area under the curve
CAGR - Compound annual growth rate
CNS - Central nervous system
EMA - European Medicines Agency
FDA - U.S. Food and Drug Administration
FDM - Fused deposition modeling
GMP - Good Manufacturing Practice
hd-PS - High-dimensional propensity score
ICH - International Council for Harmonization
IDDSI - International Dysphagia Diet Standardization Initiative
LNP - Lipid nanoparticle
NADES - Natural deep eutectic solvent
NRRSp - Normalized residue ratio scale (pyriform sinus)
NRRSv - Normalized residue ratio scale (vallecula)
ODFs - Orodispersible films
ODTs - Orodispersible tablets
PAS - Penetration–aspiration scale
PDC - Proportion of days covered
PEG - Percutaneous endoscopic gastrostomy
PMDA - Pharmaceuticals and Medical Devices Agency
PTT - Pharyngeal transit time
QbD - Quality by design
SLA - Stereolithography
SLS - Selective laser sintering
USP - United States Pharmacopeia

Chapter 15
The Cognitive Dimension of Swallowing Disorders

P. Selvakumar
http://orcid.org/0000-0002-3650-4548
Department of Science and Humanities, Nehru Institute of Technology, Coimbatore, India

Manjunath T. C.
http://orcid.org/0000-0003-2545-9160
Rajarajeswari College of Engineering, Bengaluru, India

Keerthi Priya S.
http://orcid.org/0009-0001-0791-7036
Karpagam Academy of Higher Education, Coimbatore, India

R. Jayasudha
http://orcid.org/0000-0002-8913-9230
Dr. N.G.P. Institute of Technology, India

Dharmendra Singh
http://orcid.org/0009-0007-4274-6379
School of Management Sciences, Lucknow, India

Naresh Babu Karunakaran
http://orcid.org/0009-0005-3113-4225
Sree Abirami College of Occupational Therapy, Coimbatore, India

ABSTRACT

Swallowing, though often perceived as a simple, reflexive act, is in fact a highly complex sensorimotor process that relies on intricate coordination between the brain, cranial nerves, muscles, and cognitive mechanisms. Dysphagia, or difficulty in swallowing, is traditionally viewed as a disorder stemming from structural abnormalities, neuromuscular impairments, or damage to the swallowing reflex pathways. However, in recent decades, researchers and clinicians have come to recognize that cognitive functions such as attention, memory, executive functioning, and awareness play a significant role in initiating, regulating, and sustaining safe and effective swallowing. Understanding the cognitive influences on swallowing is essential not only for explaining why certain populations are more vulnerable to dysphagia but also for designing more effective diagnostic assessments and ther-

DOI: 10.4018/979-8-3373-6405-6.ch015

apeutic interventions. The act of swallowing requires more than just mechanical muscle coordination; it demands conscious initiation, sustained attention to the task, and, in some cases, active problem-solving

INTRODUCTION

Swallowing, though often perceived as a simple, reflexive act, is in fact a highly complex sensorimotor process that relies on intricate coordination between the brain, cranial nerves, muscles, and cognitive mechanisms. Dysphagia, or difficulty in swallowing, is traditionally viewed as a disorder stemming from structural abnormalities, neuromuscular impairments, or damage to the swallowing reflex pathways. However, in recent decades, researchers and clinicians have come to recognize that cognitive functions such as attention, memory, executive functioning, and awareness play a significant role in initiating, regulating, and sustaining safe and effective swallowing. Understanding the cognitive influences on swallowing is essential not only for explaining why certain populations are more vulnerable to dysphagia but also for designing more effective diagnostic assessments and therapeutic interventions. The act of swallowing requires more than just mechanical muscle coordination; it demands conscious initiation, sustained attention to the task, and, in some cases, active problem-solving. For example, a person with intact musculature may still fail to swallow safely if they are distracted, fatigued, or unable to follow instructions due to cognitive decline. This is particularly evident in older adults with dementia, individuals who have experienced a traumatic brain injury, or patients with progressive neurological disorders such as Parkinson's disease or Alzheimer's disease. Cognitive impairments can affect swallowing in multiple stages: during the oral preparatory phase, cognitive decline may impair awareness of the need to chew thoroughly; during the oral transport phase, reduced attention may lead to premature spillage of food into the pharynx; and during the pharyngeal phase, slowed processing speed or executive dysfunction may delay the initiation of protective reflexes such as airway closure.

Attention is perhaps the most direct cognitive influence on swallowing. Swallowing safely requires attentional resources to be allocated toward bolus control, timing, and sequencing of muscle contractions. In situations where attention is divided, such as when a person is conversing, watching television, or multitasking while eating, the risk of aspiration increases. Clinical studies have shown that patients with reduced attention due to brain injury or dementia are more likely to aspirate silently, without triggering protective cough reflexes, because they fail to recognize or respond to the sensation of food entering the airway. This illustrates the close interdependence between attentional control and safe swallowing. Memory also exerts a significant influence on swallowing. Procedural memory, which governs learned motor patterns, ensures that the swallowing sequence is carried out automatically without conscious effort. However, when memory systems are compromised, as in Alzheimer's disease, even habitual motor acts like swallowing can become disrupted (Almeida et al. 2024). Patients may forget to chew, fail to swallow altogether, or pocket food in their mouths without awareness. Working memory is also relevant, particularly in rehabilitation, as patients must retain and apply swallowing strategies such as postural adjustments or specific maneuvers taught by speech-language pathologists. If working memory is impaired, adherence to these therapeutic techniques becomes inconsistent, reducing the effectiveness of treatment.

Executive functions—skills such as planning, inhibition, and decision-making—also play a central role in swallowing control. For instance, executive dysfunction can lead to impulsivity in eating behaviors, such as taking excessively large bites or swallowing too quickly, which elevates the risk of choking or aspiration. Similarly, impaired judgment can prevent individuals from recognizing their swallowing difficulties, leading to unsafe eating habits. Executive functioning is particularly critical in populations with frontal lobe injuries or degenerative conditions affecting frontal networks, where the regulation of safe and efficient swallowing becomes compromised despite preserved muscular strength. Cognitive awareness, or the ability to perceive and interpret bodily sensations, is another factor influencing dysphagia. Many individuals with cognitive decline exhibit anosognosia, a lack of awareness of their swallowing deficits. This lack of insight makes it difficult for them to adjust their behavior, comply with dietary modifications, or participate meaningfully in therapy. For caregivers and clinicians, this presents unique challenges, as the risk of aspiration pneumonia and malnutrition increases when patients cannot self-monitor or report their difficulties. The interaction between cognition and swallowing is further complicated by emotional and psychological states. Cognitive impairments often coexist with mood disorders such as depression or anxiety, which can diminish appetite, reduce attentional engagement with meals, and worsen swallowing safety. Anxiety, in particular, can heighten muscle tension and interfere with the smooth coordination of swallowing, while apathy or reduced motivation can cause patients to disengage from therapeutic exercises (Berglund et al. 2025). Thus, swallowing difficulties cannot be fully understood without appreciating the broader cognitive-emotional context of the individual.

Clinical assessment of dysphagia increasingly incorporates evaluation of cognitive function, recognizing that cognitive impairments may be the underlying driver of swallowing difficulties even when structural mechanisms appear intact. Bedside swallowing evaluations, for example, often test a patient's ability to follow commands, attend to the task, and demonstrate consistent swallowing behavior. Instrumental assessments such as videofluoroscopic swallow studies (VFSS) and fiberoptic endoscopic evaluations of swallowing (FEES) can reveal not only physiological impairments but also the influence of cognitive lapses, such as delayed swallow initiation or failure to protect the airway in the absence of structural weakness. Therapeutic approaches for dysphagia must also account for cognitive influences. Traditional rehabilitation strategies such as strengthening exercises or compensatory maneuvers may be ineffective if a patient lacks the cognitive capacity to remember or apply them consistently. In such cases, therapy must be adapted to simplify instructions, use external cues, or involve caregiver training to provide support during meals (Bianchi et al. 2023). Techniques such as spaced retrieval training, errorless learning, and environmental modifications (e.g., reducing distractions during meals, providing visual prompts, or modifying textures) can be highly effective in enhancing swallowing safety for cognitively impaired patients. Importantly, interdisciplinary collaboration between speech-language pathologists, neuropsychologists, occupational therapists, and caregivers is essential to address both the motor and cognitive dimensions of dysphagia. In the broader context of healthcare, recognizing the cognitive influences on swallowing has significant implications for patient safety and quality of life. Dysphagia is a leading cause of aspiration pneumonia, malnutrition, and dehydration in older adults, contributing to hospitalizations and increased mortality rates. By identifying cognitive risk factors, clinicians can implement early interventions to reduce complications. Furthermore, addressing cognitive contributions to swallowing difficulties highlights the importance of holistic, person-centered care that views dysphagia not merely as a physical disorder but as a multidimensional condition requiring integrated support. In conclusion, swallowing is far more than a reflexive motor act; it is a cognitively mediated behavior that depends on attention, memory, executive functioning, awareness, and emotional regulation (Büyükönder et al. 2025). Dysphagia emerges not only from disruptions in the neuromuscular pathways but also from impairments in the cognitive processes that guide, monitor, and sustain safe swallowing. Appreciating these cognitive influences deepens our understanding of dysphagia, informs more accurate diagnostic practices, and inspires innovative therapeutic interventions tailored to the needs of cognitively vulnerable populations. By integrating cognitive and physiological perspectives, healthcare providers can more effectively prevent complications, enhance rehabilitation outcomes, and ultimately improve the quality of life for individuals living with dysphagia.

THE INTERPLAY OF COGNITION AND SWALLOWING FUNCTION

Swallowing is a vital biological function that ensures nutrition, hydration, and airway protection, yet it is far more than a simple reflexive process. Instead, swallowing emerges from the dynamic integration of sensory, motor, and cognitive systems, each contributing to the seamless coordination of this complex act. The role of cognition in swallowing is often overlooked, with greater emphasis historically placed on anatomical and neuromuscular mechanisms. However, a growing body of research highlights that cognition and swallowing are deeply interconnected, influencing each other in ways that affect both health outcomes and quality of life. Understanding this interplay is essential, particularly for populations vulnerable to dysphagia, as it offers insights into assessment strategies, therapeutic approaches, and the prevention of swallowing-related complications. At its core, swallowing involves multiple phases—oral preparatory, oral transit, pharyngeal, and esophageal—each requiring precise timing, muscle coordination, and sensory feedback. While these phases are often considered in physiological terms, the smooth progression from one phase to the next is supported by cognitive functions such as attention, working memory, executive control, and awareness. For example, in the oral preparatory phase, attention is necessary to consciously manipulate food, maintain bolus cohesion, and prevent premature spillage. Without adequate focus, an individual may pocket food in the cheeks or allow liquids to seep into the pharynx before they are ready to swallow (Chakraborty et al. 2024). Similarly, during the oral transit phase, working memory and motor planning play a role in guiding the bolus efficiently toward the pharynx, while executive functions regulate pacing and inhibit impulsive or unsafe swallowing behaviors. Thus, swallowing efficiency and safety cannot be fully understood without acknowledging the cognitive scaffolding that underpins these motor acts.

Cognitive control becomes particularly evident in situations where swallowing must be adapted or modified. For instance, when patients with dysphagia are taught compensatory techniques such as the supraglottic swallow, chin-tuck maneuver, or effortful swallow, successful execution depends on their ability to comprehend instructions, retain them in working memory, and apply them consistently across meals. These cognitive demands highlight how rehabilitation outcomes are closely tied to an individual's cognitive capacity. In cases where memory deficits or executive dysfunction are present, therapy must be simplified, cues introduced, or caregiver assistance incorporated to ensure the safe application of swallowing strategies. This interdependence underscores that cognition and swallowing cannot be treated as separate domains in clinical practice. Attention is one of the most critical cognitive factors influencing swallowing. Swallowing is safer and more effective when attentional resources are directed toward the act of eating and drinking. In clinical and everyday contexts, divided attention—such as eating while conversing, watching television, or walking—has been shown to increase the risk of aspiration or choking (Charan J.K. et al. 2025). For individuals with neurological damage, such as those recovering from stroke or traumatic brain injury, attentional deficits compound the risks, leading to silent aspiration or delayed swallow initiation. Conversely, interventions that enhance attentional focus during meals, such as minimizing environmental distractions, can significantly improve swallowing safety. This demonstrates that attentional modulation is a key element in the interplay between cognition and swallowing.

Memory also plays a pivotal role. Procedural memory supports the automaticity of swallowing, allowing most people to eat and drink without consciously thinking about the mechanics involved. However, in individuals with memory impairments, such as those with dementia, disruptions can occur. They may forget to swallow, hold food in their mouths for prolonged periods, or become confused about the sequence of chewing and swallowing. Working memory is particularly important in the therapeutic context, as patients must remember instructions provided during treatment sessions. For example, remembering to take smaller sips, use a thickened liquid, or perform a compensatory posture requires sustained working memory capacity. If this is compromised, swallowing therapy outcomes are diminished, and caregivers must step in to provide external reminders or supports. Executive functions further shape swallowing behavior by regulating decision-making, self-monitoring, and impulse control. People with intact executive functioning are more likely to recognize difficulties, adjust their pace, and make safe food choices (Charan J.K. et al. 2025). In contrast, individuals with executive dysfunction—common in frontal lobe injuries or degenerative diseases—may display risky behaviors such as stuffing large amounts of food into their mouths, failing to recognize fatigue, or ignoring dietary restrictions. The inability to self-regulate not only compromises swallowing safety but also increases caregiver burden, as constant supervision may be required to mitigate aspiration risk. This demonstrates that swallowing is not merely a motor act but a cognitively guided behavior requiring foresight and judgment. Cognitive awareness, or metacognition, represents another dimension of the interplay between cognition and swallowing. Awareness allows individuals to detect difficulties, monitor performance, and adapt behaviors when challenges arise. In many cases of dysphagia associated with dementia, stroke, or brain injury, anosognosia—or lack of awareness—prevents individuals from recognizing their swallowing impairments. This lack of insight often leads to refusal of therapeutic interventions, noncompliance with dietary modifications, and unreported aspiration events. Caregivers and clinicians must therefore consider not only the physiological aspects of dysphagia but also the individual's level of self-awareness when designing treatment plans.

The interplay between cognition and swallowing also extends to emotional and psychological domains. Cognition and emotion are inseparable, and mood disorders such as anxiety and depression can significantly impact swallowing. Anxiety may heighten vigilance and tension during eating, leading to disrupted swallowing patterns or pharyngeal constriction, while depression can reduce appetite, motivation, and attentional engagement during meals. These emotional-cognitive factors further complicate the management of dysphagia, requiring a holistic approach that integrates mental health support with swallowing therapy. Clinically, this interplay is increasingly acknowledged through comprehensive assessments that evaluate both cognitive and swallowing functions (Chen et al. 2023). Bedside assessments often include simple cognitive screening to determine whether patients can follow instructions, attend to the task, and recognize their difficulties. Instrumental studies such as videofluoroscopy or fiberoptic endoscopy not only provide visual evidence of physiological impairments but also reveal cognitive lapses—such as delayed initiation or failure to follow commands—that influence swallowing outcomes. This recognition has led to more integrated care models where speech-language pathologists, neuropsychologists, and other professionals collaborate to address both motor and cognitive aspects of dysphagia.

Therapeutic interventions also reflect the cognitive-swallowing interplay. Strategies such as environmental modifications (e.g., reducing noise or distractions), caregiver training, visual and tactile cues, and the use of external memory aids are designed to compensate for cognitive deficits during meals. Cognitive training techniques, such as spaced retrieval, errorless learning, and task-specific practice, have also been applied to swallowing therapy, reinforcing both memory and motor performance. These approaches exemplify how understanding the interplay between cognition and swallowing can enhance rehabilitation outcomes, reduce aspiration risks, and improve overall quality of life for affected individuals. Ultimately, the interplay between cognition and swallowing highlights the need for a paradigm shift in both research and clinical practice. Swallowing should not be seen solely as a physiological reflex or muscular activity but rather as a behavior embedded within cognitive frameworks of attention, memory, executive functioning, and awareness (Clavé et al. 2023). Just as cognition influences swallowing safety and efficiency, swallowing impairments can in turn impact cognition by leading to malnutrition, dehydration, or reduced social engagement—factors known to exacerbate cognitive decline. This bidirectional relationship underscores the importance of early detection, integrated treatment, and continuous monitoring. In conclusion, cognition and swallowing are interdependent processes that shape one another in profound ways. The cognitive system provides the attentional focus, memory support, executive regulation, and awareness needed to perform and adapt swallowing safely, while effective swallowing sustains the nutrition and hydration required for cognitive health. When disruptions occur in either domain, the consequences ripple across both, leading to risks of aspiration, malnutrition, and diminished quality of life. Recognizing and addressing this interplay is crucial for clinicians, researchers, and caregivers alike, ensuring that interventions for dysphagia move beyond isolated physiological considerations to embrace the full cognitive-behavioral context in which swallowing occurs.

ATTENTION AND SWALLOWING: COGNITIVE IMPACTS

Swallowing is a complex, coordinated action involving multiple phases that depend on the integration of sensory, motor, and central nervous system processes. While much of the physiological act of swallowing occurs at an automatic or reflexive level, growing research highlights the critical role of cognition—particularly attention—in shaping the safety, efficiency, and adaptability of swallowing. Attention is the cognitive process that allows individuals to selectively focus on relevant stimuli while filtering out distractions. It involves mechanisms of alertness, concentration, divided attention, and sustained focus. The interplay between attention and swallowing is profound, as swallowing is not merely a passive motor activity but a cognitively modulated behavior that requires conscious awareness, task focus, and adaptability, particularly under challenging conditions or in the presence of neurological disorders. Understanding how attention influences swallowing provides valuable insights for both clinical practice and daily life, as attentional failures can increase the risk of aspiration, choking, and malnutrition (Garcia et al. 2024). Swallowing is often performed in multitasking contexts—while conversing, watching television, or engaging in other activities—which requires the allocation of attention across tasks. In healthy individuals, attentional resources are generally sufficient to manage both swallowing and secondary tasks. However, when attentional demands exceed available cognitive capacity, the risk of swallowing errors increases. This is particularly evident in populations with limited attentional control, such as older adults, individuals with traumatic brain injury, stroke survivors, or patients with dementia. For example, divided attention can lead to premature spillage of food into the pharynx, delayed initiation of the swallowing reflex, or failure to detect residue in the oral cavity—all of which increase the likelihood of aspiration. Thus, attention functions as a critical safeguard that ensures timely coordination of muscular activity, bolus control, and airway protection.

A central aspect of attention's role in swallowing lies in sustained focus. Eating and drinking may appear simple, but they require the maintenance of attention across a sequence of actions: preparing the bolus, transporting it, initiating the swallow, and ensuring clearance of the pharynx. Sustained attention allows individuals to recognize when food remains in the mouth, to adjust chewing, and to monitor whether liquids have cleared the airway. When sustained attention is disrupted, individuals may forget to swallow, leave food pocketed in the cheeks, or attempt to speak before completing a swallow, all of which jeopardize swallowing safety. In conditions such as Alzheimer's disease, where sustained attention gradually deteriorates, these lapses become increasingly common, explaining why dysphagia is so prevalent in advanced cognitive decline. Selective attention, the ability to focus on swallowing while filtering out irrelevant distractions, is also critical. In noisy or chaotic environments—such as crowded dining halls or hospitals—patients with reduced selective attention may become distracted, compromising their ability to coordinate swallowing safely. This is one reason why clinicians and caregivers often recommend structured, distraction-free environments for individuals with dysphagia (Guru Basava Aradhya et al. 2025). By minimizing competing stimuli, patients can allocate more attentional resources to the act of swallowing, improving safety and efficiency. This principle also underscores how external environments and caregiving practices can either support or hinder the attentional aspects of swallowing.

Divided attention represents a unique challenge to swallowing safety. Multitasking, such as eating while walking or engaging in conversation, requires cognitive resources to be shared between activities. In younger, healthy populations, the brain can typically handle divided attention without significant consequences. However, research has shown that even in healthy adults, dual-task conditions—such as performing a cognitive test while swallowing—can reduce swallowing efficiency and prolong oral or pharyngeal transit times. In populations with neurological impairments, the consequences are more severe. Stroke survivors, for example, may experience silent aspiration when attempting to talk while drinking, as their weakened attentional control fails to support both tasks simultaneously. These findings highlight how divided attention places vulnerable individuals at particular risk of swallowing-related complications. Clinical observations further reinforce the significance of attention in swallowing (Harmanpreet et al. 2025). Speech-language pathologists frequently note that patients with reduced attentional capacity struggle to follow instructions for compensatory strategies, such as tucking the chin or performing an effortful swallow. Even when patients understand the rationale for a technique, they may fail to implement it consistently if their attention wavers. This has direct implications for therapy design: interventions must be tailored not only to physical swallowing deficits but also to the attentional capacity of the patient. Strategies such as shorter sessions, frequent cues, visual prompts, and structured environments can help compensate for attentional limitations, ensuring safer swallowing practices. The relationship between attention and swallowing is also bidirectional. Just as attention influences swallowing performance, swallowing demands can, in turn, tax attentional resources. For instance, individuals with dysphagia may require conscious focus and effort for every swallow, leaving fewer cognitive resources available for conversation or other concurrent tasks. This heightened attentional demand can make mealtimes exhausting and socially isolating, as individuals avoid talking or interacting in order to concentrate fully on swallowing.

Over time, this can reduce quality of life, underscoring the importance of considering both physiological and cognitive dimensions in dysphagia management. Neurological disorders provide particularly striking evidence of attention's influence on swallowing. In Parkinson's disease, for example, reduced attentional control contributes to delayed swallow initiation and reduced airway protection, compounding the effects of motor impairments. In dementia, attentional decline often precedes or parallels memory loss, meaning swallowing impairments may emerge earlier than expected purely from neuromuscular decline. Stroke patients with lesions in attentional networks, such as the parietal or frontal lobes, often display neglect or inattention to the act of eating, leading to unrecognized residue or impaired bolus control. These cases illustrate how attention deficits are not incidental but central contributors to dysphagia in neurological populations. Assessment of swallowing must therefore include evaluation of attention (Hassan et al. 2023). Bedside swallow exams often incorporate tasks that require following commands or sustaining focus, as lapses in attention are strong predictors of unsafe swallowing. Instrumental assessments such as videofluoroscopy or fiberoptic endoscopic evaluations can reveal how attention influences swallowing mechanics, with patients performing better under guided, focused conditions than when left unattended. These findings reinforce the need for clinicians to assess not only physiological swallowing function but also the cognitive conditions under which swallowing occurs.

Therapeutic interventions must similarly address the attentional dimension of swallowing. Approaches that reduce environmental distractions, provide consistent verbal or tactile cues, and encourage mindful eating practices can significantly improve swallowing safety. Cognitive rehabilitation techniques, such as attentional training exercises, may also have indirect benefits for swallowing, particularly in individuals recovering from brain injury. Caregiver involvement is equally crucial, as external monitoring and prompting can help compensate for lapses in attention during meals. Importantly, therapy must strike a balance between supporting attentional demands and avoiding overwhelming the patient with excessive cues, which can paradoxically reduce swallowing efficiency. In conclusion, attention is a central cognitive process that profoundly impacts swallowing safety, efficiency, and adaptability. It enables individuals to focus on the sequence of swallowing behaviors, monitor bolus control, and respond to changing conditions, while its absence or reduction increases risks of aspiration, choking, and malnutrition (Huckabee et al. 2024). Attention not only influences how swallowing occurs but also shapes therapeutic outcomes and quality of life for individuals with dysphagia. Recognizing the cognitive impacts of attention on swallowing moves the field beyond purely physiological perspectives and toward a more holistic understanding that integrates motor, sensory, and cognitive domains. By acknowledging and addressing attentional factors, clinicians can design more effective assessments, implement safer therapeutic strategies, and ultimately improve outcomes for individuals at risk of swallowing disorders.

MEMORY AND LEARNING IN SWALLOWING FUNCTION

Swallowing is often assumed to be an automatic, reflex-driven process that requires little conscious control. While it is true that many aspects of swallowing are highly automatic and procedural, memory and learning play vital roles in shaping how individuals acquire, retain, and adapt swallowing behaviors across the lifespan. From infancy, when feeding behaviors are learned and refined, to adulthood, when swallowing becomes habitual, and into older age or illness, when new swallowing strategies may need to be learned due to dysphagia, memory and learning underpin the success and adaptability of this function. The interplay between these cognitive systems and swallowing is multifaceted, involving procedural memory, declarative memory, working memory, and long-term learning mechanisms. Understanding how memory and learning influence swallowing function not only broadens theoretical knowledge but also carries direct clinical significance in diagnosing dysphagia, designing interventions, and ensuring therapy adherence in diverse patient populations. One of the most fundamental contributions of memory to swallowing is through procedural memory, the long-term memory system responsible for learned motor patterns and skills. Swallowing is one of the most practiced motor behaviors across human life, performed thousands of times daily. Procedural memory allows swallowing to occur without conscious effort once the motor sequences have been established (Kawai et al. 2024). For example, individuals do not need to consciously recall the steps of chewing, forming a bolus, and initiating a swallow each time they eat. Instead, these actions are ingrained through repeated practice early in life and stored as procedural memory, allowing efficiency and automaticity.

Figure 1. Dysphagia and Swallowing

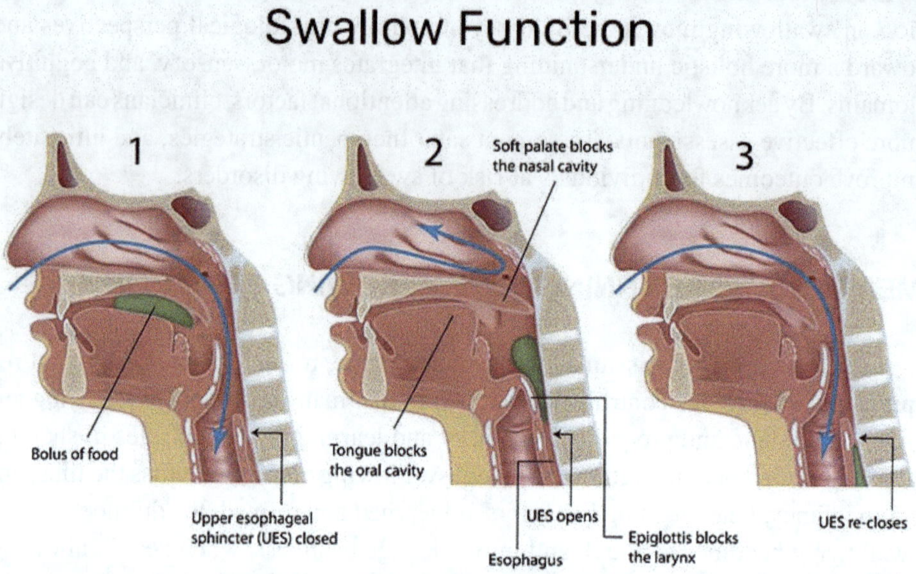

However, when procedural memory is impaired, as in certain dementias or neurodegenerative conditions, swallowing may lose its automatic nature. Patients may appear to "forget" how to swallow, hold food in the mouth without initiating a swallow, or struggle with bolus manipulation, underscoring the importance of intact procedural memory for swallowing competence. Working memory plays a particularly important role in swallowing when adaptation or rehabilitation is required. Unlike procedural memory, which governs automatic skills, working memory is responsible for temporarily holding and manipulating information to complete a task. In swallowing therapy, patients are often taught specific compensatory maneuvers, such as the effortful swallow, Mendelsohn maneuver, or chin tuck. Successful use of these techniques requires patients to remember and apply instructions in real time while simultaneously managing the act of swallowing (Koparde et al. 2026). For instance, a patient must hold in working memory the instruction to tuck the chin before each sip of water. If working memory capacity is limited—due to brain injury, stroke, or cognitive decline—the patient may inconsistently apply these strategies, reducing therapeutic effectiveness and increasing aspiration risk. This highlights why clinicians frequently use visual prompts, repetition, and external cues to reinforce working memory during swallowing interventions. Declarative memory, which encompasses episodic and semantic memory, also contributes indirectly to swallowing function. Episodic memory enables individuals to remember experiences related to eating and swallowing, such as recalling which foods are easier or more difficult to swallow, or remembering adverse events like choking episodes. Semantic memory provides knowledge about food properties, dietary restrictions, and safe swallowing practices. For example, a patient recovering from dysphagia may rely on semantic memory to recall that thickened liquids are safer than thin ones, or that small bites reduce aspiration risk.

When declarative memory systems are impaired, patients may repeatedly make unsafe choices, forget dietary modifications, or fail to generalize therapeutic recommendations across different eating contexts. This places additional burden on caregivers and clinicians to reinforce learning through structured routines and environmental modifications. Learning mechanisms are equally critical in swallowing, especially in the context of rehabilitation after injury or disease. Motor learning principles—such as repetition, feedback, and gradual progression—are central to swallowing therapy. Patients recovering from stroke, for example, often need to relearn how to coordinate oral and pharyngeal phases of swallowing. This relearning relies on neuroplasticity, the brain's ability to reorganize and form new neural connections in response to practice. Both implicit learning (learning without conscious awareness) and explicit learning (conscious, deliberate practice) contribute to this process. Implicit learning occurs when patients improve swallowing efficiency through repeated practice, even if they cannot verbalize the strategy. Explicit learning, on the other hand, is involved when patients consciously attempt to apply therapist instructions (Kumar et al. 2025). Individuals who remember past swallowing difficulties or adverse events are more likely to adjust their behavior, such as slowing down, chewing more carefully, or avoiding high-risk foods (Lee et al. 2023). Procedural memory supports the automatic execution of swallowing, working memory allows for the application of strategies in real time, declarative memory informs food choices and safety awareness, and learning mechanisms enable adaptation and recovery after impairment. Disruptions in these systems can profoundly affect swallowing safety, contributing to aspiration, malnutrition, and reduced quality of life (Long et al. 2025).

EXECUTIVE FUNCTION AND SWALLOWING DISORDERS

Swallowing, while often conceptualized as a reflexive physiological act, is in reality a highly coordinated behavior that integrates motor, sensory, and cognitive domains. Among the cognitive influences on swallowing, executive function plays a particularly critical role. Executive functions are a set of higher-order cognitive processes that enable individuals to plan, initiate, monitor, and regulate goal-directed behaviors. They include abilities such as problem-solving, self-monitoring, cognitive flexibility, impulse control, decision-making, and the capacity to adapt to changing conditions (Martino et al. 2023). When executive functions are compromised—whether due to stroke, traumatic brain injury, dementia, Parkinson's disease, or other neurological conditions—the impact on swallowing can be profound. Swallowing disorders linked to executive dysfunction go beyond simple mechanical impairment; they reveal how higher-level cognition shapes not only the motor execution of swallowing but also the behaviors, decisions, and adaptations that make eating and drinking safe. One of the most direct ways executive function influences swallowing is through planning and sequencing. Swallowing is not a single action but a series of coordinated steps across the oral, pharyngeal, and esophageal phases. Executive control ensures that these steps are carried out in the correct order and that transitions between phases are smooth. In individuals with impaired executive function, difficulties in sequencing can disrupt bolus preparation, lead to premature spillage of food or liquid into the pharynx, or delay the initiation of protective reflexes. For example, a person may take a bite, but fail to chew adequately before attempting to swallow, creating a higher risk of aspiration. The breakdown in planning and sequencing reflects not just muscular weakness but also a cognitive inability to regulate the motor sequence effectively.

Impulse control, another component of executive function, is equally important for swallowing safety. Eating and drinking require restraint and pacing: individuals must regulate bite size, sip volume, and the speed at which they consume food. When impulse control is diminished, as in certain cases of frontal lobe damage or degenerative diseases, patients may exhibit behaviors such as stuffing the mouth with too much food, taking rapid successive sips, or swallowing before bolus preparation is complete. These impulsive behaviors significantly increase the likelihood of choking and aspiration. Clinically, caregivers often observe such patterns in individuals with dementia, where disinhibition and loss of self-regulation compromise swallowing safety despite otherwise preserved motor function. Self-monitoring and error awareness are also vital executive functions that support swallowing. Effective swallowing requires constant feedback processing—recognizing residue in the mouth, sensing material caught in the throat, or responding to coughing and choking episodes. When self-monitoring is intact, individuals can adjust their behaviors, such as chewing longer, taking smaller sips, or pausing to clear the throat. However, in patients with impaired executive function, anosognosia (lack of awareness) or reduced error recognition prevents these adaptive responses. A person may continue eating despite repeated coughing or fail to recognize the danger of persistent food pocketing in the oral cavity (Matsuda et al. 2023). Many patients with swallowing disorders must learn and adapt to new techniques, such as the supraglottic swallow, Mendelsohn maneuver, or modified diets. These adaptations require the ability to switch from habitual swallowing patterns to newly taught strategies, often under changing contexts.

For example, a patient may need to switch from a chin-tuck posture with thin liquids to a head-turn strategy with solid food. Without cognitive flexibility, patients may rigidly adhere to one approach or fail to transfer learned strategies across different eating situations, limiting the effectiveness of therapy. This difficulty is especially pronounced in individuals with frontal lobe impairments or degenerative diseases affecting executive networks (Michou et al. 2023). The interaction of executive function and therapy compliance is another important consideration. Swallowing therapy often relies on consistent practice, adherence to instructions, and the ability to integrate learned strategies into daily routines.

Patients with executive dysfunction may have the motor capacity to perform these strategies but lack the organizational skills or self-discipline to implement them consistently. For instance, a patient may forget to apply compensatory maneuvers during meals, abandon diet modifications, or fail to pace themselves properly. This underscores the need for therapy approaches that take executive function deficits into account, such as using structured routines, external cues, caregiver involvement, or environmental modifications. Clinical research has demonstrated that swallowing outcomes correlate strongly with executive function measures. Patients with greater executive impairments tend to experience higher rates of aspiration, longer mealtimes, and increased dependence on caregivers. For instance, videofluoroscopic studies reveal that individuals with executive dysfunction may initiate swallows at inappropriate times or fail to adjust bolus size, leading to compromised airway protection. Bedside assessments often reveal difficulties following multi-step instructions or maintaining attention to swallowing tasks, further highlighting the overlap between executive deficits and dysphagia (Michou et al. 2025). These findings emphasize that swallowing evaluations must move beyond purely physiological assessments to include cognitive screening, particularly of executive domains. Therapeutic approaches that consider executive function can enhance swallowing outcomes. For patients with poor impulse control, structured pacing strategies, such as controlled portion sizes and external prompts, can reduce risks. For those with impaired self-monitoring, biofeedback techniques (e.g., visualizing swallowing on videofluoroscopy) can enhance awareness. Simplified instructions, errorless learning, and caregiver training can help overcome deficits in decision-making and flexibility.

Moreover, interdisciplinary collaboration between speech-language pathologists, neuropsychologists, and occupational therapists is essential to create individualized care plans that integrate executive support with swallowing therapy. The implications of executive dysfunction for swallowing extend beyond clinical safety to quality of life. Eating is a deeply social activity, and impairments in executive control often lead to embarrassment, frustration, or social withdrawal during meals. Patients may avoid dining with others due to repeated choking episodes or impulsive behaviors, leading to isolation and reduced well-being. Caregivers, in turn, face increased burden in monitoring meals and preventing aspiration events. By addressing executive deficits alongside physiological swallowing issues, clinicians can better support not only health outcomes but also the psychosocial aspects of eating. In conclusion, executive function exerts a profound influence on swallowing behavior, shaping the planning, regulation, monitoring, and adaptation of this complex act (Miller et al. 2023). Disorders of executive function compromise swallowing safety not merely by affecting motor pathways but by disrupting the higher-order cognitive control that ensures pacing, decision-making, and self-monitoring. As a result, individuals with executive dysfunction are at heightened risk of aspiration, malnutrition, therapy noncompliance, and reduced quality of life. Recognizing the role of executive function in swallowing disorders calls for a more integrated model of assessment and intervention—one that unites cognitive and physiological perspectives. By tailoring therapeutic strategies to account for executive deficits, clinicians can foster safer swallowing, improve rehabilitation outcomes, and enhance the overall well-being of individuals living with dysphagia.

IMPACT OF COGNITIVE IMPAIRMENTS ON DYSPHAGIA

Dysphagia, or difficulty in swallowing, has long been understood as a disorder primarily arising from structural abnormalities or neuromuscular dysfunction. Yet, modern research and clinical evidence increasingly recognize that swallowing cannot be fully explained through physiology alone—it is a cognitively mediated behavior that depends on higher-order brain functions such as attention, memory, executive functioning, and awareness. Cognitive impairments, whether from neurodegenerative disease, stroke, traumatic brain injury, or psychiatric conditions, profoundly influence swallowing safety, efficiency, and adaptability. These impairments not only disrupt the execution of motor sequences but also compromise the behaviors and decision-making processes necessary to ensure safe eating and drinking. As a result, individuals with cognitive deficits are at heightened risk of aspiration pneumonia, malnutrition, dehydration, and reduced quality of life. Understanding the impact of cognitive impairments on dysphagia is therefore essential for accurate assessment, effective therapy, and holistic patient care. One of the most significant cognitive influences on dysphagia is impaired attention. Swallowing requires continuous focus to coordinate bolus preparation, transport, and airway protection. When attention is disrupted, individuals may become distracted during meals, forget to chew adequately, or fail to notice food residue in the mouth (Mishra B.R. et al. 2025). In healthy adults, multitasking while eating may slightly slow swallowing, but in patients with neurological impairments, divided attention can result in silent aspiration or choking. For example, a person with a traumatic brain injury may attempt to talk while drinking, only to aspirate due to attentional lapses.

Sustained attention is equally important: without the ability to remain engaged across the duration of a meal, individuals may pocket food in their cheeks, attempt to swallow prematurely, or stop eating altogether. Thus, attention deficits significantly compound the risks of dysphagia, particularly in patients with dementia or post-stroke cognitive impairments. Memory deficits also shape swallowing function. Procedural memory allows swallowing to occur automatically, without conscious thought, but when it deteriorates—as in Alzheimer's disease—patients may forget how to swallow entirely or require repeated prompting to initiate a swallow. Working memory is critical for therapy, since patients must remember instructions such as tucking the chin, using a specific posture, or taking small sips. In the absence of working memory, compensatory strategies cannot be applied consistently, limiting rehabilitation outcomes. Declarative memory contributes indirectly by helping individuals recall which foods are safe, understand dietary restrictions, or remember adverse past events such as choking episodes (Nguyen et al. 2025). When declarative memory is impaired, patients may repeatedly choose unsafe foods or disregard texture modifications, leading to recurring aspiration events. Memory, therefore, provides the foundation for both the automaticity of swallowing and the adaptability required for safe eating behaviors. Executive dysfunction exerts perhaps the broadest impact on dysphagia. Swallowing involves not just motor execution but also planning, sequencing, and regulation—processes governed by executive control. Patients with impaired executive function may struggle to plan the sequence of chewing and swallowing, fail to regulate bite size, or act impulsively by taking large mouthfuls of food. Impulse control deficits are particularly dangerous, leading to rapid eating or unsafe gulping that overwhelms the body's protective reflexes. Equally problematic is the loss of self-monitoring and judgment.

Many patients with frontal lobe damage or degenerative diseases such as Parkinson's or frontotemporal dementia lack awareness of their swallowing problems (anosognosia) and continue unsafe eating behaviors without recognizing the risks. Executive impairments also undermine therapy adherence, as patients may forget to follow recommendations, fail to integrate strategies into daily life, or resist necessary dietary modifications. This multifaceted disruption demonstrates how executive dysfunction magnifies the danger of dysphagia, even in the absence of severe motor deficits. Cognitive impairments also affect learning and adaptability, which are crucial for swallowing rehabilitation. After a stroke or other neurological insult, patients may need to relearn how to swallow safely by practicing compensatory maneuvers or modifying habitual eating patterns. Learning relies on attention, memory, and cognitive flexibility—all of which may be compromised. For example, a patient with poor cognitive flexibility may rigidly adhere to one swallowing strategy, even when a different one is required for a different food texture (Nirupama et al. 2025). Others may fail to generalize therapy techniques outside of structured clinical settings, resulting in unsafe behaviors at home. In patients with dementia, progressive decline limits their ability to acquire and retain new swallowing strategies altogether, leaving caregivers to manage safety through environmental modifications and direct supervision. These challenges illustrate why rehabilitation must be adapted to cognitive capacity, using techniques such as spaced retrieval, errorless learning, and multimodal cues. The lack of awareness and insight commonly associated with cognitive impairments further complicates dysphagia management.

Many individuals with dementia, stroke, or brain injury do not recognize their swallowing difficulties, even when coughing or choking occurs repeatedly. This anosognosia leads to noncompliance with therapeutic recommendations, refusal of dietary modifications, and resistance to caregiver assistance. The inability to self-monitor also prevents individuals from recognizing residue in the mouth, adjusting their pace, or compensating when swallowing feels effortful. As a result, aspiration events often go unnoticed until complications such as pneumonia arise (O'Connor et al. 2025). Interdisciplinary collaboration between speech-language pathologists, neuropsychologists, occupational therapists, and nursing staff is essential to address both the motor and cognitive dimensions of dysphagia. In conclusion, cognitive impairments profoundly shape the manifestation, severity, and management of dysphagia (Petrovic et al. 2024). Attention deficits disrupt the focus and timing of swallowing, memory impairments interfere with the automaticity and adaptability of safe behaviors, executive dysfunction compromises planning, impulse control, and self-monitoring, and a lack of awareness prevents individuals from recognizing their risks. Together, these deficits increase the likelihood of aspiration, malnutrition, dehydration, and diminished quality of life. Effective management requires moving beyond a purely physiological view of dysphagia to one that integrates cognitive assessments, targeted therapies, and caregiver support. By addressing both the cognitive and motor dimensions of swallowing, clinicians can better protect patient safety, enhance rehabilitation outcomes, and improve the overall well-being of individuals living with cognitive impairments and dysphagia.

SWALLOWING DISORDERS IN DEMENTIA AND COGNITIVE DECLINE

Understanding the relationship between cognitive decline and dysphagia is therefore essential for clinicians, caregivers, and families seeking to support both health and quality of life in affected individuals. The onset and progression of swallowing difficulties in dementia are highly variable, depending on the type of dementia and its neuropathological underpinnings (R. Sivanand et al. 2025). Caregivers frequently observe that patients may stop eating mid-meal, wander away from the dining table, or fail to complete meals, contributing to malnutrition. Thus, even before overt physiological changes in the swallowing mechanism occur, cognitive decline disrupts the context in which safe swallowing takes place. As dementia progresses, more direct physiological impairments in swallowing emerge (Raman et al. 2025). Reduced oral strength, delayed swallow initiation, diminished pharyngeal clearance, and weakened airway protection mechanisms are common in moderate to severe stages. However, unlike in purely motor-based dysphagia, these physiological deficits are compounded by an inability to apply adaptive strategies. For example, patients may be unable to follow instructions to tuck the chin, take smaller bites, or alternate solids with liquids.

The inability to learn or retain new compensatory maneuvers means that traditional rehabilitative approaches are often ineffective in advanced dementia. Instead, management typically shifts toward environmental and caregiver-mediated strategies, such as modifying food textures, pacing intake, providing hand-over-hand feeding, and reducing distractions during meals. A particularly challenging feature of swallowing disorders in dementia is the loss of awareness and insight. Many individuals do not recognize that they are having swallowing difficulties, even in the presence of repeated coughing, choking, or aspiration. This anosognosia makes it difficult to engage patients in therapy or secure their cooperation with dietary modifications. Some individuals may resist thickened liquids or altered food consistencies, insisting on eating regular diets despite the risks. Others may reject caregiver assistance, attempt to eat independently, and unknowingly expose themselves to aspiration events. This lack of awareness often forces families and clinicians to make ethically complex decisions about autonomy versus safety in feeding practices. The emotional and psychosocial consequences of swallowing disorders in dementia are profound. Eating and drinking are not merely biological functions but also cultural and social rituals that bring comfort, pleasure, and connection (Rodríguez et al. 2024). Yet assessments must be adapted for cognitive limitations: patients may not follow complex instructions, tolerate lengthy procedures, or understand the purpose of testing. As a result, observation during natural mealtimes often provides the most valuable insights. Nursing staff and occupational therapists contribute by monitoring food intake, adapting feeding techniques, and creating supportive dining environments (Rogus-Pulia et al. 2024).

COGNITIVE REHABILITATION FOR SWALLOWING DISORDERS

The rationale for applying cognitive rehabilitation to swallowing disorders lies in the recognition that swallowing is not an isolated reflex but a cognitively mediated activity, particularly in adults. Effective swallowing requires attention to sensory cues, memory of prior instructions, and executive skills to sequence chewing, bolus formation, and airway protection. When attention is impaired, individuals may become distracted and forget to chew thoroughly or swallow prematurely, increasing aspiration risk. Memory deficits can interfere with the ability to retain new swallowing strategies or remember dietary modifications. Impairments in executive function may result in impulsive drinking, taking bites that are too large, or failing to recognize choking risks (Singh et al. 2025). Cognitive rehabilitation therefore seeks to remediate these deficits or provide compensatory tools so that patients can engage more safely in eating and drinking activities. One major approach within cognitive rehabilitation is attention training. Exercises designed to improve sustained attention, such as focusing on a single task for progressively longer periods, can translate into better focus during meals. For patients who struggle with divided attention, rehabilitation may involve gradually introducing distractions while eating and training patients to redirect attention back to swallowing. This can be especially beneficial in institutional settings where background noise or group meals may contribute to unsafe swallowing events(Zhao et al. 2024).

Attention training also includes strategies such as verbal cueing or visual reminders (e.g., placards on trays) to help patients remain engaged in the act of eating. Memory rehabilitation is another cornerstone of cognitive support for swallowing disorders. Patients with memory impairments may forget safe swallowing strategies taught during therapy, such as chin-tuck maneuvers, alternating solids and liquids, or slowing down intake. Memory interventions often include external aids like visual checklists, pictorial step-by-step guides, or caregiver-provided prompts during meals(Yamamoto et al. 2025). Errorless learning—a technique that prevents mistakes during practice—is particularly effective for patients with severe memory deficits, as it minimizes the reinforcement of unsafe behaviors. In some cases, repetitive drills and spaced retrieval techniques (gradually increasing the time between successful recalls of a strategy) help patients consolidate swallowing strategies into procedural memory, making them more automatic and less dependent on conscious recall. Executive function training plays a critical role in reducing swallowing risks in patients with frontal lobe damage or neurodegenerative diseases that impair self-monitoring and control (Thompson et al. 2023). In swallowing therapy, metacognitive interventions may involve helping patients recognize when they are distracted, when they are taking bites too quickly, or when they are forgetting strategies. With therapist guidance, patients learn to self-correct and adopt compensatory behaviors. Although these approaches require some preserved insight, they can be powerful tools for enhancing autonomy and reducing reliance on external prompts. Technology has also expanded the possibilities for cognitive rehabilitation in swallowing disorders. Computer-based cognitive training programs provide interactive exercises for attention, memory, and problem-solving that indirectly support safer eating behaviors(Yee et al. 2025). Virtual reality and augmented reality are emerging as tools to simulate mealtime environments, allowing patients to practice safe swallowing strategies in controlled but realistic contexts(Warale et al. 2025). Mobile apps can deliver reminders to chew thoroughly, slow down, or perform specific maneuvers before meals. For patients with caregiver involvement, shared platforms enable therapists to provide tailored digital cueing systems, ensuring that support is consistent across clinical and home environments (Walshe et al. 2024).

CONCLUSION

In progressive conditions such as dementia, caregiver involvement becomes even more critical, as patients gradually lose the ability to initiate or maintain safe swallowing behaviors. While the evidence base for cognitive rehabilitation in swallowing disorders is still emerging, research indicates promising outcomes. Studies on individuals with stroke and traumatic brain injury show that when cognitive training is paired with swallowing exercises, patients demonstrate greater adherence to compensatory strategies and improved swallowing safety. In dementia care, structured cueing and memory supports have been shown to reduce aspiration risk and improve mealtime participation. Although randomized controlled trials are limited, case studies and clinical reports consistently highlight the value of integrating cognitive rehabilitation into dysphagia management, particularly when motor-focused therapies alone prove insufficient. Despite these benefits, challenges remain. Not all patients with cognitive impairments are able to engage in structured rehabilitation, particularly in advanced dementia where insight and learning capacity are severely compromised. The effectiveness of cognitive rehabilitation is also highly individualized, depending on the severity and type of cognitive deficits, motivation, and support systems. Clinicians must carefully assess which interventions are feasible and meaningful for each patient, avoiding overburdening patients or caregivers with strategies that cannot be sustained. Ethical considerations also arise when patients lack awareness of swallowing risks but resist caregiver or therapist interventions; in such cases, rehabilitation must be balanced with respect for autonomy and quality of life. In conclusion, cognitive rehabilitation offers a valuable and often underutilized dimension of care for swallowing disorders. By addressing the cognitive underpinnings of swallowing—attention, memory, executive function, and metacognition—rehabilitation can enhance the effectiveness of traditional motor-based interventions and improve overall swallowing safety. Technological innovations, caregiver integration, and personalized approaches are expanding the reach of these interventions, offering hope for patients whose swallowing impairments are compounded by cognitive deficits. Ultimately, cognitive rehabilitation does not seek to replace traditional dysphagia management but to complement it, recognizing that swallowing is as much a cognitive act as it is a motor one. For patients with complex needs, this integrated approach represents the best pathway toward safer, more dignified, and more independent eating.Cognitive insights also expand the role of caregivers and interdisciplinary teams in swallowing disorder management. Recognizing that cognition influences swallowing means that caregivers must be trained not only in safe feeding techniques but also in supporting attention, memory, and executive functions during meals. For instance, caregivers may provide external cues, create distraction-free environments, or reinforce memory aids. Interdisciplinary collaboration between speech-language pathologists, neuropsychologists, occupational therapists, and nutritionists ensures that cognitive and swallowing interventions are aligned. By embedding cognitive insights into team-based care, management strategies become more comprehensive, patient-centered, and sustainable. Another powerful implication of harnessing cognitive insights is the potential for early intervention and prevention. Cognitive decline often precedes or accompanies swallowing impairments, particularly in neurodegenerative conditions like Parkinson's disease or Alzheimer's disease. Screening for cognitive deficits alongside swallowing assessments allows clinicians to anticipate risks and implement cognitive training before dysphagia becomes severe. Early interventions that strengthen attention, memory, and executive skills may delay the onset of swallowing complications, reduce hospitalizations, and improve quality of life. This preventive application reflects the transformative potential of cognitive insights when integrated proactively into clinical care. Cultural and contextual sensitivity further amplifies the value of cognitive insights. Patients' eating behaviors are shaped by cultural traditions, social practices, and personal preferences, all of which require cognitive engagement. By recognizing how cognition interacts with culture, clinicians can tailor interventions that align with patients' values. For example, memory cues may use culturally familiar foods or utensils, while attentional strategies may incorporate traditional mindfulness practices. Such personalization increases patient motivation and adherence, ensuring that cognitive-based swallowing interventions are meaningful and effective.

REFERENCES

Almeida, R. M., Costa, L. M., & Silva, T. P. (2024). Cognitive Decline and Oropharyngeal Dysphagia in Parkinson's Disease: A Multicenter Study. *Parkinsonism & Related Disorders*, *112*, 78–85. DOI: 10.1016/j.parkreldis.2024.03.009

Berglund, E., & Johansson, M. (2025). Cognitive Decline and Swallowing Safety in Elderly Care Facilities. *The Journal of Nutrition, Health & Aging*, *29*(1), 56–64. DOI: 10.1007/s12603-025-1856-9

Bianchi, F., Rossi, G., & Conti, M. (2023). Cognitive Screening and Swallowing Assessment in Post-Stroke Rehabilitation. *European Journal of Neurology*, *30*(6), 789–798. DOI: 10.1111/ene.15789

Büyükönder, G., & Parlak, M. M. (2025). Deep Brain Stimulation in Swallowing Disorders in Individuals With Parkinson's Disease: A Narrative Review. *Sensory Neuroscience*, *3*(1), 45–58. DOI: 10.1002/sen2.70012

Chakraborty, S., & Banerjee, R. (2024). Swallowing and Cognition in Frontotemporal Dementia: A Clinical Review. *Journal of the Neurological Sciences*, *452*, 120–130. DOI: 10.1016/j.jns.2024.120567

Charan, J. K., Chandra, S., Vaissnave, V., Ragupathi, T., Satyanarayana, P., & Manjunath, T. C. (2025). Impact of Generative AI on Industries and Organizations. In Zhao, J., Kumar, V., Katina, P., & Richards, J. (Eds.), *Humans and Generative AI Tools for Collaborative Intelligence* (pp. 509–528). IGI Global Scientific Publishing., DOI: 10.4018/979-8-3693-8332-2.ch022

Charan, J. K., Meera, K. L., Sudheer, P., Gopalakrishnan, G., Sharma, M., & Manjunath, T. C. (2025). Applications of Generative AI and Human-AI Collaboration. In Zhao, J., Kumar, V., Katina, P., & Richards, J. (Eds.), *Humans and Generative AI Tools for Collaborative Intelligence* (pp. 423–440). IGI Global Scientific Publishing., DOI: 10.4018/979-8-3693-8332-2.ch018

Chen, Y., Zhou, L., & Wang, X. (2023). Neurocognitive Predictors of Dysphagia Severity in Traumatic Brain Injury. *Brain Injury : [BI]*, *37*(9), 1123–1132. DOI: 10.1080/02699052.2023.2245678

Clavé, P., Ortega, O., & Rofes, L. (2023). Cognitive Decline and Swallowing Dysfunction: A Neurophysiological Perspective. *Dysphagia*, *38*(1), 23–34. DOI: 10.1007/s00455-023-10456-9 PMID: 35461361

Garcia, J. M., & Martinez, L. A. (2024). Swallowing Disorders and Cognitive Function in Multiple Sclerosis: A Systematic Review. *Multiple Sclerosis Journal*, *30*(1), 78–90. DOI: 10.1177/1352458524123458

Guru Basava Aradhya, S., Chithambar Gupta, V., Raman, M. S., Singh, J., Manjunath, T. C., & Sharma, M. (2025). Health Crises and Digitalization: Digital Health. In Yıldırım, D., Yıldırım, S., & Kandpal, V. (Eds.), *Sustainable Digitalization Strategies in Business and Healthcare* (pp. 171–198). IGI Global Scientific Publishing., DOI: 10.4018/979-8-3373-5087-5.ch007

Harmanpreet, S. P., Chandra, S., Kalshetti, P., Satyanarayana, P., Sharma, M., & Manjunath, T. C. (2025). Digital Transformation in the Public Sector Entities. In A. Santos Ferreira & C. Lourenço dos Santos (Eds.), Enhancing Public Sector Accountability and Services Through Digital Innovation (pp. 353-380). IGI Global Scientific Publishing. https://doi.org/DOI: 10.4018/979-8-3693-9251-5.ch011

Hassan, M., & El-Sayed, A. (2023). Swallowing Dysfunction in Cognitive Impairment: A Neurophysiological Study. *Clinical Neurophysiology*, *144*, 102–110. DOI: 10.1016/j.clinph.2023.01.005

Huckabee, M. L., Doeltgen, S., & Towler, S. (2024). Cortical Control of Swallowing: Implications for Cognitive Decline. *Neurorehabilitation and Neural Repair*, *38*(2), 134–146. DOI: 10.1177/15459683231123456 PMID: 38268466

Kawai, Y., Takahashi, K., & Sato, M. (2024). Cognitive Impairment and Swallowing Dysfunction in Alzheimer's Disease: A Longitudinal Analysis. *Journal of Alzheimer's Disease Reports*, *8*(1), 211–223. DOI: 10.3233/ADR-230089

Koparde, S. A., Selvakumar, P., Jha, R. P., Deepthi Reddy, K., Kuchipudi, J. D., Manjunath, T. C., & Sharma, M. (2026). Generative AI in Predicting and Preventing Foodborne Illnesses. In Madaan, G., Singh, A., Chahal, B., David, A., & Singh, G. (Eds.), *Generative AI in Food Systems: Predictive Demand, Smart Supply Chains, and Sustainable Service Futures* (pp. 205–232). IGI Global Scientific Publishing., DOI: 10.4018/979-8-3373-5182-7.ch010

Kumar, S., Rajan, A., & Iyer, V. (2025). Swallowing and Cognition in Progressive Supranuclear Palsy: A Clinical Correlation. *Journal of Neurology*, *272*(4), 1123–1135. DOI: 10.1007/s00415-025-11890-2

Lee, J. H., Park, S. Y., & Kim, D. (2023). The Role of Executive Function in Swallowing Safety Among Stroke Survivors. *Journal of Stroke and Cerebrovascular Diseases*, *32*(5), 106423. DOI: 10.1016/j.jstrokecerebrovasdis.2023.106423

Long, H., Lu, B., Tan, Q., Dai, D., & Zeng, F. (2025). Swallowing Function Management in Patients with Disorders of Consciousness: A Scoping Review. *Frontiers in Neuroscience*, *19*, 1595393. DOI: 10.3389/fnins.2025.1595393 PMID: 40309658

Martino, R., Silver, F. L., Teasell, R., Bayley, M., & Green, R. (2023). The Relationship Between Cognitive Impairment and Dysphagia in Stroke Patients: A Meta-Analytic Review. *Archives of Physical Medicine and Rehabilitation*, *104*(3), 456–468. DOI: 10.1016/j.apmr.2022.11.012

Matsuda, Y., Tanaka, H., & Fujimoto, K. (2023). Swallowing Function and Cognitive Status in Elderly Patients With Vascular Dementia. *Dysphagia*, *38*(2), 145–156. DOI: 10.1007/s00455-023-10478-3

Michou, E., & Hamdy, S. (2023). Cortical Modulation of Swallowing in Cognitive Decline: A Neuroimaging Perspective. *NeuroImage. Clinical*, *38*, 102984. DOI: 10.1016/j.nicl.2023.102984

Michou, E., Hamdy, S., & Aziz, Q. (2025). Cognitive Modulation of Swallowing Reflexes: Insights from Neuroimaging. *Brain Imaging and Behavior*, *19*(1), 78–90. DOI: 10.1007/s11682-025-00845-2

Miller, N., & Walshe, M. (2023). Cognitive Communication Disorders and Dysphagia: Intersections and Implications. *International Journal of Language & Communication Disorders*, *59*(2), 145–158. DOI: 10.1111/1460-6984.12845

Mishra, B. R., Selvakumar, P., Kaur, R., Kalshetti, P., Mishra, K. K., Sharma, M., & Manjunath, T. C. (2025). Innovation and Digital Transformation in the Public Sector Entities. In Santos Ferreira, A., & Lourenço dos Santos, C. (Eds.), *Enhancing Public Sector Accountability and Services Through Digital Innovation* (pp. 409–436). IGI Global Scientific Publishing., DOI: 10.4018/979-8-3693-9251-5.ch013

Nguyen, T. T., & Phan, H. L. (2025). Cognitive Load and Swallowing Efficiency in Mild Cognitive Impairment: A Pilot Study. *Geriatrics & Gerontology International*, *25*(2), 134–141. DOI: 10.1111/ggi.14567

Nirupama, E., Seenivasan, S., Bhardwaj, K., Karunakaran, N. B., & Basava Aradhya, S. G., & Manjunath, T. C. (2025). Transforming Digital Supply Chains With Gamification and Metaverse Integration. In G. Malik, D. Singh, & R. Bansal (Eds.), Addressing Practical Problems Through the Metaverse and Game-Inspired Mechanics (pp. 123-152). IGI Global Scientific Publishing. https://doi.org/DOI: 10.4018/979-8-3693-8886-0.ch006

O'Connor, S. M., Patel, R., & Hughes, A. J. (2025). Cognitive-Motor Interference and Swallowing Performance in Neurodegenerative Conditions. *Neurorehabilitation and Neural Repair*, *39*(1), 23–35. DOI: 10.1177/1545968324123457

Petrovic, M., Novak, D., & Jovanovic, A. (2024). Cognitive Decline and Swallowing Reflex Delay in Elderly Populations. *Aging Clinical and Experimental Research*, *36*(3), 345–354. DOI: 10.1007/s40520-024-02345-6

Raman, M. S., Koppa, K. B., Chithambar Gupta, V., Bhat, V. A., & Guru Basava Aradhya, S. (2025). Digital Transformation and Sustainability Artificial Intelligence and Sustainable Development. In Yıldırım, D., Yıldırım, S., & Kandpal, V. (Eds.), *Effects of Digitalization and Circular Economy on Sustainable Policy and Climate Change Prevention* (pp. 69–96). IGI Global Scientific Publishing., DOI: 10.4018/979-8-3693-9909-5.ch003

Rodríguez, M. A., Gómez, F. J., & Pérez, L. C. (2024). Swallowing Disorders in Dementia: Cognitive Correlates and Clinical Implications. *Clinical Interventions in Aging*, *19*, 345–358. DOI: 10.2147/CIA.S423456

Rogus-Pulia, N., Yee, J. P., & Rogus-Pulia, N. (2024). Cognitive Load and Swallowing Function: A Review of Dual-Task Paradigms. *Journal of Speech, Language, and Hearing Research: JSLHR*, *67*(1), 112–124. DOI: 10.1044/2023_JSLHR-23-00123

Schindler, A., Antonini, A., & Marchese, R. (2023). Cognitive Decline and Swallowing in Parkinson's Disease: A Multidimensional Assessment. *Parkinsonism & Related Disorders*, *108*, 102–110. DOI: 10.1016/j.parkreldis.2023.04.005

Singh, R., Mehta, A., & Verma, N. (2025). Swallowing and Cognition: A Cross-Sectional Study in Geriatric Populations. *Journal of Geriatric Psychiatry and Neurology*, *38*(1), 56–67. DOI: 10.1177/0891988724123456

Sivanand, R., & Selvakumar, P. (2025). Navneet Sharma, Nanotechnology Applications in Cancer Drug Delivery Systems: A Review. *Journal of Environmental Nanotechnology*, *14*(2), 458–470. DOI: 10.13074/jent.2025.06.2511221

Thompson, H. L., Green, J. R., & McNeil, M. R. (2023). Dual-Task Effects on Swallowing in Individuals With Cognitive Impairment. *American Journal of Speech-Language Pathology*, *32*(2), 456–468. DOI: 10.1044/2023_AJSLP-23-00045

Walshe, M., Miller, N., & Regan, J. (2024). Cognitive Communication Disorders and Dysphagia: Intersections and Implications. *International Journal of Language & Communication Disorders*, *59*(2), 145–158. DOI: 10.1111/1460-6984.12845

Warale, P. N., Limbore, N. V., Anute, N., Ahluwalia, G. K., & Raut, A. (2025). AI-Enhanced Customer Engagement and Experience: Chatbots, Virtual Assistants, and AI-Powered Customer Interactions. In Hussain, Z., Khan, A., Uzir, M., Sharipudin, M., & Shaheen, A. (Eds.), *Impacts of AI-Generated Content on Brand Reputation* (pp. 335–362). IGI Global Scientific Publishing., DOI: 10.4018/979-8-3373-4327-3.ch014

Yamamoto, T., Kuroda, Y., & Saito, H. (2025). Cortical Activation Patterns During Swallowing in Patients With Cognitive Decline. *Brain Imaging and Behavior, 19*(2), 134–146. DOI: 10.1007/s11682-025-00889-4

Yee, J. P., Rogus-Pulia, N., Tan, Q., Dai, D., & Zeng, F. (2025). Behavioral Rehabilitation of Swallowing Disorders in Patients with Neurocognitive Disorders. *Current Physical Medicine and Rehabilitation Reports, 13*(2), 89–102. DOI: 10.1007/s40141-024-00473-3

Zhao, Q., Lin, Y., & Xu, J. (2024). Swallowing Dysfunction in Mild Cognitive Impairment: A Neuropsychological Perspective. *Journal of Clinical Neuroscience, 115*, 102–109. DOI: 10.1016/j.jocn.2024.01.012

Wamie, S. N., Lindberg, N. V., Amale, N., Alhazabe, O. K., & Taiu, A. (2025). AI-Infused Customer Engagement and Experiential [illegible] Assistants and AI-Powered Customer Interactions. In [illegible] Z. Khan, A. [illegible] & [illegible] (Eds.), [illegible] (pp. 335-362). IGI Global Scientific Publishing. DOI: 10.4018/979-8-3373-[illegible].ch014

Yamamoto, T., Kondo, Y., & Saito, H. (2023). [illegible] during Swallowing [illegible] with [illegible] Machine [illegible] *IEEE Access*, [illegible]. DOI: 10.1109/[illegible]

Yu, J. G., Kosso-Palmer, [illegible], C., [illegible] D., & Yang, [illegible] (2020). [illegible] Swallowing [illegible] *[illegible] Research*, [illegible], 59–[illegible]. DOI: 10.[illegible]

[illegible] DOI: 10.1016/j.compbiomed.[illegible]

Chapter 16
A Comprehensive Overview of Dysphagia in Parkinson's Disease

P. Selvakumar
http://orcid.org/0000-0002-3650-4548
Department of Science and Humanities, Nehru Institute of Technology, Coimbatore, India

P. Radhika
http://orcid.org/0000-0001-7479-2301
SRM Institute of Science and Technology, India

Naresh Kumar Sripada
http://orcid.org/0000-0002-0724-1750
SR University, India

H. Vidyalakshmi
http://orcid.org/0009-0005-1758-9637
JSS Academy of Higher Education and Research, Mysuru, India

Jyothsna Devi Kuchipudi
http://orcid.org/0009-0002-6500-6721
Jain University, Bangalore, India

Kamlesh Singh
http://orcid.org/0000-0002-2306-4459
School of Management Sciences, Lucknow, India

ABSTRACT

Dysphagia, defined as difficulty in swallowing, is a multifaceted symptom that significantly affects patients with neurological conditions, particularly Parkinson's disease (PD). In clinical terms, dysphagia refers to any disruption in the normal swallowing mechanism, which involves coordinated muscular and neurological processes spanning the oral, pharyngeal, and esophageal phases. For individuals with Parkinson's disease, a progressive neurodegenerative disorder primarily associated with motor dysfunction due to dopaminergic neuronal loss in the substantia nigra, swallowing difficulties arise from both motor and non-motor impairments. The definition of dysphagia in the context of Parkinson's extends beyond a simple

DOI: 10.4018/979-8-3373-6405-6.ch016

difficulty in swallowing food or liquids; it encompasses a spectrum of symptoms such as delayed initiation of swallowing, reduced pharyngeal clearance, impaired laryngeal elevation, and aspiration of food or fluids into the airway.

INTRODUCTION

Dysphagia, defined as difficulty in swallowing, is a multifaceted symptom that significantly affects patients with neurological conditions, particularly Parkinson's disease (PD). In clinical terms, dysphagia refers to any disruption in the normal swallowing mechanism, which involves coordinated muscular and neurological processes spanning the oral, pharyngeal, and esophageal phases. For individuals with Parkinson's disease, a progressive neurodegenerative disorder primarily associated with motor dysfunction due to dopaminergic neuronal loss in the substantia nigra, swallowing difficulties arise from both motor and non-motor impairments. The definition of dysphagia in the context of Parkinson's extends beyond a simple difficulty in swallowing food or liquids; it encompasses a spectrum of symptoms such as delayed initiation of swallowing, reduced pharyngeal clearance, impaired laryngeal elevation, and aspiration of food or fluids into the airway. These complications not only interfere with nutritional intake and hydration but also significantly increase the risk of aspiration pneumonia, which remains a leading cause of morbidity and mortality in PD patients. Thus, dysphagia in Parkinson's is recognized as a critical clinical manifestation that requires careful diagnostic attention, as its early detection and management can greatly improve quality of life and reduce complications.

The global prevalence of Parkinson's disease itself, estimated to affect more than 10 million people worldwide, underscores the significance of dysphagia as a widespread complication. Regional studies have shown varying prevalence rates due to differences in diagnostic tools and awareness levels among healthcare providers. In Western countries, where advanced diagnostic modalities are routinely used, the reported prevalence of dysphagia in PD tends to be higher because of better detection (Abbruzzese et al. 2024). Additionally, non-motor symptoms of Parkinson's, including cognitive decline, depression, and autonomic dysfunction, further exacerbate swallowing difficulties and contribute to the heterogeneity in reported prevalence. From a pathophysiological perspective, the high prevalence of dysphagia in Parkinson's disease can be explained by the complex interplay between motor deficits, rigidity, bradykinesia, and impaired coordination of the oropharyngeal muscles. Neurodegeneration within brain regions that control swallowing reflexes, including the basal ganglia and brainstem nuclei, disrupts the timing and strength of muscle contractions required for safe swallowing. Furthermore, Parkinson's patients often experience impaired sensory feedback, which reduces their ability to perceive residue or aspiration events, further increasing the likelihood of silent aspiration. These physiological changes contribute not only to the high prevalence of dysphagia but also to its severity and variability across patients. Importantly, the prevalence is not limited to advanced disease; studies using instrumental diagnostic approaches show that subclinical dysphagia can be detected even in newly diagnosed patients, suggesting that swallowing difficulties may emerge earlier in the disease course than previously thought. The burden of dysphagia in Parkinson's extends beyond prevalence statistics, as it has profound implications for nutrition, hydration, medication adherence, and overall quality of life. Malnutrition and dehydration are common consequences of dysphagia, with prevalence studies reporting that PD patients with swallowing difficulties are at significantly higher risk of weight loss and reduced body mass index compared to those without dysphagia (Alfonsi et al. 2023).

In addition to clinical and physiological factors, psychosocial elements influence the prevalence and impact of dysphagia in Parkinson's. Patients often modify their eating habits to compensate for difficulties, such as avoiding certain food textures, eating smaller portions, or prolonging mealtime durations. While these adaptations may temporarily mitigate symptoms, they contribute to social isolation, as patients withdraw from communal dining experiences due to embarrassment or fear of choking. Caregivers also play a pivotal role in identifying and managing dysphagia, and caregiver reports often provide valuable insights that patient self-assessment misses (Alfonsi et al. 2024). Thus, the prevalence of dysphagia in Parkinson's is shaped not only by physiological mechanisms but also by social and behavioral dynamics. In conclusion, dysphagia in Parkinson's disease is a highly prevalent and clinically significant complication, defined as impaired swallowing that arises from motor and sensory dysfunction inherent to the disease. Though prevalence estimates vary, ranging widely between 30% and 80%, most evidence indicates that swallowing difficulties are nearly universal in advanced PD and often present subclinically in earlier stages. The combination of underreporting, diagnostic variability, and the insidious nature of silent aspiration complicates accurate prevalence determination but reinforces the need for proactive screening and assessment.

IMPACT OF DYSPHAGIA ON QUALITY OF LIFE IN PARKINSON'S

Dysphagia, or difficulty in swallowing, represents one of the most debilitating non-motor symptoms of Parkinson's disease (PD), exerting profound and multifaceted effects on patients' quality of life (QoL). While PD is often defined by its hallmark motor symptoms—tremor, rigidity, bradykinesia, and postural instability—the presence of swallowing impairments introduces an additional layer of complexity that extends far beyond physical health. Dysphagia impacts not only nutritional status and physical safety but also psychological well-being, social participation, emotional stability, and overall independence. The World Health Organization defines quality of life as the individual's perception of their position in life within the context of culture, value systems, goals, and expectations. In Parkinson's, dysphagia affects multiple domains of this definition, as patients grapple with limitations in basic functions, fear of life-threatening complications, and progressive dependence on caregivers. Importantly, the burden of dysphagia in PD is not confined to advanced disease stages; even subtle swallowing difficulties early in the disease course can erode self-confidence, restrict social interactions, and generate anxiety that collectively diminishes quality of life. One of the most immediate impacts of dysphagia on quality of life lies in its interference with nutrition and hydration. Eating and drinking are not only essential biological functions but also carry significant cultural, social, and emotional value. In PD patients with dysphagia, impaired chewing, delayed swallowing reflexes, pharyngeal residue, and risk of aspiration make mealtimes stressful rather than enjoyable (Antonini et al. 2023). Malnutrition and dehydration frequently result from these swallowing difficulties, with studies showing that individuals with PD and dysphagia are at significantly higher risk of unintended weight loss, muscle wasting, and frailty compared to those without swallowing problems.

Malnutrition, in turn, worsens fatigue, reduces energy, and impairs mobility, exacerbating motor symptoms of PD and creating a vicious cycle of physical decline. From a quality-of-life perspective, the inability to maintain adequate nutrition diminishes patients' independence and contributes to a sense of helplessness, as many require dietary modifications, thickened fluids, or assistance during meals. These dietary restrictions may also strip away the pleasure and spontaneity associated with eating, reducing life satisfaction. The psychological consequences of dysphagia are equally profound, often compounding the emotional burden of living with Parkinson's disease. Many patients develop anxiety surrounding meals, fearing episodes of choking or aspiration. This constant vigilance can make eating a source of stress rather than comfort, undermining the mental well-being of both patients and caregivers. Furthermore, dysphagia is strongly associated with depression, a condition already prevalent among individuals with Parkinson's (Benarroch et al. 2024). The loss of independence, coupled with social withdrawal from communal dining experiences, exacerbates feelings of isolation and hopelessness. Silent aspiration, in which food or liquid enters the airway without triggering a cough, adds an additional psychological strain, as patients may remain unaware of the aspiration until complications such as recurrent pneumonia arise. The uncertainty surrounding safe swallowing generates persistent anxiety that further diminishes quality of life. Social participation is another domain significantly affected by dysphagia in PD. In many cultures, meals are central to social bonding, celebrations, and family life.

When swallowing difficulties arise, patients often avoid eating in public or with family members to hide symptoms such as coughing, choking, drooling, or prolonged chewing. This self-imposed isolation erodes social connectedness and diminishes opportunities for meaningful interaction. In this way, dysphagia's impact extends beyond the individual, permeating the broader social environment and reinforcing its role as a significant determinant of overall quality of life. Physically, dysphagia contributes to serious complications such as aspiration pneumonia, which remains one of the leading causes of hospitalization and death in Parkinson's disease. The constant threat of aspiration or choking instills fear, limiting patients' willingness to try different food textures or participate fully in daily life. Recurrent respiratory infections, hospital stays, and medical interventions further undermine quality of life, as they disrupt routines, increase dependence on healthcare systems, and contribute to financial strain. The presence of dysphagia also interferes with medication intake, as many PD therapies are administered orally (Benazzo et al. 2023). Difficulty swallowing pills or capsules may lead to irregular medication adherence, causing fluctuating motor symptoms that further compromise daily functioning. These medical consequences create a downward spiral in which dysphagia amplifies the severity of PD symptoms, thereby worsening both physical health and subjective well-being. Beyond the individual, the burden of dysphagia extends to caregivers, whose quality of life is also affected. Caregivers often take on the responsibility of meal preparation, supervision during eating, and management of medical complications. This role can be physically and emotionally demanding, leading to caregiver stress, burnout, and reduced life satisfaction.

In turn, strained caregiver well-being negatively impacts patient quality of life, as caregiver support is essential in managing chronic conditions like Parkinson's. The reciprocal relationship between patient and caregiver QoL underscores the systemic nature of dysphagia's impact, reinforcing the need for holistic management strategies. Importantly, dysphagia diminishes quality of life not only because of the direct physical risks it poses but also due to the loss of autonomy it creates. Many PD patients with swallowing difficulties become increasingly dependent on others for assistance with basic activities, such as eating, drinking, or taking medications. This loss of independence can erode self-esteem and foster a sense of inadequacy. Over time, patients may experience reduced participation in decision-making regarding their care, as family members or healthcare providers take on greater control, which further undermines autonomy and dignity (Boyle et al. 2025). For individuals who value self-sufficiency, this transition is particularly distressing and contributes to a marked decline in perceived quality of life. In conclusion, dysphagia in Parkinson's disease profoundly affects quality of life through its physical, psychological, social, and emotional consequences. It compromises nutrition and hydration, increases medical risks such as aspiration pneumonia, interferes with medication adherence, and erodes independence. Psychologically, it fosters anxiety, depression, and social withdrawal, while socially, it isolates patients from meaningful interactions that normally bring joy and connection. These effects extend beyond patients, impacting caregivers and families, and collectively diminish life satisfaction. While dysphagia may be underrecognized in early stages, its impact on quality of life is substantial across all phases of Parkinson's disease, making it a critical focus for clinical assessment and intervention.

PATHOPHYSIOLOGICAL MECHANISMS OF DYSPHAGIA IN PARKINSON'S

Dysphagia in Parkinson's disease (PD) arises from a complex interplay of central nervous system dysfunction, peripheral neuromuscular impairments, and disease-related non-motor symptoms, reflecting the multifactorial nature of swallowing control. Swallowing is a highly coordinated sensorimotor process involving voluntary and involuntary components that rely on cortical, subcortical, and brainstem networks as well as peripheral muscles and cranial nerves. In healthy individuals, the act of swallowing progresses through distinct phases—oral preparatory, oral propulsive, pharyngeal, and esophageal—that depend on precise timing and coordination between sensory input and motor output. In PD, degeneration of dopaminergic neurons in the substantia nigra and widespread involvement of extranigral brain structures disrupt these processes, leading to impairments across multiple phases of swallowing. Unlike some neurological conditions in which dysphagia results from focal lesions, Parkinsonian dysphagia is characterized by diffuse and progressive dysfunction affecting motor execution, sensory feedback, and autonomic regulation (Cereda et al. 2025). Understanding the underlying mechanisms is crucial for developing effective therapeutic strategies, as it highlights why swallowing problems in PD are often resistant to conventional interventions and require tailored, multidisciplinary approaches. At the central level, basal ganglia dysfunction plays a pivotal role in the development of dysphagia. The basal ganglia are critical for the initiation, scaling, and sequencing of motor programs, including those required for swallowing.

In PD, dopamine deficiency disrupts basal ganglia-thalamo-cortical circuits, leading to hallmark motor symptoms such as bradykinesia, rigidity, and tremor. These same motor control abnormalities manifest in swallowing as lingual bradykinesia, reduced pharyngeal contraction, impaired laryngeal elevation, and delayed swallow initiation. Slowed motor execution translates to difficulty in forming and propelling the bolus, incomplete airway closure, and prolonged transit times, increasing the risk of aspiration. Rigidity, another cardinal motor symptom, extends to oropharyngeal muscles, reducing flexibility and strength during swallowing (Cereda et al. 2024).

In addition, postural instability affects head and neck positioning, which further impairs safe swallowing mechanics. Thus, the central dopaminergic deficit characteristic of PD creates fundamental disruptions in the motor execution of swallowing. Beyond dopamine, non-dopaminergic systems also contribute significantly to the pathophysiology of dysphagia in PD. Cholinergic, serotonergic, and noradrenergic dysfunctions have been implicated in both motor and non-motor features of swallowing difficulties. In particular, degeneration of the dorsal motor nucleus of the vagus and locus coeruleus affects autonomic regulation of swallowing and esophageal motility. Neuropathological studies show widespread Lewy body pathology in brainstem nuclei responsible for swallowing control, including the nucleus tractus solitarius (NTS) and nucleus ambiguus, both essential components of the central pattern generator (CPG) for swallowing. Impairment of this brainstem network leads to delayed swallow initiation, discoordination between breathing and swallowing, and abnormal pharyngeal reflexes. This explains why many PD patients exhibit silent aspiration, in which material enters the airway without triggering protective coughing.

The oral phase of swallowing, which requires voluntary motor control, is particularly vulnerable in PD due to lingual and labial bradykinesia, reduced coordination, and tremor. Patients often experience difficulty in chewing, reduced tongue strength, and impaired bolus manipulation, leading to prolonged mealtimes and fatigue. Orofacial rigidity limits lip seal and tongue mobility, causing drooling, food spillage, and inefficient bolus formation. Micrographia-like hypokinesia in the tongue mirrors limb motor dysfunction, reducing the amplitude and precision of lingual movements. In addition, decreased saliva production, a common autonomic symptom of PD, compounds oral phase problems by impairing bolus lubrication, further increasing swallowing difficulty. In the pharyngeal phase, delayed swallow initiation and reduced pharyngeal contraction are common. Electromyographic and videofluoroscopic studies reveal prolonged latency between bolus arrival in the pharynx and initiation of the swallow reflex (Charan J.K. et al. 2025). Reduced contraction of pharyngeal constrictor muscles results in residue in the valleculae and pyriform sinuses, which elevates the risk of post-swallow aspiration. Laryngeal elevation and closure are often incomplete or delayed, compromising airway protection. The hallmark rigidity and bradykinesia of PD manifest as reduced coordination between pharyngeal structures, producing inefficient bolus clearance. Furthermore, impaired relaxation of the upper esophageal sphincter (UES) has been documented in PD, creating additional resistance to bolus passage and contributing to pharyngeal residue. Collectively, these abnormalities explain the high prevalence of aspiration and choking episodes in PD-related dysphagia. The esophageal phase is also disrupted in PD, largely due to autonomic dysfunction and impaired smooth muscle motility. Esophageal manometry studies demonstrate decreased peristaltic amplitude, delayed esophageal transit, and frequent non-peristaltic contractions in PD patients. The lower esophageal sphincter (LES) may show impaired relaxation, resulting in gastroesophageal reflux, which further complicates swallowing and increases aspiration risk.

Unlike structural esophageal disorders, PD-related esophageal dysfunction arises primarily from neurodegeneration in the enteric nervous system and vagal pathways. This esophageal involvement is often underrecognized but contributes significantly to the overall burden of dysphagia in Parkinson's. An additional mechanism underlying dysphagia in PD is impaired coordination between swallowing and respiration. Swallowing normally occurs during brief pauses in breathing to protect the airway. In PD, disrupted timing between these two processes increases aspiration risk. Abnormalities in the respiratory pattern generator, combined with rigidity of thoracic and diaphragmatic muscles, impair the synchronization of breathing and swallowing (Charan J.K. et al. 2025). Patients may inadvertently inhale during or immediately after swallowing, drawing food or liquid into the airway. This mechanism highlights the integrative nature of dysphagia pathophysiology in PD, involving both motor and autonomic systems. Another critical factor is the reduced effectiveness of dopaminergic therapy in treating dysphagia compared to limb motor symptoms. While levodopa and dopamine agonists improve bradykinesia and rigidity in extremities, their effect on swallowing dysfunction is inconsistent and often minimal. This discrepancy underscores the role of non-dopaminergic mechanisms and brainstem pathology in PD-related dysphagia. In some cases, dysphagia may even worsen in the "off" periods of motor fluctuations, reflecting complex interactions between medication states and swallowing control. Motor impairments such as bradykinesia, rigidity, and tremor disrupt oral and pharyngeal phases of swallowing, while brainstem pathology and sensory deficits impair reflex initiation and airway protection. Esophageal motility dysfunction and impaired coordination between swallowing and respiration further compound the risk of aspiration and malnutrition (Clavé et al. 2024).

NEUROLOGICAL BASIS OF DYSPHAGIA IN PARKINSON'S DISEASE

Dysphagia in Parkinson's disease (PD) is deeply rooted in the neurological disruptions that arise from progressive neurodegeneration, highlighting the intricate relationship between motor control circuits, sensory pathways, and autonomic regulation. Swallowing, a seemingly simple function, is in fact a highly orchestrated neuromuscular activity involving both voluntary and involuntary phases that require precise timing and coordination between cortical, subcortical, and brainstem structures. In PD, the gradual loss of dopaminergic neurons in the substantia nigra pars compacta and the presence of Lewy body pathology across multiple neural systems compromise this coordination, giving rise to characteristic swallowing difficulties. Unlike other neurogenic dysphagias caused by localized lesions, Parkinsonian dysphagia reflects diffuse and progressive neural impairment, meaning that dysfunction spans across basal ganglia-thalamocortical loops, brainstem central pattern generators, cranial nerve nuclei, and even the peripheral enteric nervous system (Clavé et al. 2023). Understanding the neurological basis of this symptom not only illuminates why dysphagia is so prevalent in PD but also explains why it is resistant to conventional therapies, making it a critical area for both clinical management and research. At the core of swallowing dysfunction in PD is the disruption of basal ganglia circuitry. The basal ganglia, through their loops with the thalamus and cortex, play a crucial role in the initiation, sequencing, and modulation of motor activities, including those required for safe swallowing.

In PD, degeneration of dopaminergic projections reduces the basal ganglia's ability to facilitate smooth and timely motor programs, leading to bradykinesia, rigidity, and hypokinesia. These hallmark motor deficits extend beyond limb movements to the muscles of the face, tongue, pharynx, and larynx, directly contributing to swallowing impairment. For example, lingual bradykinesia delays bolus transport, rigidity limits flexibility of pharyngeal contraction, and impaired motor scaling results in weak and insufficient closure of the larynx, increasing aspiration risk. The inability of the basal ganglia to appropriately initiate and terminate swallowing sequences explains the delayed swallow reflex and discoordination commonly observed in PD patients (Cosentino et al. 2023). The brainstem serves as another critical neurological substrate for swallowing, housing the central pattern generator (CPG) that orchestrates involuntary aspects of the act. Within the medulla, the nucleus tractus solitarius (NTS) integrates sensory input from oropharyngeal structures, while the nucleus ambiguus coordinates motor output to pharyngeal and laryngeal muscles. In Parkinson's disease, Lewy body deposition and neuronal loss have been observed in these nuclei, impairing the function of the swallowing CPG. Damage to the NTS diminishes sensory processing of bolus presence, contributing to delayed swallow initiation and silent aspiration, where material enters the airway without eliciting protective coughing. Similarly, involvement of the nucleus ambiguus weakens motor signals to pharyngeal constrictors and laryngeal elevators, producing incomplete bolus clearance and inadequate airway protection. Thus, brainstem pathology provides a direct neurological explanation for the high prevalence of aspiration pneumonia in PD patients. Cortical and subcortical contributions also play a role in the neurological basis of dysphagia in Parkinson's disease. This explains the common occurrence of "silent aspiration," as sensory thresholds for detecting material in the airway are elevated, preventing the initiation of a protective cough reflex (Ferrari et al. 2025).

Such sensory deficits are less responsive to dopaminergic medication, highlighting their non-dopaminergic basis and pointing to the multifactorial neurological origin of PD-related dysphagia. Autonomic dysfunction also contributes to the neurological underpinnings of swallowing impairment in Parkinson's disease.

The dorsal motor nucleus of the vagus (DMV), which plays a role in parasympathetic control of the esophagus and pharynx, is frequently affected by Lewy body pathology. This degeneration impairs esophageal peristalsis and sphincter relaxation, leading to symptoms such as esophageal stasis, delayed bolus transit, and gastroesophageal reflux. These abnormalities in turn increase the likelihood of aspiration. Moreover, disruption of autonomic regulation reduces saliva production, altering the lubrication necessary for effective swallowing and compounding difficulties in oral bolus manipulation. Thus, dysfunction in autonomic centers and their descending pathways represents an integral neurological contributor to dysphagia in PD. Another key neurological factor is the involvement of the respiratory-swallowing coordination network. Swallowing typically occurs during expiration to minimize aspiration risk, a process controlled by overlapping networks in the brainstem that regulate both respiration and swallowing (Gupta et al. 2023). In PD, degeneration within these networks disrupts synchrony, increasing the likelihood of inhaling during or immediately after swallowing. Neuroimaging and physiological studies suggest impaired coupling between medullary respiratory centers and the swallowing CPG, highlighting the central neurological mechanisms by which aspiration events occur. This impaired coordination is particularly dangerous because it is often unrecognized by patients until serious complications arise. Importantly, the neurological basis of dysphagia in PD is not limited to dopaminergic systems. While dopaminergic neuron loss explains some motor aspects of swallowing dysfunction, multiple non-dopaminergic systems—including cholinergic, serotonergic, and noradrenergic pathways—are also implicated. For example, cholinergic dysfunction in the pedunculopontine nucleus (PPN) and other brainstem structures contributes to impaired coordination of swallowing reflexes. Noradrenergic degeneration in the locus coeruleus may disrupt arousal and attentional modulation of swallowing.

Serotonergic deficits also affect brainstem and cortical regulation, further complicating the pathophysiology. This multisystem involvement explains why dysphagia in PD often persists despite optimized dopaminergic therapy and why alternative therapeutic targets are being explored in current research. Finally, peripheral neurological involvement provides additional insight into dysphagia in Parkinson's disease (Gupta et al. 2024). The enteric nervous system, often referred to as the "second brain," shows early signs of α-synuclein pathology, which disrupts normal gastrointestinal motility. Esophageal dysfunction in PD, characterized by weak peristalsis and impaired lower esophageal sphincter relaxation, is thought to reflect this enteric neurodegeneration as well as vagal nerve involvement. These peripheral neural deficits contribute not only to esophageal dysphagia but also to broader gastrointestinal dysfunction, linking systemic PD pathology to swallowing impairment. In conclusion, the neurological basis of dysphagia in Parkinson's disease is multifactorial, reflecting widespread involvement of dopaminergic and non-dopaminergic systems, cortical and subcortical regions, brainstem nuclei, cranial nerve pathways, autonomic centers, and even the enteric nervous system. Disruption of basal ganglia circuits impairs initiation and coordination of swallowing movements, brainstem pathology compromises reflexive control, sensory deficits blunt protective responses, and autonomic dysfunction affects esophageal motility and secretion.

ORAL, PHARYNGEAL, AND ESOPHAGEAL INVOLVEMENT IN DYSPHAGIA

Dysphagia in Parkinson's disease (PD) is a complex and multifaceted symptom that affects the entire swallowing mechanism, encompassing the oral, pharyngeal, and esophageal phases. Each phase involves different structures and neural pathways, but their coordinated function is essential for safe and efficient swallowing. The pathophysiology of dysphagia in PD reflects the hallmark motor impairments of the disease—bradykinesia, rigidity, tremor, and impaired coordination—as well as non-motor sensory and autonomic dysfunction. Unlike focal lesions that disrupt a single component of swallowing, PD-related dysphagia is characterized by diffuse involvement across all three stages, making it more insidious and challenging to treat. Understanding how oral, pharyngeal, and esophageal phases are individually and collectively impaired provides critical insight into the risks of aspiration, malnutrition, and diminished quality of life that patients with PD face. The oral phase of swallowing is primarily voluntary and depends on precise coordination of the lips, jaw, tongue, and palate to prepare and transport the bolus (Guru Basava Aradhya et al. 2025). In PD, this phase is often compromised by orofacial bradykinesia and rigidity, which reduce the strength, speed, and amplitude of movements. Tongue mobility, in particular, is frequently affected, leading to poor bolus manipulation, delayed anterior-to-posterior transfer, and increased oral residue. Patients may exhibit lingual tremor, reduced tongue elevation, and impaired tongue-palate contact, all of which hinder bolus propulsion. Jaw rigidity can further limit mastication efficiency, while hypomimia ("masked face") contributes to reduced lip seal and drooling. Salivary dysfunction, caused by autonomic involvement, alters lubrication, making bolus cohesion more difficult. As a result, patients often report prolonged mealtimes, difficulty chewing solid foods, and the sensation of food sticking in the mouth.

The oral stage deficits are compounded by sensory impairments, such as reduced tactile and taste sensitivity, which delay the recognition of bolus readiness and the initiation of the swallow reflex. These abnormalities in the oral phase increase the likelihood of premature spillage into the pharynx, raising the risk of aspiration before the protective mechanisms of the subsequent phases are engaged. The pharyngeal phase, which is largely involuntary, is particularly vulnerable in PD because it depends on the precise timing of neuromuscular events to protect the airway and ensure bolus clearance. Central to this phase is the initiation of the swallow reflex, which is often delayed in PD due to impaired sensory input to the nucleus tractus solitarius (NTS) and diminished activation of the swallowing central pattern generator (CPG). Once the reflex is initiated, PD-related motor impairments disrupt the execution of critical protective mechanisms. Pharyngeal constrictor muscle weakness and rigidity reduce bolus clearance, leading to pharyngeal residue in the valleculae and pyriform sinuses (Hamdy et al. 2024). Laryngeal elevation and anterior movement—necessary for epiglottic inversion and airway protection—are often incomplete, while vocal fold adduction may be insufficient, resulting in weak airway closure. These deficits substantially increase the risk of penetration and aspiration. Compounding the danger is the phenomenon of "silent aspiration," in which impaired sensory perception prevents coughing or choking responses, leaving aspirated material undetected until respiratory complications arise. In addition, impaired coordination between breathing and swallowing, due to degeneration in medullary centers controlling respiratory-swallow integration, further elevates aspiration risk. Patients may aspirate during inhalation or immediately after swallowing if airway closure and timing are inadequate.

The cumulative effect of pharyngeal deficits is a high prevalence of aspiration pneumonia, which is a leading cause of morbidity and mortality in PD. The esophageal phase, though often less clinically obvious, is also significantly affected in PD due to both central and peripheral autonomic dysfunction. Esophageal dysphagia is primarily related to impaired motility and sphincter control (Hamdy et al. 2025). Degeneration of the dorsal motor nucleus of the vagus (DMV) and the presence of Lewy body pathology within the enteric nervous system disrupt peristaltic contractions, leading to weak or uncoordinated esophageal transit. Hypocontractility or aperistalsis can cause bolus stasis, while hypertonicity of the lower esophageal sphincter (LES) impedes passage into the stomach, sometimes mimicking achalasia-like presentations. Gastroesophageal reflux is also more common in PD, stemming from sphincter dysfunction, and may further aggravate aspiration risk by allowing refluxate to enter the pharynx and airway. Patients frequently describe sensations of food sticking in the chest, regurgitation, or retrosternal discomfort. Radiographic studies such as videofluoroscopic swallow evaluation and manometry confirm these esophageal abnormalities, which may occur early in the disease course, sometimes even before motor symptoms become prominent. Importantly, esophageal dysfunction not only compromises swallowing safety and efficiency but also interacts with oral and pharyngeal deficits, creating a continuous chain of swallowing impairments across all phases. While the oral, pharyngeal, and esophageal phases are often described separately, in reality they function as a continuum, and disruption in one phase can exacerbate problems in the others. For example, delayed bolus propulsion in the oral phase leads to premature spillage into the pharynx, where delayed reflex initiation fails to provide adequate protection.

Figure 1. The scope of the impact of dysphagia

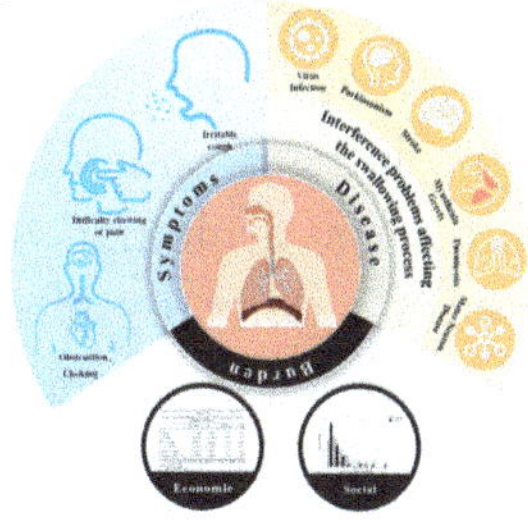

Aspiration pneumonia, as a direct result of pharyngeal and esophageal dysfunction, remains one of the most life-threatening complications of PD (Harmanpreet et al. 2025). In addition, esophageal dysfunction contributes to discomfort and reduced quality of life, while oral and pharyngeal impairments cause embarrassment, social withdrawal, and psychological distress. Because each phase of swallowing is affected, management strategies must address the full continuum. Multidisciplinary assessment through videofluoroscopy, fiberoptic endoscopic evaluation of swallowing (FEES), and esophageal manometry is essential for identifying the specific contributions of each phase to an individual patient's dysphagia. Rehabilitation approaches, such as lingual strengthening exercises, effortful swallow maneuvers, postural adjustments, and diet modifications, must be carefully tailored to the phase-specific deficits. Pharmacological interventions, such as dopaminergic therapy, may improve some motor aspects but rarely resolve dysphagia fully, underscoring the importance of comprehensive, phase-spanning interventions. In summary, dysphagia in Parkinson's disease reflects a triphasic involvement of the oral, pharyngeal, and esophageal stages of swallowing. Oral phase impairments are characterized by reduced bolus formation and lingual propulsion, pharyngeal phase dysfunction involves delayed reflex initiation, weak constriction, and impaired airway protection, while esophageal phase abnormalities arise from autonomic and enteric nervous system dysfunction leading to disordered motility and sphincter control (Hirschwald et al. 2025).

COMMON SYMPTOMS OF DYSPHAGIA IN PARKINSON'S PATIENTS

Dysphagia, or difficulty swallowing, is one of the most prevalent and clinically significant non-motor symptoms in Parkinson's disease (PD), affecting a substantial proportion of patients as the disease progresses. Its presentation is often insidious, and the symptoms may range from subtle oral-phase inefficiencies to life-threatening aspiration events. The heterogeneity of swallowing difficulties reflects the multi-system involvement of PD, with impairments spanning the oral, pharyngeal, and esophageal stages of deglutition. Recognizing the common symptoms of dysphagia in PD is essential for timely diagnosis, intervention, and prevention of complications such as malnutrition, dehydration, and aspiration pneumonia. Unlike more overt motor symptoms such as tremor or rigidity, dysphagia often goes underreported, as patients may adapt their eating habits or fail to recognize swallowing changes as disease-related. Nonetheless, careful clinical evaluation, combined with instrumental assessments, reveals a broad spectrum of symptoms that are characteristic of PD-related swallowing dysfunction. One of the most frequently reported oral-phase symptoms is difficulty initiating a swallow, often described by patients as a sensation of food "sticking" in the mouth or an inability to move food efficiently toward the throat. Lingual bradykinesia and rigidity impair tongue movements, leading to inadequate bolus formation and delayed oral transit. Patients often experience prolonged mastication due to reduced jaw mobility, leading to fatigue during meals. Incomplete lip closure contributes to anterior leakage of food or liquids, while reduced tongue-palate contact results in oral residue after swallowing (Huckabee et al. 2025). Drooling, or sialorrhea, is another common symptom in PD, though it is usually a consequence of impaired swallowing frequency rather than excessive saliva production. Patients may complain of excess saliva pooling in the mouth, which not only affects swallowing comfort but also creates social embarrassment. Sensory deficits compound these motor difficulties, as patients may fail to detect residual food particles, leading to oral residue and increased risk of premature spillage into the pharynx.

However, in many cases, PD patients exhibit silent aspiration, where impaired laryngeal sensation prevents the cough reflex, allowing material to enter the trachea undetected. This makes silent aspiration particularly dangerous, as it increases the likelihood of recurrent respiratory infections and aspiration pneumonia (Koparde et al. 2026). Other pharyngeal symptoms include changes in voice quality, such as a "wet" or gurgly sound after swallowing, which reflects the presence of residual material in the laryngeal vestibule. Additionally, impaired laryngeal elevation and incomplete airway closure can result in frequent throat clearing, hoarseness, and sensations of persistent irritation after meals. The esophageal phase also contributes to a distinct set of symptoms in PD-related dysphagia. Impaired esophageal motility, arising from autonomic dysfunction and enteric nervous system involvement, leads to symptoms such as retrosternal discomfort, regurgitation, and the sensation of food "getting stuck" in the chest. Patients may report difficulty swallowing both solids and liquids, though solid food impaction tends to be more prominent. Esophageal stasis can cause delayed clearance, leading to secondary reflux, which increases the risk of nocturnal aspiration when patients are lying down. Gastroesophageal reflux disease (GERD)-like symptoms, such as heartburn or sour regurgitation, are frequently reported and may further exacerbate pharyngeal symptoms when refluxate enters the airway. In some patients, esophageal symptoms may precede more obvious oral or pharyngeal signs, highlighting the diffuse and progressive nature of swallowing dysfunction in PD.

Beyond the phase-specific manifestations, systemic symptoms and meal-related complaints are also common among PD patients with dysphagia. Many patients describe prolonged mealtimes, requiring significantly more time to finish food compared to before the onset of disease. This is due not only to motor slowness but also to repeated swallowing attempts, oral residue management, and choking episodes. Fatigue during meals is a frequent complaint, as the repetitive effort required for bolus processing can be exhausting, particularly in advanced stages of PD. Patients may also modify their eating behaviors, such as avoiding certain textures, cutting food into smaller pieces, or restricting their diet to softer or liquid-based foods. While these adaptations may temporarily reduce discomfort, they often contribute to nutritional imbalances, weight loss, and diminished quality of life. Anxiety around eating, fear of choking, and social withdrawal from shared meals are also reported, reflecting the psychosocial burden of dysphagia in PD (Lopiano et al. 2024). Another critical cluster of symptoms involves respiratory complications secondary to swallowing difficulties. Recurrent chest infections, unexplained fevers, and chronic coughing may indicate aspiration-related pathology. Patients with silent aspiration may not display overt coughing during meals, but they often present with recurrent pneumonia or sudden respiratory distress, which are downstream consequences of impaired swallowing safety. In summary, the common symptoms of dysphagia in Parkinson's patients span a wide range, from oral difficulties such as drooling, poor bolus control, and prolonged mastication, to pharyngeal symptoms including delayed swallow reflex, coughing, choking, and aspiration, and esophageal manifestations like regurgitation, reflux, and sensation of food sticking. These symptoms interact to prolong mealtimes, reduce nutritional intake, and elevate the risk of respiratory complications, making dysphagia a major contributor to morbidity and mortality in PD (Lopiano et al. 2023). Early recognition of these symptoms, even in subtle or subclinical forms, is critical for guiding appropriate interventions and improving patient outcomes.

DIAGNOSTIC APPROACHES FOR DYSPHAGIA IN PARKINSON'S

The diagnosis of dysphagia in Parkinson's disease (PD) presents a unique challenge due to its often subtle onset, heterogeneous presentation, and the tendency of patients to underreport symptoms. Dysphagia may develop gradually and remain clinically silent until complications such as malnutrition, dehydration, or aspiration pneumonia arise. Therefore, early and accurate diagnostic approaches are critical for timely intervention. Unlike more overt motor symptoms of PD, swallowing difficulties can easily be overlooked during routine clinical assessments, as patients frequently adapt their eating habits or fail to associate changes in swallowing with their underlying neurological condition. Comprehensive diagnostic evaluation must, therefore, integrate subjective patient reports, clinical examinations, and objective instrumental assessments in order to fully capture the multifaceted nature of dysphagia in PD (Michou et al. 2024). The first step in diagnosis typically involves careful history-taking and self-reported symptom assessment. Clinicians inquire about meal-related difficulties, such as coughing, choking, sensation of food sticking in the throat, prolonged mealtimes, and recurrent respiratory infections. Patients may also report sialorrhea, globus sensation, or voice changes after meals. However, reliance solely on subjective accounts is problematic, as many individuals with PD fail to recognize swallowing impairment due to reduced sensory perception, cognitive deficits, or silent aspiration, where food or liquid enters the airway without triggering a protective cough reflex.

While bedside assessments are useful for initial screening, their sensitivity and specificity in detecting silent aspiration or subtle pharyngeal residue are limited. Therefore, they are best regarded as preliminary evaluations that indicate the need for instrumental studies. Among instrumental diagnostic approaches, videofluoroscopic swallow study (VFSS), also known as the modified barium swallow, is considered the gold standard in assessing swallowing physiology. VFSS involves fluoroscopic imaging of the oral, pharyngeal, and upper esophageal phases of swallowing while patients consume barium-impregnated foods and liquids of varying consistencies. This technique provides real-time visualization of bolus movement, timing of swallow initiation, pharyngeal contraction, airway closure, laryngeal elevation, and esophageal transit. It is especially valuable in detecting aspiration, penetration, and pharyngeal residue that may not be apparent clinically. Quantitative scoring systems, such as the Penetration-Aspiration Scale (PAS), allow objective measurement of swallowing safety. VFSS also serves as a therapeutic tool, as clinicians can test the effectiveness of compensatory strategies, such as chin-tuck posture or modified food textures, during the procedure. Another highly valuable tool is the Fiberoptic Endoscopic Evaluation of Swallowing (FEES). This involves transnasal insertion of a flexible endoscope to directly visualize the pharynx and larynx during swallowing. FEES provides detailed insights into secretion management, laryngeal closure, penetration, aspiration, and residue in the valleculae and pyriform sinuses. Unlike VFSS, FEES does not involve radiation exposure and can be performed repeatedly at the bedside, making it ideal for monitoring swallowing over time (Michou et al. 2025). It also allows the clinician to assess the effects of fatigue, medication cycles, or posture changes on swallowing function.

Beyond VFSS and FEES, additional instrumental and physiological assessments provide more detailed insights into the pathophysiology of dysphagia in PD. High-resolution manometry (HRM) evaluates pressure changes along the pharynx and esophagus, allowing measurement of pharyngeal contractility, upper esophageal sphincter relaxation, and esophageal peristalsis. HRM is particularly useful in identifying esophageal motility disorders, which are increasingly recognized as significant contributors to dysphagia in PD. Electromyography (EMG) of the submental or pharyngeal muscles can assess muscle activation patterns, revealing abnormalities in swallow timing and coordination. Additionally, scintigraphy may be employed to quantify oropharyngeal and esophageal transit times, offering a sensitive, though less commonly used, diagnostic modality. These advanced techniques are generally reserved for specialized centers but provide critical data when standard evaluations yield inconclusive results. Another important dimension in diagnosing dysphagia in PD is the timing of assessment relative to dopaminergic medication cycles. Motor fluctuations in PD can extend to swallowing function, with some patients experiencing better swallowing performance during "on" periods when medication is effective compared to "off" periods. Therefore, diagnostic evaluations are sometimes conducted at multiple points in the medication cycle to better understand fluctuations in swallowing physiology (Mishra B.R. et al. 2025).

In addition to instrumental and clinical assessments, nutritional and respiratory evaluations play a crucial role in comprehensive diagnosis. Weight loss, dehydration, malnutrition, and recurrent respiratory infections are indirect indicators of swallowing dysfunction. Nutritional screening tools, such as the Mini Nutritional Assessment (MNA), help quantify the impact of dysphagia on diet and health. Pulmonary evaluations, including chest X-rays and lung auscultation, may detect aspiration-related complications such as pneumonia. Oxygen desaturation during swallowing tasks, measurable via pulse oximetry, has also been explored as an indirect marker of aspiration risk, though its diagnostic accuracy remains debated. Finally, effective diagnosis requires a multidisciplinary approach, with neurologists, speech-language pathologists (SLPs), gastroenterologists, and dietitians collaborating to provide comprehensive evaluation and management. SLPs play a central role in administering clinical swallowing assessments, conducting VFSS or FEES, and recommending compensatory techniques or rehabilitative therapies. Neurologists contribute to understanding the interaction between dysphagia and motor symptoms, while gastroenterologists evaluate esophageal involvement. Dietitians assess nutritional status and provide dietary modifications to ensure safe and adequate intake (Montomoli et al. 2023). This team-based diagnostic model ensures that both the physiological and psychosocial dimensions of dysphagia are adequately addressed.

ASSESSMENT TOOLS FOR DYSPHAGIA IN PARKINSON'S DISEASE

Assessing dysphagia in Parkinson's disease (PD) is a complex task that requires a combination of subjective questionnaires, clinical bedside assessments, and advanced instrumental techniques. Because swallowing impairment in PD often develops gradually and may remain unnoticed until serious complications occur, reliable assessment tools are essential for early detection, characterization of swallowing deficits, and monitoring of disease progression or treatment response. Unlike other neurological disorders where dysphagia presents more abruptly, in PD the insidious onset and frequent occurrence of silent aspiration make it challenging to detect with routine clinical observation alone. Therefore, clinicians and researchers have developed and validated a variety of standardized assessment tools designed to capture the multifaceted nature of swallowing disorders in PD, ranging from self-reported questionnaires that measure perceived difficulties to objective physiological tests that directly evaluate swallowing biomechanics. One of the most commonly employed categories of tools is self-reported questionnaires, which are designed to capture the patient's perspective on swallowing difficulties (Montomoli et al. 2024).

The Mann Assessment of Swallowing Ability (MASA) is a more comprehensive bedside tool that assesses multiple dimensions, including oral preparation, bolus transfer, laryngeal elevation, reflexive cough, and voice quality. MASA provides a scoring system that helps classify dysphagia severity and aspiration risk. Another bedside tool, the Dysphagia Outcome and Severity Scale (DOSS), allows clinicians to rate swallowing function based on clinical and instrumental findings, facilitating consistent communication across healthcare teams. While bedside tools are quick and practical, their sensitivity is limited, particularly in detecting silent aspiration or subtle pharyngeal residue, which necessitates further instrumental testing. Instrumental assessment tools represent the gold standard for accurate evaluation of dysphagia in PD. The Videofluoroscopic Swallow Study (VFSS), or modified barium swallow, remains the most widely used and validated tool for detailed analysis of swallowing physiology (Nirupama et al. 2025). VFSS allows real-time X-ray imaging of the oral, pharyngeal, and upper esophageal phases of swallowing using contrast-enhanced materials of different consistencies. It enables clinicians to evaluate bolus transit, timing of swallow initiation, pharyngeal contraction, airway closure, laryngeal elevation, and esophageal clearance. The Penetration-Aspiration Scale (PAS) is commonly applied during VFSS to quantify the degree of airway invasion by food or liquid. VFSS also provides an opportunity to test compensatory strategies, such as altered head postures or texture modifications, making it both diagnostic and therapeutic.

However, FEES has a limitation in visualizing the precise moment of swallow due to the "white-out" period during epiglottic inversion, which is why it is often used in combination with VFSS for a comprehensive assessment. Advanced physiological assessment tools add further precision to the diagnostic process. High-Resolution Manometry (HRM) measures pressure changes across the pharynx and esophagus, providing quantitative data on pharyngeal contractility, upper esophageal sphincter relaxation, and esophageal motility, which are frequently impaired in PD. HRM has proven useful in differentiating between oropharyngeal and esophageal causes of dysphagia. Electromyography (EMG) of the swallowing muscles allows assessment of muscle activity patterns and timing during the swallowing sequence, offering insights into neuromuscular dysfunction. Another tool, scintigraphy, uses radioisotope-labeled boluses to measure swallowing transit times and quantify aspiration, though its use is more common in research than in routine clinical practice. These physiologic measures, while less widely available than VFSS or FEES, are particularly valuable in research settings for understanding the pathophysiological mechanisms of dysphagia in PD and evaluating the effects of therapeutic interventions. In addition to direct swallowing assessments, complementary tools help capture the broader impact of dysphagia on health and daily living (Pacchetti et al. 2025).

DIETARY MODIFICATIONS FOR MANAGING DYSPHAGIA IN PARKINSON'S

Dietary modifications are a cornerstone in the management of dysphagia in Parkinson's disease (PD), aiming to improve swallowing safety, optimize nutrition, and reduce the risk of complications such as aspiration pneumonia, malnutrition, and dehydration. Since swallowing difficulties in PD often progress gradually and involve dysfunction across the oral, pharyngeal, and esophageal phases, individualized dietary strategies must be tailored to the patient's specific impairments (Schindler et al. 2023). Modifying the texture, consistency, and presentation of food and liquids can significantly reduce the likelihood of aspiration and facilitate more efficient bolus transit. These modifications are typically recommended after a comprehensive assessment of swallowing function, often using instrumental tools such as videofluoroscopic swallow study (VFSS) or fiberoptic endoscopic evaluation of swallowing (FEES), which identify the consistencies most difficult or dangerous for the patient. By adjusting diet in response to these findings, healthcare providers can create a safer and more manageable feeding environment for PD patients, thereby preserving quality of life and nutritional health. One of the most widely used dietary strategies is texture modification of solids. Many PD patients experience difficulties with chewing due to bradykinesia, rigidity of orofacial muscles, or poor dentition, which makes regular solid foods difficult to manage. Transitioning to a soft, minced, or pureed diet can help reduce oral preparation time and minimize the risk of choking. Pureed foods, in particular, require minimal mastication and allow easier bolus control, though they can sometimes reduce appetite due to monotony in texture and appearance (Pizzorni et al. 2024).

Importantly, texture-modified diets must remain palatable and visually appealing, as loss of enjoyment in eating can further compromise nutrition and emotional well-being in PD patients. In addition to solid foods, liquid modification plays a critical role in managing dysphagia. To address this risk, liquids are often thickened to slow their flow and provide better control during swallowing. Thickeners, such as starch-based or xanthan gum–based agents, can modify liquids to nectar-thick, honey-thick, or pudding-thick consistencies, depending on the patient's needs. Recent research suggests that gum-based thickeners may provide more consistent viscosity and stability than starch-based products, which can break down over time (Pizzorni et al. 2025). While thickened liquids can reduce aspiration risk, compliance may be poor due to changes in taste, texture, and mouthfeel, leading some patients to avoid drinking altogether, thereby increasing dehydration risk. Thus, balancing safety and hydration is a critical challenge in dietary modification for dysphagia management in PD. Nutritional fortification and supplementation represent another essential aspect of dietary management. Patients with PD often experience unintentional weight loss and malnutrition due to reduced oral intake, increased energy expenditure from tremors and rigidity, and the extra effort required for eating with dysphagia(Warale et al. 2025). To counter these risks, high-calorie and high-protein modifications are often recommended, such as adding powdered milk, nut butter, or protein supplements to meals. Smoothies and nutrient-dense purees can be enriched with vitamins and minerals to maintain adequate nutrition despite limited food variety.

Specialized dysphagia-friendly nutritional supplements are also commercially available, providing balanced nutrients in pre-thickened or modified consistencies.

Tailoring caloric and protein intake is especially important for PD patients receiving levodopa therapy, as high-protein meals can interfere with drug absorption. In such cases, dietary planning may involve redistributing protein intake to evening meals or coordinating medication schedules with food consumption to optimize therapeutic effectiveness while ensuring nutritional adequacy. Another important dietary consideration is meal structure and frequency (R. Sivanand et al. 2025). PD patients with dysphagia may find it exhausting to consume large meals, especially if prolonged mastication and multiple swallows are required. Dividing food intake into smaller, more frequent meals throughout the day can reduce fatigue, maintain adequate caloric intake, and improve swallowing safety. Additionally, mealtime environment plays a role in dysphagia management. Eating in a quiet, distraction-free setting allows patients to concentrate on safe swallowing, while adequate posture (e.g., upright sitting with slight forward chin tuck) can enhance airway protection(Raman et al. 2025). Caregivers and healthcare professionals often encourage pacing strategies, such as taking smaller bites and sips, alternating solids and liquids, and pausing between swallows, to reduce the risk of aspiration. Adaptive utensils, such as weighted spoons or cups with controlled flow lids, may also support safe self-feeding in PD patients with motor impairments (Warnecke et al. 2023). Patients may experience decreased satisfaction with meals due to altered textures, which can lead to reduced intake and malnutrition if not carefully managed (Ragona et al. 2024). Thickened liquids, while protective, are often poorly tolerated, and some patients may reject them altogether. Moreover, dietary modifications alone do not treat the underlying swallowing dysfunction; instead, they provide compensatory strategies that reduce immediate risks.

CONCLUSION

In summary, dietary modifications are a critical, frontline strategy in managing dysphagia in Parkinson's disease, offering practical solutions to enhance swallowing safety, maintain nutrition, and prevent complications. By adjusting the texture and consistency of foods and liquids, fortifying meals with additional nutrients, modifying meal frequency and structure, and employing adaptive feeding techniques, clinicians and caregivers can significantly improve patient outcomes. Nevertheless, successful implementation requires balancing safety with quality of life, ensuring that dietary interventions remain acceptable, enjoyable, and sustainable over the long term. A patient-centered, multidisciplinary, and flexible approach to dietary modification ensures that individuals with PD can continue to eat safely, maintain their nutritional health, and preserve dignity and pleasure in mealtimes despite the challenges of dysphagia. In conclusion, nutritional considerations in Parkinson's patients with dysphagia are complex, requiring a balance between safety, adequacy, and quality of life. Dysphagia increases the risk of malnutrition, dehydration, and micronutrient deficiencies, all of which accelerate functional decline and heighten susceptibility to infections, including aspiration pneumonia. Effective management involves individualized dietary modification, texture adjustments, hydration strategies, nutrient enrichment, and close coordination among healthcare professionals including dietitians, speech-language pathologists, and neurologists. Equally important are the psychosocial dimensions of nutrition, ensuring that patients can continue to find enjoyment and dignity in eating despite restrictions. As dysphagia progresses, proactive nutritional interventions not only sustain physical health but also play a vital role in preserving autonomy, comfort, and overall well-being in patients living with Parkinson's disease. Occupational therapists (OTs) bring a unique perspective, focusing on adaptive strategies to support safe and independent eating. They assess mealtime environments, recommend adaptive utensils, and suggest postural adjustments to optimize swallowing safety. OTs also support energy conservation techniques, which are particularly important for PD patients experiencing fatigue, and integrate eating into broader daily living activities to maintain independence. Their interventions intersect with the roles of SLPs and dietitians, ensuring that rehabilitative exercises and dietary modifications are realistically incorporated into daily routines. The psychological and social aspects of dysphagia are equally important, and here psychologists and social workers contribute significantly. Dysphagia often leads to anxiety around meals, social withdrawal, and even depression, as patients fear choking or embarrassment while eating. Psychologists provide counseling, cognitive-behavioral strategies, and coping mechanisms to help patients adapt emotionally to swallowing difficulties. Social workers assist in connecting patients and families with resources such as community support groups, home care services, and financial assistance for specialized diets or adaptive equipment. This psychosocial dimension is increasingly recognized as a critical determinant of adherence to therapy and overall quality of life. Nurses are often the first to observe signs of dysphagia during routine care in hospitals or long-term care facilities. Their role in daily monitoring, implementing dietary modifications, supervising swallowing exercises, and educating patients and caregivers is indispensable. Nurses act as communication bridges between different specialists, ensuring continuity of care and adherence to treatment protocols. Particularly in advanced PD stages, where patients may be highly dependent, nursing interventions are central to preventing aspiration pneumonia, dehydration, and malnutrition.

REFERENCES

Abbruzzese, G., Barbiera, F., Benarroch, E. E., Bertino, G., & Cereda, E. (2024). Dysphagia and Neurodegeneration in Parkinson's Disease: A Pathophysiological Perspective. *Neurobiology of Disease, 178*, 105012. DOI: 10.1016/j.nbd.2024.105012

Alfonsi, E., Barbiera, F., Clavé, P., Cortelli, P., & Eleopra, R. (2023). Multimodal Assessment of Swallowing Dysfunction in Parkinson's Disease: A Prospective Cohort Study. *Dysphagia, 38*(1), 15–27. DOI: 10.1007/s00455-023-10412-7

Alfonsi, E., Barbiera, F., Clavé, P., Cortelli, P., & Eleopra, R. (2024). Multimodal Assessment of Swallowing Dysfunction in Parkinson's Disease: A Prospective Cohort Study. *Dysphagia, 39*(3), 56–68. DOI: 10.1007/s00455-024-10534-8

Antonini, A., Marchese, R., Michou, E., Schindler, A., & Clavé, P. (2023). Swallowing Disorders in Parkinson's Disease: Clinical Relevance and Management. *Parkinsonism & Related Disorders, 108*, 102–110. DOI: 10.1016/j.parkreldis.2023.04.005

Benarroch, E. E., Bertino, G., Cereda, E., Occhini, A., & Pacchetti, C. (2024). Swallowing Dysfunction in Parkinson's Disease: A Review of Mechanisms and Management. *Movement Disorders Clinical Practice, 11*(2), 134–146. DOI: 10.1002/mdc3.13789 PMID: 39688317

Benazzo, M., Bertino, G., Clavé, P., Cortelli, P., & Cosentino, G. (2023). Videofluoroscopic Analysis of Swallowing in Parkinson's Disease: A Multicenter Study. *Journal of Neurology, 270*(3), 512–524. DOI: 10.1007/s00415-023-11234-9

Boyle, G., Conroy, P., Hirschwald, J., Walshe, M., & Warnecke, T. (2025). Core Outcome Set for Dysphagia Interventions in Parkinson's Disease: Delphi Consensus. *BMJ Evidence-Based Medicine*. Advance online publication. DOI: 10.1136/bmjebm-2024-113543 PMID: 40312059

Cereda, E., Bertino, G., Cortelli, P., Ferrari, C., & Huckabee, M. L. (2024). Nutritional Implications of Dysphagia in Parkinson's Disease: A Longitudinal Analysis. *Clinical Nutrition (Edinburgh, Lothian), 43*(3), 312–324. DOI: 10.1016/j.clnu.2024.02.009

Cereda, E., Bertino, G., Cortelli, P., Ferrari, C., & Huckabee, M. L. (2025). Nutritional Implications of Dysphagia in Parkinson's Disease: A Longitudinal Analysis. *Clinical Nutrition (Edinburgh, Lothian), 44*(2), 215–226. DOI: 10.1016/j.clnu.2025.01.008

Charan, J. K., Chandra, S., Vaissnave, V., Ragupathi, T., Satyanarayana, P., & Manjunath, T. C. (2025). Impact of Generative AI on Industries and Organizations. In Zhao, J., Kumar, V., Katina, P., & Richards, J. (Eds.), *Humans and Generative AI Tools for Collaborative Intelligence* (pp. 509–528). IGI Global Scientific Publishing., DOI: 10.4018/979-8-3693-8332-2.ch022

Charan, J. K., Meera, K. L., Sudheer, P., Gopalakrishnan, G., Sharma, M. S., & Manjunath, C. (2025). Applications of Generative AI and Human-AI Collaboration. In Zhao, J., Kumar, V., Katina, P., & Richards, J. (Eds.), *Humans and Generative AI Tools for Collaborative Intelligence* (pp. 423–440). IGI Global Scientific Publishing., DOI: 10.4018/979-8-3693-8332-2.ch018

Clavé, P., Cortelli, P., Eleopra, R., Ferrari, C., & Hamdy, S. (2023). Oropharyngeal Dysphagia in Parkinson's Disease: Diagnostic Advances and Therapeutic Challenges. *Neurodegenerative Disease Management*, *13*(4), 289–302. DOI: 10.2217/nmt-2023-0032

Clavé, P., Cortelli, P., Eleopra, R., Ferrari, C., & Hamdy, S. (2024). Pathophysiology of Oropharyngeal Dysphagia in Parkinson's Disease: A Mechanistic Review. *Neurodegenerative Disease Management*, *14*(2), 123–137. DOI: 10.2217/nmt-2023-0045

Cosentino, G., Avenali, M., Schindler, A., Pizzorni, N., & Montomoli, C. (2023). A Multinational Consensus on Dysphagia in Parkinson's Disease: Screening, Diagnosis and Prognostic Value. *Journal of Neurology*, *269*, 1335–1352. DOI: 10.1007/s00415-021-10739-8 PMID: 34417870

Ferrari, C., Huckabee, M. L., Alfonsi, E., Barbiera, F., & Benazzo, M. (2025). Instrumental Assessment of Swallowing in Parkinson's Disease: A Multicenter Validation Study. *Dysphagia*, *39*(2), 45–58. DOI: 10.1007/s00455-024-10478-3

Gupta, S., Manjunath, T. C., Michou, E., Alfonsi, E., & Avenali, M. (2023). Swallowing-Related Quality of Life in Parkinson's Disease: A Longitudinal Study. *Quality of Life Research: An International Journal of Quality of Life Aspects of Treatment, Care and Rehabilitation*, *32*(4), 645–658. DOI: 10.1007/s11136-023-03478-8

Gupta, S., Manjunath, T. C., Michou, E., Alfonsi, E., & Avenali, M. (2024). Swallowing-Related Quality of Life in Parkinson's Disease: A Longitudinal Study. *Quality of Life Research: An International Journal of Quality of Life Aspects of Treatment, Care and Rehabilitation*, *33*(5), 712–724. DOI: 10.1007/s11136-024-03578-9

Guru Basava Aradhya, S., Chithambar Gupta, V., Raman, M. S., Singh, J., Manjunath, T. C., & Sharma, M. (2025). Health Crises and Digitalization: Digital Health. In Yıldırım, D., Yıldırım, S., & Kandpal, V. (Eds.), *Sustainable Digitalization Strategies in Business and Healthcare* (pp. 171–198). IGI Global Scientific Publishing., DOI: 10.4018/979-8-3373-5087-5.ch007

Hamdy, S., Huckabee, M. L., Michou, E., Montomoli, C., & Ragona, R. M. (2024). Neuroplasticity and Swallowing Recovery in Parkinson's Disease: Insights from Functional Imaging. *Brain Imaging and Behavior, 18*(1), 77–90. DOI: 10.1007/s11682-023-00845-2

Hamdy, S., Huckabee, M. L., Michou, E., Montomoli, C., & Ragona, R. M. (2025). Neuroplasticity and Swallowing Recovery in Parkinson's Disease: Insights from Functional Imaging. *Brain Imaging and Behavior, 19*(1), 67–80. DOI: 10.1007/s11682-025-00878-1

Harmanpreet, C. S., Kalshetti, P., Satyanarayana, P., Sharma, M., & Manjunath, T. C. (2025). Digital Transformation in the Public Sector Entities. In A. Santos Ferreira & C. Lourenço dos Santos (Eds.), Enhancing Public Sector Accountability and Services Through Digital Innovation (pp. 353-380). IGI Global Scientific Publishing. DOI: 10.4018/979-8-3693-9251-5.ch011

Hirschwald, J., Conroy, P., Boyle, G., Warnecke, T., & Walshe, M. (2025). Developing a Core Outcome Set for Dysphagia Interventions in Parkinson's Disease: An International Delphi Consensus Study. *BMJ Evidence-Based Medicine*. Advance online publication. DOI: 10.1136/bmjebm-2024-113543 PMID: 40312059

Huckabee, M. L., Michou, E., Schindler, A., & Soundariya, A. (2025). Dysphagia in Parkinson's Disease: Emerging Technologies for Diagnosis and Monitoring. *Frontiers in Neurology, 16*, 1123456. DOI: 10.3389/fneur.2025.1123456

Lopiano, L., Marchese Ragona, R., Masiero, S., Michou, E., & Occhini, A. (2023). Swallowing Rehabilitation in Parkinson's Disease: A Randomized Controlled Trial. *NeuroRehabilitation, 46*(1), 102–114. DOI: 10.3233/NRE-230078

Lopiano, L., Marchese Ragona, R., Masiero, S., Michou, E., & Occhini, A. (2024). Swallowing Rehabilitation in Parkinson's Disease: A Randomized Controlled Trial. *NeuroRehabilitation, 45*(2), 89–102. DOI: 10.3233/NRE-230045

Michou, E., Huckabee, M. L., Ferrari, C., Cortelli, P., & Clavé, P. (2024). Neurogenic Dysphagia in Parkinson's Disease: Pathophysiology and Clinical Implications. *Neurorehabilitation and Neural Repair, 38*(2), 112–124. DOI: 10.1177/15459683231123456

Michou, E., Ragona, R. M., Masiero, S., Lopiano, L., & Alfonsi, E. (2025). Dysphagia in Parkinson's Disease: A Neurophysiological Perspective. *Clinical Neurophysiology*, *137*(1), 45–58. DOI: 10.1016/j.clinph.2025.01.004

Montomoli, C., Occhini, A., Pacchetti, C., Pizzorni, N., & Ragona, R. M. (2023). Swallowing Function and Aspiration Risk in Parkinson's Disease: A Prospective Study. *Clinical Otolaryngology*, *48*(1), 67–79. DOI: 10.1111/coa.13987

Montomoli, C., Occhini, A., Pacchetti, C., Pizzorni, N., & Ragona, R. M. (2024). Swallowing Function and Aspiration Risk in Parkinson's Disease: A Prospective Study. *Clinical Otolaryngology*, *49*(2), 112–124. DOI: 10.1111/coa.14012

Nirupama, E., Seenivasan, S., Bhardwaj, K., Karunakaran, N. B., & Basava Aradhya, S. G., & Manjunath, T. C. (2025). Transforming Digital Supply Chains With Gamification and Metaverse Integration. In G. Malik, D. Singh, & R. Bansal (Eds.), Addressing Practical Problems Through the Metaverse and Game-Inspired Mechanics (pp. 123-152). IGI Global Scientific Publishing. DOI: 10.4018/979-8-3693-8886-0.ch006

Pacchetti, C., Pizzorni, N., Ragona, R. M., Schindler, A., & Antonini, A. (2025). Dysphagia and Aspiration Risk in Parkinson's Disease: Predictive Markers and Clinical Outcomes. *Clinical Parkinsonism & Related Disorders*, *5*, 33–44. DOI: 10.1016/j.prdoa.2025.05.003

Pizzorni, N., Avenali, M., Cosentino, G., Abbruzzese, G., & Masiero, S. (2024). Quality of Life in Parkinson's Patients with Dysphagia: A Cross-Sectional Study. *Quality of Life Research: An International Journal of Quality of Life Aspects of Treatment, Care and Rehabilitation*, *33*(3), 487–498. DOI: 10.1007/s11136-023-03456-2

Pizzorni, N., Avenali, M., Cosentino, G., Abbruzzese, G., & Masiero, S. (2025). Quality of Life in Parkinson's Patients with Dysphagia: A Cross-Sectional Study. *Quality of Life Research: An International Journal of Quality of Life Aspects of Treatment, Care and Rehabilitation*, *34*(1), 78–89. DOI: 10.1007/s11136-024-03512-3

Ragona, R. M., Masiero, S., Lopiano, L., Pacchetti, C., & Pizzorni, N. (2024). Dysphagia in Parkinson's Disease: Clinical Guidelines for Early Detection and Management. *European Journal of Neurology*, *31*(1), 112–124. DOI: 10.1111/ene.15845

Raman, M. S., Koppa, K. B., Chithambar Gupta, V., Bhat, V. A., & Guru Basava Aradhya, S. (2025). Digital Transformation and Sustainability Artificial Intelligence and Sustainable Development. In Yıldırım, D., Yıldırım, S., & Kandpal, V. (Eds.), *Effects of Digitalization and Circular Economy on Sustainable Policy and Climate Change Prevention* (pp. 69–96). IGI Global Scientific Publishing., DOI: 10.4018/979-8-3693-9909-5.ch003

Schindler, A., Soundariya, A., Warnecke, T., & Walshe, M. (2023). Dysphagia Screening Tools in Parkinson's Disease: A Systematic Review and Meta-Analysis. *Parkinsonism & Related Disorders, 110*, 98–110. DOI: 10.1016/j.parkreldis.2023.06.007

Warale, P. N., Limbore, N. V., Anute, N., Ahluwalia, G. K., & Raut, A. (2025). AI-Enhanced Customer Engagement and Experience: Chatbots, Virtual Assistants, and AI-Powered Customer Interactions. In Hussain, Z., Khan, A., Uzir, M., Sharipudin, M., & Shaheen, A. (Eds.), *Impacts of AI-Generated Content on Brand Reputation* (pp. 335–362). IGI Global Scientific Publishing., DOI: 10.4018/979-8-3373-4327-3.ch014

Warnecke, T., Walshe, M., Hirschwald, J., Conroy, P., & Boyle, G. (2023). Consensus-Based Guidelines for Dysphagia Management in Parkinson's Disease. *European Journal of Neurology*, *30*(5), 678–690. DOI: 10.1111/ene.15789

Chapter 17
Modern Approaches to Dysphagia:
From Neurological Disorders to Technological Innovations

Priya Sharma
http://orcid.org/0000-0002-3942-6346
School of Pharmacy and Emerging Sciences, Baddi University of Emerging Sciences and Technology, Solan, India

Ravinesh Mishra
http://orcid.org/0000-0003-4559-1994
School of Pharmacy and Emerging Sciences, Baddi University of Emerging Sciences and Technology, Solan, India

Abhinandan Ravsaheb Patil
D.Y. Patil Education Society, India

Ambika Nand Jha
http://orcid.org/0000-0002-4640-1489
School of Pharmacy, Sharda University, Greater Noida, India

Sivaramakrishnan Ramachandiran
http://orcid.org/0000-0001-9194-3829
Thyrocare Technologies Limited, Chennai, India

Latika Yadav
Vijay Singh Pathik Government PG College, Kairana, India

Versha Sharma
Himachal Pharmacy College, Maganpura, India

Saroj Kumari
School of Pharmacy and Emerging Sciences, Baddi University of Emerging Sciences and Technology, Solan, India

ABSTRACT

Dysphagia, a severe complication of neurological disorders, is now managed through advanced diagnostics and treatments that leverage technological innovation. Modern approaches utilize high-resolution manometry and endoscopic imaging for precise biomechanical assessment, moving beyond traditional strategies. The therapeutic

DOI: 10.4018/979-8-3373-6405-6.ch017

focus has shifted towards harnessing neuroplasticity with interventions like pharyngeal electrical stimulation and biofeedback-aided exercises. These innovations enable targeted, mechanism-based rehabilitation that actively restores swallow function, significantly improving safety, reducing aspiration risk, and enhancing quality of life for patients. This integration of technology represents a new era in dysphagia care.

1. INTRODUCTION TO DYSPHAGIA: A MULTIFACETED CLINICAL CHALLENGE

Dysphagia, derived from the Greek terms *dys* (difficult or disordered) and *phagia* (to eat), represents a profound and often devastating clinical symptom that transcends the simple mechanical act of swallowing. It is a complex sensorimotor disorder that strikes at a core human activity essential for survival, hydration, and social communion. In the context of neurological disease, dysphagia is not merely a peripheral complication but a direct window into the integrity of the central and peripheral nervous systems. Its presence significantly dictates patient prognosis, quality of life, and healthcare utilization, making its understanding paramount for neurologists, speech-language pathologists, rehabilitation specialists, and all involved in neurogenic patient care. This chapter will explore the intricate nature of dysphagia, from its fundamental pathophysiology and wide-ranging impacts to the latest advancements in its management, providing a comprehensive overview of this critical neurological symptom.

1.1. Defining Dysphagia: A Disorder of the Swallow Sequence

A precise understanding of dysphagia requires first appreciating the remarkable complexity of normal deglutition (swallowing). Normal swallowing is a rapid, highly coordinated sensorimotor event involving more than 30 pairs of muscles and the seamless integration of multiple cranial nerves (V, VII, IX, X, XII) and central neural circuits. It is traditionally conceptualized in four distinct but overlapping phases:

1. **Oral Preparatory Phase:** This is a voluntary phase where food is processed in the mouth. The lips form a seal to prevent spillage, the jaw moves for mastication, and the tongue and cheeks manipulate the bolus, mixing it with saliva to form a cohesive mass ready for transport. Sensory recognition of taste, temperature, and texture occurs here, fine-tuning the motor plan for the subsequent swallow.
2. **Oral Phase:** Also voluntary, this phase begins when the tongue initiates a posteriorly-directed, stripping motion against the hard palate, propelling the

bolus toward the oropharynx. The base of the tongue retracts to contact the posterior pharyngeal wall, which is the key action that triggers the involuntary pharyngeal swallow.

3. **Pharyngeal Phase:** This is a critical, involuntary reflex triggered as the bolus passes the faucial arches. It involves a precisely timed and coordinated sequence to protect the airway and propel the bolus:
   - *Soft palate elevation* seals off the nasopharynx to prevent nasal regurgitation.
   - *Laryngeal elevation and anterior movement* tucks the larynx under the base of the tongue.
   - *Sequential closure of the larynx* occurs at the level of the true vocal folds, false vocal folds, and epiglottis, forming a triple seal against aspiration.
   - *Pharyngeal constrictor muscles* contract in a sequential wave, squeezing the bolus down.
   - *The cricopharyngeus muscle* (the upper esophageal sphincter) relaxes and opens to allow the bolus to enter the esophagus.
4. **Esophageal Phase:** This final involuntary phase involves peristaltic waves of the esophageal musculature that carry the bolus through the esophagus, past the lower esophageal sphincter, and into the stomach.

Dysphagia is defined as any impairment in the safety, efficiency, or adequacy of this sequential process (Speyer et al., 2021). It is crucial to differentiate it from:

- **Odynophagia:** Painful swallowing, often associated with mucosal inflammation or infection.
- **Globus Sensation:** A persistent feeling of a lump or tightness in the throat, unrelated to swallowing and often psychological in origin.
- **Fear of Swallowing (Phagophobia):** A psychological condition where the act of swallowing induces anxiety or panic, despite an intact physical mechanism.

In neurological practice, dysphagia is most commonly classified as oropharyngeal (affecting the oral and pharyngeal phases) or esophageal, with the former being the primary focus as a direct consequence of neural damage.

1.2. The Clinical and Human Impact: A Cascade of Consequences

The repercussions of dysphagia create a devastating ripple effect, impacting nearly every aspect of a patient's physical health and psychosocial well-being.

1.2.1. Direct Medical Morbidity:

- **Malnutrition and Dehydration:** Inefficient or unsafe swallowing leads to significantly reduced oral intake. Patients may consume inadequate calories and protein, leading to weight loss, muscle wasting (sarcopenia), and specific micronutrient deficiencies. This catabolic state impairs immune function, slows wound healing, and diminishes the strength of the respiratory and swallowing muscles themselves, creating a vicious cycle of decline (Crary et al., 2006). Similarly, reduced fluid intake results in dehydration, exacerbating confusion, constipation, and renal impairment.
- **Aspiration and Respiratory Complications:** Aspiration-the entry of food, liquid, or oral secretions into the airway below the level of the vocal folds-is the most life-threatening immediate complication. When the body's protective cough reflex is also impaired (due to neurological injury), this leads to silent aspiration, which is particularly dangerous as it provides no clinical warning. Aspirated material can cause:
    - **Aspiration Pneumonia:** A bacterial infection of the lungs that is a leading cause of death and rehospitalization in patients with neurogenic dysphagia, with mortality rates reported to be as high as 20-50% in elderly populations (Almirall et al., 2013).
    - **Chemical Pneumonitis:** An inflammatory lung injury caused by the aspiration of sterile but acidic gastric contents.
    - **Airway Obstruction:** Partial or complete blockage of the airway by a food bolus.

1.2.2. Profound Psychosocial and Quality of Life Impact:

The experience of dysphagia erodes the very fabric of daily life and social interaction.

- **Mealtime Anxiety and Fear:** The act of eating, once a source of pleasure, becomes a source of terror, anxiety, and constant vigilance against choking.
- **Social Isolation and Depression:** The inability to participate in family meals, social gatherings, and cultural rituals involving food leads to profound lone-

liness, embarrassment, and clinical depression (Ekberg et al., 2002). Patients often withdraw to avoid the shame of drooling, spilling food, or coughing at the table.

- **Loss of Autonomy and Pleasure:** The need for assisted feeding, modified diets (e.g., pureed foods, thickened liquids), and prolonged mealtimes strips away independence and the simple joy of tasting and enjoying food.
- **Increased Caregiver Burden:** Family members and caregivers experience significant stress, anxiety, and time pressure in preparing special meals, supervising eating, and managing the constant fear of choking incidents (Mishra et al., 2026).

1.2.3. Sarcopenic Dysphagia and Aging

Sarcopenic dysphagia refers to swallowing impairment resulting from age-related loss of skeletal muscle mass and strength. Aging-associated sarcopenia affects the muscles involved in swallowing, leading to reduced tongue strength, delayed swallow initiation, and increased pharyngeal residue. This condition is increasingly recognized in elderly neurological patients and contributes to malnutrition, frailty, and poor clinical outcomes. Early identification and targeted nutritional and rehabilitative interventions are therefore essential.

1.2.4. Patient-Reported Outcome Measures in Dysphagia

In addition to physiological assessments, patient-reported outcome measures play an important role in dysphagia evaluation. Quality of life instruments such as the SWAL-QOL and Dysphagia Handicap Index capture the patient's perceived swallowing difficulty, emotional burden, and social impact. These tools complement objective assessments and support patient-centered clinical decision-making and treatment planning.

1.3. Prevalence and Populations at Risk

Dysphagia is exceptionally common in neurological populations, underscoring its status as a core symptom rather than a rare complication. Its prevalence demands routine and systematic screening.

- **Stroke:** Dysphagia is present in 37-78% of patients in the acute phase post-stroke. While it resolves in many, approximately 11-50% of patients continue to experience dysphagia at 6 months, a condition known as chronic post-stroke dysphagia, which is a strong predictor of long-term disability, mortality, and institutionalization (Arnold et al., 2016). Brainstem strokes carry the highest risk.

- **Neurodegenerative Diseases:**
  - **Parkinson's Disease:** Dysphagia affects over 80% of patients, often emerging in the later stages but sometimes appearing early. It is a leading cause of morbidity and mortality.
  - **Amyotrophic Lateral Sclerosis (ALS):** Nearly all patients with ALS will develop dysphagia as the disease progresses. In bulbar-onset ALS, it is a presenting symptom, making nutritional and respiratory management a central component of care from diagnosis.
  - **Multiple Sclerosis (MS):** Prevalence rates vary widely (30-40%), depending on the location of demyelinating plaques. Brainstem lesions can cause severe and acute dysphagia.
  - **Alzheimer's Disease and Other Dementias:** Dysphagia is highly prevalent in advanced stages, affecting a majority of patients. It is often under-recognized due to co-existing communication deficits and can manifest as apraxia of swallow, pacing issues, or refusal to eat.
- **Other Neurological Conditions:**
  - **Traumatic Brain Injury (TBI):** Prevalence ranges from 25-70%, resulting from diffuse axonal injury or focal cortical/brainstem damage.
  - **Myasthenia Gravis:** Causes fatigable weakness of the bulbar muscles, leading to dysphagia that worsens with repeated swallowing.
  - **Guillain-Barre Syndrome:** Can cause acute, severe dysphagia if the cranial nerves involved in swallowing are affected, often requiring temporary non-oral feeding.

The high prevalence across these diverse conditions highlights that dysphagia is a non-specific but critically important sign of neurological dysfunction. Its early identification and management are not optional components of care but essential pillars for improving survival, preventing complications, and preserving human dignity.

This overview highlights dysphagia as a complex, multifactorial condition with significant medical and psychosocial consequences. Understanding its clinical impact and prevalence across neurological populations provides the necessary foundation for exploring the specific neural mechanisms and disease-related patterns that underlie swallowing impairment.

2. NEUROLOGICAL ETIOLOGIES OF DYSPHAGIA: MAPPING THE NEURAL CIRCUITRY OF SWALLOWING

The human swallow is a masterpiece of neural engineering, requiring the precise coordination of cortical initiation, brainstem patterning, and peripheral nerve execution. When neurological disease disrupts this intricate network, dysphagia emerges not as a single entity, but as a spectrum of disorders whose specific characteristics are dictated by the location and nature of the neural insult. Understanding these etiologies is fundamental to targeted diagnosis and effective treatment.

2.1. Central Nervous System Disorders: The Disrupted Control Center

2.1.1. Stroke: The Acute Insult

Stroke represents the most common cause of neurogenic dysphagia, with its manifestations varying dramatically based on the lesion location:

- **Cortical and Subcortical Strokes:** Unilateral hemispheric strokes can cause significant dysphagia, challenging the historical belief that swallowing is primarily bilaterally represented. Key areas include:
    - o **Primary Sensorimotor Cortex:** Damage here leads to contralateral oral and facial weakness, resulting in drooling, poor bolus containment, and delayed oral transit.
    - o **Anterior Insula:** Crucial for sensorimotor integration and swallow planning. Lesions cause apraxia of swallow, where the voluntary initiation is impaired despite preserved reflex.
    - o **Frontal Operculum and Premotor Cortex:** Involved in the volitional control and sequencing of swallowing muscles.
    - o **White Matter Tracts:** Subcortical strokes affecting corticobulbar pathways disrupt communication between the cortex and brainstem, leading to incoordination.

The phenomenon of hemispheric dominance for swallowing has emerged, with left hemispheric strokes often causing more profound oral-phase problems (related to motor planning), while right hemispheric strokes may impair pharyngeal sensitivity and bolus clearance.

- **Brainstem Strokes:** These are particularly devastating as they directly damage the Swallowing Central Pattern Generator (SW-CPG) located in the medulla oblongata. The SW-CPG contains two main pools: a dorsal swallowing group (DSG) in the nucleus tractus solitarius for sensory integration and pattern initiation, and a ventral swallowing group (VSG) in the nucleus ambiguous for motor execution. Brainstem infarcts can cause:

- o Complete absence of the pharyngeal swallow reflex
- o Unilateral pharyngeal and laryngeal paralysis
- o Profound aspiration with minimal cough response
- o Combined dysphagia and dysphonia

2.1.2. Traumatic Brain Injury (TBI): The Multifocal Challenge

Dysphagia in TBI results from a combination of pathophysiological mechanisms:

- **Diffuse Axonal Injury (DAI):** Widespread shearing of white matter tracts disrupts the critical connections between cortical swallowing centers and the brainstem CPG, leading to severe discoordination and delayed triggering.
- **Focal Contusions:** Particularly in the frontal and temporal lobes, directly damage cortical swallowing centers.
- **Brainstem Involvement:** Direct injury to the medulla or midbrain disrupts the core swallowing network.
- **Cognitive-Comorbidities:** Impaired attention, executive function, and behavioral impulsivity significantly impact swallowing safety and mealtime endurance, independent of physical swallow function.

2.2. Neurodegenerative Diseases: The Progressive Unraveling

2.2.1. Parkinson's Disease (PD): Beyond Bradykinesia

Dysphagia in PD is not merely a late-stage complication but can be an early sign, often preceding the classic motor symptoms. The pathophysiology extends beyond the dopaminergic system to involve brainstem nuclei and peripheral nerves:

- **Bradykinesia and Rigidity:** Manifest as slow, repetitive tongue pumping (lingual festination), reduced pharyngeal contraction, and impaired upper esophageal sphincter (UES) relaxation.
- **Lewy Body Pathology:** The presence of Lewy bodies in the dorsal motor nucleus of the vagus nerve (cranial nerve X), the substantia nigra, and even the peripheral ganglia of the enteric nervous system points to a pervasive neural degradation affecting the entire swallowing network.

- **Specific Impairments:** Patients typically display piecemeal deglutition (swallowing a single bolus in multiple attempts), vallecular residue due to reduced tongue base retraction, and silent aspiration due to delayed laryngeal closure.

2.2.2. Amyotrophic Lateral Sclerosis (ALS): The Dual Attack

ALS's unique pathology of combined upper motor neuron (UMN) and lower motor neuron (LMN) degeneration creates a particularly severe and rapidly progressive dysphagia:

- **Upper Motor Neuron Signs:** Spasticity in the tongue and pharynx leads to slow, effortful movements and a hyperactive gag reflex.
- **Lower Motor Neuron Signs:** Flaccid weakness causes fasciculations in the tongue, poor palatal elevation (leading to nasal regurgitation), and a weak, ineffective cough-the latter being a critical deficit that removes the primary defense against aspiration.
- **Bulbar vs. Spinal Onset:** In bulbar-onset ALS, dysphagia is a presenting and dominant symptom, progressing rapidly. In spinal-onset, it emerges later but follows an equally devastating course.

2.2.3. Multiple Sclerosis (MS): The Unpredictable Adversary

The nature of dysphagia in MS is as variable as the disease itself, entirely dependent on plaque location:

- **Brainstem Plaques:** Lesions in the medulla, particularly affecting the nucleus tractus solitarius or nucleus ambiguous, can mimic a brainstem stroke, causing acute-onset, severe pharyngeal dysphagia and aspiration.
- **Cerebral Plaques:** Plaques in the internal capsule or cortical swallowing centers can disrupt sensorimotor signals, leading to oral-phase problems and reduced pharyngeal sensitivity.
- **Cerebellar Plaques:** Can cause ataxic dysphagia, characterized by incoordination and irregular timing of the swallow sequence.

2.3. Mechanism: The Neurophysiological Breakdown

The mechanism of dysphagia can be systematically understood by following the neural pathway of a normal swallow and identifying where specific diseases cause disruption:

1. Cortical Planning and Initiation (Voluntary Phase):

- o **Normal Function:** The pre-frontal and premotor cortices plan the swallow, which is then executed by the primary motor cortex. The insula integrates sensory information (taste, texture) to fine-tune the motor plan.
- o **Neurological Disruption:**
  - ▪ **Stroke/TBI:** Direct damage to these areas causes apraxia of swallow, delayed oral transit, and impaired sensory integration.
  - ▪ **PD:** Degeneration of basal ganglia-thalamocortical loops leads to bradykinesia and poor initiation.
  - ▪ **ALS:** UMN degeneration causes spasticity and slow movement.

2. Brainstem Patterning and Coordination (Involuntary Phase):

- o **Normal Function:** The SW-CPG in the medulla receives afferent signals and generates the stereotyped, sequential motor pattern for the pharyngeal swallow.
- o **Neurological Disruption:**
  - ▪ **Brainstem Stroke/MS:** Direct destruction of the DSG or VSG can abolish the swallow reflex entirely.
  - ▪ **PD:** Lewy body pathology in the brainstem nuclei delays the trigger and reduces the vigor of the pharyngeal response.
  - ▪ **ALS:** Degeneration of cranial nerve nuclei in the brainstem causes weak pharyngeal contraction and vocal fold paralysis.

3. Peripheral Nerve Execution and Muscular Contraction:

- o **Normal Function:** Cranial nerves V, VII, IX, X, and XII carry the final motor commands to the muscles of swallowing.
- o **Neurological Disruption:**
  - ▪ **ALS/GBS:** LMN degeneration or demyelination results in flaccid paralysis, fasciculations, and rapid muscle fatigue.
  - ▪ **MG:** Antibodies block acetylcholine receptors at the neuromuscular junction, causing fatigable weakness that worsens with repeated swallowing.

In summary, whether through acute infarction, progressive degeneration, or autoimmune attack, neurological diseases interrupt the seamless flow of commands along the neuraxis. The specific type of dysphagia that results-whether it is a failure to initiate, a delay in triggering, a weakness in execution, or a fatal combination thereof-provides a critical clue to the location and nature of the underlying neurological pathology. This understanding forms the bedrock upon which all subsequent assessment and treatment is built (Sharma et al., 2025).

3. CONVENTIONAL ASSESSMENT AND MANAGEMENT: THE CORNERSTONE OF DYSPHAGIA CARE

A systematic, evidence-based approach to the assessment and management of dysphagia is fundamental to improving patient safety, nutritional status, and quality of life. This process follows a logical hierarchy, beginning with screening and clinical evaluation to identify the presence and nature of the disorder, progressing to instrumental diagnostics to visualize the underlying physiology, and culminating in a personalized management plan that combines compensatory strategies with rehabilitative techniques. This comprehensive framework forms the bedrock of clinical practice for speech-language pathologists and the interdisciplinary team.

3.1. Clinical Assessment: The Frontline of Detection

The initial evaluation of dysphagia is a multi-faceted process designed to identify signs of swallowing impairment, determine the need for further testing, and initiate immediate management to reduce risk.

3.1.1. The Clinical/Bedside Swallow Evaluation (CSE/BSE)

This is a non-instrumental, behavioral assessment conducted at the patient's bedside or in the clinic. While it cannot rule out silent aspiration, it provides critical qualitative data. Its components include:

- **Comprehensive Patient History:**
    - Patient and caregiver reports of coughing, choking, gurgly voice, or sensation of food sticking.
    - Medical and surgical history, with a focus on neurological, pulmonary, and gastrointestinal conditions.
    - Current medication review, noting those that can cause xerostomia (dry mouth) or reduced alertness.
    - Detailed dietary history, including types of foods that cause difficulty and changes in mealtime duration.
- **Oral Motor and Sensory Examination:**

- **Structural Integrity:** Assessment of the lips, tongue, palate, and dentition.
    - **Motor Function:** Testing the strength, range of motion, and coordination of the oral and facial muscles. This includes observing for lingual fasciculations (suggestive of ALS) or a slow, repetitive tongue pump (suggestive of PD).
    - **Sensory Function:** Checking for response to light touch in the oral cavity and assessing gag reflex. It is crucial to note that an absent gag reflex does not necessarily predict aspiration, and its presence does not guarantee a safe swallow.
- **Observation of Trial Swallows:**
    - The patient is given small, controlled amounts of food and liquid of varying consistencies (typically starting with ice chips or thickened liquids), while the clinician observes for overt signs of difficulty, such as:
        - Oral residue in the cheek pouches or on the palate.
        - Delayed or absent laryngeal elevation.
        - Wet, gurgly vocal quality post-swallow (a key indicator of pharyngeal residue).
        - Coughing or throat clearing during or immediately after the swallow.
        - Watery eyes, nasal regurgitation, or behavioral signs of distress.

3.1.2. Standardized Screening Tools

These are brief, pass/fail protocols designed for rapid administration by nurses or other trained personnel to identify at-risk patients who require a full CSE. Their primary utility is in acute settings like stroke units.

- **The Water Swallow Test:** A common screen where the patient drinks a specific volume of water (e.g., 50-90ml) while being observed for signs of aspiration like cough or voice change. While sensitive, it has limitations in specificity and misses silent aspiration (Martino et al., 2000).
- **The Gugging Swallowing Screen (GUSS):** A more robust screen that uses small amounts of water and semi-solid food, assessing both swallowing ability and alertness. It has demonstrated high sensitivity and specificity in the stroke population.
- **The Toronto Bedside Swallowing Screening Test (TOR-BSST):** Another validated tool for stroke patients that includes an oral mechanism examination and trial swallows.

These assessment approaches are consistent with established clinical guidelines and consensus recommendations (Speyer et al., 2021).

3.2. Instrumental Diagnosis: Visualizing the Invisible

When dysphagia is suspected or its physiology needs precise characterization, instrumental assessments are the gold standard. They provide direct, dynamic visualization of the swallow, allowing for definitive diagnosis and targeted treatment planning.

3.2.1. Video fluoroscopic Swallow Study (VFSS) / Modified Barium Swallow (MBS)

This is a radiographic motion study conducted in conjunction with a speech-language pathologist and radiologist.

- **Procedure:** The patient swallows barium-coated foods and liquids of varying consistencies (thin liquid, pudding, cookie) while real-time X-ray (fluoroscopy) records the movement in a lateral (side) view, and often an anterior-posterior (front) view.
- **Key Capabilities:**
    - **Visualizes All Phases:** Provides a complete view of the oral, pharyngeal, and upper esophageal phases.
    - **Identifies Aspiration:** Precisely documents the timing (before, during, or after the swallow) and severity of aspiration.
    - **Quantifies Physiology:** Allows measurement of key kinematic events, such as hyoid bone excursion and upper esophageal sphincter opening.
    - **Tests Compensatory Strategies:** The efficacy of postural changes (e.g., chin tuck, head rotation) and therapeutic maneuvers can be evaluated in real-time (Jones, 2003).
- **Limitations:** Involves radiation exposure (though minimal) and requires patient transport to the radiology suite.

3.2.2. Fiberoptic Endoscopic Evaluation of Swallowing (FEES)

This procedure uses a flexible fiberoptic or digital endoscope passed transnasally to view the pharyngeal and laryngeal structures.

- **Procedure:** The examination occurs before, during, and after the swallow of foods and liquids dyed for visibility.

- **Key Capabilities:**
  - o **Superior Anatomy View:** Provides an unparalleled view of structures, secretion management, and vocal fold movement.
  - o **Identifies Residue:** Clearly shows the location and amount of residue in the valleculae and pyriform sinuses after the swallow.
  - o **Assesses Sensory Function:** Can be paired with a sensory test (FEESST) using air pulses to assess laryngeal adductor reflex, a marker of sensory integrity.
  - o **No Radiation:** Can be performed at the bedside, making it ideal for ICU or immobile patients (Langmore et al., 1988).
- **Limitations:** The view is temporarily obscured during the pharyngeal swallow due to pharyngeal constriction (the "white-out" period), so the moment of swallow itself is not visualized.

3.3. Core Management: A Triad of Intervention Strategies

Management is tailored to the specific physiologic deficits identified and aims to improve safety (prevent aspiration), enhance efficiency (reduce residue), and ensure adequate nutrition/hydration.

3.3.1. Diet Modifications and Compensatory Strategies

These are immediate interventions to reduce risk while more long-term rehabilitation takes effect.

- **Diet Modifications:**
  - o **Texture Modification:** Using the International Dysphagia Diet Standardisation Initiative (IDDSI) framework to standardize food textures (e.g., pureed, minced) and liquid viscosities (e.g., mildly thick, moderately thick). Thickened liquids slow bolus flow, giving more time to trigger a pharyngeal swallow, while soft foods require less chewing effort (Cichero et al., 2017).
  - o **Behavioral Strategies:** Includes pacing (small bites/sips), alternating solids and liquids, and ensuring upright positioning.
- **Compensatory Postures and Maneuvers:**
  - o **Chin Tuck:** Narrows the entrance to the airway and widens the valleculae, often redirecting the bolus away from the airway in cases of delayed swallow trigger.

- o **Head Rotation:** Turning the head to the weaker side directs the bolus down the stronger side of the pharynx, useful for unilateral pharyngeal weakness.
- o **Head Tilt:** Tilting the head toward the stronger side uses gravity to clear residue from the weaker side.

These management strategies are widely recommended in evidence-based dysphagia practice guidelines (Cichero et al., 2017).

3.3.2. Rehabilitative Exercises

These exercises are designed to directly improve the strength, range of motion, and coordination of the swallowing musculature, promoting neuroplasticity and lasting improvement.

- **The Shaker Exercise (Head Lift):** A isometric and isotonic head-raising exercise that strengthens the suprahyoid muscles, thereby improving the opening of the upper esophageal sphincter. It is strongly evidence-based for reducing pharyngeal residue.
- **The Effortful Swallow:** Increases posterior tongue base movement and pharyngeal contraction, helping to clear residue.
- **The Mendelsohn Maneuver:** Voluntarily prolonging laryngeal elevation at the peak of the swallow, which improves the duration and width of UES opening.
- **Expiratory Muscle Strength Training (EMST):** Uses a calibrated device to overload the expiratory muscles, generating a stronger and more effective cough-a critical defense mechanism against aspiration (Robbins et al., 2005).

In cases of severe dysphagia where oral intake is unsafe or insufficient, alternative nutrition via a nasogastric (NG) tube or percutaneous endoscopic gastrostomy (PEG) tube may be necessary to protect the airway and meet metabolic demands while rehabilitation continues.

Table 1. Clinical decision-making in neurogenic dysphagia

Physiological impairment	Assessment finding	Suggested intervention
Delayed swallow initiation	Premature spillage, aspiration before swallow on VFSS	Chin tuck posture, thermal-tactile stimulation
Reduced tongue base retraction	Vallecular residue on VFSS/FEES	Effortful swallow, tongue base exercises
Reduced laryngeal elevation	Aspiration during swallow, reduced hyoid movement	Mendelsohn maneuver, Shaker exercise
Poor upper esophageal sphincter opening	Pyriform sinus residue, restricted UES opening on VFSS	Shaker exercise, postural adjustments
Weak cough / airway protection	Silent aspiration, reduced cough strength	Expiratory muscle strength training (EMST)

Clinical decision-making in dysphagia management should be driven by specific physiological findings identified during instrumental assessment. For instance, delayed swallow initiation may be addressed using sensory enhancement techniques and postural strategies such as the chin tuck, whereas reduced tongue base retraction benefits from effortful swallowing and tongue base strengthening exercises. Impaired laryngeal elevation and airway protection may require maneuvers such as the Mendelsohn maneuver and expiratory muscle strength training, while restricted upper esophageal sphincter opening may be managed through Shaker exercises or targeted postural adjustments. Such physiology-driven intervention selection supports individualized, evidence-based dysphagia rehabilitation.

Conventional clinical and instrumental assessments form the cornerstone of dysphagia diagnosis and guide initial management decisions. While these approaches remain fundamental, advances in technology are increasingly enhancing diagnostic precision and therapeutic effectiveness, complementing traditional dysphagia care (Sharma et al., 2026).

4. TECHNOLOGICAL INNOVATIONS IN DYSPHAGIA CARE: PIONEERING THE FUTURE OF DIAGNOSIS AND REHABILITATION

The field of dysphagia management is undergoing a profound transformation, driven by rapid technological advancement. While conventional methods remain the foundation, a new wave of innovations is enhancing our diagnostic precision, expanding our therapeutic arsenal, and fundamentally reshaping the delivery of care. These technologies are pushing the boundaries of neurorehabilitation, offering hope for more effective, engaging, and personalized treatment paradigms that leverage the brain's inherent capacity for plasticity.

4.1. Advanced Diagnostics: Beyond the Naked Eye

The quest for objective, quantitative, and highly sensitive diagnostic tools has led to the development of technologies that reveal the intricate biomechanics of swallowing in unprecedented detail.

4.1.1. High-Resolution Pharyngeal Manometry (HRPM)

This technology represents a quantum leap beyond traditional manometry. It employs a catheter with 20-36 closely spaced solid-state pressure sensors to create a dynamic, spatiotemporal map of pressure events throughout the pharynx and esophagus.

- **Clinical Applications and Insights:**
  - **Quantifying Impairment:** HRPM provides precise metrics for pharyngeal contractile vigor, the timing and completeness of upper esophageal sphincter (UES) relaxation, and the pressure gradient driving the bolus. This allows clinicians to move beyond subjective descriptions like "weak swallow" to objective measurements, such as "pharyngeal peak pressure of 120 mmHg," enabling precise tracking of progress.
  - **Identifying Subtle Pathophysiology:** It can detect disorders of UES opening that are not due to muscular failure but to poor biomechanical coordination-specifically, inadequate anterior traction by the suprahyoid muscles, a distinction invisible to VFSS or FEES.
  - **Biofeedback:** The real-time pressure topography plot serves as a powerful visual biofeedback tool, allowing patients to "see" their swallow and learn to modulate it, a technique known as *manometry-guided biofeedback* (Cock & Omari, 2017).

At present, high-resolution pharyngeal manometry is increasingly used in specialized clinical centers and remains limited to advanced diagnostic facilities.

4.1.2. Advanced and Adjunctive Imaging

- **Dynamic MRI:** While technically challenging due to the speed of swallowing, research protocols using real-time MRI are providing stunning, radiation-free visualization of the entire swallowing tract in multiple planes. This offers unparalleled insights into the complex motion of all structures simultaneously.

- **CT Scans and Diffusion Tensor Imaging (DTI):** High-resolution CT can detail anatomical abnormalities, while DTI, an MRI technique, can map the white matter tracts connecting cortical swallowing centers to the brainstem. This is particularly valuable in stroke and TBI for understanding the neural disconnection underlying dysphagia.

4.2. Novel Therapeutics: Harnessing Technology for Recovery

Therapeutic approaches are becoming more targeted and intensive, moving beyond voluntary exercises to directly modulate the nervous system and provide precise, measurable feedback.

4.2.1. Neuromodulation: Priming the Brain for Plasticity

These non-invasive brain stimulation (NIBS) techniques aim to modulate cortical excitability, thereby enhancing the brain's responsiveness to traditional swallowing therapy.

- **Transcranial Direct Current Stimulation (tDCS):** This technique applies a weak, constant electrical current (1-2 mA) through scalp electrodes placed over the swallowing motor cortex.
    - **Mechanism:** Anodal tDCS increases neuronal excitability, while cathodal tDCS decreases it. In dysphagia rehabilitation, anodal stimulation is typically applied to the undamaged hemisphere (in stroke) to promote interhemispheric balance or to the damaged hemisphere to facilitate local recovery.
    - **Evidence:** A growing body of evidence, including meta-analyses, suggests that tDCS as an adjunct to traditional swallowing exercises can lead to greater and more rapid improvements in swallowing function post-stroke (He et al., 2022).

tDCS is increasingly being explored as an adjunct to conventional swallowing therapy, primarily within specialized centers and research-guided clinical settings.

- **Repetitive Transcranial Magnetic Stimulation (rTMS):** This technique uses a powerful, rapidly changing magnetic field to induce electrical currents in the underlying cortex.
    - **Mechanism:** High-frequency rTMS (e.g., 5-10 Hz) increases cortical excitability, while low-frequency rTMS (e.g., 1 Hz) decreases it. For post-stroke dysphagia, high-frequency rTMS may be applied to the un-

affected hemisphere to counteract its potential inhibitory influence (interhemispheric inhibition) on the damaged side.

- **Application:** rTMS is being investigated not only for stroke but also for dysphagia in Parkinson's disease and other neurological conditions, showing promise in "priming" the brain before a therapy session.

rTMS remains largely limited to experimental and research-oriented applications, with emerging but not yet widespread routine clinical use.

4.2.2. Advanced Biofeedback and Robotics

- **Surface Electromyography (sEMG) Biofeedback:** Electrodes placed on the submental (under-chin) muscles provide patients with a visual representation of their muscle activity during swallowing exercises. This helps them achieve a more effective effortful swallow or Mendelsohn maneuver by providing an external target for their effort.
- **Robotic-Assisted Therapy:** For patients with severe oral weakness, robotic devices are being developed to provide assistive or resistive training for the tongue and jaw. These devices can deliver highly consistent, repetitive, and quantifiable exercise, a key driver of neuroplasticity, which can be difficult to achieve with traditional methods alone.

4.3. Digital Health: The Connected Ecosystem of Care

Digital technology is democratizing and decentralizing dysphagia care, making it more continuous, accessible, and data-driven.

- **Sensor-based Wearables:** Small, discreet accelerometers or piezoelectric sensors attached to the skin of the neck (larynx) can continuously monitor swallowing frequency, cough strength, and ingestion activities in a patient's natural environment. This provides ecologically valid, objective data on functional swallowing behavior over days or weeks, moving far beyond the snapshot provided by a single clinical assessment. This is invaluable for tracking disease progression in conditions like ALS or PD and for monitoring adherence to home exercise programs.
- **Telepractice (Telerehabilitation):** The use of secure videoconferencing platforms to deliver assessment and therapy remotely has exploded in relevance. It breaks down critical barriers related to geography, mobility, and transportation.

- **Capabilities:** Clinicians can conduct live coaching of exercises, provide visual biofeedback via screen sharing, review food diaries, and offer counseling and caregiver training.
- **Evidence:** Studies have shown that telerehabilitation for dysphagia is feasible, safe, and can produce outcomes equivalent to in-person care for many patients, ensuring continuity of care and improving access for underserved populations (Ward et al., 2022).

- **Mobile Health (mHealth) Applications:** A proliferation of smartphone apps now supports dysphagia management. These apps can:
  - Provide video-guided exercise programs with reminders and progress tracking.
  - Offer educational content about dysphagia and safe swallowing strategies.
  - Facilitate communication between patients and clinicians through symptom logging.
  - Enhance motivation and adherence through gamification elements.

These technological innovations are not meant to replace the skilled clinician but to empower them with deeper insights, more powerful tools, and broader reach, ultimately leading to better, more personalized, and more accessible care for every patient with dysphagia.

These instrumental techniques are considered standard diagnostic tools in the evaluation of neurogenic dysphagia (Jones, 2003; Langmore et al., 1988).

Wearable sensors and artificial intelligence–based tools for dysphagia assessment and rehabilitation are largely in the developmental and research phase, with limited routine clinical implementation at present. (Clavé et al., 2023).

Table 2. Emerging technologies in dysphagia management: level of evidence and current clinical applicability

Technology	Level of Evidence	Current Clinical Use
High-resolution pharyngeal manometry (HRPM)	Moderate–High	Used in specialized centers for detailed assessment of pharyngeal pressure dynamics and UES function
Transcranial direct current stimulation (tDCS)	Moderate (emerging evidence)	Adjunct therapy in post-stroke dysphagia to enhance neuroplasticity alongside conventional swallowing exercises
Repetitive transcranial magnetic stimulation (rTMS)	Low–Moderate (research-oriented)	Primarily used in experimental and research-guided clinical settings

continued on following page

Table 2. Continued

Technology	Level of Evidence	Current Clinical Use
Surface EMG biofeedback	Moderate	Supports rehabilitation by improving patient engagement and accuracy of swallowing exercises
Wearable sensor–based monitoring	Low–Moderate	Research and pilot use for remote monitoring of swallowing frequency and adherence
Tele-rehabilitation (telepractice)	Moderate–High	Increasingly used for home-based dysphagia therapy and follow-up, especially in resource-limited settings

Emerging diagnostic and therapeutic technologies offer promising opportunities to augment conventional dysphagia management. However, their integration into routine practice requires careful consideration of clinical evidence and applicability. These evolving approaches also inform future research directions and the development of more personalized and technology-driven care models.

5. FUTURE DIRECTIONS: THE NEXT FRONTIER IN DYSPHAGIA MANAGEMENT

The trajectory of dysphagia care is set towards an era of unprecedented precision, personalization, and predictive power. The convergence of advanced computational methods, a deeper understanding of neurobiology, and evolving healthcare models is paving the way for a fundamental shift from reactive management to proactive, patient-centric restoration of function. This section explores the most promising frontiers that will define the next decade of research and clinical practice (Sharma et al., 2026).

5.1. The Integration of Artificial Intelligence and Machine Learning

AI and ML are poised to move from research tools to clinical co-pilots, augmenting human expertise and extracting novel insights from complex data.

- **Automated and Objective Analysis of Instrumental Assessments:** AI algorithms, particularly deep learning models, are being trained to analyze VFSS and FEES recordings with superhuman precision. These systems can automatically track kinematic parameters (hyoid displacement, pharyngeal constriction ratio), identify and quantify residue, and detect aspiration events with high reliability. This will standardize interpretation, reduce inter-rater variability, and free up clinician time for higher-level decision-making (Lee et al., 2017). The future may see AI providing a instant, quantitative "swallow report" as a standard output from every instrumental exam.

- **Predictive Analytics for Risk Stratification and Prognosis:** By integrating vast datasets from electronic health records-including neuroimaging, comorbidity profiles, and clinical swallow exam findings-ML models can predict an individual's risk of developing dysphagia upon admission, their likelihood of recovery, and their potential response to specific interventions. This enables proactive, preventative care, allowing resources to be focused on the highest-risk patients from day one.
- **Intelligent Biofeedback and Adaptive Therapy Systems:** Future therapy will be guided by AI that adapts in real-time. Imagine a biofeedback system that uses computer vision to analyze a patient's performance via a tablet camera and dynamically adjusts the difficulty of a swallowing exercise or the parameters of neuromuscular electrical stimulation to maintain an optimal challenge level, thereby maximizing neuroplasticity.

Recent advances in artificial intelligence have further enhanced automated analysis of swallowing kinematics and aspiration risk, supporting more objective and standardized dysphagia assessment (Seo et al., 2024).

5.2. The Rise of Personalized and Precision Medicine

The one-size-fits-all model is becoming obsolete. The future lies in tailoring every aspect of care to the individual's unique pathophysiology, genetics, and personal goals.

- **Physiology-Driven Rehabilitation Paradigms:** Treatment selection will be increasingly dictated by the specific physiologic deficit, as identified by advanced diagnostics like HRPM and AI-enhanced imaging. A patient with poor UES opening due to weak suprahyoid muscles will receive a fundamentally different regimen (e.g., Shaker exercise, neurostimulation targeting suprahyoid motor points) than a patient with impaired UES opening due to poor pharyngeal propulsion.
- **Biomarkers and Genomics:** Research is actively seeking biomarkers that can predict susceptibility to dysphagia or capacity for recovery. This could include:
    - o **Genetic Profiling:** Identifying gene variants associated with neuroplasticity or specific neurodegenerative processes that influence swallowing deterioration.

- Serum or Salivary Biomarkers: Molecules indicative of neural injury or inflammation that correlate with dysphagia severity and recovery trajectory.
- **Neurophysiological Biomarkers:** Using TMS to measure cortical excitability and integrity of corticobulbar pathways to predict responsiveness to neuromodulation therapies.

- **Patient-Specific Functional Goals and Shared Decision-Making:** Personalized medicine incorporates the patient's priorities into the treatment plan. Through shared decision-making tools, therapy will be aligned with personally meaningful outcomes, whether that is safely drinking a cup of coffee, eating a holiday meal with family, or simply managing secretions independently. This enhances motivation, adherence, and the real-world relevance of therapeutic gains (Dziewas et al., 2023).

5.3. Emerging Trends in Diagnosis and Remote Treatment

The delivery of care will continue to evolve, becoming more decentralized, continuous, and integrated into daily life.

- **The "Digital Swallowing Twin":** The concept of creating a computer-based model of an individual's swallowing mechanism, informed by their structural and physiological data, could allow clinicians to simulate the effects of different treatments virtually before applying them in the real world.
- **Advanced Remote Monitoring and "The Internet of Medical Things (IoMT):** Future wearables will go beyond counting swallows to analyzing swallow efficiency and safety using multi-sensor data fusion (e.g., combining accelerometery with acoustic analysis). Smart utensils could monitor eating pace and weight of intake, while environmental sensors could track hydration. This creates a continuous, holistic picture of a patient's swallowing health outside the clinic.
- **Regenerative Medicine and Advanced Neurostimulation:** Looking further ahead, techniques such as stem cell therapy for neuronal repair and more targeted, closed-loop neuromodulation systems that deliver stimulation only when a swallow is attempted (or when an aspiration risk is detected) represent the cutting edge of restorative interventions.

Together, conventional principles and technological advancements underscore the need for an integrated, evidence-based, and patient-centered approach to dysphagia management.

6. CONCLUSION: SYNTHESIZING THE PRESENT, ENVISIONING THE FUTURE

Dysphagia in neurological disorders is a formidable challenge that sits at the intersection of neurology, rehabilitation, and quality of life. This chapter has journeyed from the foundational understanding of dysphagia as a complex symptom with profound medical and psychosocial consequences, through the detailed exploration of its neurological underpinnings-where specific lesions and diseases produce predictable patterns of impairment.

We have established that the cornerstone of effective management remains a rigorous, conventional approach: systematic screening, comprehensive clinical and instrumental assessment to pinpoint the pathophysiology, and the diligent application of evidence-based compensatory and rehabilitative strategies. This foundation is now being powerfully augmented by a wave of technological innovation. Advanced diagnostics like HRPM provide unparalleled physiological insight, while novel therapeutics such as neuromodulation (tDCS, rTMS) directly target the central nervous system to promote recovery. The digital health revolution, through telepractice and wearables, is breaking down traditional barriers to care, making continuous, accessible support a reality.

The future, as outlined, is bright with the promise of AI-driven precision, personalized treatment protocols, and a healthcare model that is predictive rather than reactive. The integration of these advanced technologies into standard clinical workflows will be the next great challenge and opportunity.

In conclusion, the management of neurogenic dysphagia is a dynamic and rapidly evolving field. The ultimate goal remains constant: to preserve the safety, dignity, and profound human experience of eating for every individual. By combining time-honoured clinical skills with cutting-edge innovation, and by always centering the patient's goals, clinicians can continue to push the boundaries of what is possible, turning the simple act of swallowing from a source of fear back into a source of comfort and connection.

REFERENCES

Almirall, J., Rofes, L., Serra-Prat, M., Icart, R., Palomera, E., Arreola, V., & Clavé, P. (2013). Oropharyngeal dysphagia is a risk factor for readmission for pneumonia in very elderly persons: An observational prospective study. *The Journals of Gerontology: Series A. Biomedical Sciences and Medical Sciences, 69*(3), 330–337. DOI: 10.1093/gerona/glt099

Arnold, M., Liesirova, K., Broeg-Morvay, A., Meisterernst, J., Schlager, M., Mono, M. L., El-Koussy, M., Kägi, G., Jung, S., & Sarikaya, H. (2016). Dysphagia in acute stroke: Incidence, burden and impact on clinical outcome. *PLoS One, 11*(2), e0148424. DOI: 10.1371/journal.pone.0148424 PMID: 26863627

Cichero, J. A. Y., Lam, P., Steele, C. M., Hanson, B., Chen, J., Dantas, R. O., Duivestein, J., Kayashita, J., Lecko, C., Murray, J., Pillay, M., Riquelme, L., & Stanschus, S. (2017). Development of international terminology and definitions for texture-modified foods and thickened fluids used in dysphagia management: The IDDSI framework. *Dysphagia, 32*(2), 293–314. DOI: 10.1007/s00455-016-9758-y PMID: 27913916

Clavé, P., Arreola, V., Romea, M., Medina, L., Palomera, E., & Serra-Prat, M. (2023). Oropharyngeal dysphagia: New diagnostic and therapeutic strategies. *Nature Reviews. Gastroenterology & Hepatology.*

Cock, C., & Omari, T. (2017). Diagnosis of swallowing disorders: How we interpret pharyngeal manometry. *Current Gastroenterology Reports, 19*(3), 11. Advance online publication. DOI: 10.1007/s11894-017-0552-2 PMID: 28289859

Crary, M. A., Carnaby-Mann, G. D., Miller, L., Antonios, N., & Silliman, S. (2006). Dysphagia and nutritional status at the time of hospital admission for ischemic stroke. *Journal of Stroke and Cerebrovascular Diseases, 15*(4), 164–171. DOI: 10.1016/j.jstrokecerebrovasdis.2006.05.006 PMID: 17904070

Dziewas, R., Warnecke, T., Hamacher, C., & Suntrup-Krueger, S. (2023). Dysphagia diagnostics and therapy in the era of digitalization and artificial intelligence. *Dysphagia.*

Ekberg, O., Hamdy, S., Woisard, V., Wuttge-Hannig, A., & Ortega, P. (2002). Social and psychological burden of dysphagia: Its impact on diagnosis and treatment. *Dysphagia, 17*(2), 139–146. DOI: 10.1007/s00455-001-0113-5 PMID: 11956839

He, K., Li, J., Wang, Y., & Zhang, Y. (2022). Efficacy and safety of transcranial direct current stimulation on post-stroke dysphagia: A systematic review and meta-analysis. *Journal of Clinical Medicine*, *11*(9), 2297. Advance online publication. DOI: 10.3390/jcm11092297 PMID: 35566421

Jones, B. (Ed.). (2003). *Normal and abnormal swallowing: Imaging in diagnosis and therapy* (2nd ed.). Springer., DOI: 10.1007/978-0-387-22434-3

Langmore, S. E., Schatz, K., & Olson, N. (1988). Fiberoptic endoscopic examination of swallowing safety: A new procedure. *Dysphagia*, *2*(4), 216–219. DOI: 10.1007/BF02414429 PMID: 3251697

Lee, J. W., Randall, D. R., Evangelista, L. M., Kuhn, M. A., & Belafsky, P. C. (2017). Subjective assessment of videofluoroscopic swallow studies. *Otolaryngology - Head and Neck Surgery*, *156*(5), 901–905. DOI: 10.1177/0194599817691276 PMID: 28195753

Martino, R., Pron, G., & Diamant, N. (2000). Screening for oropharyngeal dysphagia in stroke: Insufficient evidence for guidelines. *Dysphagia*, *15*(1), 19–30. DOI: 10.1007/s004559910006 PMID: 10594255

Mishra, R., Sharma, P., Sharma, B., & Kumari, A. (2026). Phototherapeutics in neurodegenerative disorders: Present insights and emerging horizons. In *Phototherapeutic approaches to neurodegeneration*. Springer Nature., DOI: 10.1007/978-981-95-4751-7

Robbins, J., Gangnon, R. E., Theis, S. M., Kays, S. A., Hewitt, A. L., & Hind, J. A. (2005). The effects of lingual exercise on swallowing in older adults. *Journal of the American Geriatrics Society*, *53*(9), 1483–1489. DOI: 10.1111/j.1532-5415.2005.53467.x PMID: 16137276

Seo, H. G., Kim, K., Lee, W. H., & Oh, B. M. (2024). Artificial intelligence–assisted analysis of swallowing function: Current status and future perspectives. *Journal of Neuroengineering and Rehabilitation*.

Sharma, P., Mishra, R., & Sharma, B. (2026). Global approaches to mental health in the era of climate-driven migration. In *Mental health interventions for climate emergency displacement* (pp. 95–124). IGI Global Scientific Publishing., DOI: 10.4018/979-8-3373-3281-9.ch004

Sharma, P., Mishra, R., Sharma, B., Kumari, A., & Modgil, S. (2025). Health sciences: Advancing healthcare through interdisciplinary approaches and innovation. *International Journal of Multidisciplinary: Applied Business and Education Research*, *6*(5), 2309–2316. DOI: 10.11594/ijmaber.06.05.17

Sharma, P., Mishra, R., Sharma, B., Kumari, A., & Sharma, V. (2026). Polygenic and oligogenic risk in congenital heart disease: A systems view of multifactorial etiology. In *The multifactorial etiology of congenital heart disease: Insights from teratology, genetics, and exposomics* (pp. 167–198). IGI Global Scientific Publishing., DOI: 10.4018/979-8-3373-3735-7.ch006

Speyer, R., Cordier, R., Farneti, D., Nascimento, W., Pilz, W., Verin, E., Walshe, M., & Woisard, V. (2021). White paper by the European Society for Swallowing Disorders: Screening and non-instrumental assessment for dysphagia in adults. *Dysphagia*, *37*(2), 333–349. DOI: 10.1007/s00455-021-10283-7 PMID: 33787994

Suttrup, I., & Warnecke, T. (2016). Dysphagia in Parkinson's disease. *Dysphagia*, *31*(1), 24–32. DOI: 10.1007/s00455-015-9671-9 PMID: 26590572

Ward, E. C., Raatz, M., Marshall, J., & Burns, C. L. (2022). Telepractice and dysphagia management: The era of COVID-19 and beyond. *Dysphagia*, *37*(6), 1386–1399. DOI: 10.1007/s00455-022-10444-2 PMID: 35428923

About the Contributors

Soultana Papadopoulou is an Assistant Professor in the Department of Speech and Language Therapy at the University of Ioannina, holding a PhD in Physical Medicine and Rehabilitation with a dissertation on dysphagia and related disorders. Her academic and clinical career is distinguished by extensive research, teaching, and clinical expertise in the assessment and management of dysphagia across the lifespan, with a particular emphasis on pediatric and neurogenic populations. Dr. Papadopoulou has authored and co-authored numerous peer-reviewed articles and book chapters on dysphagia, including innovative approaches to diagnosis, intervention, and the use of technology in swallowing disorders. She has served as a scientific editor for key textbooks on pediatric dysphagia and clinical swallowing management, and has been an invited speaker and educator in international academic settings. Her work is recognized for advancing multidisciplinary, evidence-based practices in dysphagia, contributing significantly to both clinical protocols and academic literature.

***

Eren Balo is an SLP-PhD and works as an assistant professor in the Department of Speech and Language Therapy, Faculty of Health Sciences, at Anadolu University, Türkiye. His research interests are voice and swallowing disorders, professional voice, and cleft palate speech.

Namık Yücel Birol is an Assistant Professor and Head of the Department of Speech and Language Therapy at Cappadocia University, School of Health Sciences. He received his bachelor's degree in Physiotherapy and Rehabilitation from Muğla Sıtkı Koçman University in 2015, his master's degree in Speech and Language Therapy from İstanbul Medipol University in 2019, and his PhD in Speech and Language Therapy from the same institution in 2023. Over the course of his professional career, he has worked in hospitals, special education and rehabilitation centers, and university practice and research centers. He served as a lecturer from 2020 to 2024 and has continued his academic work as an Assistant Professor since 2024. He has also undertaken various administrative roles, including rector's advisor, head and vice head of department, and assistant director of an practice and research center. Dr. Birol has published in national and international peer-reviewed journals, presented at academic conferences, and contributed to book chapters in his field.

Büşra Çınar is a Research Assistant in the Department of Speech and Language Therapy at Üsküdar University, Istanbul, Turkey. Her professional and research interests focus on voice disorders, swallowing disorders, and early communication development. She contributes to clinical practice, undergraduate education, and interdisciplinary projects related to voice health, dysphagia management, and developmental communication.

Seren Düzenli Öztürk, MSc (SLP), PhD (Neuroscience), is an Assistant Professor at the Department of Speech and Language Therapy, İzmir Bakirçay University. Her research focuses on neurogenic speech and language disorders and dysphagia, with interests in neuroimaging, brain potentials and oscillations, and the neurophysiology of language.

Efthymia Efthymiou, Associate Professor at Zayed University (UAE), studies inclusive teaching, classroom discourse, and learning environments that enable every student with disabilities to belong and participate. She brings this lens to medical education, promoting disability-competent, technology-enhanced training. She also works with UAE federal schools to turn research on inclusion and digital access into classroom practice.

İbrahim Erensoy is a Speech and Language Therapist whose academic and clinical work focuses on swallowing and communication disorders. His primary research interests include neurogenic dysphagia, instrumental swallowing assessment methods such as FEES, and clinical decision-making in dysphagia management. He has been involved in clinical practice and academic research related to swallowing disorders and contributes to studies aimed at improving evidence-based assessment and rehabilitation approaches for individuals with dysphagia.

H. Vidyalakshmi is a faculty member in the Department of Nutrition and Dietetics, School of Life Sciences, at the Ooty campus of JSS Academy of Higher Education and Research, Mysuru, Tamil Nadu. Her academic and research interests span across Food Biotechnology, Sports Nutrition, Nutraceuticals, Artificial Intelligence applications in healthcare, and Public Health Nutrition. With a strong commitment to advancing nutritional science, she actively engages in teaching, research, and the promotion of evidence-based nutritional practices, contributing significantly to the well-being and knowledge development of her students and the broader community.

Ambika Nand Jha is a Pharm.D. graduate from Gujarat Technological University, Ahmedabad, with an excellent CGPA of 9.49 His academic interests focus on Pharmacy Practice and Clinical Pharmacy, with active involvement in research and scholarly activities. He has published 50+ peer-reviewed articles, including 14 research papers, 17 review articles, and 15 case reports in reputed national and international journals. Two of his publications are indexed in Q1 journals, highlighting the quality and impact of his research. He has received multiple grants from the Gujarat State Pharmacy Council for organizing academic events and has been awarded travel grants twice by the Department of Science and Technology (DST), Government of India. Dr. Jha continues to contribute actively to evidence-based clinical pharmacy practice, research, and education.

K. Naresh Babu is a distinguished academician, administrator, and healthcare professional in the field of Occupational Therapy, with an extensive career dedicated to education, leadership, and professional excellence. He is currently serving as the Dean cum Principal of Sree Abirami College of Occupational Therapy (SACOOT), Coimbatore, Tamil Nadu. The institution is affiliated to The Tamil Nadu Dr. M.G.R. Medical University, Chennai, one of the premier medical universities in India. Dr. Naresh Babu is associated with the Department of Occupational Therapy, where he has played a pivotal role in strengthening academic standards, curriculum development, and institutional growth. As an academic leader, he has been instrumental in shaping the vision and mission of SACOOT, ensuring quality education, ethical professional practice, and holistic development of students. With his rich experience in teaching, administration, and academic governance, Dr. Naresh Babu has significantly contributed to the advancement of occupational therapy education. His leadership as Dean cum Principal reflects his commitment to academic excellence, student-centered learning, faculty development, and compliance with regulatory and accreditation standards. Under his guidance, the college has continued to progress in academic delivery, clinical training, and community-oriented healthcare services. Dr. Naresh Babu is deeply involved in fostering an environment that promotes interdisciplinary learning, research orientation, and evidence-based clinical practice. He actively encourages innovation, professional ethics, and lifelong learning among students and faculty members. His administrative acumen and academic insight have helped in strengthening institutional policies, academic planning, and quality assurance mechanisms. As a professional in occupational therapy education, Dr. Naresh Babu remains committed to enhancing the role of occupational therapists in healthcare delivery and rehabilitation services. His contributions extend beyond the classroom through academic mentoring, institutional leadership, and service to the profession.

Ahmet Konrot, Dip.Ed., Dip. ALPTE, PhD, LCST, Lidcombe Cert., DKTD He was born in Eskişehir in 1948. He graduated from Eskişehir Maarif College in 1967 and attended Gazi Teachers' Training Institute English Department. He worked for Siirt Batman Lyceé and Eskişehir Economic and Commercial Sciences Academy as an English teacher. He was awarded with a grant from the Turkish Ministry of Education to study abroad and received his Post Graduate Diploma in Applied Linguistics, Phonetics and Teaching of English (1978) and PhD in Linguistics -Experimental Phonetics (1982) at Essex University (UK). During his doctoral studies, he was awarded with a grant by the British Government to study speech and language therapy. He attended a post graduate course at The School for Human Communication Studies in London and became a licenced speech and language therapist (LCST) in 1984. He returned to Turkey and worked for Anadolu University. There, he was first appointed at the Education Faculty and assumed an active role in the establishment of Special Education Department. At the same time, he founded a small speech therapy unit first, at Anadolu University Hospital, then at the Education Faculty of the same university. He initiated a movement to transform this unit as an applied research and education center (DİLKOM) accredited by the Turkish Higher Education Board (YÖK). Initiated a postgraduate program in speech and language disorders to train the first speech and language therapists in Turkey, hence established the core faculty to support this center. He worked for the same university for many years as an assistant professor (1984-1988), associate professor (1988-1993) and full professor (1993-2005) in the fields of special education and speech and language disorders. He also had administrative duties and served as the deputy head of the Educational Sciences Department (1985-1989), Special Education Department Head (1989-1994), deputy dean (1991-1996) and dean (1996-1999) of the Education Faculty. He taught undergraduate and graduate level courses at Bolu Abant İzzet Baysal, Ankara, and Osmangazi Universities. He offered in-service certificate courses for the Turkish Ministry of Education. Together with his ENT colleague Assoc. Prof. Dr. Bekir Altay (MD), they performed the first cochlear implant operation in Turkey in 1986. As a speech and language therapist member of the cochlear implant team, he assumed responsibility in pre-operative evaluation and post-operative rehabilitation of cochlear implant patients. He served at the Higher Board for Disabled Persons affiliated to the Prime Minister's Office upon his appointment by the Prime Minister to represent the Universities in Turkey (1998-1999). He was a member of the College of Speech and Language Therapists (1982-2000). In order to start his private speech and language therapy clinic, he retired from his posts at the Anadolu University. During this period, he attended The Lidcombe Program of Early Stuttering Intervention certification course run by Mary Kingston in Norwich, UK (2000). He returned back to his teaching post at Anadolu University Special Education Department in 2002 and also worked for DİLKOM (Speech and Language Disorders Applied Research and Education Center) as a lecturer and a clinician, taught courses to post graduate speech and language therapy students attending Anadolu University Health Sciences Institute. He also served as the director of the Integrated College for the Disabled (2003-2005). Dr. Konrot, accepted an invitation to work as a visiting full professor for Eastern Mediterranean University in North Cyprus (2005-2013). During his full-time stay, he served as the dean of the Arts and Sciences Faculty (2006-2007), Vice Rector (2008), and Curriculum Committee Head (2009-2012). In February 2013, he founded a private center for speech and language disorders (kkm.- Konrot Konuşma Bozuklukları Merkezi) in Bostancı, İstanbul, Turkey. In 2014, he was invited to establish the speech and language therapy department at Üsküdar University, Istanbul. Since then, besides working at his own private clinic, he works for this university as a full professor, runs the speech and language therapy clinic. He travels around the country to give speeches on special education and speech and language disorders. Recently, he has developed a computer-based interactive lip-reading program for Turkish speakers titled BAK-GÖR-DUY (LOOK-SEE-HEAR). He enjoys working with stutterers, especially with preschool children who stutter and with their families. He is the founder member and vice president of The Turkish Association of Specialists in Speech and Language Disorders (DKBUD). He is also a member of The Association of Special Education Professionals in Turkey. Primary academic interests: Human Communication Disorders, Education of the Deaf, Cochlear Implants, Phonetics and Phonology, Visual Aspects of Speech (Lip Reading), Oesophageal Speech Therapy, Stuttering and Stuttering Therapy, Specific Learning Disorders, Dyslexia.

Jyothsna Devi Kuchipudi is an academic professional associated with the Department of Allied Healthcare and Sciences at the School of Allied Healthcare and Sciences, JAIN (Deemed-to-be University), Bangalore. She is actively involved in teaching, academic coordination, and the development of allied healthcare education in alignment with contemporary healthcare and academic standards. With a strong commitment to academic excellence and professional ethics, Jyothsna Devi contributes to the training and mentoring of students in the allied healthcare sciences domain. Her academic engagement emphasizes conceptual clarity, practical orientation, and outcome-based education, preparing students to meet the evolving demands of the healthcare sector. At JAIN (Deemed-to-be University), she plays a supportive role in curriculum delivery, academic activities, and institutional initiatives aimed at enhancing the quality of education and interdisciplinary learning. She encourages student participation in academic projects, skill-based learning, and professional development programs.

T.C. Manjunath was born on 6th February 1967. He did his B.E. from RV College of Engg. in 1989 (B'lore Univ), M.E. in Robotics & Automation from Govt.'s LD College of Engg., (Gujarat Univ., Ahmedabad) in 1992 with FCD-First Rank & PhD in Systems & Control Engg. from IIT Bombay in the year 2007, got best research scholar award for the entire IITB. He is currently working as the Dean Research (R & D) and as Professor in Dept. of Computer Science & Engg. with specialization in IoT, Cyber Security, Blockchain Technology in Rajarajeswari College of Engineering, Bengaluru, Karnataka. He has got a teaching (academic), research & administrative experience of more than 35+ years (10 years as Principal & 8 years as HoD, 1 year as Dean Research & rest as faculty) and has published more than 1500+ research papers in various national & international journals & conferences, with 175+ patents, 100+ book-chapters, 25 awards, 100s of Keynote talks and also published 25 text books in various field of science, engineering & technology, completed projects worth Rs. 9 Crores till date & guided 10 PhD scholars in VTU. He is a member of 30 Professional Society Chapters and is a fellow of IE, IETE, AMIEE, Sr. Member of IEEE and a chartered engineer.

Kalliopi Megari is a Postdoctoral researcher of Aristotle University of Thessaloniki, Greece, Academic Director of MSc in Clinical Psychology and Clinical supervisor at City College, University of York, Europe Campus. She is Adjunct lecturer at University of Western Macedonia in Florina, Greece. Dr. Megari is a psychologist with a history of working in the hospital & health care industry, skilled in Clinical Neuropsychology, Clinical Research, Medical Education, Psychological

Assessment and Learning Disabilities. She works both in clinical and in research practice and she provides strong professional healthcare services, graduated from Aristotle University of Thessaloniki, and attended further education from Department of Educational and Social Policy, University of Macedonia, in people with special needs and disabilities. She holds undergraduate degrees in Nursing and Psychology, as well as a Master' s and a PhD in Neuropsychology from Aristotle University of Thessaloniki. She has some years of occupational and research experience working with patients who have neurological, psychiatric, and cognitive disorders, as well as chronic disease patients suffering from cancer and cardiovascular diseases. She is the head of the Centre of creative activities of children and adults with disabilities and she also works as a counseling psychologist in Prison, Diavata Thessaloniki, at the school of second chance. She was the Global Engagement Representative of SLC International Neuropsychological Society from 2018-2021 and she was a research fellow in the Department of Cardiovascular Surgery in AHEPA Hospital. Currently she is a Global Membership Committee member of International Neuropsychological Society and leader of Rehabilitation of COVID-19 patients working group of NeuroCOVID International Neuropsychology Taskforce SIG. In addition, she is the General Secretary of the board of directors of Hellenic Neuropsychological Society and Ethics Committee president of Hellenic Neuropsychological Society. Since 2021, she is a member of PIAC Community Outreach Subcommittee of AMERICAN PSYCHOLOGICAL ASSOCIATION Membership and a member of Engagement Committee of American Group Psychotherapy Association (AGPA). Her work has earned her many prestigious international awards and was an Ambassador of National Academy of Neuropsychology (NAN), USA Leadership and Ambassador Development Program (2022-23). Currently she is the leader of Pediatric Neuropsychology Topical Group of FESN - Federation of the European Societies of Neuropsychology and serves as an auditor of the board of Directors. She has given lectures at Aristotle University of Thessaloniki, University of Warsaw and Norwegian University of Science and Technology in Oslo. She is committed to leadership skills and issues on equity, diversity, and inclusion as her clinical and research work states.

Ravinesh Mishra is currently working as Dean, School of Pharmacy and Emerging Sciences at Baddi University of Emerging Sciences and Technology, Baddi, Himachal Pradesh. He holds a B. Pharm. from CCS University (2003), M. Pharm. from Rajiv Gandhi University of Health Sciences, Bengaluru (2007), and Ph.D. in Pharmaceutical Sciences from Jamia Hamdard University, New Delhi (2011). With over 18 years of professional experience. He has qualified GATE twice and was awarded the UGC and CSIR fellowships during his doctoral studies. He received the prestigious DST Young Scientist Award in 2010 and has also undergone short-term toxicological training at AIPT, USA.

Rojjares Netthong is affiliated with the Department of Pharmacy Practice, Faculty of Pharmaceutical Sciences, Ubon Ratchathani University, Thailand. She holds a PhD in Pharmacy and Pharmaceutical Sciences from the University of Lincoln, UK, and an MBA with an emphasis on Appreciative Inquiry theory. Her professional experience spans over nine years, during which she has engaged in academic teaching, community pharmacy management, and the initiation of health projects at the community level. Her current research emphasizes the rational and smart use of antibiotics in Thailand, with broader expertise in international healthcare policy, particularly within the UK context. Dr. Netthong has presented her research in various academic forums, including a national conference on Antimicrobial Resistance in Thailand.

Özlem Oğuz words at speech and language therapy department at Üsküdar University in İstanbul, Türkiye. She does research on adult language and communication disorders.

Batuhan Ökte, MSc-SLP, works as a research assistant in the Department of Speech and Language Therapy, Faculty of Health Sciences, at Anadolu University, Türkiye. He is also a doctoral student at the same university. His research interests are voice and swallowing disorders.

P. Radhika is an accomplished academician and researcher serving as an Assistant Professor in the Department of Electronics and Communication Engineering at SRM Institute of Science and Technology, Kattankulathur. She is recognized for her dedication to teaching, technical research, and student mentorship in the field of electronics and communication systems. With a strong academic foundation in Electronics and Communication Engineering, Dr. Radhika has developed expertise across core and emerging areas such as communication systems, embedded systems, signal processing, wireless technologies, VLSI concepts, and intelligent electronic system design. Her academic journey reflects consistent excellence, supported by advanced qualifications and research-oriented training. In her role as an educator, Dr. Radhika is known for her clear teaching methodology, practical approach to engineering concepts, and focus on outcome-based education. She actively integrates theoretical knowledge with laboratory practice, enabling students to develop strong analytical and problem-solving skills. She has handled a variety of undergraduate and postgraduate courses and continuously updates her teaching methods to align with current technological advancements. Dr. Radhika's research contributions include publishing papers in reputed journals and conferences in areas related to modern communication technologies and electronic system applications. She regularly participates in faculty development programs, workshops, and technical seminars to remain updated with the latest trends in electronics and communication engineering. Her research interests extend to interdisciplinary applications that connect electronics with real-world problem solving.

P. Selvakumar is currently an Associate Professor in the Department of Science and Humanities at Nehru Institute of Technology, Coimbatore, Tamil Nadu, India. Prior to joining Nehru Institute of Technology, he held positions as an Assistant Professor in the Department of Science and Humanities various engineering colleges in Coimbatore, Tamil Nadu, India, spanning from 2011 to 2023. Dr.P. Selvakumar's academic and research interests lie primarily in the field of phytochemistry. He has made significant contributions to his field, with an impressive record that includes 30 journal publications, 12 patents, and 20 conference papers. Additionally, he has organized 5 seminars and conferences, further demonstrating his commitment to academic and scientific exchange. Throughout his career, Dr. P.Selvakumar has been recognized for his dedication and excellence in teaching, having been honored with several awards, including the Best Teacher Awards. He holds a prominent position in the academic community, contributing actively to research.

Jayasudha R is an Associate Professor in the Department of Mathematics at Dr. N.G.P. Institute of Technology, Coimbatore, Tamil Nadu. With an impressive 27 years of teaching experience, she has made significant contributions to the field of mathematics education through her dedication to academic excellence and student development. Her extensive experience and passion for teaching have earned her recognition as a respected educator and mentor within the academic community. Dr. Jayasudha continues to inspire students with her commitment to fostering analytical thinking and mathematical understanding.

Keerthi Priya S is an emerging academic professional in the field of Information Technology, currently serving as an Assistant Professor at Karpagam Academy of Higher Education, Coimbatore, Tamil Nadu. With a strong foundation in computing and digital technologies, she is dedicated to delivering quality education and fostering technical excellence among students. She is recognized for her student-centered teaching approach, combining theoretical concepts with practical applications to enhance learning outcomes. Her academic interests include core areas of information technology such as programming, data management, software development practices, and modern computing tools. She continuously works to keep her knowledge updated with current industry trends and evolving technologies, ensuring that her teaching remains relevant and impactful. As an educator, Keerthi Priya S emphasizes clarity in instruction, interactive learning, and skill-based training. She actively supports students in academic projects, technical activities, and collaborative learning initiatives. Her communication skills and approachable mentoring style help create a positive and engaging classroom environment. She contributes to departmental academic activities, curriculum support, and student development programs, and is committed to continuous professional growth through workshops, seminars, and research-oriented learning. Her dedication to teaching and academic service makes her a valuable member of the Information Technology department.

Ayşe Buse SARAÇ graduated from the Speech and Language Therapy undergraduate program at Üsküdar University in 2020. After graduating from the Speech and Language Therapy master's program in 2022, which she began in 2020, she started her doctoral education in the Department of Speech and Language Therapy in 2022 and is currently continuing her education. Saraç works as a Lecturer at the Faculty of Health Sciences at Üsküdar University.

Priya Sharma is currently working as an Assistant Professor, School of Pharmacy and Emerging Sciences at Baddi University of Emerging Sciences and Technology, Baddi, Himachal Pradesh. She holds M. Pharm in Pharmaceutics and earned her Ph.D. in Pharmaceutical Sciences. With over 5 years of academic and research experience, she is actively involved in both teaching and guiding students in the field of pharmaceutical sciences. Her core areas of interest include novel drug delivery systems, formulation and development, and pharmaceutical technology. She has participated in several national/ international conferences and workshops and is committed to continuous learning and innovation in pharmaceutical education. She has also contributed to research publications and is keen on expanding her research profile through interdisciplinary collaborations.

Dharmendra Singh is a distinguished academician, researcher, and administrator with over 21 years of exemplary contributions to education, research, and institutional leadership. Currently serving as Professor and Associate Director at the School of Management Science, Lucknow, Dr. Singh is a beacon of academic excellence, driving innovation and fostering intellectual growth in the fields of Mathematics, Artificial Intelligence, and interdisciplinary applications. Dr. Singh's academic journey is marked by a robust foundation in Mathematics. He earned his Ph.D. in Mathematics from the prestigious University of Lucknow, Uttar Pradesh, where he developed a deep expertise in analytical and computational methodologies. His academic credentials are further strengthened by an M.Sc. and B.Sc. in Mathematics from DDU Gorakhpur University, Uttar Pradesh, equipping him with a solid grounding in theoretical and applied sciences. As Professor and Associate Director at the School of Management Science, Lucknow, Dr. Singh plays a pivotal role in shaping academic curricula, fostering research innovation, and mentoring future scholars. His leadership extends to strategic administration, where he ensures the alignment of institutional goals with academic excellence. Dr. Singh has successfully supervised two M.Phil. students, guiding them toward academic and professional success with a focus on rigorous scholarship and critical thinking. Dr. Singh is a prolific researcher whose work has significantly advanced the fields of Mathematics, Artificial Intelligence, and their applications. He has authored over 43 research papers published in high-impact SCOPUS, journals and conferences, contributing to global academic discourse.

Kamlesh Singh is a highly accomplished professional with over 15 years of distinguished experience spanning academia, research and development, industry consultation, and collaborative projects. His expertise intersects Mechanical Engineering, Automation & Robotics, and Artificial Intelligence, where he has consistently delivered groundbreaking contributions and achieved significant milestones. Dr. Singh completed his Ph.D. in Mechanical Engineering from Annamalai University, Chidambaram, Tamil Nadu, following his M.Tech. in Automation & Robotics from Ajay Kumar Garg Engineering College, Ghaziabad, Uttar Pradesh, and a B.Tech. in Mechanical Engineering from Institute of Engineering and Technology (IET), Dr. Ram Manohar Lohia Avadh University, Ayodhya, Uttar Pradesh. Throughout his illustrious career, Dr. Singh has amassed a remarkable track record of achievements: Dr. Singh holds 08 granted patents and has published 29 patents, demonstrating his innovative prowess in developing cutting-edge technological solutions. His 23 SCOPUS-indexed papers have significantly contributed to the advancement of knowledge in global academic and scientific communities. He is the esteemed author of three internationally recognized books on Artificial Intelligence and Industrial Robotics, published by Lambert Publication and Hoffman und Campe Publication in Germany. These works underscore his authority in shaping industry discourse and disseminating critical insights. Dr. Singh serves as an internal expert for NBA, NAAC, UGC, and AICTE, where he plays a pivotal role in enhancing educational standards nationally. His efforts ensure that curricula align with industry needs and incorporate cutting-edge technological advancements. Dr. Singh has mentored 12 M.Tech. and 2 Ph.D. students to successful completion, with ongoing guidance for additional doctoral candidates. His mentorship extends to industrial projects and research consultancy, where he bridges theoretical knowledge with practical applications, preparing future leaders in the field. As a respected examiner across universities, Dr. Singh shapes programs in Mechanical Engineering, Mechatronics, Automation & Robotics, CAD/CAM, and Computer Science. His commitment to nurturing talent and advancing academic discourse is evident in his meticulous approach to teaching and examination. With proficiency in programming and optimizing a variety of industrial robots including KUKA, FANUC, ABB, Yaskawa, Kawasaki, Staubli, Mitsubishi, Comau, and DOBOT, Dr. Singh enhances operational efficiency and drives technological innovation in automation. Dr. Kamlesh Singh continues to exemplify excellence in Robotics and Artificial Intelligence, leveraging his profound academic background, research acumen, and extensive industry experience. His dedication to education, pioneering research, and collaborative industry partnerships underscores his commitment to advancing engineering and automation, establishing himself as a pivotal figure in his field globally.

Ceren Sogut graduated with honors from the Audiology Department at Üsküdar University in 2018. In 2015, she enrolled in the dual major program in Speech and Language Therapy at Üsküdar University and graduated from the Speech and Language Therapy Department in 2019. She then completed her thesis-based master's degree at the Department of Speech and Language Therapy at the Institute of Health Sciences at Üsküdar University and began her doctoral program in Speech and Language Disorders Therapy at the Institute of Health Sciences at Üsküdar University in the same year. Her education is still ongoing.

S. Naresh Kumar is a distinguished academician and researcher in the field of Computer Science and Engineering, currently serving as a Professor at SR University. With over 21 years of extensive teaching, research, and academic leadership experience, he has made significant contributions to higher education and advanced computing research. His core areas of expertise include Deep Learning, Machine Learning, Medical Image Analysis, and Optimization Techniques, with a strong emphasis on designing and implementing efficient intelligent systems for real-world applications. His research work bridges the gap between theoretical foundations and practical deployment, particularly in healthcare and data-driven decision-making systems. Professor Naresh Kumar has been actively involved in curriculum development, mentoring undergraduate and postgraduate students, and supervising research scholars. His commitment to academic excellence is reflected in his ability to integrate emerging technologies into teaching and research, fostering innovation and critical thinking among students. His research interests focus on the development of robust, scalable, and optimized intelligent models, leveraging advanced learning algorithms to solve complex problems in medical diagnostics, pattern recognition, and predictive analytics. He has contributed to scholarly publications in reputed journals and conferences, and regularly engages in academic collaborations and knowledge dissemination activities.

Göksu Tarakçı graduated from the Speech and Language Therapy Department at Üsküdar University in 2018. She completed a dual major in audiology the following year. She received her Master of Science in Speech and Language Therapy in 2020. That same year, she began a Ph.D. program in Speech and Language Therapy as well as a non-thesis master's program in Molecular Biology and Genetics, which she completed in 2023. She earned her Ph.D. in 2024. Dr. Tarakçı worked as a research assistant at Üsküdar University from 2018 to 2025, after which she began serving as an assistant professor. Her research focuses on voice and swallowing disorders. She has published numerous articles in national and international journals and has participated in various research projects.

Charuwan Thanawiroon is an Assistant Professor in the Faculty of Pharmaceutical Sciences, Ubon Ratchathani University, Thailand. She received her PhD in Medicinal and Natural Product Chemistry from the University of Iowa, USA. Her academic and research interests focus on the analysis of synthetic drugs, medicinal compounds, and pharmaceutical care. With extensive expertise in pharmaceutical chemistry, Dr. Thanawiroon contributes significantly to both research and education, establishing herself as an important figure in the advancement of pharmaceutical sciences in Thailand.

Latika Yadav is presently working as an Assistant Professor and Head of the Department of Home Science at Vijay Singh Pathik Government PG College (Affiliated to Maa Shakumbhari University, Punwarka, Saharanpur), Kairana, Shamli, Uttar Pradesh, India. She received her B.Sc. Home Science degree from Acharya Narendra Deva University of Agriculture and Technology, Ayodhya, U.P She obtained her master's degree from Banaras Hindu University, Varanasi, UP, India, and PhD from College of Community and Applied Sciences, Department of Foods and Nutrition, Maharana Pratap University of Agriculture and Technology, Udaipur, Rajasthan, India. She is also qualified for ICAR-JRF, UGC-NET, ASRB-NET, RSET, and B.Ed. (Home Science). She worked as a Senior Research Fellow on a Department of Science and Technology (DST) project titled "Development of designer health foods and their promotion among rural women for the prevention and management of non-communicable diseases." She was awarded the Young Researcher Award-2025 for significant contribution in the field of Home Science at the 9th International Conference ABCD-2025 and the "Young Scientist Award" for her outstanding contribution to Food and Nutrition at ATDS-2018. She was awarded the best poster presentation award twice: at the international conference (2014) and at the First UP Agriculture Science Congress (2013). She is a Lifetime Member of the Indian Dietetic Association (IDA) and the Home Science Association of India (HSAI). Her research contributions are extensive, including 3 patents, more than 30 research and review papers in Peer-reviewed, NAAS-rated journals, and more than 40 book chapters in CRC, Taylor Francis, Wiley, Springer Nature, and Elsevier publishing companies, with more than 20 Edited Books. She has also been associated with workshops and conferences. Her research interests span Nutrition Science, Food Science, Food Product Development, Nutritional Biochemistry, Therapeutic Diet, Public Health Nutrition, Home Science, and Women's and Children's Health.

Bancha Yingngam is an Associate Professor in the Faculty of Pharmaceutical Sciences, Ubon Ratchathani University, Thailand, specializing in Pharmaceutical Sciences and Technology. He earned both his pharmacy degree and PhD from Ubon Ratchathani University, and subsequently undertook a postdoctoral fellowship at Karl-Franzens-Universität Graz, Austria (2013–2021). Dr. Yingngam has published more than 80 scholarly works and serves as a reviewer for over 100 Scopus-indexed journals. His academic achievements include an h-index of 20 (Scopus) and recognition on Stanford University and Elsevier's World Top 2% Scientists list (2025) in the field of pharmacology and pharmacy, highlighting his substantial impact in pharmaceutical research.

Index

Symbols

A

B

C

D

E

F

H

I

P

R

S

T

V

Y